CURRENT THERAPY IN OBSTETRICS AND GYNECOLOGY 2

EDWARD J. QUILLIGAN, M.D.
Professor of Obstetrics and Gynecology
University of California, Irvine
School of Medicine
Irvine, California

W.B. SAUNDERS COMPANY
Philadelphia London Toronto Mexico City Rio de Janeiro Sydney Tokyo

W. B. Saunders Company: West Washington Square
Philadelphia, PA   19105

1 St. Anne's Road
Eastbourne, East Sussex BN21 3UN, England

1 Goldthorne Avenue
Toronto, Ontario M8Z 5T9, Canada

Apartado 26370—Cedro 512
Mexico 4, D.F., Mexico

Rua Coronel Cabrita, 8
Sao Cristovao Caixa Postal 21176
Rio de Janeiro, Brazil

9 Waltham Street
Artarmon, N.S.W. 2064, Australia

Ichibancho, Central Bldg., 22-1 Ichibancho
Chiyoda-Ku, Tokyo 102, Japan

Library of Congress Cataloging in Publication Data
(Revised for vol. 2)

Quilligan, Edward J.
  Current therapy in obstetrics and gynecology.

  Includes index.
  1. Gynecology. 2. Generative organs, Female—
Diseases. 3. Pregnancy, Complications of. 4. Therapeu-
tics. I. Title. [DNLM: 1. Genital diseases, Female—
Therapy. 2. Infant, Newborn, Diseases—Therapy.
3. Pregnancy complications—Therapy. WP 650 C976]
RG125.Q53   618   79-65461
ISBN 0-7216-7414-3 (v. 1)
ISBN 0-7216-7413-5 (v. 2)

Current Therapy in Obstetrics and Gynecology 2   ISBN 0-7216-7413-5

© 1983 by W. B. Saunders Company. Copyright 1980 by W. B. Saunders Company. Copyright under the Uniform Copyright Convention. Simultaneously published in Canada. All rights reserved. This book is protected by copyright. No part of it may be reproduced, stored in a retrieval system, or transmitted in any form or by any means, electronic, mechanical, photocopying, recording, or otherwise, without written permission from the publisher. Made in the United States of America. Press of W. B. Saunders Company. Library of Congress catalog number 79-65461.

Last digit is the print number: 9   8   7   6   5   4   3   2

To a wonderful wife and family

Contributors

MARINA BALL, M.D.
Clinical Instructor, Department of Dermatology, University of California, Irvine, California College of Medicine, Irvine, California
Acne Vulgaris

JOSE P. BALMACEDA, M.D.
Assistant Professor, University Health Science Center at San Antonio, Physician, Medical Center Hospital, San Antonio, Texas
Secondary Amenorrhea

GERARD E. BALSLEY, M.D.
Senior Resident, Parkland Memorial Hospital, Dallas, Texas
Pulmonary Tuberculosis

HUGH R. K. BARBER, M.D.
Professor and Chairman, Department of Obstetrics and Gynecology, and Associate Dean for Cancer Programs, New York Medical College, Valhalla; Director, Department of Obstetrics and Gynecology, Lenox Hill Hospital, New York, New York
Vaginal Adenosis

WILLIAM M. BARRON, M.D.
Research Fellow, Departments of Medicine, Obstetrics and Gynecology, and Pathology, University of Chicago, Pritzker School of Medicine, Chicago, Illinois
Hypertension in Nonpregnant Patient

GERARD M. BASSELL, M.D.
Assistant Professor of Anesthesiology and Obstetrics and Gynecology, University of California, Irvine, California College of Medicine, Irvine; Director of Obstetric Anesthesia, University of California, Irvine Medical Center, Orange, California
Anesthesia for Labor and Delivery

THOMAS J. BENEDETTI, M.D.
Associate Professor, Division of Perinatal Medicine, Department of Obstetrics and Gynecology, University of Washington School of Medicine, Seattle, Washington
Rheumatic Heart Disease

ALFRED E. BENT, M.D.
Lecturer, Department of Obstetrics and Gynecology, Dalhousie University, Consultant, Victoria General Hospital, Active Staff/Consultant in Obstetrics and Gynecology, Grace Maternity Hospital, Halifax Infirmary, Halifax, Nova Scotia, Canada
Urinary Incontinence

WATSON A. BOWES, JR., M.D.
Professor, Department of Obstetrics and Gynecology, School of Medicine, University of North Carolina at Chapel Hill, Physician, University of North Carolina–Memorial Hospital, Chapel Hill, North Carolina
Pancreatitis in Pregnancy

PAUL F. BRENNER, M.D.
Associate Professor, Department of Obstetrics and Gynecology, University of Southern California School of Medicine, Attending Staff, Women's Hospital, Los Angeles County–University of Southern California Medical Center, Los Angeles, California
Contraception: Hypopituitarism

RICHARD C. BUMP, M.D.
Assistant Professor of Obstetrics and Gynecology, Ohio State University College of Medicine, Columbus, Ohio
Asherman's Syndrome

DENIS CAVANAGH, M.D.
American Cancer Society Ed. C. Wright Professor of Clinical Oncology, Director of Gynecologic Oncology, University of South Florida, Attending Staff, Tampa General Hospital, Tampa, Florida
Shock

CONTRIBUTORS

ROBERT C. CEFALO, M.D., Ph.D.

Professor, Obstetrics and Gynecology, Director, Division of Maternal and Fetal Medicine, Department of Obstetrics and Gynecology, Assistant Dean, School of Medicine, Director, Graduate Medical Education, University of North Carolina at Chapel Hill, Chapel Hill, North Carolina

Postpartum Pelvic Hematomas

THOMAS C. CESARIO, M.D.

Associate Professor, Division of Infectious Diseases, Department of Internal Medicine, University of California, Irvine, California College of Medicine, Irvine; Staff Physician, University of California, Irvine Medical Center, Orange, California

Pneumonia

DAVID CHARLES, M.D.

Professor and Chairman, Department of Obstetrics/Gynecology, Marshall University School of Medicine, Huntington, West Virginia

Sexually Transmitted Diseases

DANIEL L. CLARKE-PEARSON, M.D.

Assistant Professor, Obstetrics and Gynecology, Duke University School of Medicine, Assistant Professor, Gynecologic Oncology and Obstetrics and Gynecology, Duke University Medical Center, Durham, North Carolina

Ovarian Carcinoma

ROBERT L. CLEARY, M.D.

Professor of Obstetrics and Gynecology, Head, Section of Reproductive Endocrinology and Infertility, Indiana University School of Medicine; Head, Section of Reproductive Endocrinology and Infertility, Indiana University Hospital, Indianapolis, Indiana

Dysmenorrhea

DANIEL CLEMENT, M.D.

Assistant Professor, Department of Obstetrics and Gynecology, University of Connecticut School of Medicine, Farmington, Connecticut

Amnionitis

JOSEPH V. COLLEA, M.D.

Associate Professor, Division of Maternal-Fetal Medicine, Department of Obstetrics and Gynecology, Georgetown University School of Medicine, Attending Obstetrician, Georgetown University Hospital, Columbia Hospital for Women, Sibley Memorial Hospital, Washington, D.C.

Breech Presentation; Twin Gestation

BETH COLVIN, R.N., M.S.N.

Clinical Nurse Specialist, Gynecologic Oncology, Vanderbilt University Hospital, Nashville, Tennessee

Hydatidiform Mole

WILLIAM T. CREASMAN, M.D.

James M. Ingram Professor of Gynecologic Oncology, Duke University Medical Center, Durham, North Carolina

Ovarian Carcinoma

CHRISTOPHER P. CRUM, M.D.

Assistant Professor, Department of Pathology, Columbia University College of Physicians and Surgeons, Associate Director, Obstetrical and Gynecological Pathology and Cytology, Sloane Hospital for Women, New York, New York

Abnormal Papanicolaou Smear

F. GARY CUNNINGHAM, M.D.

Professor of Obstetrics and Gynecology, University of Texas Health Science Center, Chief of Obstetrics, Parkland Memorial Hospital, Dallas, Texas

Pulmonary Tuberculosis

VAL DAVAJAN, M.D.

Professor of Obstetrics and Gynecology, University of Southern California School of Medicine, Attending Physician, Los Angeles County–University of Southern California Medical Center, Co-Director, Center for Gynecologic Endocrinology and Infertility, Hospital of the Good Samaritan, Los Angeles, California

Galactorrhea and Hyperprolactinemia

PHILIP J. DiSAIA, M.D.

Professor and Chairman, Department of Obstetrics and Gynecology, University of California, Irvine, California College of Medicine, Irvine, California

Neoplasia of Cervix

JOHN W. DOBBINS, M.D.

Associate Professor of Medicine, Yale University School of Medicine, Attending Physician, Yale–New Haven Hospital, Consultant, West Haven Veterans Administration Hospital, New Haven, Connecticut

Gastrointestinal Disorders During Pregnancy

STAVROS G. DOUVAS, M.D.

Assistant Professor, Rush Medical College, Assistant Attending, Rush–Presbyterian St. Luke's Medical Center, Chicago, Illinois

Anemias

PATRICK DUFF, M.D.

Clinical Assistant Professor, University of Texas Health Science Center at San Antonio, Fellow, Maternal-Fetal Medicine, University of Texas Health Science Center Medical Center Hospital, San Antonio, Texas

Hypothyroidism; Hyperthyroidism

SHERMAN ELIAS, M.D.

Associate Professor, Department of Obstetrics and Gynecology, Northwestern University Medical School, Director, Medical Genetic Services and Attending Obstetrician and Gynecologist, Prentice Women's Hospital and Maternity Center of Northwestern Memorial Hospital, Chicago Illinois

Amniocentesis; Congenital Abnormalities

MICHAEL F. EPSTEIN, M.D.

Assistant Professor of Pediatrics, Harvard Medical School, Associate Chairman, Department of Newborn Medicine, Brigham and Women's Hospital, Physician-in-Charge, Newborn Intensive Care Unit, Children's Hospital Medical Center, Boston, Massachusetts

Respiratory Distress Syndrome

FREDRIC D. FRIGOLETTO, JR., M.D.

Associate Professor in Obstetrics and Gynecology, Harvard Medical School, Chief, Maternal-Fetal Medicine, Brigham and Women's Hospital, Boston, Massachusetts

Erythroblastosis Fetalis

THOMAS J. GARITE, M.D.

Assistant Professor of Obstetrics and Gynecology, University of California, Irvine, Associate Medical Director for Perinatology, Women's Hospital, Memorial Medical Center, Long Beach, California

Premature Rupture of Membranes

ALBERT B. GERBIE, M.D.

Professor of Obstetrics and Gynecology, Northwestern University Medical School, Attending Obstetrician and Gynecologist, Prentice Women's Hospital of Northwestern Memorial Hospital, Chief of Obstetrics and Gynecology, Children's Memorial Hospital, Chicago, Illinois

Amniocentesis; Congenital Abnormalities

RONALD S. GIBBS, M.D.

Professor, Obstetrics and Gynecology, University of Texas Health Science Center at San Antonio, San Antonio, Texas

Pelvic Inflammatory Disease

EDWARD A. GRABER, M.D.

Professor, Clinical Obstetrics and Gynecology, Cornell University Medical College, Attending Physician, Obstetrics and Gynecology, New York Hospital–Cornell Medical Center, New York, New York

Mastalgia

A. GERSON GREENBURG, M.D., PH.D.

Associate Professor of Surgery, University of California, San Diego, School of Medicine, Chief, Surgical Intensive Care Unit, University of California Medical Center, Staff Physician, Veterans Administration Medical Center, San Diego, California

Ileus

MICHAEL T. GYVES, M.D.

Assistant Professor, Department of Reproductive Biology, Case Western Reserve University, Cleveland, Ohio

Premature Labor

CHARLES B. HAMMOND, M.D.

Professor and Chairman, Department of Obstetrics and Gynecology, Duke University Medical Center, Durham, North Carolina

Anorexia Nervosa

ROBERT H. HAYASHI, M.D.

Associate Professor, Department of Obstetrics and Gynecology, University of Texas Health Science Center at San Antonio, Attending Staff, Medical Center Hospital, Teaching Hospital for the University of Texas, Health Science Center at San Antonio, San Antonio, Texas

Third Trimester Bleeding

DAVID L. HEMSELL, M.D.

Assistant Professor of Obstetrics and Gynecology, University of Texas Medical School, Director, Division of Gynecology, Parkland Memorial Hospital, Obstetrician/Gynecologist, Presbyterian Hospital, St. Paul's Hospital, Dallas, Texas

Female Genital Tuberculosis

WILLIAM N. P. HERBERT, M.D.

Assistant Professor, Department of Obstetrics and Gynecology, School of Medicine, University of North Carolina at Chapel Hill, Chapel Hill, North Carolina

Postpartum Pelvic Hematomas

JOSEPH P. HOLT, JR., M.D., PH.D.

Assistant Professor of Reproductive Biology, Case Western Reserve University School of Medicine, Attending Obstetrician/Gynecologist, University Hospitals of Cleveland, Cleveland, Ohio

Polycystic Ovary Syndrome

JOHN F. HUDDLESTON, M.D.

Professor of Obstetrics and Gynecology, Director, Division of Maternal and Fetal Medicine, School of Medicine, University of Alabama in Birmingham, Attending Obstetrician/Gynecologist, University Hospital, Children's Hospital, Cooper Green Hospital, Birmingham, Alabama

Intrapartum Fetal Distress; Postterm Pregnancy

CONTRIBUTORS

ROBERT W. HUFF, M.D.

Professor of Obstetrics and Gynecology and Chief, Division of Obstetrics, University of Texas Medical School at San Antonio, Chief of Obstetrics, Medical Center Hospital, San Antonio, Texas

Dysfunctional Labor; Hypothyroidism; Hyperthyroidism

GORDON K. JIMERSON, M.D.

Clinical Associate Professor, Department of Gynecology and Obstetrics, Oklahoma University Health Science Center, Chairman, Department of Obstetrics and Gynecology, Norman Municipal Hospital, Norman, Oklahoma

Fibrocystic Disease; Breast Mass and Nipple Discharge

GEORGEANNA SEEGAR JONES, M.D.

Professor of Obstetrics and Gynecology, Eastern Virginia Medical School, Medical Staff, Norfolk General Hospital, Norfolk, Virginia

Luteal Phase Defects

HOWARD W. JONES, III, M.D.

Associate Professor and Director of Gynecologic Oncology, Vanderbilt University School of Medicine, Attending Gynecologist, Vanderbilt Hospital, Metropolitan Nashville General Hospital, Nashville, Tennessee

Hydatidiform Mole

NANCY E. JUDGE, M.D.

Assistant Professor, Department of Obstetrics and Gynecology, Case Western Reserve University Medical School, Fellow in Maternal-Fetal Medicine, Cayahoga County Metropolitan General Hospital, Cleveland, Ohio

Drug Abuse; Alcohol Abuse

RAYMOND H. KAUFMAN, M.D.

Ernst Bertner Chairman and Professor, Department of Obstetrics and Gynecology, Professor of Pathology, Baylor College of Medicine, Houston, Texas

Herpes Genitalis; Condyloma Acuminatum

KIRK A. KEEGAN, M.D.

Assistant Professor, University of California, Irvine, California College of Medicine, Irvine, Attending Obstetrician-Gynecologist, University of California, Irvine Medical Center and Saint Joseph's Hospital, Orange, California

Fetal Heart Rate Monitoring

MOON H. KIM, M.D.

Professor and Director, Division of Reproductive Endocrinology and Infertility, Ohio State University College of Medicine, Vice-Chairman, Department of Obstetrics and Gynecology, and Director, Division of Reproductive Endocrinology, University Hospitals, Columbus, Ohio

Asherman's Syndrome

ROBERT W. KISTNER, M.D.

Assistant Professor, Department of Obstetrics and Gynecology, Harvard Medical School, Senior Gynecologist, Brigham and Women's Hospital, Boston, Massachusetts

Endometriosis

OSCAR A. KLETSKY, M.D.

Associate Professor of Obstetrics and Gynecology, University of Southern California School of Medicine, Associate Professor, Women's Hospital, Los Angeles County–University of Southern California Medical Center, Los Angeles, California

Galactorrhea and Hyperprolactinemia

SHELDON B. KORONES, M.D.

Professor of Pediatrics and Obstetrics and Gynecology, University of Tennessee Center for the Health Sciences, Director of Newborn Center, E. H. Crump Women's Hospital and Perinatal Center, President-Elect of Medical Staff, City of Memphis Hospital, Memphis, Tennessee

Hypoglycemia, Hypocalcemia, and Hypomagnesemia

RUSSELL K. LAROS, Jr., M.D.

Professor and Vice Chairman, Department of Obstetrics, Gynecology and Reproductive Sciences, University of California, San Francisco, San Francisco, California

Venous Thrombosis

JOHN W. LARSEN, Jr., M.D.

Associate Professor, Obstetrics, Gynecology and Genetics, George Washington University, Attending Obstetrician-Gynecologist, George Washington University Hospital, Washington, D.C.; Consultant, Interinstitute Genetics Program, National Institutes of Health, Bethesda, Maryland

Rubella

MARC R. LEBED, M.D.

Director of Maternal-Fetal Medicine, Huntington Memorial Hospital, Pasadena; Courtesy Teaching Staff, Glendale Adventist Medical Center, Glendale, California

Fetal Hydrocephaly

THOMAS B. LEBHERZ, M.D.

Professor, University of California, Los Angeles, Attending Staff, University of California, Los Angeles, California

Vesicovaginal Fistula

RAYMOND A. LEE, M.D.

Professor of Obstetrics and Gynecology, Mayo Medical School, Consultant in Gynecologic Surgery, Mayo Clinic and Mayo Foundation, Rochester, Minnesota

Disorders of Pelvic Support

CONTRIBUTORS

KENNETH J. LEVENO, M.D.
Assistant Professor of Obstetrics and Gynecology, The University of Texas Health Science Center at Dallas, Attending Staff, Parkland Hospital, Methodist Hospital, St. Paul Hospital, Dallas, Texas
Acute Hypertension in Pregnancy

JOHN L. LEWIS, Jr., M.D.
Professor, Obstetrics and Gynecology, Cornell University Medical College, Attending Surgeon and Chief of Gynecology Service, Memorial Hospital, New York, New York
Carcinoma of Endometrium

MARSHALL D. LINDHEIMER, M.D.
Professor of Medicine and Obstetrics and Gynecology, University of Chicago, Pritzker School of Medicine, Attending Physician, University of Chicago Hospital Clinics, Consultant, Medical High Risk Clinic, Chicago Lying-in Hospital, Chicago, Illinois
Hypertension in Nonpregnant Patient

E. MICHAEL LINZEY, M.D.
Assistant Professor of Obstetrics and Gynecology, Division of Maternal-Fetal Medicine, University of California, Irvine, College of Medicine, Irvine; Attending Perinatologist, University of California Medical Center, Consulting Perinatologist, St. Joseph's Hospital, Orange, California
Diabetes in Pregnancy

BRIAN LITTLE, M.D.
Professor of Reproductive Biology, Case Western Reserve University School of Medicine, Attending Obstetrician/Gynecologist, University Hospitals of Cleveland, Cleveland, Ohio
Polycystic Ovary Syndrome

STEVE N. LONDON, M.D.
Assistant Professor, Department of Obstetrics and Gynecology, Division of Reproductive Endocrinology, Duke University School of Medicine, Durham, North Carolina
Anorexia Nervosa

EDGAR L. MAKOWSKI, M.D.
Professor and Chairman, Department of Obstetrics and Gynecology, University of Colorado School of Medicine, Attending Staff, University of Colorado Hospital, Denver General Hospital, Denver, Colorado
Chronic Renal Disease

PAUL D. MANGANIELLO, M.D.
Assistant Professor, Maternal-Child Health and Surgery, Dartmouth Medical School, Reproductive Endocrinologist, Mary Hitchcock Memorial Hospital, Hanover, New Hampshire
Precocious Puberty

DOUGLAS J. MARCHANT, M.D.
Professor of Obstetrics and Gynecology and Professor of Surgery, Tufts University School of Medicine, Director, Cancer Institute, Tufts New England Medical Center, Gynecologic Oncology and Breast Health Center, New England Medical Center, Boston, Massachusetts
Breast Cancer

DONALD E. MARSDEN, M.D.
Assistant Professor of Obstetrics and Gynecology, University of South Florida College of Medicine, Fellow in Gynecologic Oncology, Tampa General Hospital, Tampa, Florida
Shock

G. ROBERT MASON, M.D., Ph.D.
Professor and Chairman, Department of Surgery, University of California, Irvine, College of Medicine, Irvine; Surgeon-in-Chief, University of California Medical Center, Senior Staff Surgeon, Long Beach Veterans Administration Medical Center, Orange, California
Atelectasis

THOMAS A. McCARTHY, M.D.
Assistant Clinical Professor, Department of Obstetrics, Gynecology and Reproductive Sciences, University of California, San Francisco, School of Medicine, San Francisco, California
Pruritus Vulvae

PAUL G. McDONOUGH, M.D.
Professor, Obstetrics and Gynecology, Endocrinology and Pediatrics, Chief, Reproductive Endocrine Division, Medical College of Georgia, Attending Obstetrician-Gynecologist, Eugene Talmadge Memorial Hospital, Augusta, Georgia
Spontaneous and Recurrent Abortion

PAUL R. MEIER, M.D.
Assistant Professor, Obstetrics and Gynecology, University of Colorado, School of Medicine, Attending Staff, University of Colorado Health Science Center, Denver, Colorado
Chronic Renal Disease

DAVID R. MELDRUM, M.D.
Associate Professor, Obstetrics and Gynecology, University of California, Los Angeles, School of Medicine, Los Angeles, California
Menopause

IRWIN R. MERKATZ, M.D.
Professor and Chairman, Department of Obstetrics and Gynecology, Albert Einstein College of Medicine, Attending, Montefiore Medical Center, New York, New York
Premature Labor

JAMES A. MERRILL, M.D.

Professor of Gynecology-Obstetrics and Professor of Pathology, University of Oklahoma College of Medicine, Attending Staff, University of Oklahoma Hospital, Oklahoma City, Oklahoma

Uterine Myomas

WALTER L. MILLAR, M.D.

Assistant Clinical Professor of Anesthesiology, University of California Medical Center, San Diego, School of Medicine, Attending Anesthesiologist, San Diego, University Hospital, San Diego, California

Resuscitation of the Newborn

FRANK C. MILLER, M.D.

Associate Professor, Department of Obstetrics and Gynecology, University of Southern California School of Medicine, Los Angeles, California

Fetal Hydrocephaly

R. DAVID MILLER, M.D.

Assistant Professor, University of California, Irvine, College of Medicine, Irvine Attending Staff, University of California Medical Center, St. Joseph's Hospital, Orange, California

Urinary Tract Infections

DANIEL R. MISHELL, Jr, M.D.

Professor and Chairman, Department of Gynecology, University of Southern California School of Medicine, Los Angeles, California

Induction of Ovulation

GEORGE W. MORLEY, M.D.

Professor, University of Michigan, Chief of Gynecology, University of Michigan Hospitals, Ann Arbor, Michigan

Uterine and Vaginal Anomalies

JOHN C. MORRISON, M.D.

Professor and Director, Division of Maternal-Fetal Medicine, Department of Obstetrics and Gynecology, University of Mississippi Medical Center, Jackson, Mississippi

Anemias

C. PAUL MORROW, M.D.

Professor of Obstetrics and Gynecology, Director, Gynecologic Oncology, University of Southern California School of Medicine, Los Angeles, California

Gestational Trophoblastic Disease

DAVID J. NOCHIMSON, M.D.

Associate Professor, Obstetrics and Gynecology, Director of Maternal-Fetal Medicine, University of Connecticut School of Medicine, Farmington, Connecticut

Amnionitis

KENNETH L. NOLLER, M.D., M.S.

Associate Professor of Obstetrics and Gynecology, Mayo Medical School, Consultant, Division of Obstetrics and Medical Gynecology, Mayo Clinic and Mayo Foundation, Rochester, Minnesota

Infectious Vaginitis

DONALD R. OSTERGARD, M.D.

Professor of Obstetrics and Gynecology, Department of Obstetrics and Gynecology, University of California, Irvine, College of Medicine, Irvine; Associate Medical Director, Women's Hospital, Memorial Hospital Medical Center, Long Beach, California

Urinary Incontinence

DAVID PENT, M.D.

Associate, Department of Obstetrics and Gynecology, University of Arizona College of Medicine, Tucson; Director, Urodynamics Laboratory, St. Joseph's Hospital and Medical Center, Phoenix, Arizona

Cervicitis

ROY H. PETRIE, M.D.

Associate Professor, Department of Obstetrics and Gynecology, College of Physicians and Surgeons of Columbia University, Associate Attending Obstetrician-Gynecologist, Sloane Hospital for Women, Presbyterian Hospital, Columbia–Presbyterian Medical Center, New York, New York

Postpartum Hemorrhage

ROY M. PITKIN, M.D.

Professor and Head, Department of Obstetrics and Gynecology, College of Medicine, University of Iowa, Chief of Obstetrics and Gynecology, University of Iowa Hospitals and Clinics, Iowa City, Iowa

Fetal Death Syndrome

RICHARD P. PORRECO, M.D.

Clinical Assistant Professor of Obstetrics and Gynecology, University of Colorado Health Sciences Center, Director of Perinatal Services, St. Lukes–Presbyterian Medical Center, Denver, Colorado

Asthma and Rhinitis During Pregnancy

EDWARD J. QUILLIGAN, M.D.

Professor of Obstetrics and Gynecology, University of California, Irvine, School of Medicine, Irvine, California

Ectopic Pregnancy

ROBERT RESNIK, M.D.

Professor of Reproductive Medicine, Director, Division of Perinatal Medicine, University of California, San Diego, School of Medicine, San Diego, California

Immune Thrombocytopenic Purpura

CONTRIBUTORS

RALPH M. RICHART, M.D.

Professor of Pathology, Columbia University College of Physicians and Surgeons, Director, Division of Obstetrical and Gynecological Pathology and Cytology Laboratory, Sloane Hospital for Women, New York, New York

Abnormal Papanicolaou Smear

MORTIMER G. ROSEN, M.D.

Professor, Department of Reproductive Biology, Case Western Reserve University, Director, Department of Obstetrics and Gynecology, Cleveland Metropolitan General Hospital, Cleveland, Ohio

Seizure Disorders

KEITH P. RUSSELL, M.D.

Clinical Professor of Obstetrics and Gynecology, University of Southern California School of Medicine, Director of Obstetrics-Gynecology, Department of Medical Education, California Hospital Medical Center, Senior Attending Obstetrician-Gynecologist, Women's Hospital, Los Angeles County–University of Southern California Medical Center, Los Angeles, California

Female Sterilization

EDWARD W. SAVAGE, M.D.

Professor, Charles R. Drew Postgraduate Medical School, Professor and Chief, Division of Gynecology, Martin Luther King, Jr. General Hospital, Los Angeles, California

Bartholin Cysts and Abscesses

GEORGE SCHAEFER, M.D.

Emeritus Professor, New York Hospital–Cornell Medical College, New York, New York; Director, Obstetric and Gynecology Residency Training Program, Mercy Hospital and Medical Center, San Diego, California

Pelvic Tuberculosis

MICHAEL SCHATZ, M.D.

Clinical Assistant Professor of Medicine and Pediatrics, University of California, San Diego, School of Medicine, La Jolla; Attending Staff, Department of Allergy-Immunology, Kaiser-Permanente Medical Center, San Diego, California

Asthma and Rhinitis During Pregnancy

JOHN B. SCHLAERTH, M.D.

Assistant Professor of Obstetrics and Gynecology, Associate Director, Division of Gynecologic Oncology, University of Southern California School of Medicine, Los Angeles, California

Hyperalimentation for the Cancer Patient; Gestational Trophoblastic Disease

PATRICIA L. SCHMIDT, M.D.

Assistant Professor of Obstetrics and Gynecology, University of California, Irvine, College of Medicine, Irvine; Attending Physician, University of California Irvine Medical Center, St. Joseph's Hospital, Orange California

Intrauterine Growth Retardation

JACK M. SCHNEIDER, M.D.

Clinical Professor, Obstetrics and Gynecology, University of California, Davis, School of Medicine, Davis; Director, The Perinatal Center, Sutter Memorial Hospital, Sacramento, California

Collagen Diseases in Pregnancy

PETER E. SCHWARTZ, M.D.

Associate Professor of Obstetrics and Gynecology, Director, Gynecologic Oncology, Yale University School of Medicine Attending Physician, Yale–New Haven Hospital, New Haven, Connecticut

Carcinoma of Vulva

ANTONIO SCOMMEGNA, M.D.

Professor, Pritzker School of Medicine, University of Chicago, Chairman, Department of Obstetrics and Gynecology, Michael Reese Hospital and Medical Center, Chicago, Illinois

Dysfunctional Uterine Bleeding

JOSEPH C. SCOTT, JR., M.D.

Professor and Chairman, Department of Obstetrics and Gynecology, University of Nebraska College of Medicine, Attending Staff, University Hospital, Clarkson Hospital, Methodist Hospital, Bergan Mercy Hospital, Veterans Administration Hospital, Omaha, Nebraska

The Adnexal Mass

JOSEPH SEITCHIK, M.D.

Professor of Obstetrics and Gynecology, University of Texas Health Science Center at San Antonio, San Antonio, Texas

Dysfunctional Labor

JAMES P. SEMMENS, M.D.

Professor, Obstetrics and Gynecology, Medical University of South Carolina, Charleston, South Carolina

Dyspareunia and Vaginismus

JOHN L. SEVER, M.D., PH.D.

Chief, Infectious Disease Branch, National Institute of Neurological and Communicative Disorders and Stroke, National Institutes of Health, Bethesda, Maryland

Rubella

JOE LEIGH SIMPSON, M.D.

Head, Section on Human Genetics, Professor, Obstetrics and Gynecology, Northwestern University Medical School, Chicago, Illinois

XY Gonadal Dysgenesis; Testicular Feminization

ROBERT J. SOKOL, M.D.

Professor of Obstetrics and Gynecology, Department of Obstetrics and Gynecology, Cleveland Metropolitan General Hospital/Case Western Reserve University School of Medicine, Program Director, Perinatal Clinical Research Center, Associate Director, Department of Obstetrics and Gynecology, Cleveland Metropolitan General Hospital/Case Western Reserve University, Cleveland, Ohio

Drug Abuse in Pregnancy; Alcohol Abuse in Pregnancy

YORAM SOROKIN, M.D.

Assistant Professor, Reproductive Biology, Case Western Reserve University School of Medicine, Obstetrician-Gynecologist-Staff, Department of Obstetrics and Gynecology, Cleveland Metropolitan General Hospital, Cleveland, Ohio

Seizure Disorders

HOWARD M. SPIRO, M.D.

Professor of Medicine, Yale University School of Medicine, Chief of Gastroenterology, Yale–New Haven Hospital, New Haven, Connecticut

Gastrointestinal Disorders

LEO STERN, M.D.

Professor and Chairman of Pediatrics, Brown University, Pediatrician-in-Chief, Rhode Island Hospital, Providence, Rhode Island

Hyperbilirubinemia of the Neonate

SERGIO C. STONE, M.D.

Associate Professor, University of California, Irvine, College of Medicine, Irvine; Attending Staff, University of California Irvine Medical Center, Orange, California

Androgen Excess of Adrenal Origin

MARY C. TAYLOR, M.D.

Assistant Adjunct Professor, Department of Neurology, University of California, Irvine, College of Medicine, Irvine, California

Headache

WILLIAM BENBOW THOMPSON, JR. M.D.

Associate Professor of Obstetrics and Gynecology, University of California, Irvine, College of Medicine, Irvine, California

Therapeutic Abortion

PAMELA J. TROPPER, M.D.

Fellow in Maternal-Fetal Medicine, Columbia Presbyterian Medical Center, New York, New York

Postpartum Hemorrhage

STANLEY VAN DEN NOORT, M.D.

Professor of Neurology, University of California, Irvine, College of Medicine, Irvine; Attending Neurologist, University of California, Irvine Medical Center, Orange, California

Myasthenia Gravis and Multiple Sclerosis

FEIZAL WAFFARN, M.B.B.S.

Assistant Professor of Pediatrics, University of California, Irvine, College of Medicine, Irvine; Associate Director, Neonatal Intensive Care Unit, University of California Irvine Medical Center, Orange, California

Seizures in Neonatal Period

JAMES C. WARREN, M.D., PH.D.

Professor, Department of Obstetrics and Gynecology and Department of Biological Chemistry, Washington University School of Medicine, Head, Department of Obstetrics and Gynecology, Barnes and Allied Hospitals, St. Louis, Missouri

Primary Amenorrhea

PEGGY J. WHALLEY, M.D.

Jack A. Pritchard Professor of Obstetrics and Gynecology, University of Texas Health Science Center, Attending Staff, Parkland Hospital, St. Paul Hospital, Methodist Hospital, Dallas, Texas

Acute Hypertension in Pregnancy

JOHN VALENTIC, M.D.

Chief Resident, Department of Dermatology, University of California, Irvine, College of Medicine, Irvine, California

Acne Vulgaris

J. DONALD WOODRUFF, M.D.

Professor of Obstetrics and Gynecology, Richard W. TeLinde Professor of Gynecologic Pathology, Johns Hopkins Hospital, Baltimore, Maryland

Dystrophy

ROBERT S. ZEIGER, M.D., PH.D.

Clinical Associate Professor of Pediatrics, University of California, San Diego, School of Medicine, La Jolla; Chief, Department of Allergy. Immunology, Kaiser-Permanente Medical Center, San Diego, California

Asthma and Rhinitis During Pregnancy

FREDERICK P. ZUSPAN, M.D.

Professor and Chairman, Department of Obstetrics and Gynecology, Ohio State University, Columbus, Ohio

Chronic Hypertension in Pregnancy; Amniotic Fluid Embolism

Preface

This is the second edition of *Current Therapy in Obstetrics and Gynecology*. It remains true to the original precepts set forth by Dr. Conn in *Current Therapy,* short articles with an emphasis on the therapy of specific entities with which the practitioner may have to cope.

In the vast majority of chapters you will find a different author discussing a given disease than appeared in the first edition. This rotation of authors has purpose: to give the readers a spectrum of opinions about any given topic. In some chapters the second edition will stress a different therapy for a given disease than the first edition. This may be due to advances in therapy over the past two years in some situations, while in others it is simply a difference of opinion when two very competent physicians approach the same topic. The readers of the book should be able to differentiate between these two reasons from the opening remarks of the author of each chapter.

Again I am indebted to the many busy people, obstetricians and gynecologists, pediatricians and surgeons and internists, who took their valuable time to write the chapters for this edition. I also want to thank my secretary, Mona Wapner, who spent hours on the telephone getting the chapters in to our office.

EDWARD J. QUILLIGAN

Contents

SECTION 1. OBSTETRICS

Acute Hypertension in Pregnancy 3
Kenneth J. Leveno and
Peggy J. Whalley

Chronic Hypertension in Pregnancy 4
Frederick P. Zuspan

Diabetes in Pregnancy 5
E. Michael Linzey

Third Trimester Bleeding 9
Robert H. Hayashi

Breech Presentation 11
Joseph V. Collea

Intrapartum Fetal Distress 13
John F. Huddleston

Antepartum Fetal Heart Rate Monitoring ... 16
Kirk A. Keegan

Premature Rupture of the Membranes 19
Thomas J. Garite

Premature Labor 21
Irwin R. Merkatz and
Michael T. Gyves

Fetal Death Syndrome 24
Roy M. Pitkin

Spontaneous and Recurrent Abortion 27
Paul G. McDonough

Therapeutic Abortion 29
William Benbow Thompson

Urinary Tract Infection 30
R. David Miller

Treatment of Herpes Genitalis 32
Raymond H. Kaufman

Ectopic Pregnancy 34
E. J. Quilligan

Dysfunctional Labor 35
Joseph Seitchik and
Robert W. Huff

Postterm Pregnancy 39
John F. Huddleston

Erythroblastosis Fetalis 41
Frederic D. Frigoletto, Jr.

Hypothyroidism 43
Robert W. Huff and
Patrick Duff

Hyperthyroidism 45
Patrick Duff and
Robert W. Huff

xv

Amniotic Fluid Embolism 49
  Frederick P. Zuspan

Venous Thrombosis 50
  Russell K. Laros, Jr.

Intrauterine Growth Retardation 55
  Patricia L. Schmidt

The Safe Conduct of Pregnancy in Patients with Rheumatic Heart Disease 57
  Thomas J. Benedetti

Seizure Disorders 60
  Yoram Sorokin and
  Mortimer G. Rosen

Treatment of Female Genital Tuberculosis .. 64
  David L. Hemsell

Pulmonary Tuberculosis in Pregnancy 66
  F. Gary Cunningham and
  Gerard E. Balsley, Jr.

Collagen Diseases in Pregnancy 68
  Jack M. Schneider

Anemias 70
  John C. Morrison and
  Stavros G. Douvas

Drug Abuse in Pregnancy 74
  Nancy E. Judge and
  Robert J. Sokol

Alcohol Abuse in Pregnancy 77
  Robert J. Sokol and
  Nancy E. Judge

Amnionitis 82
  David J. Nochimson and
  Daniel Clement

Anesthesia for Labor and Delivery 83
  Gerard M. Bassell

Postpartum Hemorrhage 87
  Pamela J. Tropper and
  Roy H. Petrie

Immune Thrombocytopenic Purpura 89
  Robert Resnik

Condyloma Acuminatum 90
  Raymond H. Kaufman

Twin Gestation 90
  Joseph V. Collea

Fetal Hydrocephaly 92
  Frank C. Miller and
  Marc R. Lebed

Postpartum Pelvic Hematomas 93
  William N. P. Herbert and
  Robert C. Cefalo

Pregnancy in the Patient with Chronic Renal Disease, on Hemodialysis, or Following Renal Transplant 94
  Paul R. Meier and
  Edgar L. Makowski

Treatment of Gastrointestinal Disorders During Pregnancy 98
  John W. Dobbins and
  Howard M. Spiro

Pancreatitis in Pregnancy 102
  Watson A. Bowes, Jr.

Myasthenia Gravis and Multiple Sclerosis in Pregnancy 103
  Stanley van den Noort

The Management of Asthma and Rhinitis During Pregnancy 105
  Michael Schatz,
  Richard P. Porreco, and
  Robert S. Zeiger

Rubella 109
  John W. Larsen, Jr., and
  John L. Sever

Amniocentesis for the Antenatal Diagnosis of Genetic Defects 111
  Albert B. Gerbie and
  Sherman Elias

SECTION 2. THE NEWBORN

Immediate Resuscitation of the Newborn Infant 117
Walter L. Millar

Respiratory Distress Syndrome 119
Michael F. Epstein

Hypoglycemia, Hypocalcemia, and Hypomagnesemia in the Newborn 123
Sheldon B. Korones

Hyperbilirubinemia of the Neonate 125
Leo Stern

Seizures in the Neonatal Period 130
Feizal Waffarn

Evaluation of the Neonate for Congenital Abnormalities 134
Sherman Elias and
Albert B. Gerbie

SECTION 3. GENERAL GYNECOLOGY

Infectious Vaginitis 141
Kenneth L. Noller

Dystrophy 143
Donald Woodruff

Vaginal Adenosis 144
Hugh R. K. Barber

Disorders of Pelvic Support 146
Raymond A. Lee

Urinary Incontinence 148
Alfred E. Bent and
Donald R. Ostergard

Dysmenorrhea 150
Robert E. Cleary

Vesicovaginal Fistula 152
Thomas B. Lebherz

Pelvic Tuberculosis and Female Genital Tuberculosis 153
George Schaefer

Pelvic Inflammatory Disease 155
Ronald S. Gibbs

Sexually Transmitted Diseases 157
David Charles

Bartholin Cysts and Abscesses 167
Edward W. Savage

Uterine Myomas 168
James A. Merrill

Endometriosis 170
Robert W. Kistner

Shock—A General Plan of Management 171
Denis Cavanagh and
Donald E. Marsden

Dyspareunia and Vaginismus 174
James P. Semmens

The Adnexal Mass 177
Joseph C. Scott, Jr.

Cervicitis 177
David Pent

Pruritus Vulvae 179
Thomas A. McCarthy

Uterine and Vaginal Anomalies 181
George W. Morley

SECTION 4. GYNECOLOGIC ONCOLOGY

Carcinoma of the Vulva 189
Peter E. Schwartz

Neoplasia of the Cervix 191
Philip J. DiSaia

Carcinoma of the Endometrium 195
John L. Lewis, Jr.

Ovarian Carcinoma 198
William T. Creasman and
Daniel L. Clarke-Pearson

Hydatidiform Mole 200
Howard W. Jones III and
Beth Colvin

Management of Gestational Trophoblastic Disease 201
C. Paul Morrow and
John B. Schlaerth

Evaluation of the Patient with an Abnormal Papanicolaou Smear 203
Christopher P. Crum and
Ralph M. Richart

SECTION 5. GYNECOLOGIC ENDOCRINOLOGY AND INFERTILITY

Primary Amenorrhea 209
James C. Warren

Secondary Amenorrhea 213
Jose P. Balmaceda

Induction of Ovulation 218
Daniel R. Mishell, Jr.

Polycystic Ovary Syndrome 220
Joseph P. Holt, Jr., and
Brian Little

Galactorrhea and Hyperprolactinemia 223
Val Davajan and
Oscar A. Kletzky

Contraception 226
Paul F. Brenner

Treatment of Dysfunctional Uterine Bleeding 233
Antonio Scommegna

Menopause 235
David R. Meldrum

Androgen Excess of Adrenal Origin 236
Sergio C. Stone

Asherman's Syndrome 238
Richard C. Bump and Moon H. Kim

Female Sterilization 239
Keith P. Russell

Anorexia Nervosa 241
Steve N. London and
Charles B. Hammond

XY Gonadal Dysgenesis 243
Joe Leigh Simpson

Testicular Feminization 244
Joe Leigh Simpson

Hypopituitarism 245
Paul F. Brenner

Luteal Phase Defects 247
Georgeanna Seegar Jones

Precocious Puberty 249
Paul D. Manganiello

SECTION 6. BREAST DISEASES

Fibrocystic Disease 255
Gordon K. Jimerson

Breast Mass and Nipple Discharge 255
Gordon K. Jimerson

Mastalgia 257
Edward A. Graber

Breast Cancer 259
Douglas J. Marchant

SECTION 7. GENERAL MEDICAL AND SURGICAL PROBLEMS

Hyperalimentation for the Cancer Patient ..265
John B. Schlaerth

Hypertension in the Non-pregnant Patient .267
William M. Barron and
Marshall D. Lindheimer

Acne Vulgaris 271
Marina Ball and
John Valentic

Ileus 274
A. Gerson Greenburg

Headache 276
Mary C. Taylor

Pneumonia 278
Thomas C. Cesario

Atelectasis 282
G. Robert Mason

Index 285

Section 1
OBSTETRICS

ACUTE HYPERTENSION IN PREGNANCY

KENNETH J. LEVENO, M.D.,
and PEGGY J. WHALLEY, M.D.

Acute hypertension is the most common serious complication of pregnancy developing prior to labor. Although its pathophysiology remains a puzzle, such hypertension is clearly a progressive systemic disease induced by pregnancy. Pregnancy-induced hypertension, or preeclampsia, encompasses a wide spectrum of severity of disease and, if unchecked, can result in maternal death as well as more frequent perinatal death. These disastrous results are unquestionably preventable by early identification, correct assessment of severity of disease, and aggressive management.

MANAGEMENT OF ECLAMPSIA

Prompt (1) treatment of convulsions, (2) control of severe hypertension, and (3) delivery are the basic principles of management of eclampsia. They have been successfully employed for more than two decades at Parkland Memorial Hospital, Dallas, Texas.

Control of Convulsions. Magnesium sulfate ($MgSO_4 \cdot 7H_2O$, USP) is used as the sole anticonvulsant for the following reasons. (1) The sensorium is not obtunded, which is in marked contrast to the effects of barbiturates, tranquilizers, or narcotics. (2) Airway problems and aspiration of stomach contents are much less likely to occur in an alert, awake patient. (3) The fetus is not depressed. (4) Magnesium sulfate therapy is easily managed with a minimum of demands upon the physicians and nurses.

The guidelines for administration of magnesium sulfate are as follows:

1. *Loading dose:* 20 ml of 20 per cent* magnesium sulfate (4 grams) is administered intravenously over a 3 minute period. This is immediately followed by 20 ml of 50 per cent magnesium sulfate, half (5 grams or 10 ml) injected deeply in the upper outer quadrant of each buttock through a 3 inch long 20-gauge needle.

2. *Maintenance dose:* 10 ml of 50 per cent magnesium sulfate (5 grams) is administered intramuscularly in alternating buttocks every 4 hours, provided (1) the patellar reflexes are present, (2) respirations are not depressed, and (3) urine output was at least 100 ml during the previous 4 hours. This dose of magnesium sulfate is continued for 24 hours after delivery. To reduce local discomfort, 1 ml of 2 per cent lidocaine is drawn into the syringe after loading with 50 per cent magnesium sulfate solution.

Magnesium sulfate, administered as described, almost invariably arrests convulsions and prevents their recurrence. Rarely, 50 mg incremental intravenous doses of amobarbital (up to a total dose of 250 mg) may be required to arrest the initial episode of convulsion or eliminate physical agitation. During the convulsion, efforts to maintain a clear airway, prevent aspiration, and protect the woman from injury are important.

Control of Blood Pressure. Antihypertensive agents are utilized only if diastolic blood pressure reaches 110 mm Hg. A safe, effective drug for this purpose is hydralazine hydrochloride. A 5 mg test dose is injected intravenously and the blood pressure monitored every 5 minutes. If the diastolic blood pressure is not lowered to about 100 mm Hg in 20 minutes, a 10 mg dose is administered and its effects monitored. Thereafter, 5 to 10 mg doses are given every 20 minutes whenever the diastolic pressure reaches 110 mm Hg.

Delivery. The return of normal sensorium following convulsions, usually in 4 to 6 hours, is an important sign that attempts at delivery can be safely begun. Vaginal delivery is preferred, and cesarean section is reserved for failed induction of labor or other obstetrical indications. Electronic fetal heart rate surveillance during labor is necessary, as is the availability of neonatal intensive care. It is important to note that fetal bradycardia occurring during a maternal convulsion typically resolves within a few minutes, and emergency cesarean section for fetal distress is both unnecessary and a serious threat to the unstable mother.

MANAGEMENT OF PREECLAMPSIA

There are two priorities in the management of preeclampsia. The first priority is assessment of severity, followed only then by the second, which is consideration of fetal age. Management based upon these priorities is summarized in Figure 1.

Women with severe preeclampsia who do not promptly respond to hospitalization are managed as described for eclampsia. Delivery is effected without procrastination and regardless of fetal maturity. During labor, delivery, and the puerperium, magnesium sulfate is used to prevent convulsions and blood pressure is con-

---

*A 20 per cent solution of magnesium sulfate is made by mixing in a syringe 8 ml of 50 per cent magnesium sulfate solution (4 grams) with 12 ml of sterile distilled water.

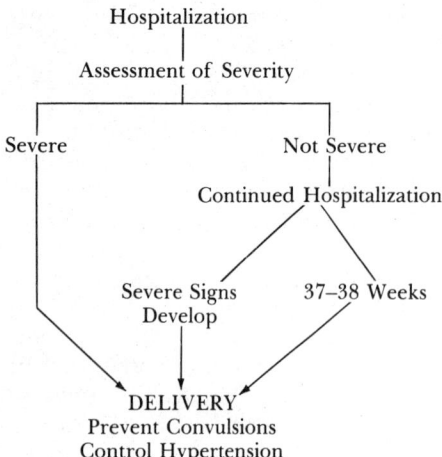

Figure 1. Management of preeclampsia.

trolled with hydralazine. It is important to emphasize that antihypertensive therapy is limited to the peripartum period and is never used in ill-advised attempts to prolong pregnancy.

When preeclampsia is not severe and the fetus is immature (less than 37 to 38 weeks' gestational age), expectant management is permissable. Continued hospitalization is mandatory. This not only lessens the intensity of hypertension by reducing physical activity, it also permits daily reassessment for worsening disease or development of signs of severe preeclampsia. Ambulation within the hospital is permitted and sedatives are avoided. Diet is not restricted and antihypertensive medications, including diuretics, are avoided. Serial measurements of renal function and fetal growth are also important.

The goal of expectant management is to delay delivery until neonatal survival is assured and the cervix is favorable for the induction of labor. In the absence of signs of severe preeclampsia, attainment of fetal maturity is the indication for delivery.

SPECIAL CONSIDERATIONS

Anesthesia. General endotracheal anesthesia using thiopental sodium, nitrous oxide plus oxygen, and succinylcholine is preferred for operative delivery. Conduction anesthesia and its attendant sympathetic blockade may precipitate hypotension in the woman with an already contracted blood volume.

Hemorrhage. Apparently normal blood pressure immediately following delivery frequently indicates hypovolemia resulting from excessive blood loss. Replacement of blood volume with whole blood is most effective in restoring circulating blood volume and maintaining renal perfusion.

Intravenous Fluids. The vasculature of women with acute hypertension is unyielding, and excessive administration of fluids to increase urine flow may precipitate heart failure. A good rule is to administer a balanced electrolyte solution at a rate no greater than 60 ml per hour.

Magnesium Sulfate Toxicity. Unless there is preexisting poor renal function, or inadvertent magnesium sulfate overdosage, the administration of magnesium sulfate as described does not cause respiratory depression. Support of ventilation, and calcium gluconate, 10 ml of a 10 per cent solution, given intravenously over a 5 minute period, are effective therapy for magnesium toxicity.

CHRONIC HYPERTENSION IN PREGNANCY

FREDERICK P. ZUSPAN, M.D.

Pregnancy may be hypertensogenic by unmasking a woman who has a tendency toward chronic hypertension. The opportunity the obstetrician has in following obstetric patients is the serial evaluation of the blood pressure; hence, the diagnosis of chronic hypertensive vascular disease, regardless of cause, can usually be made prior to the 24th week of pregnancy. The disease of chronic hypertension is seen more frequently in a multigravid individual, but the primagravid individual is not totally immune. Approximately 5 to 8 per cent of teenagers have hypertension when not pregnant, and in some of these young individuals who become pregnant chronic hypertension can be diagnosed before the 24th week of gestation.

The patient who has chronic hypertension and is pregnant is difficult to follow, since there usually is a decline in blood pressure in the middle trimester of pregnancy; hence, what one's opinion may be with regard to the final outcome will depend on when the patient is first seen. It is important that the patient be evaluated periodically during pregnancy, and that management regimens be altered as necessary. A predictive value for mean arterial pressure [(systolic − diastolic)/3 + diastolic] in which problems relate to the fetus should be considered as a value of greater than 95 mean arterial pressure in the mid-trimester of pregnancy.

If superimposed preeclampsia develops and the patient has chronic hypertension, perinatal mortality is increased by 3 to 5 times. Maternal mortality increases as well. One of the goals of therapy for the patient who has chronic hypertension is the prevention of preeclampsia.

CLASSIFICATION

Ninety-five per cent of patients have primary or essential vascular hypertension. The remainder have secondary hypertension, in which the cause is another known disease process. The essential ingredient in hypertension is vasospasm. In pregnancy this occurs in the uteroplacental bed, which means that the regulatory mechanisms and the physiologic changes that take place in normal pregnancy are no longer present.

MANAGEMENT

Before Pregnancy. If possible, women who have hypertension should be evaluated prior to pregnancy. Once pregnancy is sustained, the patient should be instructed in the following regimen: (1) a nutritious, well balanced diet containing 90 mg of protein or more per day; (2) bed rest on her side at noon for 1½ hours per day; if she works, 45 minutes at noon and an hour when she comes home from work. She must understand that it is necessary for her to visit her physician at least every two weeks throughout the pregnancy.

Care During Pregnancy. The above regimen should be instituted and consideration should be given as to whether or not antihypertensive drugs should be continued. If the woman is on any diuretic medication, it should not be continued after 20 weeks of gestation. A sedative, such as phenobarbital, is often beneficial in diminishing anxiety and may lead to increased patient compliance. It is imperative that bed rest be considered the most valuable ingredient in the pregnancy. If the diastolic blood pressure increases to 90 or more, it is essential that antihypertensive medication be given.

The only medication which has ever been subjected to any randomized study has been alpha-methyldopa (Aldomet), which can be started at 250 mg four times daily, and increased to 500 mg four times daily as needed. If the patient requires more than 2 grams of Aldomet per day, hospitalization and further evaluation are essential. The next medication to add for care is propranolol, beginning at 20 mg four times daily and increasing to 40 mg four times daily. Liberal hospitalization is necessary. Above all else, prevention of onset of acute hypertension of preeclampsia will guard against problems for both mother and fetus. Oral hydralazine (Apresoline) is of very little value during pregnancy, but if an acute hypertensive episode intervenes, intravenous Apresoline is the drug of choice to control the patient's blood pressure. If the patient has superimposed preeclampsia, then the therapeutic regimen of a loading dose of intravenous magnesium sulfate, 4 grams initially, then 1 to 2 grams per hour, should follow. Diastolic blood pressure should be controlled with the antihypertensive drug, Aldomet, and should be maintained at less than 100 mm Hg.

Fetal Evaluation. All forms of fetal evaluation are necessary, and those that are most successful, which should begin at approximately 30 weeks of gestation, are nonstress testing (NST), and contraction stress testing (CST) if the nonstress test is insufficient. These evaluations should begin on a weekly basis. Urinary estriol:creatinine ratios are helpful guideposts to identify the fetoplacental unit, but even more important are serial ultrasound determinations to rule out intrauterine growth retardation. Intrauterine growth retardation can be identified by a decrease in amniotic fluid and a decrease in the estrogen:creatinine ratio.

When to Deliver. Pregnancy in patients with hypertension should not be permitted to go beyond 40 weeks of gestation. The average chance of a cesarean section being necessary is between 15 and 20 per cent at the present time, and for the patient who has chronic hypertension it will be twice that. When the patient is in labor, intensive maternal and fetal monitoring should be carried out. Most patients who have chronic hypertension which is not severe will carry an excellent prognosis for both mother and fetus, and can be followed nearly to term before the pregnancy is interrupted. If a cesarean section is done, general anesthesia is preferable, but epidural anesthesia is a viable alternative. Spinal anesthesia should not be used.

The most essential ingredient in the care of the chronic hypertensive patient who is pregnant is ample bed rest of at least 2 hours per day, and self blood pressure determinations so the actual basal pressures are known. Frequent visits to the physician are necessary, and it is not uncommon for the obstetrician to see a woman with chronic hypertension more than 25 times during pregnancy.

DIABETES IN PREGNANCY
E. MICHAEL LINZEY, M.D.

Prior to the advent of insulin, the diabetic woman presented formidable problems for the obstetrician. Diabetes was rarely encountered in pregnancy, however, because many women severely affected with diabetes died before childbearing age, and of those women who managed to conceive there was a 25 per cent maternal mortality in addition to a 50 per cent perinatal mortality. With the introduction of insulin, control was able to be achieved and lives of both mothers and babies were saved. The obstetrician then faced the dilemma of the fetus dying in utero, along with much of the morbidity associated with the diabetic pregnancy. Difficult decisions, such as when to deliver the fetus, arose because of the risk of intrauterine death. It was at 36 weeks when the risk of in utero or neonatal death became approximately equal. Avoiding fetal death was often followed by neonatal death from respiratory distress syndrome. In the late 1960s and early 1970s a tool was introduced which enabled the obstetrician to evaluate the fetal condition in utero by employing the oxytocin challenge test (OCT) in evaluating respiratory capacity of the placenta. In addition, urinary and plasma estriol determinations enabled the obstetrician to evaluate the fetus during the interim between oxytocin challenge tests. With these fetal evaluations the perinatal mortality rate began to decrease significantly, and death from congenital malformations then made up the greater percentage of in utero and neonatal deaths. The period of the late 1970s and early 1980s has seen a move to tightly control the diabetic to establish a euglycemic state in order to decrease the incidence of macrosomia as well as congenital malformations. It has recently been shown that strict diabetic control is particularly important in decreasing perinatal mortality, and the incidence of macrosomia, and other complications such as retinal vascular disease. Recent introduction of the glycosylated hemoglobin A_1C in the evaluation of long-term control has been proven to be useful in the prediction of congenital malformations in the fetus of the pregnant diabetic. The patient entering pregnancy with normal levels of hemoglobin A_1C is assumed to have had good diabetic control prior to and around the time of conception. With a normal level of hemoglobin A_1C, one can predict a decreased chance of congenital malformation.

CLASSIFICATION

Diabetes in pregnancy can be divided into two subtypes: Class A diabetes, characterized by a normal fasting blood sugar, but an abnormal glucose tolerance test; Classes B, C, D, F, R, and H, characterized by an abnormal fasting blood sugar and therefore requiring insulin for control. Women with Class B or C diabetes classically have large neonates, because of lack of vascular disease. Those with Class D diabetes are the juvenile onset diabetics, very often with vascular disease and sometimes hypertension. The woman with Class F diabetes is the diabetic who has renal involvement. Class R diabetes is associated with proliferative retinopathy. The woman with Class H diabetes has atherosclerotic cardiovascular disease on the basis of her diabetes and stands a significant risk of maternal mortality during gestation. The term "gestational diabetes" is confusing and has been misused. Gestational diabetes does not necessarily mean Class A diabetes but may include those diabetics who require insulin for control during gestation. The term "gestational diabetes" refers mainly to the fact that the patient is normal before pregnancy and returns to normal 6 weeks after, but says nothing about the classification of diabetes during gestation. Most diabetics who have gestational diabetes are in the Class A group, but many who begin early in gestation with Class A diabetes may require insulin during their pregnancy because of the development of an abnormal fasting blood sugar. It is important therefore to observe the woman with Class A diabetes carefully with frequent fasting blood sugar determinations.

MANAGEMENT OF INSULIN AND DIET DURING PREGNANCY

The care of the pregnant diabetic requires an obstetrician knowledgeable in the control and use of insulin during pregnancy, or a combination of an obstetrician, internist and dietitian to maintain glucose levels within a range considered to be normal for pregnancy, usually between 60 and 100 mg per dl for fasting and no more than 140 mg per dl 2 hours after a meal. Oral hypoglycemic agents must not be used during pregnancy because of the potential risk of teratogenesis and also the severe hypoglycemia that can occur in the infant born to a mother taking oral hypoglycemic agents in the neonatal period. The patient's diet should contain approximately 15 Calories per lb of ideal body weight, or 30 Calories per kg, and usually consists of 45 to 50 per cent carbohydrates, 30 per cent fat, and 25 per cent protein. These meals are usually distributed as breakfast, lunch, dinner, and pre-bedtime snack. The caloric distribution of these meals consists of 2/7 at breakfast, 2/7 at lunch, 2/7 at dinner, and 1/7 taken as a pre-bedtime snack. Careful evaluation of the patient's weight gain and observation for the presence of acetone in the urine must be continued. The diet can be varied accordingly, that is if the patient gains excessive weight, the number of calories must be decreased so that the patient will gain no more than 24 lb during her gestation. If the patient experiences acetonuria, however, the caloric content must be increased, or if the patient is gaining weight normally, a shift in calories away from fats and proteins and toward carbohydrates may achieve a clearing of the urine acetone.

For those patients requiring insulin (Classes B through H), insulin is usually best administered by injection as a combination of short- and intermediate-acting insulin, that is, regular or semi-lente and NPH or lente insulin. Approximately two thirds of the total dose is administered in the morning and one third prior to the evening meal. The goal is to maintain a fasting and 4:00 P.M. blood sugar level (a blood sugar level measured 4 hours after the noon meal) between 60 and 100 mg per dl, and a 2 hour postprandial value of less than 140 mg per dl, preferably close to 120. One must be careful not to be too vigorous in the control of diabetes, so that the patient will not experience frequent hypoglycemic episodes.

The requirements for insulin during pregnancy vary according to the gestational age of the fetus. In the first trimester, insulin requirements typically drop, thus necessitating a reduction in insulin dose below that which was required before pregnancy began. This will be exhibited by the patient as frequent hypoglycemic episodes, which the patient may often be causing by adjusting her own insulin according to her urine spill of sugar. The patient must be aware that she may spill glucose in pregnancy at levels lower than she has been used to prior to the onset of gestation. During the second and third trimesters, insulin requirements begin to rise and may eventually increase by more than twice the normal pre-pregnancy insulin need. Immediately after delivery, insulin requirements fall and, depending upon diet, breast feeding, and activity of the patient may take one to two weeks or longer to return to pre-pregnancy values.

The classic approach to control of insulin during pregnancy using double-voided urine specimens collected before meals and at bedtime as a reflection of blood sugar is inadequate. Glycosuria occurs frequently, even in normal pregnancies, because of the increase in the glomerular filtration rate. The only satisfactory method for control of glucose during pregnancy is frequent evaluations of the blood glucose or plasma glucose by laboratory means, or at home using glucose oxidase–impregnated sticks (Dextrostix) and a reflectance meter (Dextrometer or glucometer, Ames Company, Ames, IA). By using such a meter at home, the patient will be able to achieve very tight control of her diabetes and can be taught to adjust her insulin levels by herself, so that she becomes active in the management of her pregnancy. This gives the patient a feeling of having some control over her diabetes, as well as participating in her care. A protocol can be given to the patient so that she may adjust her insulin at home as shown in Table 1.

TABLE 1. **Dextrometer Reading Adjustment of Insulin Dose at Home**

ONE A.M. DOSE OF INSULIN

Fasting Blood Sugar (FBS)
- Less than 60 – Call doctor for adjustment
- 60–110 – No change
- 110–150 – Increase insulin, NPH 2U, and obtain a FBS next day
- 150–200 – Increase insulin, NPH 4U, and obtain a FBS next day
- above 200 – Call doctor for adjustment

4 P.M. Blood Sugar–Same as above

SPLIT DOSE OF INSULIN

Fasting Blood Sugar
- Less than 60 – Call doctor for adjustment
- 60–110 – No change in 4 P.M. dose
- 110–150 – Increase evening NPH by 2U and obtain a FBS next day
- 150–200 – Increase evening NPH by 4U and obtain a FBS next day
- above 200 – Call doctor for adjustment

4 P.M. Blood Sugar
- Less than 60 – Call doctor for adjustment
- 60–130 – No change in the morning dose
- 130–150 – Increase morning NPH by 2U and obtain a 4 P.M. BS next day
- 150–200 – Increase morning NPH by 4U and obtain a 4 P.M. BS next day
- 200–250 – Increase morning NPH by 6U and obtain a 4 P.M. BS next day
- above 250 – Call doctor for adjustment

Evaluation of the hemoglobin A_1C level during pregnancy at monthly or two-monthly intervals has demonstrated good control with this method. Thus the rigid control of blood sugar during pregnancy is achieved, and the incidence of macrosomia is decreased using this method.

MANAGEMENT OF CLASS A DIABETES

The woman with Class A diabetes is not at increased risk for perinatal mortality compared with the normal obstetrical population, but morbidity in the neonatal period may be increased. In the antepartum period the patient should be seen in a high-risk clinic every two weeks, with fasting blood sugar levels evaluated at each visit. As long as the fasting blood sugar level remains normal, the patient can be followed to term without increased risk of intrauterine death. The patient is also asked to follow her urine sugar and acetone levels at home, and if she exhibits a fasting glycosuria, the fasting blood sugar level must be evaluated to rule in or rule out overt diabetes. If the fasting blood sugar exceeds normal, the patient must then be managed as a Class B diabetic, and may require insulin. Provided that the Class A patient has no history of previous stillbirth, does not have hypertension before the onset of pregnancy, and does not develop hypertension during pregnancy, she may safely be followed to 40 weeks of gestation before antepartum fetal surveillance is required. If the patient falls into the above categories she must be followed as a Class B diabetic with early and frequent evaluations of fetal status. Once the Class A patient reaches 40 weeks of gestation, fetal surveillance must be undertaken either in the form of weekly oxytocin challenge tests or twice weekly nonstress tests, provided vaginal delivery will be anticipated. If, however, the patient is suspected of having a macrosomic fetus, which can be further elucidated by the ultrasound measurement of biparietal diameter and transabdominal or transthoracic measurements, primary cesarean section for macrosomia should be done after evaluation of fetal lung maturity by means of a lecithin:sphingomyelin ratio obtained via amniocentesis. The purpose of this method of delivery in a Class A diabetic with macrosomia is to avoid traumatic vaginal delivery resulting in shoulder dystocia, which occurs with higher incidence in those infants exceeding 4000 grams of weight. If labor is permitted, the patient must be carefully evaluated for progress and shoulder dystocia should be anticipated. The fetal heart rate must be continuously monitored during the intrapartum period and a neonatologist must be available at delivery for management of the neonate.

MANAGEMENT OF INSULIN-DEPENDENT DIABETES (CLASSES B THROUGH H)

The obstetrician and the internist or the perinatologist should work with the patient even prior to the onset of gestation to achieve optimal diabetic control. The diabetic should have counseling before conception to inform her completely of the need for strict diabetic control, the potential cost of a diabetic pregnancy, the emotional demands of a pregnancy, and the inherent risks in beginning a pregnancy in the presence of a pre-existing medical condition. During the antepartum period, frequent visits are essential and should be made no less frequently than every two weeks until 28 weeks of gestation, and then weekly thereafter. Renal function should be carefully evaluated by BUN and creatinine determinations and a 24 hour urine specimen evaluated for creatinine clearance and total protein. Urine cultures should also be obtained to investigate for asymptomatic bacteriuria. If a patient has been a diabetic for 10 years or longer (Class C or more), an electrocardiogram and ophthalmological examination are required. The patient must evaluate a double-voided urine specimen before meals and at bedtime for glucose and acetone, and record these carefully in a book provided by her obstetrician. The patient should also evaluate her glucose levels, by obtaining both fasting and 4 P.M. levels twice weekly, in addition to a panel obtained before meals and at bedtime, once a week. This should be recorded carefully in her book and be discussed with the obstetrician at each visit.

Fetal surveillance is initiated at 32 to 34 weeks of gestation in patients without evidence of hypertensive or vascular disease. Surveillance may be begun as early as 26 weeks in patients exhibiting evidence of intrauterine growth retardation, hypertension, or other medical complications in addition to diabetes. The classic management of diabetes in pregnancy has included daily plasma estriol determinations and weekly oxytocin challenge testing. Because plasma estriols levels have been found to add little to the care of the pregnant diabetic in general and add considerable cost to her care, they may be employed in those situations in which the other antepartum tests become borderline or suspicious. Weekly oxytocin challenge testing and a midweek nonstress test may be employed, or twice weekly nonstress testing utilized for evaluation of fetal well-being. These evaluations, however, are most predictive of a healthy fetus and may show many false-positive results.

These patients may be managed at home, provided no intercurrent problems are observed and the patient is reliable. The timing of delivery must be individualized for every patient, to achieve maximum maturity while minimizing the chance of intrauterine fetal demise. Once 38 weeks of gestation is reached, delivery must be considered. A lecithin:sphingomyelin (L:S) ratio must be obtained to evaluate fetal lung maturity. An L:S ratio of 2:0 or greater and the presence of amniotic fluid phosphatidylglycerol (PG) indicates fetal lung maturity. If macrosomia is evident, primary cesarean section should be carried out. Macrosomia can be evaluated by comparing the biparietal diameter with a measurement of the fetal thorax or trunk. If the transabdominal or transthoracic measurement exceeds the biparietal diameter by more than 1.5 cm, macrosomia can be expected and shoulder dystocia anticipated. With such measurements, cesarean section would be a reasonable alternative.

Pregnancy may be prolonged beyond 38 weeks' gestation to permit successful induction of labor and vaginal delivery if macrosomia or hypertension is not present and the fetal condition is satisfactory as demonstrated by antepartum testing. If fetal jeopardy is suspected prior to 38 weeks of gestation, an L:S ratio should be obtained. If fetal lungs are mature, the pregnancy may safely be terminated. In the face of an immature L:S ratio, indicating possible fetal lung immaturity, delivery of the fetus should be undertaken only when all parameters of fetal well-being indicate deterioration, that is, if the oxytocin challenge test is positive, the nonstress test is minimally to non-reactive, and the estriol levels, if utilized, are low or falling.

Prior to delivery by cesarean section, or during the intrapartum period if labor is induced, diabetes may be controlled by continuous insulin infusion rather than by the classic method of giving half the daily dose of long-acting insulin prior to induction and then following blood and urine sugar levels, necessitating stat doses of regular insulin for control. The continuous insulin infusion may be administered as a solution of 500 cc of normal saline, 50 units of regular insulin, and 10 cc of salt-poor albumin to avoid adsorption of the insulin to glass and plastic tubing. The continuous infusion may be "piggybacked" into a dextrose and half-normal saline solution which is used as a maintenance IV and usually begun at between one-half and one unit per hour. The patient's blood sugar levels are frequently evaluated either by the Dextrostix method using the reflectance meter or by laboratory evaluation every 1 or 2 hours, using specimens drawn through a separate heparin lock tubing placed in the opposite arm of the patient. Using this method, serial induction can be carried out provided there is no evidence of fetal jeopardy and the patient does not exhibit other complications of pregnancy such as pregnancy-induced hypertension.

Once delivery is achieved, insulin control becomes less of a problem but the patient's sensitivity to insulin rises. Once the patient begins to eat and displays a need for insulin by having an abnormal fasting or postprandial blood sugar level, her long-acting insulin dose can be resumed at one-half of her *pre-pregnancy* dose. The patient's insulin requirements will slowly increase for the next one to two weeks. Women with insulin-dependent diabetes should be encouraged to breast feed if desired, provided adequate dietary supplementation, usually equal to that which was added to the diet during pregnancy, is continued.

THIRD TRIMESTER BLEEDING

ROBERT H. HAYASHI, M.D.

The incidence of significant vaginal bleeding in the last half of pregnancy is approximately 3 per cent. Several of the conditions that produce vaginal bleeding carry significant risk for the mother and fetus. Over half of these instances of significant bleeding are associated with placenta previa, the implantation of the placenta low in the uterus either overlying or reaching the vicinity of the cervical os, and abruptio placentae, separation of the normally implanted placenta between 20 weeks' gestation and birth of the infant.

Significant vaginal bleeding is the exit per vagina of bright red blood, not mixed in mucus as in a "bloody show," and equivalent in amount to menstrual bleeding or more. A physician who encounters a patient with third trimester bleeding as described should quickly obtain an accurate history to determine the onset of bleeding and activity occurring at that time, the presence or absence of abdominal or low back pain and its character, or possible trauma. Vital signs, including auscultation of fetal heart tones, should be initially obtained. If signs of maternal hypovolemic shock or fetal distress are found, an intravenous infusion of a crystalloid solution should be quickly begun and blood drawn for a hemogram and crossmatch. Lowered maternal cardiac output can impair placental blood flow, placing the fetus in jeopardy.

When the patient is stable, a careful and limited vaginal speculum examination should be performed to determine whether the bleeding is from within the uterus, and to rule out obvious causes of bleeding such as cervical or vaginal trauma, cervicitis, cervical cancer or polyps, or bleeding from cervical, vaginal, or labial varicosities. If the bleeding is painless or silent, the presumptive diagnosis is placenta previa and the placenta should be localized by ultrasonography. Ultrasonography has a diagnostic accuracy of 95 per cent in experienced hands. If the bleeding is associated with pain, the presumptive diagnosis is abruptio placentae. If the pain is intermittent and the resting tone of the uterus is normal, the patient might be in labor with a placenta previa. Ultrasonography would be diagnostically helpful in this case.

PLACENTA PREVIA

Placental implantation in the lower uterus associated with significant vaginal bleeding occurs in about 0.5 per cent or 1 in 200 pregnancies. The incidence increases with the age and parity of the patient, and if the patient has a past history of a low segment cesarean section or placenta previa.

Two basic principles used in the management of placenta previa involve the timing and route of delivery.

Once the diagnosis of placenta previa is confirmed by ultrasonography, continuing management depends on the gestational age of the fetus and the amount of bleeding. Since bleeding from a placenta previa is rarely fatal unless the placenta is disrupted by labor or by a transcervical examining finger or object, and since the high perinatal mortality in placenta previa is due to prematurity, a logical course to follow when the fetus is premature is one of expectant management. The goal of expectant management is to safely delay delivery until the fetus is mature. Management is usually carried out in the hospital. A hematocrit above 30 ml per dl is maintained by administration of hematinics or blood transfusions if necessary. Once the bleeding has subsided, an occasional patient may be managed at home provided that the following criteria are met:

1. The patient must be intelligent and reliable, and understands the ramifications of her condition; she must be willing to remain at bed rest and avoid coitus.

2. Round-the-clock transportation and communication must be available, and the patient must live within reasonable distance from the hospital.

3. The hematocrit must be above 30 ml per dl.

The expectant management program is contraindicated or terminated when:

1. The patient is in labor;
2. The fetus is mature (determined most reliably by the L:S ratio);
3. The fetus is dead;
4. An intrauterine infection develops;
5. The membranes rupture; or
6. The bleeding is excessive or life threatening.

Usually about one third of patients with placenta previa can be managed expectantly, since over half are near term when the first bleeding episode is experienced. The remainder go into labor or have profuse bleeding.

The diagnosis of a placenta previa also includes partial covering of the cervical os and marginal low-lying placenta. Under certain circumstances a vaginal delivery may be allowed with these conditions. Although the placenta can be localized in the lower uterus quite accurately by ultrasonography, determination of the exact relationship of the lower placental edge to the cervical os is less accurate. Also, during the interval of initial diagnosis to delivery, the development of the lower uterine segment from cervical tissue can result in the upward shift of the lower edge of the placenta from the cervical os.

The most accurate method of determining the relationship of the placenta to the cervical os is palpation. This should be done only after termination of expectant management and under "double set-up" conditions, that is, in the operating room with blood ready, anesthesia standby, and all preparations completed for an immediate cesarean section. The palpation of a placenta covering the cervical os or part of it mandates proceeding to an abdominal delivery. If the placenta is not palpated over the cervical os, the examining finger is inserted through the cervical os to palpate several centimeters of the lower uterine segment. A posterior low-lying placenta will usually warrant an abdominal delivery because this situation can be associated with intrapartum fetal distress and soft tissue dystocia. With an anterior low-lying placenta, on the other hand, a trial of vaginal delivery may be allowed. The goal of the "double set-up" examination is only to determine the route of delivery. If vaginal delivery is to be allowed, the need for induction of labor should be dictated by the ripeness of the cervix.

Maternal death from placenta previa is rare, but the perinatal mortality is still over 5 per cent.

ABRUPTIO PLACENTAE

The incidence of clinically diagnosed abruptio placentae varies from 0.4 to almost 2 per cent. It is usually associated with maternal hypertension (47 per cent), high parity, and a past history of an abruption (1 in 10).

The management of abruptio placentae depends on the degree of severity, defined as follows: Abruption is considered mild when the separation leads to external bleeding, mild uterine hypertonus, but not maternal shock or fetal distress. This condition may even be dismissed by the patient, only to recur. Abruption is moderate when there is no maternal shock, but fetal distress or death, uterine tetany, or external or concealed bleeding is present. Abruption is said to be severe when maternal shock, fetal death, uterine tetany, and usually a coagulopathy (30 per cent) occur. The incidence of severe abruption is 1 in 500 pregnancies.

As the placenta prematurely separates, the bleeding site extends, since the uterus cannot effectively contract to shut off the spiral arteries. The blood travels between the fetal membranes and decidua to find its way out of the cervix. The blood may also remain concealed within the uterus (20 per cent), causing an increase in uterine volume, often resulting in tearing of the fetal membranes with minimal or no external bleeding. A small placental separation can proceed to a larger one. The blood irritates the uterine muscles, causing tenderness, labor, and eventually tetany. The patient usually enters active labor rapidly, and delivers within several hours. With a severe abruption the patient can lose up to half of her blood volume (2500 ml). The thromboplastin material in the amniotic fluid can find its way into the maternal blood stream to initiate an acute disseminated intravascular coagulopathy.

Management of a patient with an abruptio placenta requires adherence to these basic tenets:

1. Rule of 30's. Maintenance of a minimum urine output of 30 ml per hour and a hematocrit of 30 ml per dl at all times by intravenous infusion of crystalloid solutions or blood as required.

2. Effect delivery as quickly and safely as possible. The goal is a vaginal delivery without a set time limit if the fetus is healthy or dead. A cesarean section may be required if fetal distress is present. The use of oxytocin is not contraindicated, although it is rarely necessary.

3. Early amniotomy to decrease amnioinfusion into the maternal blood stream.

4. Intensive maternal and fetal monitoring of vital signs and circulating volume status.

In any patient diagnosed as having an abruption (even mild, since it may progress), a reliable, large bore intravenous line should be established (two or more in severe abruption); 6 or more units of blood should be cross-matched; the bladder should be drained by catheter; an amniotomy should be done; internal fetal monitoring is done if the fetus is alive; blood coagulation studies are performed. A central venous pressure line or Swan-Ganz balloon flotation catheter may help in the fluid management of a patient in shock. A timed peripheral venous blood sample placed in a red-topped tube taped to the wall and checked in 7 to 10 minutes will indicate the coagulation status of the patient. If the clot is not formed or is fragile, the patient has a coagulopathy. If vaginal delivery is anticipated, correction of the coagulopathy is not necessary and will not alter the outcome. Careful hemostasis for an episiotomy will be required. The coagulopathy will usually be present when the patient first enters the hospital and will be restored to normal in 12 to 24 hours postpartum by a normally functioning liver. If the patient requires an abdominal delivery for obstetric indications, the coagulopathy will have to be corrected with fresh frozen plasma and cryoprecipitate (15 to 20 bags will increase fibrinogen 100 mg per dl). At the time of laparotomy, one may encounter a bruised-appearing uterus (Couvelaire uterus). This appearance should not belie the ability of the uterus to contract sufficiently to control bleeding after delivery. A coagulopathy developing in the presence of a live fetus would be quite unusual, but a clot should be checked before surgery.

By maintaining an adequate circulating volume (rule of 30's) during labor in a patient with a placental abruption, the not uncommon sequelae in the past, of renal damage, adult pulmonary distress syndrome, and Sheehan's syndrome, can be minimized. The perinatal mortality is over 50 per cent and the maternal mortality is 1 per cent or less.

BREECH PRESENTATION

JOSEPH V. COLLEA, M. D.

The management of singleton breech presentation has changed over the past decade. Prior to 1970, most patients with breech presentation were allowed to labor and deliver vaginally. Since 1970, however, the majority of patients with breech presentation are delivered electively by cesarean section.

The primary reason for the dramatic change in the route of breech delivery is the fact that infants delivered vaginally from breech presentation have five times the perinatal mortality rate of comparable infants delivered from cephalic presentations. Analysis of data published over the past 25 years reveals four major causes of this increased perinatal loss with breech presentation:

1. *Prematurity*: 25 per cent of all breech deliveries in any institution are low birth weight (less than 2500 grams).

2. *Congenital malformations*: 6 per cent of all breech infants have congenital malformations.

3. *Umbilical cord prolapse*: 10 per cent of footling breech presentations and 5 per cent of complete breech presentations are associated with intrapartum umbilical cord prolapse. Frank breech presentations, however, have a cord prolapse incidence of only 0.5 per cent, identical to that of cephalic presentations.

4. *Birth trauma*: brachial plexus palsies, clavicular and long bone fractures, soft-tissue injuries, and intracerebral hemorrhage from tentorial tears are related to difficult breech extraction or to vaginal delivery of a significantly premature infant. Vaginal delivery of a breech fetus with a deflexed head in utero is also associated with significant perinatal morbidity and mortality.

Until relatively recently, obstetricians have attempted to decrease this excessive breech perinatal mortality rate by perfecting the techniques of vaginal breech extraction, by performing external cephalic version to prevent or decrease the occurrence of breech deliveries, by using x-ray pelvimetry to avoid extracting the fetal after-coming head through an inadequate or frankly contracted maternal pelvis, and by applying Piper forceps for controlled delivery of the after-coming head. Unfortunately, none of these methods, used alone or in combination, has ever been credited with significantly decreasing the breech perinatal mortality rate. Cesarean section, on the other hand, by avoiding the problems of umbilical cord compression and birth trauma, has resulted in significantly lowered breech perinatal morbidity and mortality. The utilization of cesarean section for breech delivery, however, will *not* eliminate the perinatal deaths attributable to severe congenital malformations or extreme prematurity (gestational age less than 26 weeks, birth weight less than 700 grams). Cesarean section itself is also a major operative procedure with significant potential anesthetic, infectious, and hemorrhagic complications.

Recently, investigators have reported that careful selection of patients with singleton breech presentation for vaginal delivery as well as cesarean section minimizes the risks to both mother and fetus.

CLINICAL MANAGEMENT

Fetal presentation should be determined during the antenatal course by performing Leopold's maneuvers at each prenatal visit after the 25th week of gestational age. It is well known that the incidence of breech presentation is inversely proportional to the gestational age of the fetus. Prior to 30 weeks gestation, the incidence approaches 35 per cent, whereas at term it drops to only 3 per cent. The vast majority of breech fetuses revert to the cephalic presentation by the 34th week of gestation.

When breech presentation persists beyond 34 weeks of gestational age, the fetus should be evaluated ultrasonographically to rule out the presence of congenital malformations such as anencephaly, hydrocephaly, and meningomyelocele. The fetus should also be evaluated for intrauterine growth retardation, since many such fetuses present at birth in the breech position.

If breech presentation is detected antenatally and the fetus is free of congenital malformations detectable by ultrasonography, some investigators would advocate external cephalic version to prevent subsequent breech delivery. External cephalic version as an obstetric procedure is at best controversial, and should be performed only by those physicians expert in its execution and aware of its complications. If this procedure is to be performed at all, it must be performed by a skilled obstetrician on one or more occasions between the 32nd and the 36th week of gestation. The type of breech presentation and placental localization should be confirmed prior to the procedure by ultrasonography to avoid attempts in women with placenta previa or with frank breech presentations. The extended legs of the frank breech make external cephalic version more difficult and consequently more hazardous to perform for both mother and fetus. For the obstetrician in clinical practice, the performance of external cephalic version today would be a rare event.

The intrapartum management of singleton breech presentations depends upon maternal obstetric history, type of presentation, gestational age, and estimated fetal weight, as well as the progress of labor. Patients in premature labor who are *not* candidates for tocolysis and who are less than 26 weeks' gestation with estimated fetal weights less than 700 grams should be delivered vaginally. Cesarean delivery in these cases will not effectively increase neonatal survival and would significantly affect the patient's future childbearing capabilities.

Patients in premature labor between 26 and 34 weeks' gestation whose labor cannot be stopped should be delivered by cesarean section, since neonatal outcome in these cases is superior to delivery by the vaginal route. Fetuses with congenital malformations incompatible with life, such as anencephaly, should obviously be delivered vaginally, since cesarean section offers no advantage to either mother or fetus.

The management of patients of 34 or more weeks' gestation depends upon fetal presentation and estimated fetal weight. Footling and complete breech presentations should be delivered by cesarean section to avoid the significant incidence of umbilical cord prolapse associated with such cases. Again, ultrasonography, abdominal x-ray or both should be used prior to surgery to detect fetal malformations.

Patients with frank breech presentations, whose fetuses are free of congenital malformations, with estimated weights between 2000 and 3800 grams, are candidates for vaginal delivery provided there are no obstetric contraindications such as fetal distress or inadequate pelvic mensuration. Adequate dimensions in all maternal pelvic planes should be documented by x-ray pelvimetry prior to vaginal delivery. The minimal measurements acceptable for vaginal delivery are:

Pelvic inlet
    Transverse 11.5 cm
    Anteroposterior 10.5 cm

Midpelvis
    Transverse 10 cm
    Anteroposterior 11.5 cm

Any candidate for vaginal delivery but who presents with a deflexed fetal head on ultrasonographic or radiologic examination should be delivered by cesarean section to avoid significant injury to the fetal central nervous system. If the estimated fetal weight exceeds 3800 grams, delivery should be by cesarean section.

Lastly, patients with a history of previous difficult or traumatic deliveries should not be allowed to deliver vaginally.

Patients allowed to labor should be monitored closely for uterine contractions and for fetal heart rate in order to detect intrapartum fetal distress. Intractable fetal distress should be managed by immediate cesarean section. Dysfunctional labor patterns should be managed as in cephalic presentations.

DELIVERY PROCEDURES

Partial breech extraction is the method of choice for vaginal delivery candidates. Total breech extraction should be avoided unless the fetus is in jeopardy and cesarean section cannot be performed immediately. Appropriate anesthetic techniques for vaginal delivery include the continuous epidural block or the pudendal nerve block for delivery of the fetal body, combined with a general anesthetic, if needed, for delivery of the after-coming head. Whenever possible, Piper forceps should be applied for a more controlled delivery of the fetal head.

A second obstetrician should be present in the delivery room, to help with delivery of the fetus, particularly during application of the Piper forceps. An anesthesiologist should be in attendance to insure adequate maternal comfort for the delivery and to administer a general anesthetic if needed for delivery of the fetal head. A pediatrician should be in attendance to resuscitate the newborn if necessary.

Patients who are not candidates for vaginal delivery should be delivered by low-segment cesarean section. In most cases a transverse incision in the lower uterine segment will effect an atraumatic delivery. However, if the fetus is significantly premature or if the lower uterine segment is not well developed, a low vertical incision in the uterus may be necessary to accomplish an atraumatic delivery. Every obstetrician should be thoroughly familiar with the manual art of breech extraction before attempting to perform an abdominal breech delivery, for the manual techniques of breech delivery performed at cesarean section require the same dexterity that is essential for a safe vaginal delivery.

The method of management described here limits the candidates for vaginal delivery and essentially results in a high rate of cesarean section for breech presentation. The careful selection of patients who can be offered a trial of labor and vaginal delivery will provide a minimum risk for both mother and fetus at delivery.

INTRAPARTUM FETAL DISTRESS

JOHN F. HUDDLESTON, M.D.

Myometrial contractions of usual intensity severely diminish uterine blood flow and thus interfere with placental intervillous-space perfusion. Therefore, during the peak of normal contractions, the transplacental passage of oxygen is seriously impeded, and the fetus—which has little capacity to store this gas—is subjected to temporary decreases in its pO_2 levels. Under usual conditions without contractions, umbilical venous pO_2 levels are only 25 to 30 torr, levels which would be intolerable to adults. The fetus, however, has mechanisms (high concentration and favorable dissociation curve of fetal hemoglobin, advantageous oxygen-binding resulting from a slight differential in pH, and high umbilical flow-rate) that allow it to thrive under these seemingly adverse conditions. On the other hand, the fetus has little buffer against the rather abrupt falls in pO_2 levels whenever its oxygen supply is compromised.

Chronic reduction in oxygen delivery to the fetus may occur with those conditions known to place the fetus at risk for uteroplacental insufficiency, such as insulin-dependent diabetes mellitus, chronic hypertensive disease, and cigarette smoking. Acute reduction, in addition to its periodic recurrence with normal contractions, may also accompany such intrapartum events as hypotension (hemorrhage, supine position, sympathetic paralysis due to conduction anesthesia), cord compression (intrauterine or due to prolapse), or uterine hypertonus (placental abruption or administration of oxytocin).

DISTRESS PATTERNS OF THE FETAL HEART RATE

Studies in both animals and humans have demonstrated that *repetitive* late decelerations of the fetal heart rate (FHR) reliably imply suboptimal basal oxygenation of the fetus, at least at that time. No matter how shallow, then, late decelerations, when repetitive, should be regarded as ominous. Variable decelerations, which are relatively more common, imply cord compression but generally can be improved or abolished by maternal positional changes. Severe variable decelerations generally refer to cases in which the FHR is below 70 per minute for more than 30 seconds or in which recovery to the FHR baseline (late deceleration component) is slow.

VARIABILITY OF THE FETAL HEART RATE

Prolonged reduction in oxygen availability to the fetus results in anerobic metabolism with the eventual consequence of metabolic acidosis. This acidosis, which after membrane rupture and partial cervical dilatation can be appreciated by pH assessments of fetal capillary blood, will depress the autonomic modulation of the otherwise monotonous baseline FHR. Clinically, such modulation is apparent as FHR reactivity (evaluated antepartally in the nonstress test or with *external* FHR monitoring during labor) and as FHR variability (used during labor with the more precise FHR signals derived from an *internal* fetal electrode). Depressed FHR variability, along with fetal tachycardia, may seriously heighten the degree of concern for the fetus demonstrating repetitive late or severe variable decelerations.

Unfortunately, depression of FHR variability frequently may be seen whenever drugs that alter maternal sensorium (e.g., tranquilizers, barbiturates, narcotics) are administered. Such drugs regularly cross the placenta and may temporarily alter fetal neurologic function sufficiently to depress the autonomic influences on the FHR. Although loss of FHR variability under these conditions is not generally cause for alarm, use of such drugs (particularly in large doses) can remove for some time a most valuable tool for fetal assessment.

DIAGNOSIS AND MANAGEMENT OF FETAL DISTRESS

A reasonable diagnosis of fetal distress should be one that can be made early in the course of an observable abnormal FHR response, at a time *before* any serious likelihood of fetal damage and when measures designed for intrauterine resuscitation are likely to be successful. Repetitive late decelerations, repetitive severe variable decelerations, and prolonged decelerations generally imply distress due to fetal hypoxia and should be followed at once by intrauterine resuscitation. Persistence of these abnormal FHR patterns may lead to fetal acidosis, which is associated with an increased risk of abnormal outcome. To require that fetal acidosis be demonstrated by fetal-blood sampling before a definitive diagnosis of distress is accepted would thus seem counterproductive to the goal of delivering infants in the best possible condition. To delay instituting intrauterine resuscitation for that duration would seem totally unreasonable.

Intrauterine resuscitation is designed to increase fetal oxygenation and has as its components an augmentation of placental intervillous-space blood flow and an increase in maternal-fetal oxygen gradient. Clinically, intrauterine resuscitation is effected by maintaining the mother in the left-lateral position (to avoid aortocaval compression), ceasing the delivery of any oxytocic drugs, increasing the infusion rate of intravenous fluids, correcting any hypotension (sometimes resulting from conduction anesthetics given without adequately preloading with intravenous fluids), and administering oxygen to the mother by mask. If variable decelerations are part of the FHR pattern of distress, other maternal positions (right-lateral, Trendelenburg) may be successful in resolving the pattern. Deep variable decelerations (and especially prolonged decelerations) may be due to cord prolapse, and this diagnosis should be specifically sought by immediate digital examination, palpating for the cord and (to detect occult prolapse) elevating the presenting part while observing the fetal-monitor output. It follows that in order to detect fetal distress at the earliest possible time, *ideally* all laboring women should be electronically monitored for the duration of labor. Although so-called high-risk pregnancies are more likely to manifest patterns of late decelerations, the prediction of cord compression will prove far more elusive.

DELIVERY OF THE FETUS WITH PERSISTENT DISTRESS

Treatment of the fetus by intrauterine resuscitation will generally lead to resolution of the distress pattern(s) (transient fetal distress). In that minority of cases in which the abnormality does not resolve, the diagnosis is persistent fetal distress, a condition which should evoke a strong consideration for immediate delivery. The timing and route of delivery are of paramount concern. If a multiparous woman making rapid progress in labor is dilated 8 cm, the vertex is at +2 station, and the FHR variability is acceptable when persistent distress is diagnosed, then considerable justification exists for the continuation of this labor, which would be expected to come to a rapid and spontaneous conclusion. Alternatively, if fetal distress is persistent in a primigravida who is dilated only 2 cm and the vertex is at station −3, there may be little to be gained by delaying delivery until the FHR variability becomes flattened and the fetal pH acidotic. The management of these two examples is more obvious than that of the majority of cases of persistent distress, which fall between these extremes.

The choice of delivery route should be predicated on the perceived need for rapid extrication but, most especially, on the need to avoid further insult by inflicting unnecessary trauma on a fetus already in suboptimal condition. Following this reasoning, a delivery philosophy of "easy from below or else easy from above" should prevail. It follows that all personnel and equipment necessary to effect cesarean delivery and neonatal resuscitation should be mobilized whenever fetal distress is diagnosed and while intrauterine resuscitation is being instituted. To delay such mobilization until intrauterine resuscitation fails and immediate operative management is indicated wastes precious time for a fetus in peril. Although intrauterine resuscitation is usually successful, practicing obstetrics in a hospital where the administrator refuses to cooperate with early mobilization for such *possible* operative deliveries is perhaps to prejudice fetal outcome.

Figure 1 embodies many of the points already made. If hypoxic fetal distress is diagnosed, intrauterine resuscitation is instituted and usually results in resolution of the distress

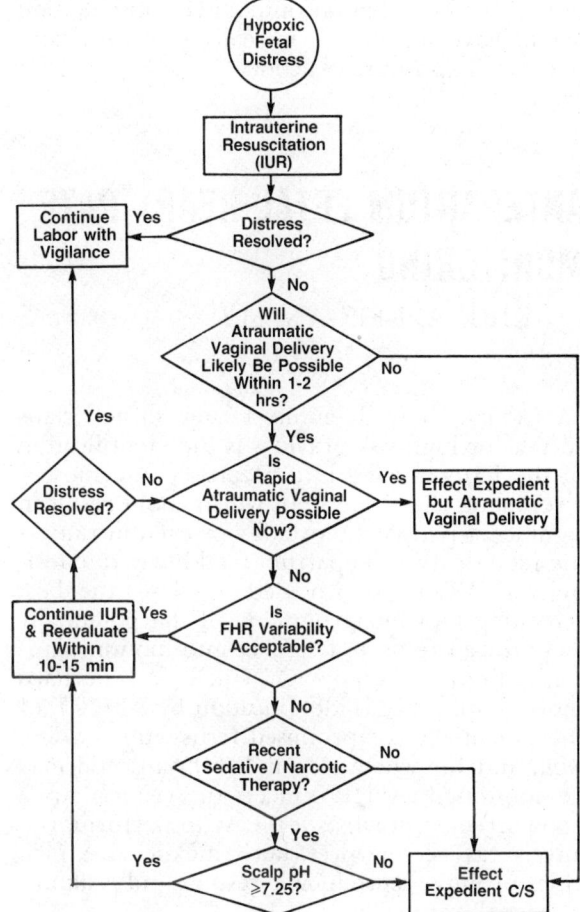

Figure 1. Flow chart for management of intrapartum fetal distress.

pattern(s); labor can then be continued with vigilance. If distress does not resolve within a reasonable time, the question of safety of vaginal delivery is raised. If vaginal delivery can be effected atraumatically, it is accomplished at once. If the labor has not progressed sufficiently to justify an attempt at vaginal delivery, then the questions concerning FHR variability, recent drug therapy that may have altered this variability, and perhaps scalp-blood pH assessment become important. (Normal FHR variability, derived from an *internal* FHR electrode, nearly always excludes significant fetal metabolic acidosis). In these latter situations in which continuation of labor is elected, the clinician is obliged continually to reevaluate the fetus and, if the distress patterns persist, to reevaluate the possibilities for atraumatic delivery.

The careful use of electronic FHR and contraction monitoring is associated with a cesarean delivery rate for fetal distress of only 1 to 2 per cent. Cesarean delivery is probably avoided for a greater percentage by the accurate interpretation of patterns that on simple FHR auscultation would have resulted in unrealistic concern and perhaps inappropriate action.

ANTEPARTUM FETAL HEART RATE MONITORING

KIRK A. KEEGAN, M.D.

A common dilemma facing obstetricians caring for high-risk gravidas is the identification of the fetus existing in a hazardous uterine environment, the sequelae of which could result in significant perinatal morbidity or even intrauterine fetal death. Antepartum fetal heart rate testing (AFHRT) has provided, to date, the best screening tool for recognition of the potentially jeopardized fetus and can set into motion plans for definitive therapy. Of equal and perhaps more significance is identification by AFHRT of the potentially compromised fetus who is doing well, and for whom a "hands-off" attitude may be continued. AFHRT meets the criteria for a good screening tool, as it is easy to perform, relatively easy to interpret, fairly inexpensive, provides prompt, reproducible results, and is almost universally available.

TESTING RATIONALE AND METHODOLOGY

The two primary modes of AFHRT in current use are the contraction stress test (CST), and the nonstress test (NST). The rationale for the CST, based on intrapartum monitoring observations during the 1960s, is that uterine contractions provide a transient stress to the fetus, interrupting the nutritive and respiratory functions of the placenta, which is poorly tolerated by the compromised fetus and results in late decelerations of the fetal heart rate. Absence of late decelerations is indicative of good fetal reserve and an uncompromised fetus.

The CST is performed using standard fetal monitoring equipment in the external mode with an ultrasound transducer for fetal heart rate (FHR) and a tokodynamometer for recording uterine contractions. The patient is placed in a semi-reclining position with left lateral tilt (to avoid aortocaval compression), and baseline blood pressure and fetal heart rate are then recorded. An intravenous line is inserted and a solution of 5 units of oxytocin in 250 ml of 5 per cent glucose is infused "piggy-back" by infusion pump.

Infusion rates should start at 0.5 to 1.0 mU per minute increasing by 1 to 2 mU every 10 minutes until a contraction frequency of three contractions is reached. The test is then interpreted and the infusions are discontinued. Not infrequently the patient may be having contractions which she does not appreciate, e.g., post-dates or post-amniocentesis, and a spontaneous CST can be achieved without the use of oxytocin.

The rationale for the NST was based on both observations of intrapartum recordings and CST results. Invariably, if FHR accelerations associated with fetal movement were present during the CST, the CST was interpreted as negative. The presence of fetal movement and FHR acceleration implies intact autonomic, central, and reflex nervous systems not blunted by hypoxia.

The NST is performed using the same maternal position and monitoring equipment as the CST but without intravenous lines or oxytocin. In some circumstances, fetuses which fail to exhibit FHR accelerations are stimulated by maternal abdominal wall manipulations or by giving the mother orange juice. Interpretation and management are described below.

Many AFHRT facilities are located in the labor and delivery setting. This may result in conflicting duties for nursing personnel and simultaneous need for monitoring equipment. A facility separate from the labor area, whose only function is AFHRT, frequently results in more efficient scheduling, shorter testing times, and more easily interpretable tracings. The use of oxytocin requires some moderate proximity to the labor and delivery area, although oxytocin-related problems are quite rare. The NST is well adapted to the non–hospital based clinic or private setting.

CHOICE AND TIMING OF TESTING

The choice of primary mode of AFHRT screening, CST or NST, remains controversial. Advocates of primary NST testing stress its ease, rapid performance, simpler interpretation, reduced cost, and absence of contraindications (premature labor, ruptured membranes, unknown uterine scar, placenta previa) when compared with the CST. Proponents of primary CST screening feel it is a more physiologic testing scheme. They suggest that detection of the fetus with a persistent pattern of late decelerations associated with FHR accelerations (a reasonably infrequent event) may allow intervention or therapy at an earlier point, resulting in a less compromised infant. Regardless of the primary method chosen, the absence of late decelerator–negative CST or the presence of acceleration–reactive NST has proved to be highly predictive of a favorable perinatal outcome. False-negative results (intrauterine fetal death with a normal test result) occur in less than 1 per cent of cases. Because of the aforementioned advantages, most perinatal units use a primary screening NST with follow-up CST for patterns which fail to show FHR acceleration.

AFHRT is generally begun at 32 to 34 weeks of gestation or thereafter if a risk factor is subsequently identified. In some circumstances, such as intrauterine growth retardation or premature rupture of membranes, testing may begin earlier if intervention for an abnormal test might be considered. Thus, timing of testing may be reflected in the availability and capability of one's neonatal intensive care unit.

PATTERN IDENTIFICATION AND MANAGEMENT

Nonstress Test. A *reactive* NST (Fig. 1A) is dependent on FHR acceleration associated with fetal movement. Numerous criteria and time limits with virtually equal prognostic ability have been proposed. At our institution a reactive pattern is defined as the presence of two accelerations lasting 15 seconds, achieving a zenith of 15 beats per minute (bpm) in one of two 20 minute periods. Fetal manipulation through the maternal abdominal wall is employed for 60 seconds, presumably to awaken the "sleeping" fetus if these criteria have not been met in the initial 20 minutes. Reactive patterns in most cases are repeated in one week if the initiating risk factor is still present. Deterioration of maternal or fetal condition would mandate earlier testing. In conditions in which fetal condition may change rapidly, most commonly diabetes and true postdates (42 weeks), testing should be done twice weekly.

A *nonreactive* NST (Fig. 1B) is one in which the criteria for reactivity are not met. Nonreactive patterns may result from fetal hypoxia, maternal drug ingestion (barbiturates, narcotics), congenital anomalies, and normal fetal wake-sleep cycles, the latter of which is the most common. To more clearly elucidate fetal status and subsequent management, a CST should be performed immediately. In approximately 75 per cent, results will be normal or negative. An alternative to an immediate CST is to repeat NST testing the same day, preferably after a meal. Again, 75 per cent will be normal or reactive with management described above. Repeat nonreactive patterns require a CST.

Contraction Stress Test. A *negative* CST (Fig. 1C) is defined as the achievement of three palpable and demonstrable contractions in 10 minutes without evidence of late deceleration or other periodic change during the test. As with reactive NSTs, negative CSTs, arbitrarily and by convention, are repeated in one week. Our policy is to terminate the CST prior to completion if criteria for reactivity by a NST definition are met. Most patterns destined to be CST-negative will achieve reactivity by the time three contractions in 10 minutes are achieved. When patterns remain nonreactive by NST definition but are interpreted as CST-negative, testing is repeated in 24 to 48 hours. There is some evidence to suggest that this group of patients may have a higher incidence of perinatal morbidity and mortality when compared with patients with reactive patterns or negative CSTs defined as nonreactive.

A *suspicious* CST is characterized by the presence of any periodic change in the absence of uterine hyperstimulation noted during the test. These periodic changes are usually nonrepetitive late decelerations, frequent variable decelerations, or a prolonged bradycardia. The suspicious CST should be continued for 30 to 40 minutes to insure that it is not positive. Some authors advocate that suspicious CSTs with a "negative window" (three contractions without late deceleration) should be termed negative even if late deceleration is noted elsewhere in the test. While it is true that most of these patients have a good perinatal outcome, they would best be benefited by repeat testing within 24 hours.

A *hyperstimulation pattern* is defined as a pattern in which late deceleration or prolonged deceleration follows a prolonged contraction (longer than 60 to 90 seconds) or a pattern of contractions more frequent than 3 per 10 minutes. Following a hyperstimulation pattern, the testing protocol should be repeated in 24 hours. FHR patterns without deceleration, despite excess uterine activity, are defined as negative and testing is repeated in one week.

A *positive* CST (Fig. 1D) is characterized by three contractions in 10 minutes associated with persistent, repetitive, late deceleration. Management is dependent on maternal condition and gestational age and pulmonary maturity of the fetus. At term or with L:S-proven lung maturity, delivery is warranted. Pre-term or with an immature L:S ratio, consideration could be given to further fetal evaluation such as estriol determinations or induction of pulmonary maturity by means of corticosteroids. In the hospital, continuous fetal monitoring should be employed if the latter mode of therapy is chosen. The preferred method of delivery following a positive

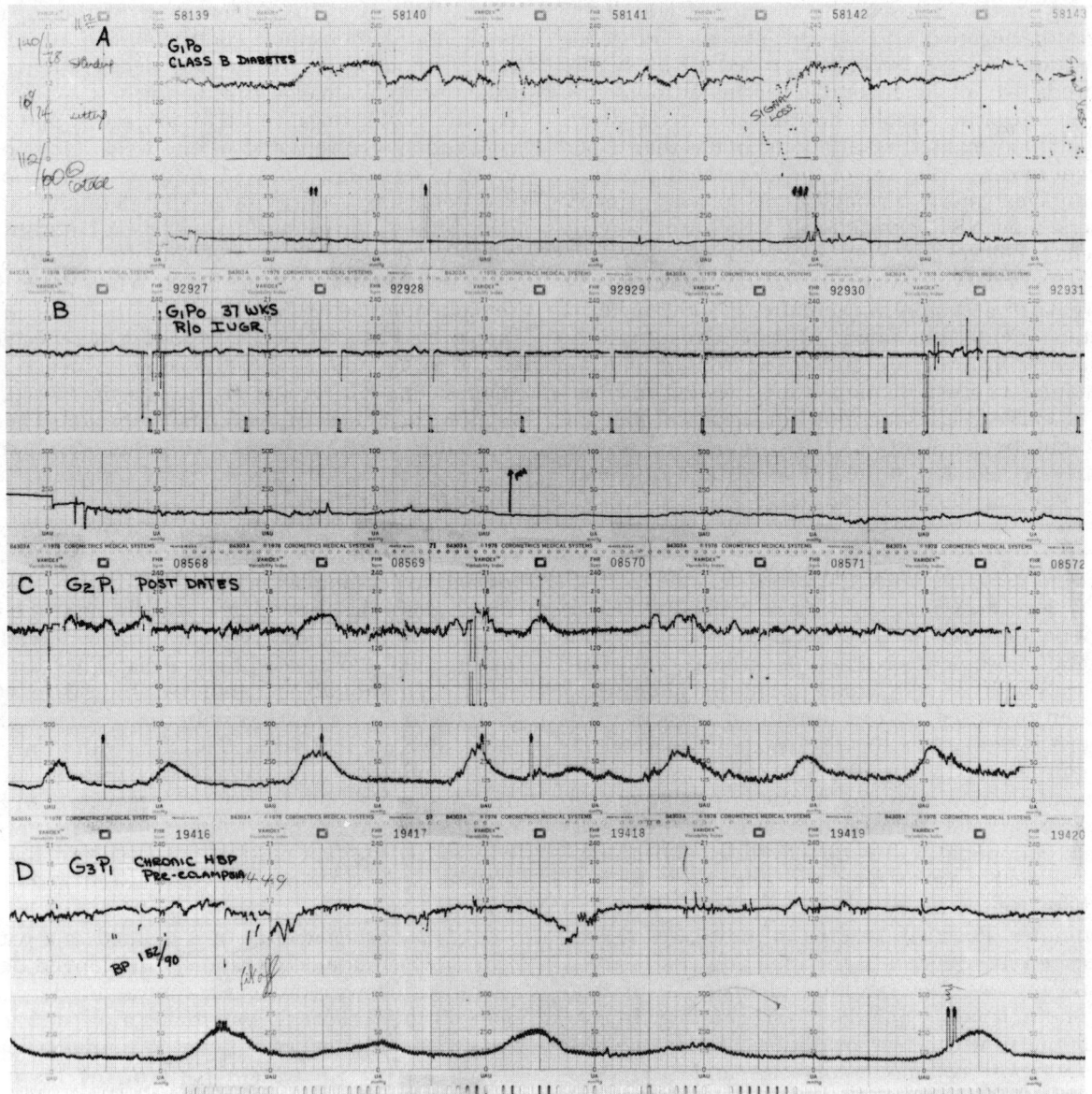

Figure 1. *A*, Reactive NST. Note FHR accelerations with fetal movement (arrows). *B*, Nonreactive pattern. Scant movement, no accelerations. *C*, Negative CST. No decelerations with contractions. Note concomitant reactivity. *D*, Positive CST. Repetitive late decelerations after each contraction. Note more subtle late contraction after last two contractions.

CST remains somewhat controversial. Regardless of reactivity noted during the CST, 30 to 50 per cent of patients can be delivered vaginally without evidence of persistent late deceleration following a positive CST. An attempt at induction and vaginal delivery should be considered if the cervix is favorable, internal FHR monitoring can be achieved, and prompt cesarean section capability is available.

Miscellaneous decelerations such as variable deceleration and prolonged bradycardia are occasionally noted during AFHRT. Repetitive variable decelerations, regardless of the NST or CST result, warrant more frequent testing. Consideration should be given to delivery if variable deceleration is present in the face of oligohydramnios and term or post-dates pregnancy or during conservative therapy for premature rupture of the membranes. Consideration for induction and attempted vaginal delivery should be given to patients who, at term, demonstrate prolonged deceleration during AFHRT regardless of test result. A protocol for the use of AFHRT is summarized in Figure 2.

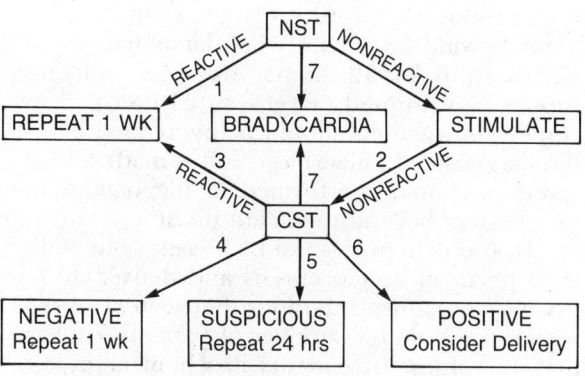

Figure 2. Management of AFHRT:
1. When:
   a. Premature rupture of membranes, diabetes, post-dates (≥ 42 weeks), repeat biweekly.
   b. Reactive, spontaneous, suspicious, positive, repeat in 24 hours
2. Nonreactive pattern following stimulation, proceed to CST or repeat NST same day
3. Terminate CST for reactive pattern
4. Repeat negative CSTs without two accelerations in 20 minutes in 24 to 48 hours
5. Continue suspicious test 30 to 45 minutes to rule out positive test
6. Next:
   a. Consider gestational age/pulmonary maturity
   b. L:S ratio >1.8 consider vaginal delivery with reactive CST, internal monitoring
   c. Markedly premature, L:S ratio <1.8, evaluate maternal condition, consider estriol, steroids for 48 hours, continuous monitoring
7. Miscellaneous:
   a. Consider attempted vaginal delivery if fetus is mature when deceleration prolonged, regardless of NST/CST result
   b. Test every 2 to 3 weeks if repetitive variable decelerations
   c. Consider delivery if variable decelerations during management of premature rupture of membranes
   d. Hyperstimulation resulting in late deceleration, repeat in 24 hours.

PREMATURE RUPTURE OF THE MEMBRANES

THOMAS J. GARITE, M.D.

Premature rupture of the membranes (PROM) is generally defined as rupture of the membranes prior to the onset of labor. This occurs in approximately 12 per cent of all pregnancies. PROM is responsible for approximately 30 per cent of all premature deliveries. At term, the risks involved with PROM are maternal and fetal/neonatal infection and fetal distress (occult cord compression and frank cord prolapse). In the preterm gestation, premature labor is an additional and probably more substantial risk, since over two-thirds of the patients with PROM prior to 36 weeks are delivered within 4 days of rupture, and nearly 90 per cent within a week.

Before a decision about management is made, five principal factors must be evaluated. These include:
1. Confirming the diagnosis;
2. Ruling out associated chorioamnionitis;
3. Ruling out fetal distress;
4. Establishing gestational age and fetal maturity; and
5. Evaluating for the presence or absence of uterine contractions.

Confirming the Diagnosis. Any patient with a history consistent with PROM should be evaluated immediately to confirm or reject this diagnosis. The first step in confirming the diagnosis is an aseptic speculum examination. Fluid from the posterior fornix, if present, should be evaluated for alkaline pH by Nitrazine paper. If there is any question of the diagnosis, the fluid should be smeared on a slide, allowed to dry and checked under the microscope for ferning. Fluid from the cervix or vulva should not be used for these tests since false-negative and false-positive results may occur. When no fluid is seen, fundal pressure may be applied while the cervix is being visualized. If this fails and the history is suspicious, the patient should be ambulated and re-examined if symptoms recur. Ultrasonographic determination of amniotic fluid volume is also useful when the diagnosis is in question. The speculum examination also allows visualization of the cervix to rule out a prolapsed umbilical cord or fetal extremity. It is extremely important in the premature patient that a digital examination NOT BE DONE when there is consideration for delay in delivery, as this may introduce bacteria and incite intra-amniotic infection. Cervical cultures for group B streptococcus and gonorrhea may be obtained at this time.

Evaluation for Infection. Chorioamnionitis is a diagnosis of exclusion made in the patient with PROM and fever without other apparent explanation. Patients with clinical chorioamnionitis should be started on antibiotics and delivered expeditiously regardless of gestational age. A single broad-spectrum antibiotic, such as ampicillin or cephalothin, with which good amniotic fluid levels can be achieved, is appropriate, and an aminoglycoside should be added in the patient who appears septic. There is no evidence that indications for cesarean section or the duration of labor allowed should be altered in the presence of chorioamnionitis. Therefore, cesarean section should be done only for usual obstetric indications. In the patient less than 35 weeks' gestation, neonatal outcome is significantly worsened in the presence of frank chorioamnionitis. Therefore, our policy is to perform amniocentesis between 28 and 35 weeks in clinically uninfected patients not in active labor to detect occult infection. Gram stains of unspun amniotic fluid showing bacteria or positive cultures correlate highly with subsequent development of maternal infection. Therefore, patients with Gram stains positive for bacteria or positive cultures are induced or delivered immediately. White blood cells on a Gram stain in the absence of bacteria do not correlate with subsequent infection and are not acted upon. Prophylactic antibiotics have not been shown to be of benefit in patients with ruptured membranes in preventing the development of chorioamnionitis or subsequent neonatal infection.

Ruling Out Fetal Distress. Significantly more fetal distress in labor, mainly in terms of cord compression patterns, is seen in patients with PROM. Direct fetal heart rate (FHR) monitoring throughout delivery should be carried out. When a delay in delivery is anticipated, continuous external FHR monitoring should be done for 12 to 24 hours following confirmation of the diagnosis. In the absence of fetal distress this may be discontinued, but should be reinstituted immediately when labor begins.

Establishing Gestational Age and Fetal Maturity. It is important to establish gestational age accurately by means of a careful menstrual history and records of early evaluation. Ultrasonography is useful in confirming dates. Patients at or beyond 35 weeks should be delivered expeditiously with the aim of being delivered by 24 hours following rupture of membranes. In patients beyond 35 weeks, when labor has not yet begun in 6 to 12 hours, oxytocin induction should be instituted. Twelve to 24 hours of adequate contractions should be demanded before the diagnosis of failed induction is made and cesarean section is performed in the patient not progressing beyond the latent phase.

In the patient less than 35 weeks, our policy is to perform amniocentesis and deliver all patients with mature L:S ratios. Between 30 and 35 weeks, a substantial number of patients will have mature values. In patients in whom amniocentesis cannot be performed, fluid from the vaginal pool may be obtained and analyzed for phosphatidylglycerol (PG). If PG is present, the patient can be induced.

Obviously patients at term with PROM, or patients beyond 35 weeks' gestation who are in labor, present no dilemma. Patients less than 35 weeks are a threat to deliver prematurely whether or not they are in labor on admission. There is substantial controversy over whether or not patients in premature labor should be given tocolytic agents and/or corticosteroids to accelerate fetal pulmonary maturity. Our current policy is to use neither, as there remains doubt over whether either is of benefit in PROM.

The management scheme is summarized in Figure 1.

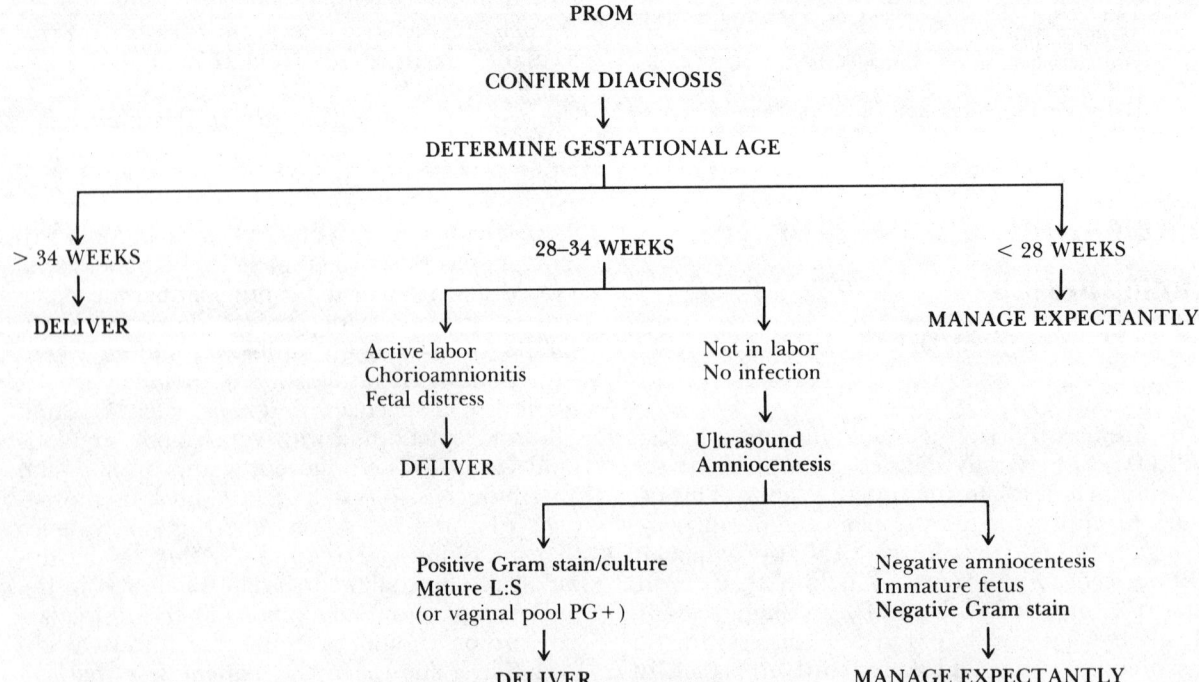

Figure 1. Management scheme for patients with premature rupture of membranes.

PREMATURE LABOR

IRWIN R. MERKATZ, M.D.,
and MICHAEL T. GYVES, M.D.

Preterm birth remains the principal factor contributing toward neonatal death and illness. Despite continued improvements in these two measures of pregnancy outcome as the result of recent perinatal advances, there has as yet been no associated underlying decline in the prematurity rate. The cost and toll of neonatal intensive care remain extremely high and it has now become even more evident that the most important unresolved issue facing obstetricians is the need for a reduction in the number of preterm births. Although the overall incidence of premature deliveries in the United States averages about 8 per cent, this rate may still be doubled among high-risk populations.

The pharmacologic control of premature labor presently offers the greatest medically based opportunity for reducing the incidence of preterm birth. Over the past decade an array of treatment modalities has been promulgated for the inhibition of uncomplicated preterm labor. Each has its potential advantages and disadvantages. It has, however, been consistently demonstrated that selectivity needs to be employed in the utilization of any of the modalities. In many cases of premature labor, the in utero environment may actually be hostile to the fetus, making preterm delivery preferable to futile and potentially dangerous attempts at inhibiting uterine activity.

Most studies have suggested that only about 25 per cent of preterm labors are uncomplicated enough to be amenable to tocolytic therapy. In many instances, delays in diagnosing preterm labor lead to excessive cervical dilatation or rupture of the membranes, either of which may make therapy ineffective. It has been postulated that part of the failure of tocolytic agents to reduce the incidence of prematurity has been such delays in instituting their use. Thus a current emphasis is on identification of the woman at risk for preterm delivery and on systematic programs of prevention rather than on the mere episodic treatment of premature labor. Clinical trials are now in progress and the results of such programs of prevention will be eagerly awaited.

HIGH RISK POPULATIONS

Uniform tools for assessing risk are now accepted as the basis for good obstetrical practice and record keeping. These instruments have been incorporated into a number of regional perinatal information systems, the more advanced of which have been developed with a capacity to ensure appropriate data acquisition, physician feedback, and population-based analyses. Examples of historical and current risk factors are listed in Tables 1 and 2.

TABLE 1. Historical Risk Factors for Preterm Labor Identified at the Initial Pregnancy Visit

Low socioeconomic status
Maternal age <17
Maternal heart disease
Low pre-pregnancy weight (<45 kg)
Prior preterm delivery
Recurrent genitourinary infections
Smoking
Maternal anxiety or excessive fatigue
Uterine anomaly or myomata; cervical conization or exposure to DES

PREVENTION

When such risk factors accumulate and compound to create a clinically higher likelihood of preterm labor, emphasis must be placed on intensified and individual prenatal care. More frequent pregnancy visits, closer maternal and fetal assessments, and a heightened sense of physician awareness must be complemented by programs of specific and detailed patient education. The pregnant woman has to be aided to truly understand the importance of avoiding unnecessary stress and fatigue, or maintaining a good diet and improved hygiene, of ensuring regular periods of bed rest at home, and of detecting the earliest signs and symptoms of preterm labor. In this context, fatigue has been identified as a specific contributor to preterm labor. Bed rest in a lateral recumbent position helps to reduce fatigue and to improve uteroplacental blood flow, which in turn helps to maximize the hormonal and physiologic milieu of the uterus. A team approach including appropriate utilization of social services and health counselors is essential to achieve these objectives.

TABLE 2. Examples of Risk Factors for Preterm Labor Related to Current Pregnancy (Developing Problems)

Multiple gestation
Hydramnios
Pregnancy-induced hypertension
Uterine bleeding
Premature cervical dilatation or effacement
Abdominal surgery
Poor maternal weight gain
Febrile illness

In addition to employing patient education as a prime tool, the physician may choose from among several therapeutic alternatives in the prevention of premature labor. Asymptomatic bacteriuria should be detected and adequately treated throughout gestation. Cervical cerclage should be reserved for those few instances in which relative cervical incompetence is felt to be a likely etiology. During pregnancy the cervix may be followed closely by frequent digital examinations or by ultrasonography to detect a progressive shortening or an unfolding of the lower uterine segment. Ideally, a pre-pregnancy evaluation of the cervix with dilator testing, hysterosalpingography, or newer biophysical technology is routinely performed following prior mid-trimester losses or preterm labors, particularly when there has been painless cervical dilatation or early premature rupture of the membranes. In some instances of clinically discernible "short cervix" occurring in women exposed to diethylstilbestrol, there may be a rationale for a more liberal approach to cerclage, but once again, a prior evaluation in the nonpregnant state is preferable.

Progestational agents have been employed successfully in controlled trials with apparent reductions in premature births. Ideally, such therapy should be monitored with serum progesterone assays. Some investigators currently insist upon a documentation of low maternal serum progesterone levels prior to drug usage, while other physicians are more empirical. Conclusive evidence of the safety and efficacy of these progestational treatments still awaits confirmatory study.

Finally, the use of oral beta-sympathomimetics is being tested on a prospective preventive basis. The effectiveness of such treatment has yet to be satisfactorily demonstrated by randomized controlled clinical trials. Ritodrine hydrochloride, developed specifically for obstetric use, is the only FDA-approved uterine relaxant. The oral form of the drug is administered every 2 to 3 hours in order to reduce uterine contractions. Such oral therapy has previously proved successful in diminishing the recurrence rate of overt preterm labor following initial episodes treated parenterally. The question is whether or not its selective mid-pregnancy use in specific high risk populations will reduce the eventual need for parenteral interventions and contribute primarily to a prolongation of pregnancy.

In trials abroad, in which prevention has appeared to have worked, most of the above interventions have been employed simultaneously. The relative contributions of each have not yet been well delineated, so it remains to be determined how they can best be coordinated programatically and utilized selectively in order to obtain optimal results.

TREATMENT REGIMENS

When preterm labor develops despite all efforts at prevention, the earlier the treatment, the greater the likelihood of success. However, such an approach entails the risk of overtreating patients in false labor. An initial period of assessment and observation is advisable following hospitalization with the patient maintained in a lateral recumbent position. The recommended criteria for qualifying and disqualifying patients should be adhered to irrespective of the tocolytic agent comtemplated for use (Table 3).

In approximately 40 per cent of threatened premature labors, a placebo response can be anticipated. Uterine activity will diminish spontaneously or respond to bed rest alone. The correction of hypovolemia may also serve to decrease spontaneous uterine contractions, so fluid loading via an initial rapid infusion with 500ml of normal saline or Ringer's lactate solution has potential merit. Subsequently, the intravenous infusion should be slowed to a maintenance rate (100–125 ml/hr) and, thereafter, care exercised to avoid circulatory fluid overload as a complication of treatment. Narcotics and barbiturates do not relax the myometrium and should not be employed on a routine basis. Such drugs depress the premature infant and thus could prove deleterious if treatment fails. Careful monitoring of maternal vital signs and biochemical status, uterine activity, and fetal condition is an essential component of care.

TABLE 3. **Selecting Patients for Treatment of Preterm Labor**

QUALIFYING CRITERIA
Gestation of 20 to 36 weeks
Fetal weight greater than 500 grams but less than 2500 grams
Regular contractions documented with a frequency of 4 in 20 minutes

DISQUALIFYING CRITERIA
Active vaginal bleeding
Eclampsia or severe preeclampsia
Dead fetus or major malformation
Intrauterine infection
Maternal cardiac disease or hyperthyroidism
Obstetric or medical conditions contraindicating prolongation of pregnancy

CONDITIONS LIMITING CHANCES OF SUCCESS
Incompetent cervix
Ruptured fetal membranes
Advanced labor (cervix dilated >4 cm)
Untreated urinary tract infections

CHOICE OF THERAPEUTIC AGENT

Each of the available treatment regimens has its own advocates and it is clear that experience and a greater familiarity with a specific agent enhances outcome. Worldwide the beta-sympathomimetic drugs have become the most popular and most frequently employed therapy, but clinical research continues in a variety of other directions.

Ethanol. Alcohol inhibits the release of endogenous oxytocin from the pituitary and also appears to have a direct effect on the myometrium. It has been subjected to clinical trials and has been shown to be an effective inhibitor of labor. Its use, however, is no longer acceptable as a prime approach because of distressing maternal side effects including disorientation, incontinence, emesis, and possible aspiration. Adverse depressive effects have been reported in the premature neonate, and the psychological interference with maternal-infant attachment is also important. With expanding knowledge regarding the effects of long-term maternal alcohol ingestion upon fetal development, the wisdom of administering ethanol to a pregnant woman must now be seriously questioned.

Magnesium Sulfate. It has long been known that an infusion of magnesium sulfate will interfere with progressive labor accompanied by nonspecific neuromuscular blockade. Reported trials for the treatment of preterm labor have been small and not totally conclusive, but nevertheless widespread clinical use of magnesium sulfate for this purpose has followed. Maternal status must be carefully monitored for loss of reflexes and for respiratory depression. The pediatrician must be particularly alert to signs of hypermagnesemia such as flaccidity, loss of muscle tone, and drowsiness in the newborn. The neonate does not excrete the magnesium load as well as the adult.

The drug is always administered with a controlled infusion device, as it has traditionally been for the treatment of preeclampsia. Typically a 4 gram loading dose with a 10 per cent solution is followed by a maintenance infusion of 2 grams per hour.

Prostaglandin Inhibitors. Since prostaglandins influence organ systems throughout the body, inhibition of prostaglandin synthesis can have many adverse effects as well as the sought-after effect of uterine relaxation. Although drugs such as aspirin and indomethacin have been shown to successfully inhibit preterm labor, a variety of potentially serious maternal and neonatal complications have been identified. These include bleeding problems, changes in newborn renal function, and the risk of premature closure of the fetal ductus arteriosus. Therefore, carefully monitored basic and clinical research is still needed before indomethacin or other prostaglandin synthetase inhibitors can be recommended for application in the treatment of preterm labor.

Beta-Adrenergic Agonists. The United States Food and Drug Administration has approved ritodrine hydrochloride for treatment of preterm labor, and since 1980 this has been the reference tocolytic agent. Other beta agonists have similar properties and comparable activity for the inhibition of uterine contractility. Isoxuprine, terbutaline, and hexoprenaline have been the most widely employed in the United States, while salbutamol, buphenin, and fenoterol have also been used abroad. Each of these agents has its own range of side effects and difficulties with administration. Therefore, experience gained with ritodrine can not be totally generalized.

Beta-adrenergic receptors are not limited to the myometrium. $Beta_2$ receptors can also be found in the smooth muscle cells of bronchi and blood vessels, while $beta_1$ receptors are present in myocardial cells, small intestine, and adipose tissue. In addition to inducing myometrial relaxation, all currently available beta-adrenergic compounds exhibit degrees of both $beta_1$ and $beta_2$ stimulation resulting in an increased rate and force of cardiac activity, vasodilatation, bronchodilatation, and metabolic changes associated with glycogenolysis and lipolysis. Familiarity with these cardiovascular and metabolic side effects is essential in employing any of the agents and it makes little sense to switch from one to another in the course of an individual patient's therapy.

Ritodrine (Yutopar) as the prototypical agent is administered intravenously with a starting dose of 50 to 100 µg per minute. The infusion rate is then increased in 50 µg per minute increments every 10 to 20 minutes until labor stops, unacceptable side effects develop, or the maximum allowable infusion rate of 350 µg per minute is reached. The dose at which labor stops is termed the effective dose and this intravenous infusion rate should be maintained for 12 hours after the cessation of labor. Oral ritodrine therapy is begun 30 minutes prior to discontinuation of the intravenous drug and continued at 10 mg every 2 hours for the first 24 hours. Subsequently, doses are titered to patient symptoms and pulse rate, usually at 10 to 20 mg every 4 to 6 hours.

Side effects with intravenous therapy are common and sometimes distressing. Maternal tachycardia is usually dose related and should not be permitted to exceed 140 beats per minute. Palpitations and tightness in the chest should be treated by reducing the dosage, sedation, and ample patient reassurance. If an electrocardiogram has not been routine prior to initiation of therapy, one should properly be obtained at this time. Serum potassium levels typically fall during therapy as the result of potassium being driven intracellularly. Potassium supplementation is not usually required except to maintain normal daily requirements. Serum electrolyte and blood glucose levels are checked at 12 hour intervals. Hyperglycemia is typical but usually transient and without impact on the fetus. Special care must of course be exercised in the case of a diabetic patient. Prolonged therapy and inadequate attention to the biochemical parameters may on rare occasions lead to an accumulation of organic acids and ketones with the development of metabolic acidosis.

A rare but serious complication of therapy is the development of maternal pulmonary edema. Most of the isolated case reports of pulmonary edema have been in association with multiple gestations or with concomitant corticosteroid treatment to induce fetal lung maturation. The risks and benefits of such concomitant therapy must be individually considered. Careful fluid restriction and accurate recording of intake and output should be standard components of all tocolytic regimens. Periodic auscultation of the lungs can aid in the early diagnosis of developing pulmonary edema and facilitate prompt treatment by diuretics, fluid restriction, and cessation of beta-mimetic therapy.

Maternal side effects or complications with continuous oral therapy are rare. The newborn may on occasion exhibit metabolic changes similar to those of an infant of a diabetic mother, i.e., the development of hyperglycemia and hypocalcemia. Infrequently, hypotension of intestinal ileus may also develop. Whereas some clinicians will use a mature lecithin/sphingomyelin ratio as the end-point of therapy, others will seek to avoid all of the potential complications of prematurity. Under optimal circumstances, oral maintenance therapy is then continued until 38 weeks of gestation so that a mature, term-sized infant will be delivered.

FETAL DEATH SYNDROME

ROY M. PITKIN, M.D.

Fetal death can occur at any time during pregnancy. Only rarely (as with cord prolapse) is the exact cause of death obvious. More frequently, some maternal condition (such as diabetes mellitus) exists which is known empirically to be associated with increased propensity to fetal death, but the precise mechanism is obscure. However, in a substantial proportion of cases there is absolutely no indication of the cause or causes. Every obstetrician has had the distressing experience of caring for a patient with a perfectly normal prenatal course until, usually in late pregnancy, the fetus dies unexpectedly and inexplicably.

The diagnosis of fetal death is usually first suspected when the patient notices that the fetus has stopped moving. If the event occurs in the first half of pregnancy, this symptom will not be present but the patient may notice failure to gain weight or lack of abdominal enlargement.

Adjuncts useful in confirming the diagnosis of fetal death include clinical, radiographic, ultrasonic, and amniotic fluid findings. On *physical examination*, the fetal heart cannot be heard. The accuracy of this sign can be improved by testing on two or more occasions by different examiners. *Radiographic* signs include overriding of the cranial sutures (Spalding's sign), exaggerated curvature of the spine, and gas in the fetal heart or great vessels (Robert's sign). These radiographic indices are helpful when they are seen, but their usefulness is limited by the fact that they develop relatively late and/or are infrequently observed. Spalding's sign and collapse of the spine typically require a week or more to become evident, and Robert's sign, while it develops more rapidly, is found in a minority of cases. *Ultrasonography* provides the most useful diagnostic test, failure to observe fetal cardiac activity on real-time scanning. In the *amniotic fluid* the marked increase in creatine phosphokinase concentration (from 30 to 1000 mU per ml) within 72 hours of fetal death seems to be a reliable indicator.

The natural history varies with the timing and cause of fetal death. Overall, three fourths of patients will labor spontaneously within 2 weeks, and 90 per cent within 3 weeks of the event. The interval, however, tends to vary inversely with the length of gestation. Additionally, there are differences in interval related to the underlying cause. For example, with Rh-isoimmunization, only half the patients will labor spontaneously within 5 weeks of fetal death.

The most serious complication is a consumptive coagulopathy arising from thromboplastin liberated from the dead products of conception and released into the maternal vascular system. This condition develops relatively late after fetal death and its course is typically gradual. Some laboratory evidence of coagulopathy can be found in 25 per cent of patients who retain a dead fetus for as long as 4 weeks. Blood studies indicating its development include a falling fibrinogen concentration and platelet count and a rising level of fibrin split products. The hematologic alterations are reversed by administration of heparin, confirming that the underlying cause is disseminated intravascular coagulation (DIC).

THERAPEUTIC OPTIONS

Among the therapeutic options available in documented fetal death are expectant management, suction curettage, hypertonic saline amnioinfusion, intravenous oxytocin, and vaginal prostaglandin E_2.

Expectant Management. In view of the natural history of a marked tendency to spontaneous delivery, simple observation is a safe and effective option. In former times it was employed much more frequently than at present. While it carries some risk of coagulopathy, this can be readily ameliorated by careful monitoring of hematologic indices (e.g., fibrinogen and platelet determinations at once or twice-weekly intervals) and prompt intervention at the first indication of abnormality. Expectant management, while safe medically, is often intolerable or unacceptable psychologically. Many women, on learning that their fetus is dead, insist on early evacuation of the uterus.

Suction Curettage. Dilation of the cervix and vacuum aspiration of the uterine contents is safe as long as pregnancy is not too far advanced. When the uterus is no larger than that of a 14 week gestation, suction curettage is usually the method of choice, assuming the surgeon is skilled in the technique. With more advanced gestations, the risk of uterine perforation and other complications increases sufficiently to contraindicate this procedure.

Suction curettage following fetal death is associated with greater risk than the same operation for interruption of normal pregnancy. The likelihood of hemorrhage is increased, and technical difficulties in dilating the cervix and removing the products of conception are more likely. Therefore, the procedure should be done in an operating room with appropriate anesthesia, an intravenous infusion established, and blood available for transfusion. The patient should be observed continuously for a minimum of 12 hours afterwards.

Insertion of laminaria tents into the cervical canal 12 hours or so prior to suction curettage may be a useful adjunct in lessening the need for cervical dilatation.

Hypertonic Saline Amnioinfusion. Intra-amniotic infusion of 20 per cent sodium chloride solution is effective in promoting the onset of uterine contractions and ultimately delivery. An additional advantage of the technique is the opportunity afforded by amniocentesis to confirm fetal death by observing characteristic changes in the color and consistency of the amniotic fluid. Most serious among its disadvantages is the risk of inadvertent intravascular injection. This catastrophic complication is probably more likely with a dead fetus, with its tendency to oligohydramnios, than with normal pregnancy.

Extreme care in technique is essential. The saline should be infused by gravity and not by injection, and only when there is absolute certainty that the needle is in the amniotic sac. The system should be checked for return of fluid repeatedly during the amnioinfusion, and the patient should be monitored continuously with regard to pulse rate, blood pressure, and any unusual subjective symptoms. The proper volume of infusion varies from 150 to 250 ml, depending on the size of the uterus.

Intravenous Oxytocin. Oxytocin is a familiar and relatively safe drug. Unfortunately, the uterus is often insensitive to oxytocin, particularly prior to term, and the failure rate in cases of fetal death is quite high. Moreover, oxytocin in doses of 40 mU per minute or higher has an antidiuretic effect, and the large amounts required in such cases, particularly when given in electrolyte-free solutions, carry a risk of water intoxication.

Oxytocin should be given as a relatively concentrated solution in an electrolyte-containing medium (e.g., 50 units in 1000 ml of lactated Ringer's solution). Administration should be by constant infusion pump with an initial low dose (e.g., 0.5 or 1 mU per min), increased stepwise to the amount causing contractions of the appropriate interval, duration, and intensity. No more than 1 liter of fluid should be given per 6 hour period, and the total duration should not exceed 24 hours.

Vaginal Prostaglandin E_2. The latest development, and in many ways the most useful method, is prostaglandin E_2 vaginal suppositories. The technique is simple, rapid, and efficacious, but it is not a panacea. Prostaglandins carry a high incidence of undesirable side effects—fever, gastrointestinal symptoms (nausea, vomiting, and diarrhea), and cardiovascular-respiratory effects (tachycardia, hypotension, and bronchospasm). More serious complications such as uterine rupture and myocardial infarction have been reported following use of vaginal prostaglandin E_2.

A limiting factor of some considerable significance is that present United States Food and Drug Administration approval for prostaglandin

E_2 vaginal suppositories in fetal death is limited to pregnancies of 28 weeks or less in duration. Thus, while the agents are undoubtedly used in later fetal deaths, the medicolegal implications of such usage, should any complications occur, are potentially serious.

The suppositories contain 20 mg of prostaglandin E_2, and the typical dose is one suppository every 4 hours until labor is well established. Typically, 3 or 4 doses are needed. In instances in which a reduced dosage seems desirable (e.g., relatively late in pregnancy or in a patient with an irritable uterus), the suppositories may be cut in half.

SUGGESTIONS FOR MANAGEMENT

Uncomplicated Cases. In fetal death during the *first trimester,* or later in cases in which the uterus recedes to no larger than 14 weeks' gestational size, suction curettage is clearly the safest and simplest method of termination. The conditions and precautions outlined above should be observed.

During the *second trimester,* vaginal prostaglandin E_2 represents the preferred method, with saline amnioinfusion a second choice.

Third trimester fetal death presents a dilemma. Vaginal prostaglandin E_2 has probably been widely used and appears to be reasonably safe, but the fact remains that it is not specifically approved for use during this trimester. With this in mind, the safest course is probably saline amnioinfusion early in the third trimester and intravenous oxytocin (with or without amniotomy) when fetal death occurs near term.

Complicated Cases. Certain maternal diseases represent contraindications to one or another technique of termination. Saline or prostaglandins should be avoided in patients with *cardiovascular diseases*. Prostaglandins are contraindicated by a history of *asthma* or other respiratory disease, and saline should be used with caution in patients with *renal disease*. In many such circumstances the proper therapeutic approach may be that of expectancy.

Ideally, *disseminated intravascular coagulation* caused by prolonged retention of a dead fetus should be entirely preventable. However, this problem is occasionally encountered because of neglect. In such instances, proper management includes heparinization to reverse the coagulopathy (e.g., 1000 to 2000 units of heparin per hour by intravenous infusion pump for 24 to 48 hours), after which the uterus can be evacuated by means appropriate to the circumstances.

Special Diagnostic Tests. A number of diagnostic tests may be helpful in identifying the cause of an apparently unexplained fetal death. Laboratory indices of potential value in this regard include serologic tests for syphilis, Rh and other antibody titers, glucose tolerance testing, and renal function studies. Maternal viral antibody titers are often included, though experience has shown that these studies are typically difficult to interpret and of little value.

Autopsy of all stillbirths should be done. Unfortunately, unless done by an individual experienced in perinatal pathology, the results, typically reported as "macerated stillborn," are not often helpful. Occasionally, however, malformations may be identified which may prove helpful in counseling regarding subsequent pregnancies.

Karyotyping of fetal tissues should be considered. Incidences of chromosomal abnormality as high as 5 per cent have been reported in large series of stillbirths. Unfortunately, the substantial costs of karyotyping represent a deterrent to widespread use. Among conditions which seem to be particularly associated with chromosomal anomalies, and which therefore increase the yield of karyotyping, are anomalies other than those involving the nervous system, fetal growth retardation, and a previous history of fetal wastage.

Feto-maternal hemorrhage has recently been recognized as a relatively common finding in otherwise unexplained fetal death, with spontaneous fetal exsanguination accounting for approximately 10 per cent of cases. Therefore, every woman carrying a dead fetus should be tested, preferably before delivery, by Kleihauer-Betke staining of a peripheral blood smear.

Emotional Support and Care. Fetal death, particularly when it occurs unexpectedly, is an emotionally wringing experience for the prospective parents and the physician. The anxiety, hostility, guilt, and doubt generated in both parties must be acknowledged and faced squarely. It is the physician's role to be available and to resist the temptation to avoid the patient, to be reassuring in allaying any guilt feelings, and to explain the grieving process.

Formerly, patients with a dead fetus were sedated heavily during labor, not permitted to see the stillborn infant, and housed postpartum in an area other than the maternity ward. Current opinion holds that this approach is generally erroneous. These issues should be explored with the patient and her husband, and their wishes scrupulously observed. Specifically, if the parents wish, they should see, touch, or photograph the infant, even if macerated or malformed. Other questions such as naming the infant or holding services need to be explored gently and nonjudgementally.

Care During Subsequent Pregnancies. Care

during a subsequent pregnancy should be individualized in accordance with the need of the patient. Particular attention should be paid to emotional support and reassurance, in view of the high level of anxiety certain to be present. The patient should be seen more frequently than customary, and more than the usual amount of time should be spent with her at each visit.

Some types of special tests (e.g., glucose tolerance test or midtrimester amniocentesis for genetic diagnosis) may be indicated by specific events or findings of the earlier pregnancy. Fetal surveillance techniques, such as antepartum heart rate testing, are advisable in late pregnancy, if for no other reason than to provide reassurance.

SPONTANEOUS AND RECURRENT ABORTION

PAUL G. McDONOUGH, M.D.

Random spontaneous and repetitive abortion constitute two of the most common problems in gynecologic practice. The vast majority of single sporadic abortions are the result of nonrepetitive errors in fertilization and gametogenesis. Assurance of uterine evacuation, avoidance of infection, and the prevention of Rh sensitization are the cardinal points in management. Gentle aseptic outpatient minicurettage or vacuum aspiration usually insures the removal of any residual products of conception. Microscopic pathology is indicated for documentation, but cytogenetic studies of an initial spontaneous abortion are not indicated. The Rh-negative, unsensitized patient should receive Rh immune globulin, which can be given as mini-Rhogam. A subsequent three week visit is scheduled, at which time a beta-subunit human chorionic gonadotropin (HCG) assay is routinely performed to assure the absence of any active trophoblastic tissue. It is our policy to delay future conceptions for three months until normal pituitary-ovarian relationships are well established.

The causes of repetitive abortion are more diverse, constant, and uncertain. General guidelines for therapy, based upon the etiologic factors in patients studied at the Medical College of Georgia, are outlined in Table 1.

In general, decisions concerning evaluation and therapy of repetitive abortion should be made in conjunction with the couple. Unstudied couples, after two abortions, may still have a 60 to 65 per cent chance of carrying a successful pregnancy. Studied couples, depending upon the etiology of repetitive abortion, may have a prognosis for successful pregnancy ranging from 30 to 90 per cent. The medical expense and the emotional frustration of two pregnancy losses are prime factors in motivating many couples to seek early evaluation and possible therapy.

Therapy is directed toward a known cause, whenever possible. In a large percentage of couples, a genetic and less frequently an endocrine etiology can only be suspected. In these couples, therapy must be empirically directed toward eliminating experimental conditions that may predispose to gametogenic and fertilization errors.

At the time of the initial visit, careful pedi-

TABLE 1. **Management and Therapy of Recurrent Abortion (Medical College of Georgia)**

ETIOLOGY	PROGNOSIS FOR NORMAL CHILD (%) AND THERAPY

Known genetic factors
  Parental translocation
  Multifactorial genetic disorder
	Normal child, 30%
	No specific therapy
	Prenatal diagnosis necessary

Anatomical factors
  Uterus subseptus (severe)
  Incompetent cervix (rare)
  Uterine fibroids—only if severe intracavitary distortion
	Normal child, 60–70%
	Metroplasty
	Cerclage
	Myomectomy

Endocrine factors Corpus luteum defect	Normal child, 90% Prenidation progesterone suppositories, 50 mg/day, starting postovulatory day #4 Ovulation asynchrony—Clomid in increasing dosage
Maternal thyroid reserve decreased	Synthroid, 0.1 mg/daily
NORMAL NONPREGNANT STUDIES	
Recurrent aneuploidy Recurrent gamete and fertilization errors	Normal child, 40% Ovulation control Avoid gamete aging Synchronization of gametes Rarely donor male Consider prenatal diagnosis and ultrasound monitoring
Euploidic abortus Immunologic	Normal child,? Immunologic studies (HLA)
Postnidation endocrine deficiency	Serial endocrine studies during pregnancy
Infections	Empirical antimicrobial therapy

gree analysis and chromosomal studies of peripheral blood in both parents will identify known genetic factors. There is no available treatment of a detected parental chromosomal translocation, or a multifactorial genetic disorder that is operative in the production of abortions, with or without fetal malformations. Therapeutically speaking, the chance of a full-term living child is in the range of 20 to 30 per cent, depending upon the specific translocation or multifactorial genetic disorder in question. Cytogenetic studies of amniotic fluid, ultrasonography, and alpha-fetoprotein levels are indicated in any future pregnancies.

Müllerian malformations, unless the intrauterine volume is severely compromised, rarely cause first trimester wastage. An unusually thick uterus subseptus should be treated surgically, but only after other possible causes have been excluded. Multiple factors may be operative in some couples.

Corpus luteum deficiency, if diagnosed with a relatively normal constant menstrual interval and a physiologic ovulation time, should be treated with prenidation progesterone. Natural progesterone, in the form of vaginal progesterone suppositories, 50 mg daily, should be started by the fourth day after ovulation and maintained until 60 or 70 days of pregnancy. At this point in gestation steroid production should be readily assumed by the normally developing placenta. Oral micronized progesterone, with reasonable intestinal absorption, is now available in Europe and may reach American markets in the future.

Corpus luteum deficiency, associated with wide ranging menstrual intervals, varying delays in ovulation timing, and inordinate lags in endometrial development should be treated with clomiphene citrate (Clomid) therapy. Clomid therapy should be progressively increased until the serum progesterone level and the histological picture of the endometrium return to normal. Pregnancy may then be attempted. The subsequent use of postnidation progesterone in the Clomid-treated group is controversial. In general, the treatment of corpus luteum deficiency associated with synchronous ovulation is prenidation progesterone. If associated with ovulation asynchrony, Clomid therapy is more appropriate.

Therapeutically speaking, the most difficult couples to manage are those in whom no genetic, anatomical, or endocrine abnormality is detectable by current diagnostic techniques. A certain knowledge of the karyotype of the previous abortus, or sequential hormonal studies throughout an early pregnancy are rarely available to the average practitioner. One may suspect that most of these couples have aneuploidic abortuses associated with repetitive gametogenic or fertilization errors. Postnidation endocrine deficits or immunological factors might be more suspect if the previous abortus was known to be cytogenetically normal.

Any therapeutic approach to these patients with unknown factors should be designed to provide an optimal physiologic setting for normal fertilization and nidation. Antibiotic therapy, doxycycline (Vibramycin), 100 mg twice daily, may be given to both partners in the cycle preceding the planned conception. The role of infection in random sporadic abortion is well documented, but repetitive infection, unless sperm-borne, has rarely been documented in human material. Basal body temperature graphs should be scrutinized, and deposition of sperm should be as synchronous with ovulation as possible. Factors related to sperm aging in vivo, and especially in the female genitalia prior to fertilization, should be avoided. Ovulation delay, post-ovulatory egg aging, sperm aging, and gamete asynchrony are all known factors predisposing to unbalanced or aneuploidic conceptuses in experimental animals.

The biochemical diagnosis of pregnancy should be established early, especially in all couples with normal nonpregnant studies. Thyroid studies, usually normal in the nonpregnant subject with recurrent abortion, should be followed at weekly intervals during pregnancy, so that the normal increase in T_4 and thyroxine binding globulin (TBG) may be observed. A persistent low T_4 accompanied by a normal estrogen-dependent increase in TBG is suspicious of inadequate maternal thyroid reserve and is an indication for thyroid therapy. In the event of a subsequent recurrence of spontaneous abortion, fetal tissue should be obtained for cytogenetic studies. If cytogenetic studies reveal a euploidic conception with normal chromosomes, then the couple should be referred to a tertiary center for immunological studies and serial determinations of steroid levels in any subsequent pregnancy. If the abortus is cytogenetically abnormal, then subsequent therapy should focus on ovulation control, and avoidance of gamete aging and gamete asynchrony.

Apart from corpus luteum deficiency, the empirical use of postnidation progesterone with a cytogenetically normal abortus remains controversial. The combination of a lack of good double-blind efficacy studies and the tenuous link between synthetic progestins and birth defects has limited the empirical use of even natural progesterone in the United States.

Unfortunately, more detailed endocrine studies are necessary in cytogenetically normal fetuses who remain viable for a sufficient period of time to identify a precise postnidation endocrine defect. Future endocrine studies of cytogenetically normal conceptuses may expand or diminish the role of endocrine deficits in the etiology of repetitive early abortion.

THERAPEUTIC ABORTION

WILLIAM BENBOW THOMPSON, JR., M.D.

The term "therapeutic abortion" is an anachronism which remains with us from the era before the Supreme Court decision of 1973. It was used to indicate that the procedure had the approval of some local body and to distinguish it from other induced abortions which were considered illegal. It might better be replaced by "termination of pregnancy" followed by a modifier to explain the indication, be it medical, socioeconomic, or psychiatric. The more modern terms have not supplanted the older, probably because some of us feel that "therapeutic" makes everything all right.

The years before 1973 were marked by an increasing mortality associated with induced abortion. For example, the 1963 Vital Statistics show that abortion was the leading cause of maternal death, with 6.8 deaths per 100,000 live births. With the change in the prohibitions against abortion there was an immediate change which continues. The current rate, using the older comparison, is about 0.25 per 100,000 live births.

Abortion has been carefully monitored over the past 9 years. Annual statistics published by the Center for Disease Control have changed our approach to these problems, and these changes have made abortion one of the safest procedures done in the United States. The reason for this change is certainly due in part to the fact that physicians, not lay abortionists, are providing the service. The use of aseptic technique, adequately sterilized instruments, and a proper environment are all factors responsible for the increasing safety of the procedure. Probably of equal importance is our patients' acceptance of the procedure and their willingness to seek help if complications arise.

We now have the experience of over 9 million abortions. Surely, with this volume of data, we can now do the procedure which allows for the greatest margin of safety for our patient. Those of us who do abortions owe it to our patients and ourselves to be proficient in the procedures we undertake. Most of us will not be involved in the development of new techniques, but will follow those which have proven effective and have minimal risk.

Factors which seem to alter the risk ratio fall in three general categories: the experience of the physician, the period of gestation, and the level of sophistication of the equipment.

The physician's experience is probably the most important factor. Vacuum aspiration is 30 per cent safer than sharp curettage, and midtrimester abortion should not be attempted unless one is familiar with the procedures.

The period of gestation is a most important consideration when one considers the odds of death of the mother. If all abortions were done in the first trimester then one could anticipate a death rate of less than 1/100,000 operations. The relative risk is 7.7 times higher in the midtrimester for dilatation and evacuation and 12.3 times higher for intrauterine instillation of hypertonic saline and/or prostaglandins. For operative termination by hysterotomy or hysterectomy, the risk jumps to 42.8. The earlier an abortion is done, the safer the procedure, the lower the complication rate, and the shorter the recuperation period.

Advances in equipment continue to be made and these have certainly improved the overall results. Vacuum aspiration is essential for a hospital or clinic setting doing abortions. The newer units with a ½ inch interior diameter are now available and will accommodate aspirating curettes up to 16 mm without clogging tubing. This improves the safety of the D and E for midtrimester abortion. Ultrasound evaluation and dating is essential for selecting the best procedure for the patient. An operative area free of contamination is needed, be it office, surgicenter, or hospital. Laminaria may be used to safely dilate the nulliparous cervix or to achieve the dilatation necessary for D and E. More recently, prostaglandin E_2 suppositories have been used to obtain the same result.

The following schedule should be of help in selecting procedure, place of operation, and equipment:

4–6 Weeks

At this early stage "menstrual extraction" in the office using local anesthesia via a paracervical block is safe. A soft 6 mm evacuation catheter and a low velocity, nonreversible, vacuum pump which will provide about 0.5 atmosphere of pressure is used. This procedure is safe, inexpensive, and practical in most office settings. The room should be a "procedure" room that is scrubbed regularly. If this is not available, surgicenter or hospital facilities using standard equipment are equally acceptable.

7–10 Weeks

Hospital or surgicenter facilities are necessary. A vacuum pump capable of 1 atmosphere negative pressure should be used. All patients should have an IV. If local anesthesia is used, an anesthesiologist should be available. As a rule of thumb the size of the evacuation curette should be equal to the estimated gestational period; i.e., for a 9 week pregnancy, a 9 mm or larger curette is used.

11–13 Weeks

A hospital or a hospital surgicenter is required. General anesthesia is probably safest. A good vacuum pump is required, as above. An IV is mandatory. Oxytocin (10 units oxytocin/1000 cc) should be administered during procedure. Nulliparous patients should have laminaria inserted the day before.

14–15 Weeks

D and E is performed using the same equipment as above, but the patient should have preoperative laminaria to achieve at least 15 mm dilatation. This can be accomplished by placing one laminaria on the morning before surgery, and have the patient return in the afternoon, at which time the laminaria is removed and two or more are placed in the cervix overnight. One must be prepared to remove fetal parts with ovum forceps. This procedure should be learned by anyone doing a moderate number of abortions. Instillation procedures are not recommended at this stage. If hypertonic saline or prostaglandin must be used, wait until 16–18 weeks. This gives a larger target and makes the procedure safer.

16–18 Weeks

D and E is statistically safer. The large diameter vacuum pump with appropriate tubing and evacuation curettes should be used. Instillation procedures are acceptable if there is no one in the community who is competent at D and E.

If an instillation procedure is necessary, it should be done after 16 weeks. Ultrasound confirmation of gestational age and localization of the placenta is advisable. The procedure is similar to the technique used for amniocentesis, with the patient supine and the abdomen surgically clean. A point of the abdomen about two fifths of the distance from pubis to fundus is selected at the midline or slightly to the right of the midline. A skin wheal is made using 1 percent lidocaine. The needle is then directed at right angles and the parietal peritoneum blocked as well as the visceral peritoneum of the uterus. This is easily accomplished using a 1¾ inch 20 gauge needle.

Following a minute or two wait, a Touhey needle is inserted in a slightly cephalad direction. With experience the various layers can be detected as encountered. The stylet is removed. A proper end point is the appearance of yellow fluid under pressure. We use the barbotage method, withdrawing 50 cc of fluid and injecting 50 cc of hypertonic saline (23 percent). The needle is left in place and the procedure is repeated. If saline alone is used, about 200 cc of a hypertonic solution is required. If saline is combined with prostaglandin F_2 then 100 cc or less of saline is adequate. The prostaglandin dosage used is 40 mg. Care should be taken to ensure that there is free fluid flow between withdrawal and injection. If fluid stops, then the needle must be repositioned.

The patient is returned to her bed and contractions will begin. With saline alone our mean abortion time was 49 hours. With prostaglandin and saline it was 19 hours. If the placenta does not promptly detach, the patient should be taken to the operating room for surgical completion.

19–20 Weeks

D and E is still statistically safer. Instillation is almost as safe. If an experienced person is not available for this patient, she should be referred to a center where one is available. The procedure is probably safest done as an inpatient procedure. Blood type and crossmatch is advised.

20–24 Weeks

D and E is still favored. An in-hospital instillation procedure is acceptable. Blood type and crossmatch is advised.

Laboratory data are necessary on all patients undergoing abortion. Rh and group are essential. Post abortal use of Microgam to 12 weeks and a standard dose of Rhogam after 12 weeks should be given to Rh-negative, Du-negative patients.

URINARY TRACT INFECTION

R. DAVID MILLER, M.D.

Urinary tract infections are second only to those of the respiratory tract in overall frequency. Urinary tract infections are best defined by the presence of replicating organisms within the urinary tract, excluding the distal urethral meatus. In order to avoid the problem of false-positive cultures, a urine specimen is said to be infected when there is growth of more than 100,000 organisms per ml of urine. A contaminated specimen will usually yield a count below 10,000 organisms.

False-negative cultures may arise in the presence of a highly alkaline urine. One may well be alerted to this by the presence of pyuria which is defined as more than 10 leukocytes per cubic millimeter in unspun urine associated with a negative culture.

Eighty-five per cent of all urinary tract infections are caused by *Escherichia coli*, while the remaining 15 per cent are due either to Proteus, Pseudomonas, Klebsiella, or occasionally the enterococci. Accurate diagnosis is frequently difficult in female infants but should be attempted utilizing collection bags. Maternal education with regard to normal hygiene and cleansing the vulva area from the front and back, and appropriate antibiotic therapy are all that are required at this stage. The peak associated with sexual activity is invariably localized and with appropriate diagnosis will usually respond to short-term antibiotic therapy.

Bacteriuria associated with pregnancy is a significant disease with regard to the risk of the patient developing acute pyelonephritis and the possibility of intrauterine growth retardation and prematurity. In view of the fact that the infection is frequently recurrent, prolonged periods of treatment may be required.

The urinary tract infections associated with menopause require both correction of any structural abnormalities and appropriate antibiotic therapy.

Recurrent Urinary Tract Infection. Where initial cure with several recurrences is documented, the patient should be evaluated for ureteric reflux. While this condition is infrequent, if uncorrected, it can result in almost total destruction of the kidney. Any woman who has more than three confirmed episodes of urinary tract infections should be investigated by means of intravenous urograms as the initial evaluation, with particular attention being paid to possible kidney scarring and a request made for evidence of ureteric reflux.

ANTIBIOTIC MANAGEMENT

The selection of appropriate antibiotic agents is based both on the possible site of the lesion and the presence or absence of pregnancy. Since all women in the reproductive years have the potential to be pregnant, and since, in addition, pregnancy may well precipitate urinary tract infection, caution is required in the prescription of any medication to women in the reproductive age groups.

A clear distinction must be made between what are essentially urinary tract antiseptics and definitive antibiotics. The former will frequently eradicate localized infection in the bladder but will have no effect on the treatment of renal parenchymal infection. Antibiotics, in general, will be active both in the renal parenchymal area and within the bladder.

The interpretation of culture sensitivity results and alterations in treatment require some caution. Since all antibiotics used in the treatment of urinary tract infection are concentrated in the urine, high concentrations of the drug will be present within the bladder. An essential example of this is the fact that most standard laboratory disks test for a minimum inhibitory concentration (MIC) of approximately 25 mcg per ml. The concentration of any drug in the urine may be in excess of 200 to 300 mcg per ml. The latter accounts for the frequently observed fact that although a culture sensitivity result shows an organism resistant, for example, to ampicillin, the patient is already asymptomatic and frequently has a negative culture thereafter. In view of the fact that 85 per cent of all urinary tract infections are due to *E. coli*, very few of these organisms are resistant above 100 mcg per ml. Conversely, the patient in whom ampicillin is given as initial therapy and who fails to respond probably has a resistant renal parenchymal infection as opposed to cystitis.

SPECIFIC THERAPEUTIC AGENTS

The semisynthetic penicillins, ampicillin, amoxicillin, and cyclicillin, are probably the safest antibiotics for women in the reproductive years. Recent evidence has shown that most patients with cystitis would have a favorable response to an initial dose of 3.5 grams of amoxicillin. Amoxicillin and cyclicillin have the advantage of requiring a 3 times a day dosage and are well absorbed in the presence of food. In view of the fact that they are almost totally absorbed, the risks of diarrhea are, therefore, minimized. Initial treatment in the presence of urinary tract infections may either be based on amoxicillin or cyclicillin, 500 mg 3 times a day, or ampicillin, 500 mg four times a day. In the presence of severe nausea, vomiting, or inability to retain all medication, the patient should be admitted to hospital and the antibiotics administered intravenously.

Cephalosporins. The range of cephalosporins is ever increasing, and overall these agents have demonstrable safety equal to that of the semisynthetic penicillins. A number of these, such as cefaclor, may be utilized on a three times daily basis in a dosage of 250 to 500 mg. Cephalosporins have the advantage of being alternative therapy for patients with penicillin sensitivity and are less likely to cause sensitivity reactions. On the other hand, they are considerably more expensive.

In the presence of resistant parenchymal infections, particularly those associated with pregnancy, therapy may well have to consist of one of the aminoglycosides such as tobramycin or gentamicin. Since the glomerular filtration rate in pregnancy is in excess of 150 per cent of normal, the risks of toxicity are small. However, caution is nevertheless required to avoid accumulation of the drug on the one hand, or lower than normal dosage on the other. Close observation of both peak and trough levels is required. In all cases, patients should be cautioned with regard to the fact that there is a small risk of an effect on the eighth nerve of the fetus, and the reason for utilizing potentially teratogenic therapy explained to the patient. Neonatal deafness has to date been reported only with kanamycin and streptomycin. The family of sulfonamides produces favorable responses in most cases. Sulfonamides act by the inhibition of folic acid metabolism. While they should not be used near term, they have been shown, in general, to be safe after the first trimester. Sulfisoxazole (Gantrisin), 2 grams four times daily, is preferable to the long-acting sulfonamides.

Nitrofurantoin is not of value in the management of any associated parenchymal abscess. It should largely be viewed as a locally acting substance at this time. Nitrofurantoin works by inhibiting various bacteriologic enzymes; its safety in pregnancy is uncertain, and there is an associated risk of hemolytic anemia in the newborn if used close to term. It should preferably be regarded as alternative therapy in the management of resistant infections in women of the reproductive years. When nitrofurantoin is utilized, the macrocrystals should preferably be used in a dose of 50 to 100 mg four times daily.

Mandelamine should be viewed purely as a urinary antiseptic with no renal parenchymal action. It is useful in treating localized infection or as a prophylaxis. It is active only in an acid medium. The dosage is 1 gram four times daily after meals.

TREATMENT OF HERPES GENITALIS

RAYMOND H. KAUFMAN, M.D.

One of the most devastating sexually-transmitted infections, both physically and emotionally, is herpes genitalis. Not only are the physical discomforts considerable, but the virus responsible for this infection has been implicated in the development of lower genital tract carcinoma. In addition, the effects upon the newborn infant are devastating, the majority of infants with neonatal herpes genitalis either dying of the infection or surviving with severe neurologic damage. In the United States, between 85 and 90 per cent of genital infection is caused by the Type II virus and the remaining genital infections are caused by the Type I virus. The disease is sexually transmitted, with symptoms beginning approximately 3 to 7 days after contact with infected individuals. Recent data suggest the possibility that individuals with prior infection may be subject to reinfection with different strains of the virus. One of the significant factors related to the lack of success of treatment in preventing recurrent infection is the fact that after primary infection, the virus is harbored in the dorsal nerve root ganglia of the segment of tissue initially infected. Thus, local treatment is of no value in eradicating the virus from its location in the ganglion. In addition, virus present within the dorsal nerve root ganglia is probably not replicating actively and thus cannot be effectively eradicated by systemic medications.

Unfortunately, despite the numerous proposed therapeutic regimens, no satisfactory treatment is currently available for genital herpes virus infection. Numerous approaches have been advocated, including the use of bacillus Calmette-Guérin (BCG), Betadine solution, photoinactivation, topically applied ether, chloroform, 5 iodo-2-6 deoxyuridine (IDU), adenine arabinoside, 2-deoxy-D-glucose, and, more recently, acyclovir. None of these approaches, however, has proved to be completely effective in treating either primary or recurrent infection. Initially, photoinactivation using neutral red or proflavine was thought to be of some benefit in shortening the duration of clinical infection and preventing recurrence. More recent randomized double-blind studies, however, have demonstrated that these medications are no more efficacious than control nonactive dyes.

On the assumption that the viruses of smallpox and herpes are related immunologically, repeated inoculations with smallpox vaccine had been advocated for the prevention of herpes genitalis. The results of such treatments have been disputed repeatedly by numerous investigators. A well-controlled study was also conducted to evaluate a specific vaccine prepared from inactive herpes virus. The results from the control material and vaccine were essentially identical. Vaccines prepared from heat-inactivated chorioallantoic membrane cultures of embryonic hen eggs consisting of Type I vaccine (Lupidon H) and Type II vaccine (Lupidon G) were prepared by Hermal-Chemie Kurt Hermann Laboratories of Hamburg. Reports on the use of this vaccine, like the results with so many therapeutic agents, were initially glowing, but to date we have not seen a well-conducted double-blind randomized study to demonstrate that this therapy is of any greater benefit than other methods currently available. Furthermore, considering the potential oncogenic effects of HSV Type II, there is some question regarding the safety of using the whole inactivated virus in a vaccine.

One reason, already alluded to above, for the ineffectiveness of most therapies in the treatment of this infection is the fact that between recurrences the virus is harbored in a latent fashion in the sensory ganglion supplying the area affected. Thus, local treatment may eradicate or inactivate virus on the vulva or cervix but does not eradicate the latent virus still present in the nerve root ganglia. Acyclovir ointment, 5 per cent (Zovirax) has recently become available for the treatment of herpes genitalis. When acyclovir is applied locally to the primary lesions in the form of an ointment, there is some evidence to suggest that the duration of the primary episode as well as duration of viral shedding may be slightly shortened if treatment is started early in the course of infection. The systemic use of acyclovir in primary infection has just been approved for use. Potentially, one would anticipate that its use early in the course of the disease might be more effective than topical application of the ointment in shortening the duration of infection and viral shedding. In treating severe primary infection the Zovirax solution is administered IV at a dose of 5 mg per kg every 8 hours for 5 days.

When the ointment is used, it should be applied liberally to the area of involvement every 3 hours at least six times during a 24-hour period. Treatment should be continued at least 7 days with primary infection, or for as long as new lesions continue to recur. Recurrent lesions should be treated for as long as open lesions persist. There is, however, no conclusive evidence indicating a shortening of the clinical course or viral shedding in individuals with recurrent infection except in immunocompromised individuals. In addition, there is no evidence to indicate that the use of acyclovir is of any benefit in the prevention of recurrent infection.

Lacking a specific treatment, palliative measures become necessary. Symptomatic relief is often obtained by hot sitz baths, wet dressings, or various shake lotions. Wet dressings are quite difficult to use because of the necessity of almost constant application. Such dressings as Burrow's solution diluted 1/20 parts in water or a saturated solution of boric acid afford some relief of symptoms. Various antibiotic ointments (Neosporin G) may expedite healing in some persons, presumably by preventing secondary infection. Some believe that topically applied corticosteroids relieve symptoms and hasten healing; however, the use of corticosteroids, even topically, in the presence of a viral infection should be cautioned against. The application of various local anesthetic ointments such as lidocaine gel has been advocated, but it has been our experience that this can occasionally result in a severe contact dermatitis. Thus, this approach is seldom recommended. Thymol, 4 per cent (an antiviral agent) in chloroform, has been reported to shorten the course of the acute infection. In our experience, it has somewhat enhanced lesion healing and decreased the duration of pain, but the drug has been of no benefit in preventing recurrent infection.

Primary genital herpes infections are frequently associated with severe vulvar pain. This usually requires the use of strong analgesics to provide the patient with relief of symptoms. Patients also report dysuria and urinary frequency that is usually related to a viral urethritis and cystitis. Use of a medication as pyridium, 100 mg, two tablets three times daily, affords some relief of these symptoms. Occasionally, a patient must be maintained on catheter drainage for several days, and the use of a suprapubic catheter is recommended.

Sometimes the symptoms associated with primary genital herpes infection are severe enough to require hospitalization. In such cases, the patient frequently has urinary retention and experiences excruciating vulvar and pelvic pain. In many instances, pelvic pain is related to pelvic lymphadenopathy secondary to severe vulvar and cervical infection. It can be relieved only by such drugs as meperidine or opiates. Frequent hot sitz baths to speed healing of vulvar lesions and to relieve local symptoms are often beneficial. The use of acyclovir as outlined above may be of some help in shortening the duration of the infection and the viral shedding. Hospitalization may be necessary until pain decreases and the patient is able to void spontaneously.

Recurrent herpes genitalis is extremely distressing to the patient, and every effort should be made to discover and control factors responsible for recurrence. An understanding of the patient's emotional problems is helpful. At times, counselling may be of some benefit in helping the patient deal with stress and thus decrease the frequency of recurrences. In some individuals, recurrences appear at the onset of menses or following sexual intercourse. In these individuals there is little that can be done to prevent recurrence except to offer assurance that in most instances, as time passes, the frequency of recurrence tends to decrease.

Genital herpes virus infection is transmitted sexually, and a question of great concern to the individual with recurrent infection is the likelihood of transmission of the infection to a sexual partner. During the acute infection, disease is transmitted to the consort by direct sexual contact in a large percentage of instances. Thus, it is wise to recommend abstinence from sexual contact during the period of active infection. Once the lesions are completely healed, the likelihood of transmitting the disease is small. The probability of transmitting the infection in the absence of clinical disease, although remote, is still possible as indicated by the fact that the virus has been recovered from the cervix of asymptomatic women and from the urethra and prostate of asymptomatic men. If coitus is engaged in during the course of active infection, the use of a condom by the man may offer some degree of protection, although this certainly will not guarantee against transmission of infection to him from an infected female or to the female from him. Singh et al. have demonstrated the viricidal effects of various intravaginal contraceptive agents, and theoretically one might suggest their use if coitus is engaged in during the acute infection. Certainly, the male partner with active lesions should avoid any sexual contact with his female partner during pregnancy.

ECTOPIC PREGNANCY

E. J. QUILLIGAN, M.D.

The adage that anyone in the childbearing years who has lower abdominal pain has an ectopic pregnancy until proven otherwise is as true today as it was over 35 years ago. At that time it was one of the major causes of maternal mortality, and it remains so today, accounting for 10 per cent of maternal deaths. Ninety-eight per cent of ectopic pregnancies are located in the fallopian tube, although they may occur in the ovary, at the cervix, or on the peritoneal surface of the abdominal cavity. Since the overwhelming majority of ectopic pregnancies are tubal, they will be the primary focus of this article.

The frequency of occurrence of ectopic pregnancy depends somewhat on the population being observed. In some indigent groups, the frequency is 1 in 100 pregnancies, while in more affluent groups the rate is 1 in 300. This difference may in part be due to a higher incidence of tubal infection in the indigent population, since the incidence of abnormal tubal architecture as a result of inflammation is very high (around 90 per cent) in those tubes removed for ruptured ectopic pregnancy. The increased frequency of ectopic pregnancy in the remaining tube after one ectopic pregnancy, 1 in 50 to 100 pregnancies, also speaks to the bilaterality of the abnormal tubal architecture.

The most frequent symptom of ectopic pregnancy is lower abdominal pain, occurring in over 90 per cent of cases. The pain may be unilateral or bilateral and may vary from the dull ache occasionally found with an unruptured ectopic pregnancy to the severe stabbing abdominal pain associated with rupture of the tube and intraperitoneal bleeding. In some instances intraperitoneal bleeding will cause shoulder pain; however, this is not always the case. The next most common symptom is some abnormality in the menstrual cycle, usually amenorrhea of 6 to 8 weeks' duration followed by uterine bleeding. The bleeding is usually light and spotty but may be as heavy as a menstrual period and associated with cramping abdominal pain, leading the physician to suspect an impending abortion. Other symptoms are those of any pregnant patient: nausea, vomiting, breast fullness, and fatigue.

The signs of ectopic pregnancy include abdominal tenderness, rebound tenderness, and an adnexal mass. The abdominal tenderness is most frequently found in the lower quadrants and is usually more severe on the affected side. Rebound tenderness will be present following intraperitoneal bleeding. An adnexal mass is palpated on pelvic examination in about 50 per cent of cases. The uterus may seem slightly enlarged and softened, causing confusion between intrauterine and tubal pregnancy. In some cases the intra-abdominal bleeding will be of sufficient magnitude to cause shock, with either a tachycardia, a drop in the blood pressure, or both.

The laboratory findings in many respects reflect the pregnant state—leukocytosis and an increase in the sedimentation rate. The hematocrit or hemoglobin may be normal or significantly reduced. The pregnancy test will almost always be positive if a sensitive test such as the radioreceptor assay of the beta subunit of human chorionic gonadotropin (HCG) is performed. If, however, a slide agglutination test for HCG is performed it will be positive only about 40 to 50 per cent of the time. A very helpful test in making the diagnosis of ectopic pregnancy is the ultrasound examination. The characteristic gestational sac found in the uterus at 6 to 8 weeks of pregnancy will usually not be found, and one may see the ectopic gestation in the adnexal area. However, on rare occasions the uterine decidua formed during an ectopic pregnancy may appear as a false intrauterine gestational sac on ultrasonography.

Another test performed less frequently today but still of value is the diagnostic culdocentesis. An 18 or 20 gauge needle inserted into the posterior fornix of the vagina will frequently encounter blood which can be aspirated from the cul-de-sac. The blood, when expressed onto a sponge, will show small clots when intra-abdominal bleeding is present. The clots will not be found if the needle is inadvertently placed in an artery or a vein.

If any question remains after thorough evaluation of the patient, a laparoscopic examination will clarify the issue; however, if a ruptured ectopic pregnancy is obvious, then one should proceed immediately to laparotomy.

Prior to surgery an intravenous infusion should be started with an 18 gauge needle and two or more units of packed red cells, typed and crossmatched. The abdomen is usually entered through either a Pfannenstiel or a midline incision. The ectopic pregnancy can be removed by doing a salpingo-oophorectomy, a salpingectomy, or a salpingostomy. If the opposite tube is open, a salpingo-oophorectomy is preferred. This optimizes the patient's chance to conceive again, because she will ovulate monthly from her remaining ovary. If any disease is apparent in the ovary on the unaffected side, then only a salpingectomy is done. If the patient has only one tube, or the opposite tube is diseased and the ectopic pregnancy is not ruptured, then a salpingostomy can be performed with the full realization that the incidence of repeat ectopic gestation is quite high. If the ectopic pregnancy has ruptured and only one tube is remaining, the ruptured segment may be resected with a view to reanastomosing the two segments of the tube at a later date. Even if both tubes are totally destroyed, the ovaries and uterus should not be removed, because recent successes with in vitro fertilization offer hope to the patient that she may carry a pregnancy in the future.

Ectopic pregnancy is a serious illness that threatens two of the most precious aspects of a woman, her life and her reproductive ability. To safeguard both requires thought, vigilance, and conservation.

DYSFUNCTIONAL LABOR

JOSEPH SEITCHIK, M.D.,
and ROBERT W. HUFF, M.D.

Dysfunctional labor is diagnosed when the woman in active labor fails to accomplish cervical effacement or dilation at an acceptable rate in the first stage of labor or fails to accomplish descent of the presenting part at an acceptable rate in the second stage of labor. Before treating dysfunctional labor, a series of diagnostic questions must be answered (Table 1).

FALSE LABOR AND PRE-LABOR

The transition from pre-labor to true labor cannot be identified precisely. If the woman's cervix is dilated at least 3 cm and well effaced on her arrival at the labor suite, and if it further dilates and effaces over the next 2 hours, the diagnosis of labor can be made with certainty. If the woman does not meet these criteria she is not in active labor and should be transferred from the labor suite. This plan avoids the inadvertent and inappropriate induction of labor in women who are in pre-labor or false labor.

RUPTURED MEMBRANES

Women with ruptured membranes should have a sterile vaginal examination to confirm amniorrhexis and check for the possibility of a prolapsed cord. If the pregnancy is at term, the vast majority of these women will be in active labor within 12 hours and will be delivered within 24 hours. Oxytocin induction of labor is usually successful if the cervix is favorable. If the cervix is unfavorable for induction, aggressive management by oxytocin induction may result in an unnecessarily high incidence of cesarean delivery because of "failure to progress in labor." The unfavorable cervix will not change rapidly in response to uterine contractions.

Chorioamnionitis is a serious but infrequent occurrence. The woman's vital signs should be taken at least every 4 hours prior to labor. Temperature above 99.6° F, maternal heart rate above 100, or fetal heart rate above 160 indicate a diagnosis of chorioamnionitis unless some other obvious source of infection is present. The diagnosis of chorioamnionitis requires prompt action. If the cervix is favorable for induction, oxytocin and antibiotic therapy should be initiated. If the cervix is unfavorable for induction, cesarean delivery and antibiotic therapy are appropriate. Broad spectrum antibiotic coverage such as penicillin plus an aminoglycoside is usually favored for chorioamnionitis. The uterus may be unresponsive to oxytocin stimulation if chorioamnionitis has been present for several hours.

MULTIPLE PREGNANCY AND ABNORMAL POSITIONS AND PRESENTATIONS

Multiple pregnancy suspected by examination at the onset of labor should be confirmed radiographically. This accurately identifies the

TABLE 1. **Diagnostic Questions in Suspected Dysfunctional Labor**

QUESTIONS	EXAMPLES OF POSSIBLE PATHOLOGY
1. Is the patient in labor?	False labor, pre-labor.
2. What phase of the first stage? Are the rates of effacement, dilatation, or descent abnormal?	Prolonged latent phase, arrest of dilatation, arrest of descent.
3. Are the membranes ruptured?	Chorioamnionitis, prolapsed cord.
4. Is the fetus singleton, in cephalic presentation and occipital position?	Multiple gestation, face, brow, transverse lie, compound presentation, occipitoposterior position.
5. Is the fetus macrosomic in the whole or locally?	Estimated fetal weight ≥4000 grams, hydrocephalus, sacral tumor, distended fetal bladder.
6. Is the birth canal obstructed?	Distended maternal bladder, inspissated feces, low-lying posterior placenta previa, abnormal pelvic shape or size, uterus didelphys, cervical myoma, ovarian cyst.
7. Does the fetus have a reasonable chance for extrauterine existence?	<27 weeks gestation (biparietal diameter <70 mm), anencephaly.
8. Are uterine contractions frequent and strong?	Hypocontractility.

number of fetuses and their position and presentation. If the fetus entering the pelvis is not in cephalic presentation and if the gestational age is greater than 26 weeks, neonatal outcome is better when delivery is by cesarean section. In cases with an uncertain gestational age, a fetal biparietal diameter (BPD) greater than 65 mm when measured ultrasonographically indicates viability of the fetus.

Face presentations are managed expectantly. Spontaneous vaginal delivery is anticipated when the fetus is in the mentum anterior position. Failure of mentum anterior rotation or of descent are indications for cesarean delivery. Prior to cesarean section, however, a diagnosis of anencephaly should be excluded. All brow presentations during labor with fetuses estimated to weigh over 1200 grams should be managed by cesarean delivery.

Transverse lie with a fetus older than 26 weeks (BPD >65 mm) should be managed by an attempt at external version if the woman has intact membranes and is not in active labor. If the gestational age is less than 26 weeks, vaginal delivery should be allowed. At this gestational age the chance for fetal salvage seems too small to expose the mother to the risks of cesarean section. When cesarean delivery is necessary for a transverse lie, an attempt at version should be made once the abdomen is open. Manipulating the "back down" fetus into a breech or cephalic position allows for a low cervical transverse incision rather than a classical incision in the uterus.

FETAL MACROSOMIA

The heavier the fetus, the more likely the need for abdominal delivery. If the patient manifests good progress in the first and second stages of labor, uncomplicated vaginal delivery is the usual result. When macrosomia is associated with dysfunctional labor, the characteristic finding is failure to descend in the second stage. It is tempting, particularly in multiparous patients, to attempt mid or low forceps delivery of the fetal head. This is usually achieved easily but unfortunately, this clinical set is associated with a 5 per cent incidence of marked shoulder dystocia. If the woman's failure to effect spontaneous vaginal delivery is not the result of weak contractions or inadequate bearing down efforts because of regional anesthesia, the safest treatment is abdominal delivery. After the patient is anesthetized, the fetal head should be disengaged from the pelvis to facilitate delivery.

Hydrocephalus may not be recognized until after labor is established. The diagnosis should be confirmed by x-ray or ultrasound (BPD ≥ 10.8 cm) examination. Therapy consists of transabdominal suprapubic needle drainage of cerebrospinal fluid to reduce the head circumference and permit vaginal delivery. If the fetus is a breech presentation and hydrocephalus is not diagnosed until after delivery of the body, drainage can be accomplished by either suprapubic aspiration or by transvaginal aspiration through the foramen magnum. If hydrocephalus is not recognized until labor, every effort should be made to achieve vaginal delivery and to avoid cesarean section. At the present state of ultrasonography, it is doubtful that the width of the cerebral mantle can be determined with certainty. Thus the potential of the fetus for extrauterine life cannot be assessed with any certainty in that emergency situation. Further, delivery of a huge fetal head by cesarean will require either a very long classical uterine incision, a vertical low cervical incision which requires extension into the upper uterine segment, or a transverse low segment incision which lacerates into the uterine blood supply at delivery of the head. These are unreasonable hazards to the mother for the delivery of a fetus of very questionable potential for extended extrauterine life.

OBSTRUCTION TO THE BIRTH CANAL

Soft tissue enlargements which hold the presenting part out of the pelvis are identified by abdominal and vaginal examination. A distended bladder or inspissated feces are easily treated by evacuation. Cervical leiomyomas, cul-de-sac masses, and uterus didelphys require abdominal delivery. The posterior lowlying placenta provides a more subtle form of pathology. It is usually found in multiparas who labor with normal uterine contractility, excessive "bloody show," slow cervical dilatation, and a floating fetal head. The leading edge of the placenta can be palpated after the cervix is dilated over 5 cm. Cesarean section is the treatment.

Contraction of the bony pelvis sufficient to predict dysfunctional labor is rarely found in natives of the United States. Exceptions to this general statement include women with unusually short stature for their racial group, prior pelvic fracture, or abnormal gait and weight-bearing in childhood. Minor contractions of the bony pelvis are of little predictive value for dysfunctional labor. X-ray pelvimetry is of no use in the management of dysfunctional labor with a cephalic presentation. Most patients labeled "possible cephalopelvic disproportion" actually suffer inadequate uterine contractility and warrant a trial of oxytocin therapy.

UTERINE HYPOCONTRACTILITY

Uterine hypocontractility is the most common cause of dysfunctional labor. It is diagnosed clinically by assessing uterine contractions for at least 10 minutes. A woman in normal active labor should have three or more firm contractions in this period of time.

Amniotomy is a useful tool to enchance contractility, provided the potential dangers are appreciated. The patient should be examined carefully prior to rupture of the membranes for identification of any pulsations (funic presentation, vasa previa) between the examining fingers and the presenting fetal head. If any vaginal bleeding occurs following amniotomy, an Apt test must be performed to insure that the fetus is not hemorrhaging. Following amniotomy, the examiner should determine how easily the vertex descends on fundal pressure and what the precise occipital position is. The examination is completed by attaching a scalp electrode and monitoring the fetus for bradycardia which is suggestive of cord blood flow obstruction.

In hypocontractile labor, amniotomy usually does not enhance the quality of uterine contractility for the first half-hour. Commonly, contractions become stronger and more frequent during the second half-hour following amniotomy. Thus, it is useful to wait at least an hour after amniotomy to identify cases that will not respond to amniotomy and will require oxytocin.

If amniotomy fails to initiate adequate uterine contractility, a trial of oxytocin therapy is warranted. Contraindications to oxytocin therapy are: gross pelvic deformities arising from trauma or developmental defects, upper uterine segment surgical scars, irremediable soft tissue obstruction, and positions of the fetus other than occipital. Relative contraindications include estimated fetal weight over 4500 grams and parity over 5. Twins are not a contraindication provided that the first fetus is in a cephalic presentation.

Oxytocin therapy requires monitoring of the uterine contractility and the fetal heart rate. This can be accomplished by a professional attendant at the bedside palpating the intensity and frequency of each contraction, obtaining the average fetal heart rate for 20 seconds immediately after each contraction and recording these observations. An alternative is continuous electronic recording of the intrauterine pressure and the fetal heart rate with review of the oscillographic record every 15 minutes by a professional attendant. The oxytocin is given intravenously by means of a calibrated pump whose output is infused into an intravenous infusion line. Oxytocin is never infused directly into the patient from the pump. The patient should be kept in the right or left lateral recumbent position.

The initial dose is 1 mU/min. The dose may be increased by 1 mU per minute at intervals not more frequent than 30 minutes. It requires at least half an hour, perhaps longer and certainly not less, for the blood level of any particular dose of oxytocin infused to reach a steady value and to manifest its maximum effect. With this regimen, we can anticipate that more than 80 per cent of patients will effect progressive cervical dilatation with infusions of 4 mU per minute or less. Patients with large blood volumes (twins, obese) or those receiving magnesium sulfate concomitantly for the treatment of pre-eclampsia may require higher infusion rates.

What is the appropriate goal of oxytocin therapy, particularly if internal pressure monitoring is used for measuring the effect of oxytocin on uterine contractility? Because 90 to 95 per cent of nulliparous patients with hypocontractility achieve cervical dilatation if contractions occur at a rate of 3½ to 5 per 10 minutes and average 30 to 60 mm Hg in amplitude, and the contractions produce 150 to 250 Montevideo units of activity, it is recommended that uterine contractility within these ranges should be achieved. However, about 5 to 10 per cent of nulliparous patients will require more activity than this to effect cervical change. Because rupture of the uterus does not occur in nulliparas with or without oxytocin unless labor is grossly prolonged, there is no harm in attempting to obtain contractions as frequent as 5 to 6 per 10 minutes or at least 60 mm Hg, and >250 Montevideo units provided that monitoring does not reveal late decelerations in fetal heart rate. Because the dose response curve for oxytocin is curvilinear, if the patient does not respond to 4 mU per minute it is probably best to double the dose (8 then 16 mU per minute) over ½ to 1 hour intervals in an attempt to obtain the strength and frequency of contractions that these patients may require. Approximately 15 per cent of patients with hypocontractility will require doses above 4 mU per minute.

An occasional patient will manifest an unusual form of hypocontractility characterized by frequent painful contractions of low intensity, with elevated baseline intrauterine pressure. Such contractility is associated frequently with abruptio placentae and some cases of polyhydramnios or untreated preeclampsia. Appropriate treatment of these underlying conditions will resolve the problem. For patients with this quality of contractility, failure of progressive effacement and dilation, and no associated disease, treatment can be very difficult. The cervix is usually poorly effaced and dilated and the amnion intact. The use of morphine, 10 mg intramuscularly, to relieve pain allows periods of rest, and the patient will occasionally be found to be more effaced and dilated and having a normal contractile pattern on awakening. If the membranes are ruptured, epidural anesthesia and a trial of oxytocin as previously described should be attempted. However, it is our observation that amniotomy has usually preceded the diagnosis of this unusual form of hypocontractility, and oxytocin therapy, rather than analgesia, is required.

DYSFUNCTIONAL LABOR IN THE SECOND STAGE

The hallmark of success in the second stage is progressive descent of the presenting part, although no specific acceptable minimal rate of descent has been identified. As long as the fetal heart rate is in the normal range for the 20 seconds of measurement immediately following a contraction, or there are no late or severe variable decelerations if the fetus is electronically monitored, or the pH of the fetal blood scalp sample remains above 7.20, slow rates of descent are acceptable.

If the rate of descent is slow, however, careful reassessment of pelvic size and shape and the precise cephalic position is necessary. The common abnormalities usually found if the head is at least at zero station include: uterine hypocontractility, inadequate maternal bearing down effort, posterior positions of the occiput, minor deflexion attitudes, and minor abnormalities of the bony pelvis such as prominent spines, short sacrospinous ligament, flat sacrum, or narrow pubic arch.

Uterine hypocontractility is managed with oxytocin. Inadequate bearing down is treated by use of the semi-Fowler or squatting position. If the patient finds bearing down painful, analgesia with nitrous oxide may be helpful. Under these circumstances, as long as the fetal rate is not abnormal and is measured after each contraction and the patient achieves some progress in descent, delay of the second stage well beyond the usual 1 to 1½ hours is entirely acceptable in the nullipara. If hypocontractility or inadequate voluntary bearing down are the only abnormalities, spontaneous or outlet forceps delivery should be achieved.

The vacuum extractor is useful for the treatment of a few specific situations in the second stage: (1) the multipara with a barely engaged head who cannot or will not push, (2) the exhausted patient with station about +2, and (3) the fetus with a deflexed transverse position. In all these circumstances, when the patient fails to manifest progressive descent in spite of the therapeutic efforts described in the preceding paragraph, a trial delivery by the vacuum extractor is indicated.

Mid-forceps delivery is an acceptable therapeutic procedure provided that there are no pelvic abnormalities, there is no macrosomia, labor has arrested in a plus station, the physician thinks that correction of the malposition by rotation or traction will resolve the patient's dysfunctional labor problem, and facilities are available for immediate cesarean if the trial forceps delivery fails.

The use of forceps for other than lifting the fetal head over the perineum from the occiput anterior position or use of the vacuum extractor has been rejected by some because it is claimed that physicians cannot avoid the occasional poor fetal result. However, review of these poor result cases reveals that the vacuum extractor was applied more than once, was not applied to the fetal occiput, was used when the patient was having no uterine contractions and little or no bearing down effort, or was used incorrectly as a rotating instrument. The vacuum extractor is a tool designed to flex the fetal head and add to the mother's forces. It is not effective if uterine contractions are absent or very weak, or if the therapeutic requirement is rotation of the fetal head.

Similarly, the use of mid-forceps today is not appropriate for patients with arrested second stage who have a less than ideal pelvis, or macrosomia. If an attempt to achieve maximum uterine and bearing down forces in the second stage fails and the progress of labor is arrested, and it is the physician's judgment that this result obtains solely because of malposition (left occiput posterior, right occiput posterior, occiput posterior), a single trial of forceps is indicated. If a single attempt at application, or rotation, or traction fails, cesarean section is the treatment of choice.

POSTTERM PREGNANCY

JOHN F. HUDDLESTON, M.D.

A gestation exceeding 42 (menstrual) weeks is known as a postterm, postdate, or prolonged pregnancy. Since the mechanism by which labor is ordinarily triggered at 38 to 42 weeks is poorly understood, it is even less clear why, in 4 to 10 per cent of pregnancies, this mechanism fails to occur by the expected time. In up to 25 per cent of these postterm pregnancies, fetal nutrition and growth seem to be maintained, as the birthweights exceed 4000 grams. However, in a similar percentage, fetal nutrition seems to have been subacutely impaired and the infants at birth show various elements of the postmaturity syndrome: loss of subcutaneous fat, abundant scalp hair, absence of lanugo and of vernix caseosa, long fingernails, peeling of the skin, and (frequently) meconium staining. In the nursery, hypoglycemia is commonly found, as the poorly nourished fetus has depleted glycogen stores. This postmaturity syndrome is probably an exaggeration of a decline in placental function frequently present in late pregnancy and is accompanied by progressive oligohydramnios and a decrease in uteroplacental respiratory function, as manifested by an increased tendency toward fetal death and intrapartum fetal distress. The meconium aspiration syndrome, generally preventable by appropriate management at delivery, can be lethal to the newborn.

DIAGNOSIS

The diagnosis of postterm pregnancy would seem to be easily made whenever any gestation exceeds 294 days. However, accuracy in this diagnosis depends upon the care with which data necessary for precise dating were *collected in early pregnancy*, and errors are common unless strict care is taken with such assessments in *all pregnancies*. For example, if a woman has regular cycles of 35 days' duration, she probably ovulates about 7 days later than would be expected if her cycles were 28 days in length; her expected date of confinement (EDC) would reasonably then be 287 days after the onset of her last menstrual period (LMP), and her pregnancy should not be considered postterm until 301 days. Since the use of oral contraceptives may delay the ovulation occurring after their discontinuance, pregnancies for which the LMP resulted from withdrawal of oral contraceptives should be suspect for the possibility of ovulation delay. Careful menstrual history, bimanual examination in early pregnancy, and ability to hear fetal heart tones with a standard (DeLee) fetoscope at about 20 weeks (when the uterine fundus is about at umbilical level) together form a clinical triad that, if internally consistent, form a reasonable basis for firmly assigning an EDC. Quickening is less reliable and is especially poor unless prospectively requested by the physician and recorded by the mother.

If the elements of the above triad are not in agreement, ultrasonic assessment of gestational age is indicated and for best accuracy should be done by 26 weeks. In the third trimester, the growth rates of fetal biparietal diameter and femoral length slow and the confidence intervals about their means increase. Both of these factors tend to amplify the degree of error in gestational-age assessments done late in pregnancy. Although evaluation of amniotic-fluid volume and placental consistency can be valuable in the management of postterm pregnancies, ultrasonic evaluation in late gestation is essentially worthless in establishing that a suspected postterm pregnancy is indeed prolonged.

Reasonable diagnostic criteria for prolonged pregnancy include:

1. reliable menstrual history (including timing, normalcy of flow and duration for that patient, and whether LMP resulted from withdrawal of oral contraceptives);

2. first trimester bimanual examination;

3. auscultation of *unamplified* fetal heart tones by 20 weeks. In the absence of agreement among the above three criteria that 42 weeks have been exceeded, a single examination by ultrasound having been done *prior* to 26 weeks and agreeing with at least one of the three should suffice.

MANAGEMENT PROTOCOL

Figure 1 delineates a suggested method of managing a postdate or postterm pregnancy and is based upon several considerations: (1) despite the fact that most such fetuses are doing well, if one is certain of the diagnosis and the conditions

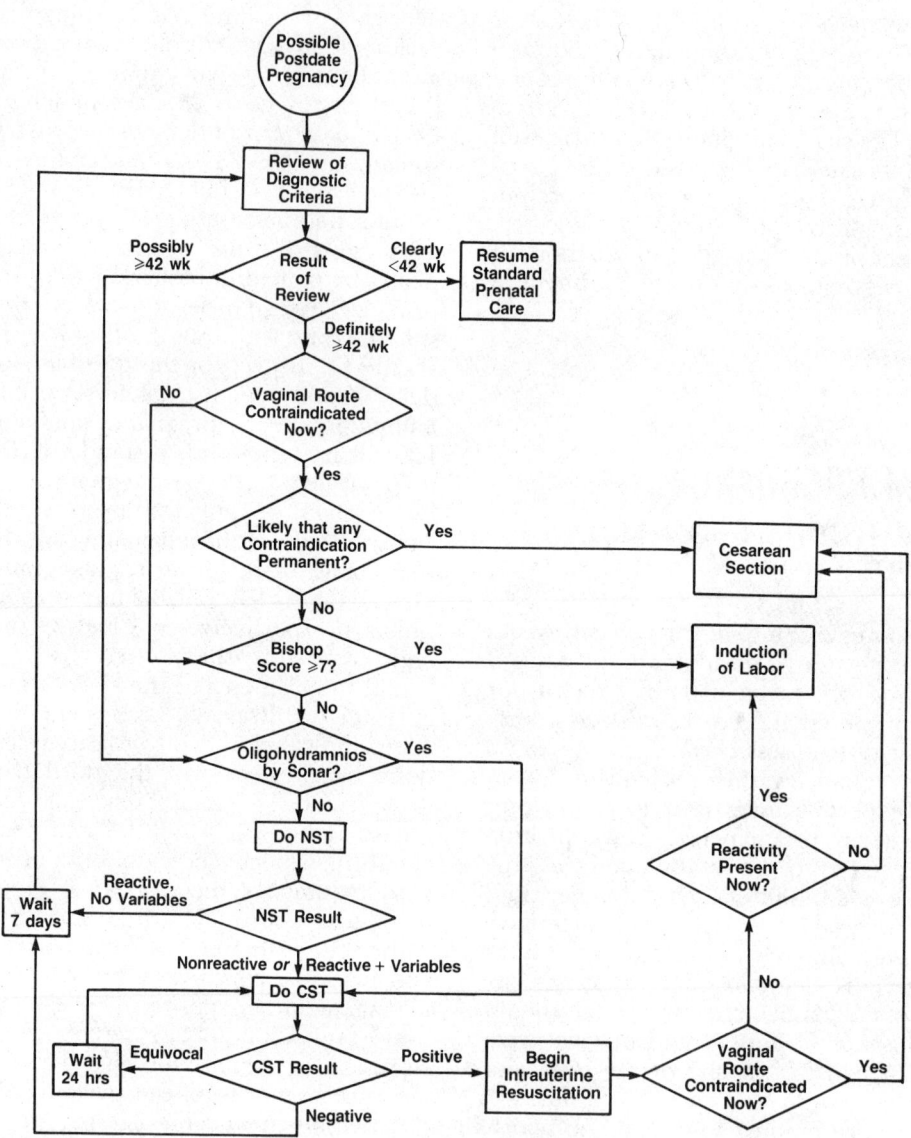

Figure 1. Flow chart for management of postterm pregnancy.

are favorable for induction of labor, induction generally should be pursued; (2) if review of the diagnostic criteria reveals a possible but not definitive diagnosis, induction should be bypassed in favor of the noninvasive (ultrasonic and fetal monitoring) tests; (3) contraindications to inducing labor may or may not be permanent (e.g., absolute disproportion versus breech presentation); (4) the Bishop score is a reasonable way to assess cervical readiness for induction of labor, but the Bishop score is usually *low* in postdate pregnancies; (5) a finding of oligohydramnios on real-time ultrasound (no pocket of fluid with greatest diameter 1 cm or more) is associated with a higher incidence of antepartum death, intrapartum distress, and neonatal risk; (6) therefore, if oligohydramnios is present, a contraction stress test (CST), with careful attention to the presence of reactivity (concurrent nonstress test), should be done primarily, rather than relying only upon the results of a nonstress test (NST); (7) variable decelerations seen during either test also suggest oligohydramnios; (8) a positive CST, for which late decelerations have been resolved by intrauterine resuscitation (expansion of maternal vascular volume, maintenance of left-lateral recumbency, and administration of oxygen by mask), does not contraindicate an attempt at vaginal delivery; (9) a reactive NST without variable decelerations (in the absence of oligohydramnios) or a negative CST (whenever indicated) will justify waiting a week before repeating the test; (10) such a 7 day wait should (because of the postterm state) frequently result in spontaneous labor; (11) prior to repeating the antepartum test, a reevaluation for delivery should be done.

In addition, the presence of reactivity in a patient with a positive CST considerably heightens the possibility that, with intrauterine resuscitation, induction of labor will be tolerated by the fetus. If reactivity is absent in a postterm pregnancy and the CST is positive, cesarean delivery probably should be accomplished forthwith.

SIGNIFICANCE AND MANAGEMENT OF MECONIUM

Meconium in the amniotic fluid is a frequent concomitant of prolonged gestation. However, there seems little justification in attempting to document its presence by amniocentesis or to consider its presence an indication for prompt delivery. Meconium is generally managed best by aggressive tracheal toilet at the moment of delivery: DeLee suction of the oropharynx and nasopharynx before delivery of the shoulders and then performing endotracheal intubation, repetitively if necessary, until the tracheal return is clear. Meconium may also represent a problem in management if severe, intrapartum distress results in fetal gasping. Gasping may result in meconium being forced peripherally so that such tracheal toilet at delivery is ineffective in preventing the frequently fatal meconium aspiration syndrome. However, unless there are abnormal fetal heart rate patterns on antepartum or intrapartum monitoring, meconium alone is probably not cause for serious alarm.

ERYTHROBLASTOSIS FETALIS

FREDRIC D. FRIGOLETTO, JR., M.D.

Isoimmune hemolytic disease of the fetus is caused by a fetal-maternal blood group incompatibility, with maternal immunization against fetal blood group antigen. ABO incompatibility accounts for approximately two thirds of cases of this disease; however, $Rh_O(D)$ is by far the most important antigen being responsible for almost all the cases of stillbirth due to erythroblastosis. A small number of cases are the result of incompatibility with respect to other blood factors such as Kell, c, E, C, C^w, JK^a, S, M, k, Fy^a and a few others, which, although less antigenic, do not differ significantly in other respects from Rh so far as erythroblastosis fetalis is concerned. ABO incompatibility does not result in severe fetal erythroblastosis or in stillbirth. Because of the mild nature of ABO disease in utero, no antenatal testing either by titer level or amniocentesis is necessary or indicated. These infants usually have a weakly positive (Coombs) direct antiglobulin test, are blood group A or B, and are born to group O mothers. The aspects of isoimmunization which require constant surveillance are:

1. Identification of patients at risk of becoming sensitized,
2. Prevention of sensitization in this group, and
3. Identification and management of the sensitized patient.

SCREENING AND PREVENTION

No controversy exists regarding the fact that the most important aspect of this disease is prevention. This should begin at the first prenatal visit by testing each patient's blood for ABO and Rh type as well as for irregular antibodies. Since it is well established that antibodies other than anti-Rh can cause serious erythroblastosis, these antibodies must be sought out. It is no longer logical to orient a work-up solely toward the identification of the $Rh_O(D)$-negative female and the possible development of anti-$Rh_O(D)$ in her circulation. On this basis, all pregnant women, both Rh-positive and Rh-negative, should have antibody screening done in early pregnancy. Rh-negative–unsensitized women should have antibody screening repeated at least two more times during pregnancy.

When an irregular antibody is present it must be specifically identified and appropriate titers obtained. We are not concerned merely with whether or not the patient is "Rh-positive" or "Rh-negative"; we are concerned with whether or not an antibody is present, and whether that antibody can harm the fetus. Anti-Lewis^a (Le^a) and anti-Lewis^b (Le^b) are antibodies detected fairly frequently. Both are of no clinical significance because they are usually of the IgM type which does not cross the placenta. In addition, the Lewis antigens are not yet present on fetal red cells.

Obstetrical care becomes more complicated when the patient has anti-Rh(D) antibodies or another antibody capable of causing erythroblastosis fetalis. Starting at 20 weeks of gestation, titers of all sensitized women are repeated at 2 to 4 week intervals until 34 weeks, and then at 1 to 2 week intervals thereafter, provided the titer remains below the "critical titer level."

Ideally, antibody identification and serial titer determinations should be performed in a laboratory that has long and extensive experience with erythroblastosis fetalis. Such a laboratory should have a well-established protocol for doing anti-Rh titers by a standardized method, using the same Rh-positive blood cells for the titers so that maximal reproducibility is achieved. In addition the outcome of many pregnancies should be known, so that a logical and reasonable correlation between titer and pregnancy outcome can be made. In this manner many laboratories have been able to establish the concept of a "critical titer level," which is defined as the titer below which there have been no stillbirths or severely affected infants. Since test cells, technicians, and details of titration methods differ, titer results in one laboratory may differ from those in another, and therefore, each laboratory must establish its own critical titer level according to its own experience.

Amniocentesis is not initiated until the critical titer level is met or exceeded. In this manner, unnecessary amniocentesis can be avoided, and many mildly sensitized patients can complete their pregnancies without having to accept the risks of an invasive procedure. In a situation where a patient has had a previous erythroblastotic stillbirth or seriously affected infant, amniocentesis is warranted no matter what the titer. When amniocentesis is indicated, the time of the first amniotic tap can be as early as 20 to 21 weeks of gestation, depending upon the titer and past history of erythroblastosis. The amniotic fluid specimen should be centrifuged and separated promptly in order to remove any contaminating blood cells, and it should also be protected from light which can break down the bilirubin pigments to be evaluated. The fluid is then filtered and the $.OD_{450}$ is determined by spectrophotometric analysis and interpretation by the method of Liley. The $.OD_{450}$ is plotted on Liley's three-zone chart (the top zone is the dangerous zone), and the degree of disease of the fetus can then be estimated from the height of the $.OD_{450}$ on the chart. Of the many amniotic fluid analysis methods in the literature, Liley's is probably the one most widely used around the world, and also the most reliable.

Amniotic taps are usually repeated at 2 week intervals; serial determinations of the OD_{450} make possible a more reliable evaluation of fetal condition than a single tap alone. The interval between amniocentesis can vary, however, depending on the previous test result. An upper middle zone result would indicate repeat amniocentesis in one week, while a very low result would permit an interval of three or possibly even four weeks, depending on the findings. Since intrauterine fetal transfusion can be beneficial, when indicated, from 21 weeks of gestation onward, one should be ready to employ amniocentesis and spectrophotometric analysis of amniotic fluid as early as 20 to 21 weeks of gestation, when the titer and past history so indicate.

The ultrasound technique of using a phased array sector scanner to localize the insertion site for intrauterine fetal transfusion allows the operator to directly view the needle advancement and entry into the fetal abdomen. It is generally agreed that this is a highly specialized technical procedure which should be carried out in a center by appropriately trained and experienced personnel.

Previous obstetric history, optical density measurements, ultrasound findings, and antibody titers supply data concerning the condition of the fetus with respect to erythroblastosis. Gestational age and the degree of pulmonary maturity as determined by lecithin:sphingomyelin (L:S) measurements establish whether efforts should be directed at intrauterine treatment or premature delivery. Because of the constant advancement and improvement in neonatal care and survival rate, the latest gestational age at which intrauterine treatment is started has been lowered, and needs to be continually evaluated at each center to establish relative risk benefit ratios for the alternatives.

As mentioned previously the most important aspect of this disease is prevention. This begins with blood group typing whereby each $Rh_O(D)$-negative patient is identified. The next step is to understand those situations in which sensitization can occur, and thus where prophylaxis must be given. These sources of maternal sensitization in order of risk per event are:

1. Sensitization associated with birth (13 per cent), abortion, and ectopic pregnancy (2 to 5 per cent);
2. Sensitization occurring during pregnancy (prior to birth) (1 to 1.8 per cent);
3. Sensitization associated with amniocentesis (?1 to 2 per cent);
4. Sensitization associated with antepartum hemorrhage (?);
5. Sensitization due to excess fetomaternal hemorrhage (?).

The recommended dose of $Rh_O(D)$ immune globulin for all pregnancy indicated situations at 12 weeks or less is 50 mcg. This includes therapeutic abortion, spontaneous abortion, and ectopic pregnancy. After 12 weeks, the standard dose of 300 mcg is used for amniocentesis, late induced or spontaneous abortion, and term delivery. Ideally, following delivery of every $Rh_O(D)$-negative patient a Kleihauer-Betke test is done to determine if more than the standard 300 mcg dose is needed because of a fetomaternal bleed in excess of 15 ml of fetal red blood cells or 30 ml of whole blood. When this or a similar test is not available, the obstetrician will have to know those situations which are associated with excess bleeding (i.e., manual removal of the placenta) and determine the need on clinical grounds. The individual's risk of becoming sensitized because of excess fetomaternal bleeding appears to be exceedingly low.

By understanding the risk factors in each of these instances and by utilizing $Rh_O(D)$ immune globulin prophylaxis, the ultimate goal of eradication of erythroblastosis fetalis secondary to Rh sensitization will be reached.

HYPOTHYROIDISM

ROBERT W. HUFF, M.D.,
and PATRICK DUFF, M.D.

Hypothyroidism is a relatively rare disorder that is responsible for approximately 1 in every 1500 hospital admissions. It occurs four to five times more frequently in women than in men, and usually develops in the fourth to sixth decades of life. Hypothyroidism may be either primary or secondary. In the former, the endocrine disorder is due to failure of the thyroid gland itself; in the latter, the metabolic derangement is due to hypothalamic or pituitary disease. Hypothyroidism may be subclassified further as in Table 1.

PRIMARY HYPOTHYROIDISM

The most common cause of primary hypothyroidism is prior ablative treatment of thyrotoxicosis with either surgery or radioactive iodine. The next most frequent cause of hypothyroidism is idiopathic atrophy of the gland. The latter disorder is most likely to occur in women toward the end of the reproductive age range. The majority of patients with idiopathic hypothyroidism have evidence of circulating antithyroid antibodies directed against the thyroglobulin molecule or against the microsomal fraction of the cell. Because of the presence of these antithyroid antibodies, it is believed that most cases of apparent idiopathic hypothyroidism represent endstage autoimmune thyroiditis.

The other causes of primary hypothyroidism outlined in Table 1 are rare. Despite their rarity, however, several deserve special mention. Hypothyroidism may result from the administration of medications such as lithium carbonate, thiocyanates, sulfonylureas, and thiourea drugs used for the treatment of hyperthyroidism. Hypothyroidism also may result from chronic thyroiditis (Hashimoto's disease), a disorder which occurs primarily in middle-aged women. It is characterized by a firm, rubbery, lobular enlargement of the gland which simulates multinodular goiter, and by the presence of antithyroid antibodies in the patient's serum.

Finally, both endemic and sporadic goitrous hypothyroidism may develop as a result of dietary deficiency of iodide. This entity is of special interest to the obstetrician because relative iodide deficiency may develop in pregnancy as a result of increased volume of distribution of iodide within the body and increased renal clearance of iodide.

SECONDARY HYPOTHYROIDISM

Secondary hypothyroidism may be the result of deficient production of thyroid-stimulating hormone (TSH) by the anterior pituitary or diminished synthesis of thyrotropin-releasing hormone (TRH) by the hypothalamus. Decreases in TSH synthesis and release by the pituitary are usually accompanied by other tropic hormone deficiencies, and may be due to pituitary tumor, ablative surgery, pituitary irradiation, or postpartum pituitary necrosis. Derangements in hypothalamic release of TRH may be the result of hypothalamic tumor, head injury, central nervous system infection, or granulomatous disease.

CLINICAL MANIFESTATIONS OF HYPOTHYROIDISM

Hypothyroidism in the adult may present with a wide variety of clinical symptoms and signs. Common symptoms include profound lethargy, fatigue, weight gain, change in hair texture, hair loss in the outer third of the eyebrow, constipation, and increased sensitivity to

TABLE 1. **Classification of Hypothyroidism**

I. Primary Hypothyroidism
  A. Goiter not present
    1. Idiopathic
    2. Postablative
    3. Postinflammatory
  B. Goiter present
    1. Congenital and hereditary defects in iodide trapping and thyroid hormone synthesis and release
    2. Acquired defects due to ingestion of goitrogens or antithyroid drugs
    3. Acquired defects due to iodide excess or lack
    4. Hashimoto's thyroiditis
II. Secondary Hypothyroidism
  A. Pituitary failure
  B. Hypothalamic disorder

cold. Patients may also report arthralgias without frank arthritis, increased bruising, persistent rhinorrhea, coryza, and decreased auditory acuity. Of particular interest to the obstetrician-gynecologist is the fact that some patients with hypothyroidism may present for evaluation of recurrent abortion, recurrent prematurity, menometrorrhagia, or amenorrhea-galactorrhea. In addition to the clinical manifestations noted above, patients with secondary hypothyroidism may have symptoms associated with defects in synthesis of other tropic hormones.

Prominent physical findings in hypothyroidism include facial pallor, alopecia affecting primarily the eyebrows, dryness and roughening of the skin, and brittleness and dryness of the hair. The tongue and larynx may be edematous, with resultant slurring of speech. There may be pronounced slowing of the patient's physical and mental activity. Galactorrhea may be present. There may also be evidence of peripheral muscle weakness, disturbance in cerebellar function, and marked slowing of the deep tendon reflexes, especially the Achilles tendon reflex. In isolated instances, actual psychosis may be present.

Myxedema coma is a rare, potentially life-threatening complication of severe hypothyroidism. Manifestations of this disorder include the symptoms and signs previously reviewed plus hypothermia, respiratory depression, and loss of consciousness. Hydrothorax, ascites, pericardial effusion, and adynamic ileus progressing to toxic megacolon are common associated findings in myxedema coma.

DIAGNOSIS OF HYPOTHYROIDISM

The diagnosis of primary hypothyroidism is established by demonstration of an elevated TSH level. This test is especially useful in instances of early or mild hypothyroidism, when the T_4, T_3, and T_3 resin uptake levels are still in the low-normal range.

In secondary hypothyroidism, TSH will be very low or undetectable in the presence of decreased T_4, T_3, and T_3 resin uptake levels. In this clinical setting, the TRH stimulation test may be used to differentiate between a hypothalamic and a pituitary defect. If TSH levels do not increase promptly following an intravenous injection of 50 to 250 μg of TRH, it may be concluded that pituitary failure is the explanation for hypothyroidism. If the TSH response is normal, a hypothalamic defect is responsible for thyroid dysfunction.

Additional laboratory results may also be of interest in the evaluation of the hypothyroid patient, although they are not essential to the diagnosis. These include decreased protein bound iodine levels, decreased basal metabolic rate, decreased radioactive iodine uptake, and elevated cholesterol and carotene levels. Circulating antithyroid antibodies may be present. In addition, there may be a normocytic or slightly macrocytic anemia, achlorhydria, and elevated LDH, CPK, SGOT, and uric acid. The chest radiograph may demonstrate mild cardiomegaly, primarily due to pericardial effusion, and the electrocardiogram may show decreased voltage and inversion or flattening of the T waves.

TREATMENT OF HYPOTHYROIDISM

Once the diagnosis of hypothyroidism is established, it is essential to initiate therapy promptly with thyroid hormone replacement. This is particularly important in pregnant patients because of the evidence that untreated hypothyroidism results in an increased incidence of spontaneous abortion, stillbirth, and premature delivery.

There are four preparations of thyroid hormone that may be used for replacement therapy: (1) desiccated thyroid, containing a variable mixture of T_4 and T_3; (2) synthetic *l*-thyroxine (T_4); (3) *l*-triiodothyronine (T_3); and (4) liotrix, a standardized mixture of T_4 and T_3 in a ratio of 4 to 1. Of these preparations, synthetic T_4 is the preferred agent because, with a single daily dose, it provides more stable blood levels of T_4 and T_3. The average daily replacement dose of *l*-thyroxine is approximately 2.25 μg per kg of body weight per day; most patients ultimately will be well controlled on 100 to 200 μg per day.

In the healthy nonpregnant patient with mild to moderately severe hypothyroidism, replacement therapy should be initiated with 50 to 100 μg of *l*-thyroxine given as a single daily dose. The patient then should be evaluated carefully for evidence of thyroid hormone excess; the usual manifestations of toxicity are anxiety, restlessness, tremor, and palpitations. If no toxicity is apparent after 2 to 3 weeks of observation, the replacement dose may be increased to the usual maintenance dose of 150 to 200 μg daily.

Clinical improvement usually is apparent within 3 to 5 weeks. In association with resolution of the clinical signs of hypothyroidism, the T_4, TSH, and free thyroxine index (FT_4I), should return to the normal range if replacement therapy is adequate. Persistent elevation of TSH is an indication for increasing the dose of *l*-thyroxine by 50 μg per day.

Patients with advanced age, cardiovascular disease, or severe hypothyroidism may experience serious toxicity when thyroid hormone replacement is initiated. Excessively high starting doses and too rapid increases in dosage may precipitate angina, tachyarrhythmias, and congestive heart failure. Accordingly, replacement therapy should begin with 25 µg of *l*-thyroxine per day with subsequent 25 µg increases in the dose every 4 to 6 weeks.

Conversely, pregnant patients with hypothyroidism should be returned to the euthyroid state as soon as possible in order to avoid the complications of abortion, stillbirth, and prematurity. Replacement therapy should be started with 150 to 200 µg of *l*-thyroxine, and the dosage should subsequently be increased to maintenance levels of 200 to 300 µg over a 3 to 4 week period. Although there is no evidence that *l*-thyroxine crosses the placenta in concentrations great enough to suppress fetal thyroid function, infants of hypothyroid mothers should be screened for thyroid disease since they may manifest one of the rare congenital or hereditary defects in thyroid hormone synthesis and release.

The physician should be alert for the possibility of deleterious interactions between supplemental thyroid hormone and certain other medications. For example, the interaction between thyroid hormone and oral anticoagulants may result in increased anticoagulant activity. This effect appears to be mediated by displacement of anticoagulant from its protein binding sites, thereby enhancing the bioavailability of active drug. Thyroid hormone also increases catabolism of clotting factors. Similarly, simultaneous administration of cholestyramine and thyroid hormone may result in decreased effectiveness of the latter drug owing to binding of the hormone in the intestine. Finally, thyroid hormone given to the pregnant woman at the time of delivery may cross the placental barrier, causing subsequent displacement of bilirubin from protein binding sites in the newborn. Although placental passage of thyroid hormone is limited, there may be sufficient transfer to cause hyperbilirubinemia when other predisposing factors, such as hemolysis, maternal diabetes, or prematurity, also exist.

TREATMENT OF MYXEDEMA COMA

Myxedema coma is an acute emergency requiring intensive medical management. The patient should be treated initially with intravenous administration of 200 to 500 µg of *l*-thyroxine as a single dose. Following this loading dose, 50 to 100 µg of *l*-thyroxine should be given each day until the patient is able to take oral medication. At this point, the dose should be gradually increased to maintenance levels, as outlined above.

In the acute phase of the illness, the patient should also be treated with corticosteroids. In patients with secondary hypothyroidism, treatment with corticosteroids will prevent adrenal insufficiency. In patients with primary hypothyroidism, steroid treatment will compensate for the rapid increase in metabolism resulting from thyroid hormone replacement. Additional supportive therapy in the patient with myxedema coma includes mechanical ventilation, stabilization of body temperature, repletion of intravascular volume, and correction of electrolyte abnormalities.

HYPERTHYROIDISM

PATRICK DUFF, M.D.,
and ROBERT W. HUFF, M.D.

Hyperthyroidism occurs predominantly in women in the third to fourth decades of life. The most common cause of hyperthyroidism is Graves' disease, a disorder characterized by diffuse enlargement of the thyroid gland, excess thyroid hormone activity, prominent infiltrative ophthalmopathy, and localized dermopathy. The exact pathogenesis of Graves' disease is uncertain, although there is evidence that it may represent an autoimmune phenomenon. Some patients with Graves' disease have a circulating antibody (long-acting thyroid stimulator, LATS) that acts on the thyroid gland to increase iodine uptake, stimulate hyperplasia, and promote release of previously synthesized thyroid hormone. This thyroid-stimulating substance has been isolated from the serum of some infants born to hyperthyroid mothers and has been implicated as one cause of neonatal thyrotoxicosis.

Although Graves' disease is the most common cause of hyperthyroidism, there are other causes to consider in the evaluation of thyrotoxic patients—thyroid adenoma, multinodular goiter or Plummer's disease, and subacute thyroiditis. Hyperthyroidism also may result from hyperfunction of ectopic thyroid tissue and from administration of large amounts of iodine or thyroid hormone.

In addition, two unusual causes of hyperthyroidism are of special interest to the obstetrician-gynecologist. A small number of patients with gestational trophoblastic disease manifest evidence of hyperthyroidism. Recent investigation has demonstrated that the excess thyroid activity results from a TSH-like effect of circulating chorionic gonadotropin. Similarly, a small number of patients with teratoma of the ovary may have clinical signs of thyrotoxicosis. In this instance, the endocrine disorder is due to the presence of active thyroid tissue within the neoplasm (struma ovarii). In both of the above clinical situations, the hyperthyroid state will resolve with treatment of the underlying gynecologic disorder.

DIAGNOSIS OF HYPERTHYROIDISM

In the nonpregnant patient, the diagnosis of thyrotoxicosis may be confirmed by the findings of elevated thyroxine (T_4), measured by competitive protein binding or radioimmunoassay; elevated free thyroxine, usually measured indirectly by means of the free thyroxine index (FT_4I)*; and elevated T_3 resin uptake. Demonstration of an elevated basal metabolic rate (BMR) and of an increased uptake of radioactive iodine also supports the diagnosis of hyperthyroidism.

The diagnosis of T_3-thyrotoxicosis is suggested by the presence of excess thyroid hormone activity in association with normal total and free T_4 levels and normal thyroid-binding globulin (TBG) levels. The diagnosis is confirmed by the finding of elevated triiodothyronine (T_3), measured by radioimmunoassay, and by demonstration that the accelerated T_3 production is autonomous. The standard T_3 suppression test is utilized for this latter purpose.

Radioactive iodine uptake values range from low to high in T_3-thyrotoxicosis and often are completely normal. This observation may be explained by the fact that the biosynthesis of T_3 requires less iodine than does T_4. Because the values of radioactive iodine uptake are so variable, this test is helpful in establishing the diagnosis of T_3-thyrotoxicosis.

The diagnosis of hyperthyroidism in pregnancy is more difficult to establish for two principal reasons. First, many of the more common manifestations of hyperthyroidism—heat intolerance, tachycardia, palpitations, nausea, vomiting, increased skin pigmentation, and hair loss—may be observed in normal pregnant women. Second, thyroid function tests are altered in pregnancy because of estrogen-mediated increased hepatic synthesis of thyroid-binding globulin.

In the euthyroid pregnant woman, total T_4 will be normal to slightly elevated, but usually will not exceed 14 µg per dl. The T_3 resin uptake will be decreased slightly because of increased thyroid hormone binding capacity, and the FT_4I will be normal.

In hyperthyroid pregnant patients, the total T_4 may be elevated above the usual levels expected for pregnancy. T_3 resin uptake values may be in the range considered normal for the nonpregnant state; however, these values are elevated for pregnancy and result from increased saturation of binding sites by endogenous thyroid hormone. The FT_4I will be elevated, and this is the most helpful laboratory study in confirming the diagnosis of hyperthyroidism in pregnancy.

The radioactive iodine uptake test is, of course, contraindicated in pregnancy. A modified T_3 suppression test, however, may be performed without risk to the fetus. In this study, levels of T_4 are measured before and after the administration of 100 µg of triiodothyronine daily for 3 days. Failure of the T_4 level to decrease by at least 2 µg per dl confirms autonomous production of T_4 by the thyroid gland and supports the diagnosis of hyperthyroidism.

TREATMENT OF HYPERTHYROIDISM

Three therapeutic modalities are utilized for the treatment of hyperthyroidism in the patient who is not pregnant: surgery, radioactive iodine, and antithyroid medication. Even in patients scheduled for ablative procedures, the manifestations of hyperthyroidism must be controlled completely with medication before performance of thyroidectomy or administration of radioactive iodine. Effective control may be achieved by treating the patient with propylthiouracil or methimazole in combination with iodide and propranolol, as outlined below.

The principal candidates for subtotal thyroidectomy are women of childbearing age and younger who have not achieved remission of symptoms during treatment with antithyroid drugs and pregnant women who have experienced a recent episode of thyroid storm. The major complications of thyroid surgery are injury to the recurrent laryngeal nerves; removal of parathyroid tissue resulting in hypoparathyroidism; postoperative thyroid storm; and postoperative hypothyroidism.

Prevention of the first two complications requires careful surgical technique. Postoperative thyroid crisis may be prevented by continuation of antithyroid medication throughout the perioperative period. Patients undergoing thyroidectomy also must be followed closely for the development of hypothyroidism; treatment with thyroid hormone replacement must be initiated promptly if clinical manifestations of thyroid dysfunction appear.

---

*$FT_4I = T_4 \times \dfrac{T_3 \text{ resin uptake}}{\text{normal } T_3 \text{ resin uptake}}$

Radioactive iodine ablation of the thyroid gland is indicated in women beyond the childbearing years who have not experienced remission of disease after an initial course of antithyroid drug therapy and who have concurrent medical illnesses that make them poor candidates for surgery. Radioactive iodine treatment also is indicated in patients who have developed an exacerbation of symptoms despite prior thyroid surgery.

The major complication of radioiodine therapy is the development of hypothyroidism following treatment. Another minor problem is that control of symptoms may not be achieved for several weeks following administration of the drug. For this reason, it is appropriate to continue medical therapy with propranolol (40 to 200 mg per day) until the patient clearly is in remission.

TREATMENT OF HYPERTHYROIDISM IN PREGNANCY

The pregnant patient with untreated hyperthyroidism is at increased risk for several major complications, including intrauterine growth retardation, preeclampsia, premature labor, and thyroid storm, all of which predispose to increased perinatal and maternal morbidity and mortality. Therefore, treatment is indicated for all pregnant patients with thyrotoxicosis. Therapy for hyperthyroidism in pregnancy is primarily medical. Surgery is indicated for patients whose disease cannot be controlled by antithyroid medication. Radioactive iodine therapy is contraindicated in pregnancy because of the risk of radiation-induced injury to the fetus, specifically the risk of ablation of fetal thyroid tissue with resultant cretinism.

Medical therapy of hyperthyroidism in pregnancy should be initiated with one of the thioureas, propylthiouracil or methimazole (Tapazole). These drugs exert their antithyroid effect by blocking the formation of diiodotyrosine (DIT) and monoiodotyrosine and by inhibiting the coupling of tyrosine residues. Propylthiouracil should be given initially in a dose of 100 mg orally every 8 hours, methimazole in a dose of 10 mg every 8 hours. The patient then should be followed carefully with serial physical examinations and measurements of FT_4I. As the clinical manifestations of thyrotoxicosis improve and as the FT_4I decreases toward normal, dosage of the antithyroid drug should be reduced in stepwise fashion. In certain patients, it ultimately may be possible to discontinue the medication entirely. In the remaining patients, every effort should be made to reduce the dose of propylthiouracil or methimazole to the lowest possible level consistent with control of the disease process. If clinical or laboratory evidence of hypothyroidism develops, replacement therapy with l-thyroxine should be instituted immediately.

The most common side-effects of thiourea therapy are a purpuric skin rash, pruritus, drug fever, and nausea. Such effects occur in approximately 2 to 8 per cent of patients receiving treatment with one of these agents. If a side-effect occurs with one of the drugs, it usually is possible to continue therapy with the other medication, since cross-reactivity is rare. The most serious complication of thiourea administration is the development of agranulocytosis. This complication occurs in 0.03 to 0.6 per cent of patients taking antithyroid drugs, and it usually is reversible if the drug is discontinued immediately. Breast feeding may be contraindicated in patients receiving thioureas because the drugs may pass into the breast milk and cause thyroid suppression in the neonate. Additional research is needed to establish the safety of antithyroid medications in the breastfed infant.

The major concern with use of antithyroid drugs in pregnancy is the effect of the medications on the fetus. Localized scalp defects have occurred in fetuses of mothers receiving thiourea drugs. Although rare, such defects appear to occur more often with methimazole; for this reason, some investigators have suggested that propylthiouracil is the preferred agent in pregnancy. More importantly, both drugs may cause hypothyroidism and goiter in the fetus, even when dosages are maintained at low levels. Concurrent administration of thyroid hormone to the mother does not consistently prevent fetal hypothyroidism and may interfere with efforts to reduce antithyroid drug dosage to lower levels. In the near future, it may be possible to reliably predict the development of fetal hypothyroidism in utero by measurement of $3,3',5'$ triiodothyronine (reverse T_3) levels in amniotic fluid. If fetal hypothyroidism is documented in this manner, it may then be possible to correct the disorder by administering l-thyroxine into the amniotic cavity.

Because of concern about the rare occurrence of fetal hypothyroidism as a result of thiourea therapy, some investigators have recommended the use of propranolol as the sole treatment for hyperthyroidism in pregnancy. The initial enthusiasm for this treatment regimen has decreased, however, for two principal reasons. First, although propranolol controls the cardiovascular and neurologic manifestations of thyrotoxicosis, it does not correct the underlying metabolic derangement. Therefore, excess thyroid hormone synthesis and release continues unchecked. There are, in fact, reports of patients who have developed overt thyroid storm while receiving propranolol as single agent therapy. Second, propranolol now has been shown to have several potentially harmful effects on the fetus and neonate, including intrauterine growth retardation, impaired response to hypoxia, respiratory depression at birth, postnatal hypoglycemia and prolonged postnatal bradycardia.

Because of these possible untoward effects on the fetus, propranolol is not the drug of choice for the long-term management of hyperthyroidism in pregnancy. Propranolol administration is indicated, however, in the acute management of patients with severe symptoms and in the preoperative preparation of patients for thyroidectomy.

Similarly, although iodide therapy may be indicated in the initial treatment of thyrotoxic crisis, long-term administration of iodide is contraindicated in pregnancy. Prolonged administration of even relatively small doses of iodides may cause massive goitrous enlargement of the fetal thyroid gland. There are reports of infants who have developed acute respiratory failure as a result of compression of the trachea by a large iodine-induced goiter.

THYROID STORM

Thyroid storm is a clinical syndrome characterized by an increase in the signs and symptoms of hyperthyroidism. The disorder is an acute medical emergency. Mortality may be as high as 40 to 50 per cent, with an average rate of 20 to 25 per cent even in the most recent surveys.

In the past, most cases of thyroid storm have occurred in the immediate postoperative period in patients whose hyperthyroidism was not well controlled before ablation of the gland by surgery or radioactive iodine. With improved methods for preoperative treatment of hyperthyroidism, thyroid storm following thyroidectomy has become increasingly rare. Most cases of thyroid storm now occur in undiagnosed or inadequately treated patients who have experienced complications such as serious systemic infection, diabetic ketoacidosis, trauma, or nonthyroidal surgery. In the obstetric patient, thyroid storm has occurred in association with preeclampsia, cesarean section, and forceps delivery.

The diagnosis of thyroid storm must be made on the basis of the patient's clinical symptoms and physical examination; rarely will there be time to await confirmatory laboratory tests prior to initiation of treatment. The single most important feature of the patient's evaluation is a prior history of hyperthyroidism; almost invariably, thyroid storm is preceded by a well-defined antecedent history of thyrotoxicosis.

In its most extreme manifestation, the physical signs of thyroid storm will include hyperpyrexia, with temperatures exceeding 106°F; extreme irritability and restlessness; confusion and disorientation; hypotension; profound muscle weakness; congestive heart failure; cardiac arrhythmia; vomiting; diarrhea; and jaundice. In isolated instances, patients with thyroid storm may present with more subtle manifestations such as apathy, prostration, loss of consciousness, and only mild temperature elevation. The differential diagnosis of thyroid storm includes septic shock, hypovolemic shock, transfusion or drug reaction, and acute adrenal insufficiency.

Once the diagnosis of thyroid storm is established, treatment must begin promptly and must fulfill several essential objectives. First, an effort must be made to diagnose and treat any underlying medical or surgical disorder that may have precipitated the thyrotoxic crisis. In particular, a careful search must be made for any source of infection such as bacterial endocarditis, pneumonia, perforated appendix, intra-amniotic infection, pelvic abscess, and any source of metabolic abnormality such as diabetic ketoacidosis.

Second, effective treatment of thyroid storm must include drugs that reduce the production and secretion of thyroid hormones. Propylthiouracil, 600 to 1000 mg, or methimazole, 60 to 100 mg, given orally or by nasogastric tube, will prevent organic binding of iodide in the thyroid gland within one hour. After this loading dose has been administered, 800 mg of propylthiouracil or 60 mg of methimazole should be given daily in 3 or 4 divided doses.

Although propylthiouracil and methimazole begin to act immediately to block thyroid hormone synthesis, they do not prevent secretion of hormone that already is stored in the thyroid gland. Therefore, it is necessary to administer iodide in conjunction with antithyroid drug therapy in order to block release of previously synthesized hormone. Iodide may be given in the form of Lugol's solution, 30 drops by mouth each day; SSKI, 5 drops orally every 8 hours; or sodium iodide, 1 gram intravenously every 8 hours. Therapy with iodide should be initiated 1 hour after propylthiouracil or methimazole is given.

Third, treatment must be directed at neutralization of the metabolic effects of excess thyroid hormone. A hypothermic blanket should be used to lower the hyperpyrexic patient's temperature; aspirin is contraindicated in this clinical setting since it may increase the metabolic rate even further. Diuretics, cardiac glycosides, and oxygen should be employed when the patient has evidence of congestive heart failure. Corticosteroids appear to improve survival in thyroid storm, although it is rare for an affected patient to have documented evidence of adrenal insufficiency.

Finally, propranolol should be administered to control the hemodynamic and psychomotor manifestations of thyroid storm. This drug should be given intravenously at a rate of 1 mg per minute for a total dose of 2 to 10 mg. Oral therapy then should be instituted in a dosage of 40 to 120 mg every 6 hours. Propranolol must be used with extreme caution in patients with diminished cardiac reserve, conduction blocks, atrial arrhythmias, and asthma. Moreover, in diabetic patients receiving insulin, propranolol may obscure the early manifestations of hypoglycemia.

Once the extreme derangements precipitated by thyroid storm have been corrected, ablative therapy with either surgery or radioactive iodine should be considered. In pregnant patients, surgical treatment is preferred to radioactive iodine therapy for the reasons outlined previously.

AMNIOTIC FLUID EMBOLISM

FREDERICK P. ZUSPAN, M.D.

Amniotic fluid embolism is fortunately a rare entity (1 in 8,000 to 20,000 deliveries) which is associated with a high maternal mortality (84 per cent). The diagnosis is made at the time of autopsy by the presence of fetal squames and mucin within pulmonary capillaries, as well as fetal hair within the pulmonary vasculature. These findings have become the hallmark of the diagnosis of amniotic fluid embolism.

PATHOGENESIS

The syndrome of amniotic fluid embolism was first described by Meyer in 1926, and further reported by Steiner and Lushbaugh in 1941. The English literature contains less than 400 reported cases of amniotic fluid embolism. There are probably many more cases than this, but they have not been reported. Cases in which the diagnosis is suspected but never proven are also never reported. Many misconceptions exist in relation to amniotic fluid embolism, but the one factor that is common in the disease is an open communication between the maternal blood stream and the contents of the amniotic sac, with the extrusion of amniotic fluid to the maternal circulation. The common misconception in the disease describes an elderly woman who is pregnant, with ruptured membranes, tetanic contractions, and tumultuous or rapid labor from the use of oxytocin stimulation, whose amniotic fluid is meconium stained. In actuality, tetanic contractions and tumultuous labor have been present in only 27 per cent of all documented cases, along with 24 per cent of patients who have been stimulated with oxytocin. (Nine patients with amniotic fluid embolism had no labor at all.) The mean age of the patients reported with amniotic fluid embolism is 32, in a multiparous patient. It is often said that infants born to women suffering from amniotic fluid embolism are unusually large, but in actuality only 19 per cent of patients had infants weighing above 3400 grams. Additionally, postmaturity has been suggested as a typical picture of amniotic fluid embolism, but in actuality only 10 per cent of the cases reported gestational ages of greater than 42 weeks. Meconium staining has been found in only 22 per cent of cases. Interestingly, there have been cases reported with the association of pregnancy and an intrauterine device. Abnormal implantations of the placenta, such as placental abruption and placenta accreta with the presence of polyhydramnios, are associated with amniotic fluid embolism.

In amniotic fluid embolism amniotic fluid and its contents are extruded into the maternal vasculature and cause an anaphylactoid reaction, most notably in the pulmonary cardiovascular system. Experimental studies have shown that injection of filtered amniotic fluid fails to produce a similar response. Weiner et al. have further noted that amniotic fluid has a hemostatic activity which results in maternal disseminated intravascular coagulation (DIC), with resulting hypofibrinogenemia. Furthermore, they found that the shock-like syndrome presented following the administration of heparin to the experimental animal. The most common cause of death is the anaphylactic shock–like reaction, which is due to the particulate matter found in amniotic fluid. Whether a woman can withstand the insult of the extrusion of amniotic fluid into her vascular circulation depends to a great degree upon the amount of particulate matter, and the volume of amniotic fluid infused. The immediate maternal death may be due to a mechanical blockage of the maternal pulmonary vasculature, pulmonary hypertension from the liberation of prostaglandin and resulting anaphylactoid shock. If the mother survives the initial insult, then profuse hemorrhage may develop owing to DIC and hypofibrinogenemia, with resultant thrombocytopenia and hypovolemia.

TREATMENT

The single most important event in therapy is the recognition that amniotic fluid embolism has occurred, with prompt and heroic methods of supporting the cardiovascular-pulmonary system. The following should be immediately instituted if this is suspected:

1. Open at least two vessels with large bore needles.
2. Infuse fluid support of Ringer's lactate or, more preferably, polyoxypropylene-polyoxyethylene glycol (PPG), or low molecular weight dextran if PPG is unavailable.
3. Place the patient in a semi-Fowler's position.
4. Institute positive pressure oxygen therapy. An endotracheal tube is usually necessary.
5. Use cardiopulmonary resuscitation as necessary.
6. Correct hypotension. Infuse fluids and vasopressors, of which dopamine is the treatment of choice.
7. Alter bronchospasm. Intravenous terbutaline sulfate is the appropriate drug.
8. Modify pulmonary edema. Restrict fluids except as necessary; use morphine (16 mg), digoxin if necessary, and tourniquets.
9. Control the hemostatic system. Correct DIC by use of cryoprecipitate, and consider the use of heparin for a bolus injection of 2000 units.
10. Correct fibrinolysis if present, using epsilon-aminocaproic acid.
11. Use intravenous steroids to counteract the stress reaction. Use hydrocortisone, 2 to 4 grams intravenously.

VENOUS THROMBOSIS

RUSSELL K. LAROS, JR., M.D.

Pulmonary embolism is the leading nonobstetric cause of postpartum death. Fortunately, it is also a disease in which early recognition and proper treatment can markedly improve the outcome. The incidence of pulmonary embolism depends on whether deep venous thrombosis is adequately treated. Untreated, as many as 24 per cent of patients with antenatal deep venous thrombosis will have pulmonary embolism, with a mortality of approximately 15 per cent. If treated with anticoagulants, embolization will occur in only 4.5 per cent of patients, with a mortality of less than 1 per cent. The importance of diagnosis and early proper treatment by anticoagulation is clear.

The association of pregnancy and thromboembolism is relatively common (0.2 per cent during pregnancy and 0.6 per cent postpartum). Puerperal patients outnumber antepartum patients by approximately three to one. Although thrombophlebitis can be seen at any stage of gestation, it appears to increase in frequency as pregnancy advances. After delivery, deep venous thrombosis is most frequently seen on the second postpartum day (deep venous thrombosis appears in 55 per cent of patients within the first 3 days) but may occur up to 4 weeks after delivery.

Proper diagnosis and careful anticoagulation are the cornerstones of management of thromboembolic disease. While the gravida is peculiarly susceptible to thromboembolism, her management differs little from that used for nonpregnant individuals. Coumarin agents (and other vitamin K antagonists) are contraindicated during pregnancy and lactation, and heparin is the preferred agent for both the acute and the long-term management of pregnant patients. While specific regimens for anticoagulation will be discussed in detail and guidelines for length of therapy will be given, each case must be individualized and a balance achieved between therapeutic efficacy and the risks of further treatment.

SYMPTOMATIC TREATMENT

Anticoagulation therapy is the mainstay of therapy for deep thrombophlebitis with or without pulmonary embolism. However, a number of additional modalities are useful in achieving symptomatic relief for both entities.

Deep Venous Thrombosis. Bed rest with elevation of the involved extremity is valuable initially, as it promotes venous return and decreases edema. The Trendelenburg position, obtained by elevating the foot of the bed approximately 8 inches, is preferable to using pillows, which, because they flex the hip, may impede femoral flow. The patient should be supplied with a foot board and instructed in the performance of hourly flexion and extension exercises of both lower extremities. However, as soon as symptoms permit, the patient should be encouraged to ambulate, since bed rest itself may enhance venous stasis. There is no evidence that bed rest prevents embolus detachment. Sitting with the legs dependent is contraindicated.

Application of moist heat to involved areas

can be beneficial. Although moist heat is more effective then dry heat, it is useless unless hot packs are replaced as soon as they cool.

Analgesic drugs may be required, but those which affect platelet function (such as aspirin) must be avoided while anticoagulants are being used. Anti-inflammatory drugs, although useful agents, are generally contraindicated during pregnancy. By decreasing prostaglandin levels, indomethacin can cause premature closure of the ductus arteriosus and pulmonary hypertension. In animal studies, phenylbutazone exhibits evidence of embryotoxicity and appears in breast milk. In addition, it potentiates the effects of the coumarin anticoagulants.

When correctly designed, elastic stockings increase the velocity of venous flow. The pressure gradient should decrease from ankle to thigh without a constricting garter at the top. Certain brands designed for ambulatory patients may be overly compressive in the recumbent position. Elastic bandages, once in vogue, are best avoided since they are easily wrapped incorrectly, with the greatest pressure ending up at the top and thus impeding venous return.

Pulmonary Embolism. If an embolic source can be traced to the lower extremities, the above measures can be employed. In addition, specific treatment of the embolus is required. Oxygen therapy is particularly important during pregnancy, because even if the mother survives, the fetus may die or be damaged secondary to maternal hypoxia. The maternal PaO_2 should be maintained above 70 mm Hg. Positive-pressure therapy may be required if pulmonary edema is present. Meperidine or morphine may be used for pain and apprehension. Bed rest is indicated for at least 5 to 7 days, allowing time for the initial organization of the clot. Straining at stool is best avoided, and stool softeners may prove helpful.

A vasoactive amine such as isoproterenol or dopamine is indicated for treatment of shock. The objective is to increase the mean arterial pressure and the flow through the pulmonary vasculature. Isoproterenol (mix 1 mg in 500 ml of normal saline; 2 μg per ml) is given in a dose of 2 to 8 μg per minute, and dopamine (200 mg in 500 ml of normal saline; 400 μg per ml) is started at 200 μg per minute and increased to a maximum dose of 2000 to 3000 μg per minute. Administration of both fluids and vasoactive amines should be monitored via a central line measuring either pulmonary artery and wedge pressures or central venous pressures.

Aminophylline and digoxin may also be useful. Aminophylline decreases reflex bronchospasm and has a diuretic action, which is particularly beneficial if pulmonary edema is present.

Digoxin is administered if cardiac failure appears, but it is rarely of benefit. The initial dose of aminophylline should be 4 to 5 mg per kg of body weight, infused over 20 minutes, followed by 12 to 15 μg per kg per minute (250 mg in 500 ml of normal saline; 500 μg per ml). The dosage should be adjusted to achieve a serum concentration of 10 to 20 μg per ml. Antibiotics are not indicated unless a septic embolus is suspected.

ANTICOAGULANT THERAPY

Three major types of therapeutic agents are available for treating thrombosis, and each is directed at a different portion of the coagulation process. They consist of (1) agents that interfere with platelet adhesion and aggregation, (2) agents that interfere with fibrin formation, and (3) agents that facilitate clot lysis.

Agents that interfere with fibrin formation are by far the most important in treating thromboembolism; in the United States these agents are heparin and the coumarin derivatives. Heparin is the preferred drug in the initial treatment of thromboembolism, while for long-term management in the nonpregnant state, conversion to a coumarin derivative is usually ideal. For reasons to be discussed later, we feel that heparin should be the preferred drug throughout pregnancy.

Heparin. Heparin is a naturally occurring mucopolysaccharide organic base found in the mast cells of most mammals. In plasma, it combines with an alpha-globulin known as antithrombin III to become a potent inhibitor of thrombin (hence preventing conversion of fibrinogen to fibrin) and to increase the circulating level of activated factor X (X_a) inhibitor. Heparin does not have a direct antiplatelet effect; nor will it stimulate fibrinolysis or directly lyse thrombi. Because of its large size and negative charge, it does not cross the placenta or appear in breast milk, both advantages for its use in pregnancy. If necessary, the effects of heparin can be reversed rapidly by administering protamine sulfate, 1 mg per 100 units of heparin administered. (When using constant-infusion methods, twice the amount necessary to neutralize the hourly dose should be sufficient. No more than 50 mg should be given over any 10-minute period, since protamine itself can cause bleeding.)

The major risk of heparin therapy is hemorrhage. In one review, hemorrhage was found to be a complication in 8 to 33 per cent of the patients. However, with careful monitoring and use of the intravenous-drip technique, this incidence can be reduced to 4 per cent. Heparin causes osteoporosis when administered in doses greater than 15,000 units per day for more than 6 months. This is not a problem during pregnancy, since patients rarely require antepartum therapy for periods this long and the effect can be prevented by administration of calcium gluconate (12 grams daily). Other rare effects of heparin include hypotension, alopecia, allergic reactions, pain at the injection site, and thrombocytopenia. The latter, apparently an immune phenomenon, is characterized by a decline in platelets between the third and eighth days following initiation of therapy, the platelet level reaching its nadir in 2 or 3 days, with recovery usually following within 5 days of discontinuing heparin. Heparin is contraindicated in threatened abortion or if suspicion of significant risk of intracranial hemorrhage exists (e.g., in the eclamptic patient or the patient with severe hypertension). Hemoptysis from pulmonary infarction is not a contraindication.

There is now clear evidence that monitoring the dosage of heparin affects the recurrence rate of thrombotic events. It is less clear that monitoring affects hemorrhagic complications, though it is presumed to do so. A variety of techniques for monitoring circulating heparin levels have been studied. After reviewing the literature on control of heparin therapy, we prefer either partial thromboplastin times (PTT, aPTT, WBPTT) or the thrombin clotting time (TCT).

Optimal anticoagulation is usually obtained with a circulating heparin level of 0.3 units per ml (TCT, 2.5 × control; aPTT, 2 to 3 × control). Spontaneous hemorrhage frequently occurs if the concentration exceeds 0.6 units per ml for periods of time greater than 12 hours. The circulating level is a balance between input of new drug, rapid metabolism, and excretion either directly by the kidneys or indirectly by diffusion into extravascular spaces to be metabolized slowly. The half-life of heparin is 1.5 hours, and a stable circulating level is most easily achieved by giving a loading dose followed by a continuous intravenous infusion. Because normal individuals vary widely in their responses to a given dose, the rate of infusion should be varied to achieve a TCT or a PTT within the therapeutic range regardless of the amount of heparin this requires. Our schemes for continuous intravenous infusion for deep venous thrombosis are as follows:

Loading dose—5,000 units IV push.

Continuous infusion—hourly rate of 15 to 20 units per kg per hr.

Adjust infusion rate to achieve TCT of 2 to 3 × control (aPTT, 1.5 to 2.5 × control).

For pulmonary emboli, a higher loading dose should be used (10,000 to 15,000 units intravenously) since high doses of heparin may have the benefit of relieving vasospasm as well as inhibiting the larger amounts of protease clotting factors involved. In patients with renal disease, heparin clearance is reduced and lower doses are used.

The maintenance dose is best delivered by an infusion pump or electronic drop counter attached to a 250 ml infusion bag. No more than a 6-hour dose should be utilized at any one time to protect against accidental overdosage.

Although ineffective orally, heparin is well absorbed after subcutaneous administration. The intramuscular route should not be used because of the high incidence of hematoma formation at the injection site. While a steady circulating level can most easily be obtained by continuous intravenous administration, either the intermittent intravenous or the subcutaneous route can be used. However, intermittent administration produces peaks and valleys in the circulating heparin activity and this can lead to seven times as many major bleeding complications as does continuous infusion. When an intermittent regimen is chosen, the total daily dose is 400 to 500 units per kg per day in divided doses. The intravenous dose should be given every 6 hours and the subcutaneous dose every 8 or 12 hours. In most cases, this will provide an average anticoagulant activity of 0.3 units per ml. Initially, monitoring should be performed frequently (three or four times daily). Blood samples should be obtained just prior to the next dose and should be at the low end of the therapeutic range (0.2 units per ml; TCT, 2 × control, aPTT, 1.5 × control). Once a stable dosage is obtained, monitoring can be decreased to daily or every other day.

Before initiating heparin therapy, a baseline hematocrit, platelet count, PT, and TCT or aPTT should be obtained. Heparin should be avoided if the platelet count is less than 50,000 or if platelet function is inadequate.

Continuous intravenous heparin should be maintained for 7 to 14 days for active thromboembolic disease or until symptoms have resolved and there is no evidence of recurrence. At this point the patient may be switched to subcutaneous heparin or oral coumarin if long-term management is indicated.

Long-term heparinization is accomplished using a schedule of 120 to 170 units per kg every 8 hours for pulmonary embolism and deep venous thrombosis. The patient is instructed in self-administration using the 40,000 units per ml preparation of heparin, a tuberculin syringe, and a 25-gauge 5/8-inch needle to inject deep into the subcutaneous fat of the anterior abdominal wall. Local hematoma formation can be reduced by applying ice to the site for several minutes prior to injection, and the injection site should be changed daily. Intramuscular injections are forbidden, and the patient must be cautioned against the use of aspirin. While some have advocated an intermittent intravenous dose schedule for long-term maintenance, we see no advantage, and several disadvantages, to this technique as compared with a subcutaneous regimen.

Indications for anticoagulant therapy beyond the acute episode include recurrence and pulmonary embolization. We would usually treat an acute first episode of thrombophlebitis during pregnancy for 3 to 6 weeks and institute prophylaxis during labor, delivery, and the immediate postpartum period. If pulmonary embolization had occurred, therapy would be extended to 6 months. Similarly, therapy should be extended for patients with iliofemoral venous thrombosis and recurrent venous thrombosis, and should include either therapeutic or prophylactic doses during labor, delivery, and the early puerperium.

Coumarin. Sodium warfarin is the coumarin derivative most widely used in managing thromboembolic disease. Its therapeutic efficacy lies in its inhibition of vitamin K activity. It is a small molecule loosely bound to albumin. It easily crosses the placenta; therefore, its use during pregnancy can be extremely hazardous. If administered during the first trimester (especially the fourth through eighth weeks), a syndrome which phenotypically resembles the Conradi-Hunermann type of chondrodysplasia punctata may result. These children are born with multiple congenital anomalies, including nasal cartilage hypoplasia, stippling of bones, slight intrauterine growth retardation, and brachydactyly.

Reports indicate that warfarin may cause birth defects, even if first administered in the second and third trimesters. It is postulated that the first trimester anomalies may be secondary either to a direct teratogenic effect of warfarin or to a vitamin K–deficiency effect, whereas the second and third trimester defects could result from fetal hemorrhage.

The primary problem of warfarin administration during the last two trimesters has been fetal and placental hemorrhage resulting in fetal death. In a collected series of 214 patients, there were 25 fetal deaths, a mortality of 11.7 per cent. The great majority of such events, however, appear to be secondary to the trauma of delivery itself. In a prospective study of 23 women with heart valve prostheses who conceived 40 times, fetal wastage exceeded 80 per cent.

Although we believe that coumarin therapy is contraindicated during pregnancy, on rare occasions this may be the only means of maintaining long-term anticoagulation in patients who either are unable to master self-administration or exhibit allergic reactions. In such cases, the patient should be fully informed of the potential risks of using coumarin (and all other vitamin K antagonists) during pregnancy. In these situations, heparin should be used for the acute episode and until 14 weeks' gestation, at which time warfarin is substituted. Warfarin should be discontinued and heparin substituted well in advance of labor. The average half-life of warfarin is 44 hours. It is not known exactly how long it takes for the effects of oral anticoagulation on the fetus to wear off, but it is thought to be somewhere between 3 and 14 days. If spontaneous labor should occur while the patient is still taking warfarin, the effects of warfarin can be reversed by administering vitamin K and fresh frozen plasma. A single dose of 5 mg of vitamin K given intravenously begins to normalize the prothrombin time within 6 hours. Higher doses (e.g., 25 to 50 mg) normalize the prothrombin time a little more rapidly but also render the patient refractory to reanticoagulation for a period of 10 days to two weeks.

Because there is experimental and clinical evidence that vitamin K crosses the placenta, its administration may enhance the rate of return of fetal clotting factors as well. Immediately after delivery, the infant is given 1 mg of vitamin K intramuscularly. If the newborn shows signs of bleeding or is less than 35 weeks' gestational age, or if it was a difficult operative delivery, fresh frozen plasma, 5 mg per kg, may be required as well.

The usual anticoagulating dose of warfarin is 10 to 15 mg daily until therapeutic prolongation of the prothrombin time is achieved (1.5 to $2.5 \times$ control). Thereafter, a maintenance dose of 3 to 20 mg daily is utilized and the prothrombin time is reevaluated once or twice weekly. Heparin is continued during the first 5 to 7 days of warfarin therapy. Since heparin can prolong the prothrombin time by 2 to 4 seconds, the prothrombin time should be at least 2.5 times the control value by the time heparin is discontinued. Alternatively, heparin can be withdrawn by gradually decreasing the dosage.

A number of drugs affect the activity of the coumarin derivatives. Agents that increase the activity of warfarin include salicylates, phenothiazines, phenylbutazone, and antibiotics; ethyl alcohol and barbiturates decrease its activity. Fever, diarrhea, and change in intake of leafy green vegetables also have an effect.

Patients already taking coumarin agents and desiring to conceive (e.g., patients with prosthetic heart valves) should be switched to heparin prior to conceiving. Patients who inadvertently receive oral agents during the first trimester must be advised of the risks involved and given the option of terminating the pregnancy.

There is controversy as to the safety of allowing women taking warfarin to nurse. While some authors state that warfarin crosses into breast milk, a study by Orme and associates disputes this finding (Br. Med. J., *1*:1564, 1977). Their study of 13 mothers showed only minute levels of warfarin in breast milk (0.08 μmol per liter) and none in the plasma of the 7 infants who were breast feeding. Despite these findings, we discourage breast feeding in women taking warfarin. As more data become available, this recommendation may change.

Estrogen suppression of lactation is contraindicated because of a tenfold increase in venous thrombosis in mothers over the age of 25. Although the issue of whether or not oral contraceptives predispose to thromboembolism is still debated, we recommend that patients use an alternative method of birth control. Patients who smoke are encouraged to stop. Elastic stockings and elevation of the foot of the bed are continued at home as long as any edema of the lower extremities persists.

Intrapartum, Intraoperative, and Postpartum Therapy

Selected patients—those with recent pulmonary embolization, recent iliofemoral thrombosis, and those with heart valve prostheses—should be continued on high-dose heparin during delivery or surgery. These patients should be hospitalized in anticipation of delivery and converted to a regimen of continuous intravenous heparin. The dose should be adjusted to achieve a circulating heparin level of 0.1 to 0.2 units per ml (TCT, 1.5 to 2×control; aPTT, 1.25 to 1.5× control) during labor and delivery. Continuing this regimen does not increase the incidence of postpartum hemorrhage in a normal delivery. However, there is a slight increase in the incidence of episiotomy hematoma, and it may contribute to blood loss in patients with uterine atonia or retained placenta. Conduction anesthesia is contraindicated in these patients.

Full doses of heparin should be reinstituted 6 hours postpartum to reattain a circulating level of 0.2 to 0.4 units per ml. Warfarin may be started (if the patient is not nursing) as soon as the patient resumes oral intake. Heparin is then discontinued 5 to 7 days later as described above. Oral agents should be continued for 3 to 6 months post partum, depending on the seriousness of the condition. Clotting factors tend to return to normal approximately 8 weeks after delivery.

ALTERNATIVE THERAPIES

Fibrinolytic Agents. Two fibrinolytic agents, streptokinase and urokinase, have undergone extensive clinical trials and are now available for clinical use. Both agents act to increase plasmin formation and thus the rate of clot lysis. In acute deep venous thrombosis, streptokinase produces total clot lysis in 30 to 50 per cent of patients. Both streptokinase and urokinase produce rapid resolution of pulmonary emboli, evident on angiography, as noted by improvement in pulmonary hemodynamics. Both agents are contraindicated during pregnancy and for the first 10 days postpartum. Urokinase should not be used in patients who are anticoagulated, and streptokinase must be used with great caution, as the combination greatly enhances the risk of overanticoagulation and bleeding.

Antiplatelet Agents. These drugs may play a role in arterial thromboembolism, but there is as yet no definitive evidence that they are effective in the treatment or prophylaxis of venous thromboembolism. Dextran, the most widely used of these agents, must be administered intravenously; yet it is less effective than low-dose subcutaneous heparin for prophylaxis.

Surgical Intervention. Surgery is reserved for those patients for whom anticoagulants are contraindicated or have failed after an adequate course. Lower extremity thrombectomy is justified only if the patient is threatened by impending gangrene due to phlegmasia cerulea dolens. It does not reduce subsequent chronic venous insufficiency since the majority of vessels so treated do not remain patent on long-term follow-up. Inferior vena caval ligation, plication, clipping, or insertion of an umbrella is not indicated unless recurrent, life-threatening embolization persists despite adequate anticoagulation. A minor recurrence is observed in approximately 10 per cent of patients during the first few days of heparin therapy and should not be considered a failure of therapy. Bilateral ligation of the femoral veins is not fully protective because of the frequent involvement during pregnancy of the pelvic and gluteal veins that drain into the iliac vessels above the inguinal ligament. If a pelvic source of embolism is suspected, the left ovarian vein may also require ligation.

Pulmonary embolectomy may be life-saving but should be considered only in those patients with angiographically demonstrated massive embolization to the main pulmonary artery with persistent inadequate cardiac output refractory to appropriate measures. In such situations the maternal outcome is of primary concern.

PROPHYLACTIC THERAPY

The prophylactic use of "minidose" heparin to prevent thromboembolism has received considerable attention. The rationale for using small doses centers on the concept that a critical concentration of factor X_a (activated factor X) is required for thrombus formation. Factor X_a is the major component of the complex that activates prothrombin and lies at the point at which both intrinsic and extrinsic pathways converge to form the final common pathway of the clotting cascade. Heparin markedly enhances the action of antithrombin III, the major plasma inhibitor of factor X_a. It takes much less heparin to inhibit factor X_a than to prevent clotting once thrombin has been formed.

Standard regimens employ only 5000 units subcutaneously every 8 to 12 hours. This dose is insufficient to do more than minimally prolong the aPTT or TCT; consequently, there is no need to monitor dosage and there is no increase in hemorrhagic complications or intraoperative transfusion requirements. The only adverse effect reported is a slight increase in the number of wound hematomas. Multiple studies confirm that low-dose heparin prophylaxis in patients undergoing abdominothoracic surgery markedly decreases the incidence of deep venous thrombosis. More important, a multicenter trial has demonstrated that the incidence of fatal pulmonary emboli is reduced as well.

Following baseline hematologic studies, the prophylactic regimen we prefer is 5000 units subcutaneously 2 hours prior to surgery and then repeated every 12 hours until the patient is fully ambulatory. Available evidence in general abdominal surgery shows no greater efficacy using an every-8-hour regimen and a higher incidence of bleeding complications. If possible, the patient should not receive antiplatelet-aggregating agents (dipyridamole, clofibrate, acetylsalicylic acid) for 5 days prior to surgery.

If a woman has had one pregnancy complicated by a pulmonary embolus, a strong argument can be made for the necessity of prophylaxis during subsequent pregnancies. In one study, 2 of every 20 patients with pregnancy-related pulmonary emboli had a history of this complication.

We believe that prophylactic doses of heparin should be used at the time of labor and delivery under the following circumstances: in patients who have had (1) previous pulmonary emboli or (2) previous thrombophlebitis; and (3) in patients at high risk for phlebitis, i.e., individuals with severe varicosities undergoing cesarean section.

When conduction anesthesia is anticipated for delivery, the regimen is changed so that the first dose is given in early labor. The epidural catheter is placed when appropriate, after obtaining a TCT in the normal range. The second dose of heparin is not given until after the catheter is removed.

INTRAUTERINE GROWTH RETARDATION

PATRICIA L. SCHMIDT, M.D.

Intrauterine growth retardation (IUGR) refers to the process which produces a baby who is small for gestational age. Such a child weighs less than two standard deviations from the mean weight for its gestational age, or less than the 10th percentile.

The growth-retarded or small-for-gestational-age fetus or newborn has a perinatal mortality five to eight times that seen in normally grown babies. There is an increased incidence of antepartum, intrapartum, and neonatal deaths in these pregnancies. Up to 48 per cent of these babies will have some degree of demonstrable intrapartum asphyxia. Neonatal problems include meconium aspiration, hypoglycemia, hypocalcemia, polycythemia, and temperature instability.

The long-term prognosis for small-for-gestational-age babies depends upon (1) the extent of the intrauterine growth retardation; (2) the presence and extent of antepartum and/or intrapartum asphyxia; (3) the presence or absence of prompt and appropriate neonatal care; (4) the presence or absence of fetal anomalies, chromosomal abnormalities, or congenital infection.

In the absence of fetal anomalies, known chromosomal abnormalities, or congenital infections, the prognosis for the small-for-gestational-age infant is most significantly correlated with the extent of intrapartum asphyxia. Approximately 35 to 38 per cent of IUGR pregnancies will be delivered by cesarean section, primarily because of demonstrable fetal distress by fetal heart rate determination and/or fetal acidosis.

CLASSIFICATION

Although intrauterine growth retardation is a heterogeneous process, two major classifications are used. The symmetrically growth-retarded fetus is uniformly small and may not appear wasted. This type is frequently associated with chromosomal defects and congenital anomalies in up to 33 per cent of cases. In the asymmetrically growth-retarded fetus, the placenta is usually able to supply fetal needs and thus allow normal growth until about the 25th week of gestation. Thereafter there is a slowing of the fetal body growth compared with the fetal head growth. Fetal anomalies occur in this latter group but are one tenth as frequent as in the symmetrically growth retarded group.

DIAGNOSIS AND MANAGEMENT

The clinical diagnosis of IUGR has been notoriously inaccurate. The physician must be cognizant of some fundamental parameters in order to suspect the presence of IUGR in otherwise "normal pregnancies" and also in those pregnancies at risk for this problem.

Pregnancy Dating. Clinical information on gestational age is important for all patients, but it is imperative in patients at risk for or suspected of having intrauterine growth retardation. For example, one of the most helpful parameters in evaluating a patient at 36 weeks' gestation for IUGR, when fetal biparietal diameter (BPD) is consistent with 32 weeks, is a record of a first trimester pelvic examination with an estimate of uterine size and notation of consistency with menstrual dating. Certainly any gestational age inconsistency in the first or second trimesters can be resolved by an ultrasound evaluation at that time.

An ultrasound examination for dating of the pregnancy early in pregnancy is extremely helpful in the management of complications which present in the mid to late third trimester, when ultrasound dating is much less accurate.

Risk Factors for IUGR. Certain risk factors for IUGR can be identified on the first prenatal visit. They include:
1. History of previous small-for-gestational-age infant;
2. Maternal illnesses, such as hypertension, diabetes mellitus with vascular involvement, cyanotic heart disease, or sickle cell disease;
3. Substance abuse: drugs, tobacco, alcohol;
4. Poor maternal nutrition;
5. High altitude;
6. Teenaged mother.

Other clinical factors may be identified as the pregnancy progresses to alert the clinician to the possibility of IUGR. These factors include:
1. Multiple gestation;
2. Suspected congenital infection;
3. Weight gain less than 10 lbs at the onset of the third trimester or less than 2 lbs in four weeks after 30 weeks gestation;
4. Poor fundal growth: less than 2 cm per 4 weeks after 30 weeks.

Surveillance of Pregnancies with Suspected IUGR. Surveillance for suspected IUGR includes:
1. Fetal heart rate (FHR) evaluation;
2. Twice weekly plasma unconjugated estriol (E_3) determinations; and
3. Ultrasound evaluations at 2 to 3 week intervals to evaluate for fetal growth and anomalies.

Controversy surrounds which type of FHR test is superior. The oxytocin challenge test (OCT) is performed weekly, whereas the nonstress test (NST) is performed twice weekly if this latter test is preferred. Recently the breast stimulation test (BST) has replaced to a great extent the need for exogenous oxytocin. This test is performed weekly in patients with suspected IUGR. Concurrent use of estriols (E_3) merely provides additional information. Here again, gestational age is important to evaluate the E_3 results completely. However, if the values are rising, this is a good sign. Conversely, if the estriol values fail to rise or decrease slowly, this suggests poor fetoplacental growth. Serial ultrasound determinations have been very helpful when performed at 2 to 3 week intervals. More frequent examinations are not helpful since the error of the procedure may skew the results.

TREATMENT OF INTRAUTERINE GROWTH RETARDATION

Treatment includes:
1. Elimination of abused substance(s);
2. Bed rest to improve placental flow;
3. Adequate diet to promote 1 lb per week weight gain;
4. Stabilization of maternal illness if possible;
5. Hospitalized supervision of the above if outpatient management is unsuccessful.

DELIVERY

Timing. Once IUGR has been diagnosed, the fetus should be delivered when the L:S ratio indicates lung maturity. There is some controversy regarding the delivery of the growth-retarded fetus who has a mature L:S but is preterm (less than 37 weeks' gestational age). Some clinicians would advise continued fetal surveillance until the fetal heart rate test became abnormal. However, when lack of fetal growth has been unequivocally demonstrated on serial ultrasound examinations, fetal nutrition must be presumed to be inadequate. Under these circumstances and with a mature L:S ratio, such babies can be better nourished in the nursery. Timing of delivery for such babies must take into consideration the extent of growth retardation and the degree of immaturity of the fetus even with a mature fetal lung profile.

In the presence of an immature L:S ratio, FHR surveillance continues, with the patient following the treatment guidelines until either the L:S becomes mature or the OCT becomes positive.

Each patient's care must be individualized, but in the patient with a positive OCT (especially if nonreactive) delivery should be the first consideration regardless of the L:S value.

Route. Since IUGR infants have an increased incidence of intrapartum asphyxia, careful intrapartum surveillance by persons experienced in fetal monitoring is indicated.

With a favorable cervix and vertex presentation, vaginal delivery with direct fetal and uterine activity monitoring should be attempted. At the first sign of fetal distress, delivery should be expedited, usually by cesarean section.

In the patient with an unfavorable cervix and a normal FHR evaluation, induction may be attempted provided the patient surveillance and monitoring of the fetus is scrupulous! The technique of external monitoring must be continuously good in order to proceed with the induction.

When the patient has a positive OCT and an unfavorable cervix, cesarean section is the delivery route of choice in most cases.

PRECAUTIONS

1. The patient's pediatrician or neonatologist must be alerted so that initial resuscitation and care of the newborn in the delivery room can be expedited.
2. Meconium should be expected and, if present, the oropharynx aspirated prior to delivery of the shoulders, whether a vaginal or cesarean section delivery is performed.
3. Remember that long-term outcome relates to a greater extent to the degree of intrapartum fetal asphyxia than to the degree of fetal growth retardation.

THE SAFE CONDUCT OF PREGNANCY IN PATIENTS WITH RHEUMATIC HEART DISEASE

THOMAS J. BENEDETTI, M.D.

In order to provide optimal care for patients with rheumatic heart disease, the obstetrician must be aware of (1) the physiologic adaptations of the maternal cardiovascular system to pregnancy, (2) the influence of the labor process on maternal cardiovascular parameters, (3) the effect of cardioactive medications and anesthetics on the mother and the fetus, and (4) the methods and indications for assessing cardiovascular performance during labor and delivery. It is the purpose of this article to review the care of the pregnant patient with reference to these four subjects.

PHYSIOLOGIC ADAPTATIONS TO PREGNANCY

Cardiac output is significantly elevated as early as 12 weeks' gestation and reaches a 50 per cent increase by 24 weeks. If measured in the lateral recumbent position, this elevation is maintained until term. The resting heart rate shows a progressive rise from early gestation until term. The heart rate at term is usually 15 beats per minute greater than in the nonpregnant state. Stroke volume also increases in early gestation but may decline somewhat near term. Blood volume increases rapidly during the first 20 to 30 weeks and then slower expansion continues until term. The total blood volume expansion can range from 20 to 100 per cent with a mean of 40 to 50 per cent in normal pregnancies. Multiple gestations tend to have a larger increase in blood volume. Pregnancy complicated by preeclampsia and chronic hypertension is associated with a lesser expansion in blood volume than pregnancy in normotensive patients.

With this basic information in mind, one can begin to formulate an approach to the management of patients with cardiovascular alterations. The skillful management of a patient during her prenatal visits will often make the process of labor and delivery less complicated for the patient and the physician. The principles of antepartum care include: (1) limitation of physical activity, (2) supplemental oral iron and folate, and (3) minimal to moderate sodium restriction (4 grams per day). During prenatal visits, three parameters are especially helpful in monitoring cardiovascular status: heart rate, weight, and vital capacity. Heart rates of greater than 100 beats per minute, rapid weight gain, or decreasing vital capacity should alert the obstetrician to the possibility of early cardiac decompensation. Patients with New York Hospital Association Class 2 or 3 cardiovascular disease should be considered candidates for admission to the hospital prior to the onset of labor. A few days at bed rest in the hospital setting are often accompanied by the spontaneous diuresis of 1 to 3 kilograms. In general, if the mother is stable, one should await the spontaneous onset of labor unless fetal indications for earlier delivery arise.

CARDIOVASCULAR ALTERATIONS DURING LABOR AND DELIVERY

From the viewpoint of the cardiovascular system, labor and delivery is a type of involuntary exercise. Even in patients with cardiac disease, this is usually well tolerated if the patient has been ambulatory prior to the onset of labor. During labor and delivery, maternal position is of vital importance to the maternal cardiovascular system. During the first stage of labor in the supine position, uterine contractions have the following cardiovascular effects: (1) increased right atrial pressure, (2) increased pulmonary artery pressure, (3) increased cardiac output, (4) increased arterial pressure, and (5) slightly decreased pulse rate. This combination of factors results in a 54 per cent increase in the left ventricular stroke work. (Left ventricular stroke work equals the mean systemic pressure times the stroke volume.) However, when the patient is on her side, there is a smaller change in each of these factors. As a result, there is only a 24 per cent increase in the left ventricular stroke work with each contraction. Thus, over 50 per cent less cardiac work is expanded during each contraction in the lateral recumbent position than is expended in the supine position.

When the patient enters the second stage of labor, even greater fluctuations in maternal hemodynamics occur. The Valsalva maneuver is accompanied by a large increase in central venous pressure and pulmonary artery pressure and large increases in the mean arterial pressure. The second stage of labor, then, imposes an even greater increase in left ventricular work than uterine contractions did during the first stage of labor. In the patient with cardiovascular disease, it would appear advantageous for the mother to shorten the second stage of labor. However, midforceps procedures impose some risk to both mother and fetus. Laceration of maternal soft tissue and subsequent hemorrhage must be avoided. The second stage of labor is probably best managed in this circumstance by awaiting the descent of the head on or near the perineal floor without voluntary Valsalva maneuvers. Using this strategy, one is often able to avoid potentially traumatic midforceps procedures in favor of the low forceps delivery.

Although its use in this situation is unfamiliar to most obstetricians, the Sims' position would seem to offer some advantages for delivery of the cardiac patient. While cardiac output is decreased in the supine position, it is even further reduced by the lithotomy position. The Sims' position should reduce the incidence of aortic and vena caval compression which occurs with uterine contractions in the supine and presumably dorsal lithotomy positions. Continuous monitoring of patients with valvular heart disease during a low forceps delivery in the Sims' position has shown only a small rise in pulmonary artery pressure and cardiac output with delivery.

CARDIOVASCULAR MEDICATIONS

Many patients with valvular cardiovascular disease will require either therapeutic or prophylactic administration of various medications during the course of pregnancy, during labor, and in the puerperium. An understanding of the indications, contraindications, and maternal and fetal effects should facilitate the safe use of these compounds.

Uterine Stimulants. The use of oxytocin in patients with significant cardiac disease can require some finesse not usually required in the normal pregnant patient. In patients at risk for congestive heart failure, one would like to limit the use of intravenous fluids containing sodium. One liter of normal saline contains 150 mEq of sodium. This amount is equivalent to a 4 gram sodium or a 9 gram table salt diet. The use of oxytocin, however, at infusion rates of greater than 15 mU per minute is associated with a significant antidiuretic effect. Prolonged use of oxytocin without electrolyte-containing fluids has resulted in water intoxication. Other factors which may contribute to the development of hyponatremia in the cardiac patient are (1) diuretic therapy which decreases the urinary diluting ability and (2) decreased renal perfusion in patients with clinical or subclinical congestive heart failure. The optimum use of oxytocin in this instance involves the frequent monitoring of serum sodium levels and appropriate intravenous fluids. Intravenous fluids in these patients would include 50 cc per hour of a solution of 5 per cent dextrose in quarter normal or half normal saline. If the serum sodium shows a serial decline to levels less than 130 mEq per liter, oxytocin should be discontinued and free water intake restricted.

The effect of oxytocin on cardiovascular dynamics is potentially hazardous if not well understood. The use of bolus oxytocin administration should be avoided. A direct infusion of 5 to 10 IU of oxytocin as a bolus results in (1) a 40 per cent decrease in mean arterial pressure, (2) a 60 per cent fall in systemic resistance, (3) a 44 per cent fall in pulmonary resistance, (4) heart rate increase of 30 per cent, and (5) increase in mean pulmonary artery and pulmonary artery wedge pressure of 35 per cent. These large fluctuations in cardiac parameters could prove disastrous for the patient with impaired cardiac reserves. The use of rapid infusions of dilute oxytocin solution at the rate of 80 mU per minute is not associated with significant systemic or pulmonary changes. An 80 mU per minute infusion is equivalent to 150 cc per hour of a solution of 1000 cc of dextrose in water containing 30 IU of oxytocin.

The use of intravenous ergot compounds is also associated with significant cardiac alterations. Femoral arterial pressure increased 11 per cent, pulmonary artery pressure increased 27 per cent, and pulmonary artery wedge pressure increased 30 per cent after the intravenous administration of 0.2 mg of methergine.

From the foregoing data, it would appear prudent to use only dilute solutions of oxytocin in the postpartum period to limit blood loss in the third stage of labor.

Digoxin. Many patients with cardiac disease will be receiving oral digoxin when they present in labor. Digoxin is used mainly in patients with rheumatic heart disease when the negative chronotropic effect is desired. This will help prevent rapid ventricular response to atrial tachyarrhythmia. It is important to prevent these patients from becoming hypokalemic during labor and in the puerperium. Digoxin intoxication can occur in the face of appropriate serum digoxin levels if the serum potassium concentration is lowered by diuretic therapy. It is also important to be aware of the effect of pregnancy and delivery on the serum digoxin level. The serum digoxin level at term using a standard dose of 0.25 mg per day is approximately 50 per cent that of the level in the nonpregnant patient. This is probably secondary to increased glomerular filtration rate and to the expanded intravascular volume present during pregnancy. If the digoxin level during pregnancy is maintained in the upper part of the optimal range (0.5 to 2.5 nanograms per ml), serious digoxin intoxication could result in the first weeks in the puerperium as the result of the decreasing glomerular filtration rate and contracting blood volume. In the puerperium, digoxin levels should be monitored or the doses reduced to levels appropriate for the nonpregnant patient.

Antibiotics. Labor and delivery, especially delivery by cesarean section, can be associated with a significant incidence of bacteremia. Patients with valvular pathology should receive prophylactic antibiotic coverage prior to delivery and for 24 to 48 hours postpartum. Ideal antibiotic coverage would include prophylaxis against Gram-positive organisms with penicillin (1.2 million units of procaine penicillin every 12 hours) and against Gram-negative organisms with an aminoglycoside (gentamicin, 80 mg every 8 hours). Despite recent recommendations to the contrary, it would appear unwise to withhold antibiotic prophylaxis in patients with valvular cardiac pathology during labor and delivery.

Anticoagulation. Patients with rheumatic heart disease are at an increased risk for thromboembolism during pregnancy. While the risk of thromboembolism in a normal pregnant patient is approximately 2 to 3 per 1000, the risk of thromboembolism in pregnant patients with rheumatic heart disease is 20 per 1000 for venous thromboembolism and 15 per 1000 for arterial embolism. Patients at highest risk for venous and arterial thromboembolism are those with cardiac chamber enlargement and atrial fibrillation. In light of the increased risk for thromboembolism in patients with rheumatic heart disease, the following seem to be appropriate indications for full-dose anticoagulation during pregnancy: (1) non-porcine prosthetic cardiac valves, (2) mitral stenosis and atrial fibrillation, (3) previous history of pulmonary embolism, deep venous thrombosis, or systemic embolization. Patients with normal sinus rhythm but cardiac chamber enlargement undergoing cesarean section are candidates to receive prophylactic low-dose heparinization preoperatively and therapeutic anticoagulation for 6 weeks postoperatively. Full anticoagulation is usually best begun after 24 to 48 hours postoperatively.

The other dilemma in pregnancy is the choice of an anticoagulant drug and management of anticoagulation at the time of labor and delivery. Oral anticoagulants, because of their low molecular weight, cross the placenta to the fetal circulation. The fetus has an immature liver enzyme system and low levels of factors II, VII, IX, and X. Appropriate anticoagulation in the mother can result in an overdose to the fetus. Thus oral anticoagulation therapy in pregnancy can result in teratogenesis in the first trimester and fetal death from hemorrhage in the second and third trimesters.

Heparin does not cross the placenta and would seem the ideal anticoagulant for pregnancy and delivery. Two factors have limited its applicability to obstetrics: (1) the lack of a good method for monitoring therapy, and (2) the necessity for self-administration by subcutaneous injections. An activated partial thromboplastin time can be measured two hours before the next dosage. Levels at this time should show a prolongation in the partial thromboplastin time 1.5 to 2 times the control value.

Anesthesia. Carefully administered anesthesia is essential to the safe conduct of labor and delivery in the cardiac patient. A combined low thoracic–low caudal block by the double catheter technique is the optimal anesthetic for these patients. This will limit the progressive rise in cardiac output as labor advances. Adequate pain relief will also eliminate the maternal tachycardiac response often seen with uterine contractions in the unmedicated patient. The lowest effective dose of local anesthesia should be used, as the amount of pre-anesthetic volume infusion in cardiac patients is usually limited.

Two groups of patients provide special problems for this general approach: (1) anticoagulated patients and (2) patients with an intracardiac shunt. Patients on full-dose anticoagulation are not candidates for regional or spinal anesthesia. If regional anesthesia is essential, the anticoagulation should be discontinued a few days before anesthesia is to be given.

There are few data available on the use of regional anesthetics and minidose heparin. Until more substantial data are available, the individual anesthesiologist and obstetrician must decide whether the risks are outweighed by the potential benefits. Patients with congenital heart disease resulting in intracardiac shunts also provide a problem for the anesthesiologist. Care must be taken to avoid systemic hypotension and reversal of a left to right shunt. These patients are candidates for regional anesthesia only with appropriate hemodynamic monitoring techniques.

Cardiovascular Monitoring. Improved cardiovascular monitoring techniques can now provide one with a dynamic description of myocardial performance and can enable one to precisely judge therapeutic interventions. The use of a flow-directed pulmonary artery catheter (Swan-Ganz) in laboring patients with cardiac disease allows one to judge the myocardial effects of labor, regional anesthesia, fluid therapy, and cardioactive medications. Indications for the use of invasive cardiac monitoring (pulmonary artery catheter and intraarterial catheter) in the pregnant patient include (1) New York Heart Association Class 3 or 4 cardiac disease, (2) significant left ventricular outflow tract obstruction, and (3) significant pulmonary hypertension.

With a triple-lumen catheter, one can measure central venous pressure (CVP), pulmonary artery pressure (PAP), pulmonary artery wedge pressure (PAWP), and cardiac output (CO). A ventricular function curve may be constructed using the cardiac output and the pulmonary artery wedge pressure. Following the dynamic changes in myocardial performance with this curve allows recognition of a worsening of myocardial performance (right and downward) or improving performance (left and upward). Often these changes may be seen graphically before clinical signs and symptoms of cardiovascular decompensation are present. Catheter-related complications can be held to a minimum by meticulous sterile technique, the use of a continuous pressure flush system, early recognition of persistent wedging, and limited number of balloon inflations.

The use of an arterial pressure catheter can provide one with continuous arterial pressure rather than the intermittent information available from a sphygmomanometer, as well as ready access to blood gas sampling without repeated arterial puncture. The arterial line is best placed in the radial artery after appropriate testing is performed to insure adequate collateral circulation from the ulnar artery. As with the Swan-Ganz catheter, a continuous pressure flush system will insure continued catheter patency while limiting the amount of fluid administered.

SEIZURE DISORDERS
YORAM SOROKIN, M.D.,
and MORTIMER G. ROSEN, M.D.

Seizure disorders affect approximately 1.5 million Americans and are serious neurological disorders which involve 0.3 per cent of pregnant women. In the majority of seizures (75 per cent) diagnostic techniques do not document structural or biochemical abnormalities. In these patients the diagnosis made is idiopathic seizure disorder. In patients with acquired seizure disorders, pathogenesis includes toxic or metabolic disorders, cerebral vascular accidents, cerebral degenerative diseases, brain tumors, congenital malformations, birth trauma, and infections. As noted, in many patients with acquired seizure disorders, the basic cause of the seizure cannot be treated directly; however, administration of anticonvulsant drugs is usually necessary.

Effect of Pregnancy on Seizure Disorders. The effect of pregnancy on the seizure disorder is unpredictable. In one large study the frequency of seizures became worse in 45 per cent, remained unchanged in 50 per cent, and decreased in 5 per cent. When seizure frequency increases, this usually begins in the first half of pregnancy, and is more likely to occur in those patients with a past history of more than one seizure a month. Maternal age and age of onset of the seizure disorder do not appear to be important factors. In subsequent pregnancies, approximately half of patients should expect the same course as occurred in the previous pregnancies.

One very important factor that may contribute to an increase in seizure frequency is the alteration in the pharmacokinetics of drugs used in the chronic treatment of seizure disorders. For example, diphenylhydantoin, at the same drug dosage, results in lower blood levels of the drug during pregnancy. Advances in monitoring of serum concentrations of anticonvulsant medications have improved seizure control during pregnancy. In addition to direct drug treatment problems, increased cerebral irritability secondary to increased water retention has been postulated as a reason for an increase in seizure frequency during pregnancy. But as noted, the change in seizure frequency is not consistent in pregnancy.

Effects of Seizure Disorders on Pregnancy. In general, the course of pregnancy is not affected by the seizure disorder. Several studies have suggested that women with seizure disorders who become pregnant are at increased risk for vaginal hemorrhage, toxemia, cesarean or difficult delivery, prematurity, and perinatal death. These problems were not found in most studies.

MANAGEMENT

General Principles

1. A woman known to have a history of a seizure disorder should be counselled early in her reproductive years, and prior to a planned conception. In most cases this counselling should include encouragement that a normal reproductive career can take place. However, drug usage, medication needs, and plans for drug changes should be carefully reviewed prior to conception. In addition, the patient should be counselled concerning the possible risks of epilepsy in the child with respect to hereditary factors, and also with respect to risks for congenital malformations.

2. Ideally, the patient should be maintained on a single drug with the serum concentration maintained in the optimal therapeutic range. Therapeutic serum concentrations should be documented before a second drug is added. The use of serum concentrations often provides objective data about lack of compliance by the patient.

3. There are patients who have a past history of seizure disorders with no relatively recent episodes. This group may benefit by review of medical treatment programs and the actual need for drug therapy. In the nonpregnant state the need for medication use may be tested more easily.

Management of a Single Seizure. Emergency care always consists of insuring a clear airway, maintaining respiration, preventing aspiration, and avoiding self-induced harm to body, tongue, and so forth. A soft object that cannot be swallowed should be placed between the teeth to protect the tongue.

During pregnancy, if a patient convulses for the first time, evaluation should include the differential diagnostic work-up for acquired convulsive disorders. However, eclampsia must always be considered the primary disease. Convulsive disorders may start at any age and they occasionally start during pregnancy.

ANTICONVULSANT MEDICATIONS

Diphenylhydantoin (Dilantin). Diphenylhydantoin (phenytoin) is useful in both major generalized (grand mal) and focal (motor) seizures. In the non-acute state it is given orally and is readily absorbed from the gastrointestinal tract. Intramuscular injections are painful and absorption may be irregular. Intravenous diphenylhydantoin should be given along with saline solutions since diphenylhydantoin is much less soluble in acid solutions, and dextrose solutions are acidic. The usual dose is 4 to 7 mg per kg or 300 to 500 mg daily. The intravenous or oral loading dose is 1 gram. The maximum safe adult intravenous dose is 50 mg per minute. The therapeutic blood level is 10 to 20 μg per ml.

Plasma protein binding of diphenylhydantoin is decreased in late pregnancy. Free unbound diphenylhydantoin probably has increased clearance in pregnancy. Total serum concentrations of diphenylhydantoin usually fall during pregnancy. Therefore, in order to protect patients with seizure disorders against seizures during pregnancy, plasma levels of diphenylhydantoin should be measured at monthly intervals, and dosages of diphenylhydantoin increased if therapeutic levels are not present. The necessary dose increment may be substantial (50 per cent or more). In the puerperium, pre-pregnancy clearance rates of diphenylhydantoin return to normal within one month; therefore adjustment of drug dosage may be necessary.

TABLE 1. Anticonvulsant Medications

GENERIC NAME	TRADE NAME	ADULT DOSAGE (mg/kg/day)	ADULT DOSAGE (mg/day)	PRINCIPAL INDICATIONS	SERUM HALF-LIFE (Hours)	THERAPEUTIC SERUM LEVEL (μg/ml)	TOXIC LEVEL (μg/ml)	TOXIC EFFECTS (Dose-Related)
Diphenylhydantoin (Phenytoin)	Dilantin	4–7	300–400	major seizures, psychomotor seizures, focal seizures	24 ± 12	10–20	>20	nystagmus, ataxia, drowsiness
Phenobarbital	Luminal	1–5	6–200	major seizures, psychomotor seizures, focal seizures, petit mal seizures	96 ± 12	15–40	>40	drowsiness, slowness, ataxia, coma
Primidone	Mysoline	10–25	750–2000	major seizures, psychomotor seizures, focal seizures	12 ± 6	5–12	>12	drowsiness, slowness, ataxia, coma
Ethosuximide	Zarontin	20–30	1000–1500	petit mal seizures	30 ± 6	40–100	>100	nausea, vomiting, anorexia, dizziness
Carbamazepine	Tegretol	10–20	1000–1200	temporal lobe seizures, focal seizures, partial seizures	12 ± 3	4–8	>8	vertigo, dizziness, drowsiness, diplopia, water intoxication
Valproic Acid	Depakene	15–25	1000–1250	petit mal seizures, myoclonic seizures	Varies 8–20	?	?	nausea, vomiting, cramps

Diphenylhydantoin readily crosses the placenta, and umbilical cord concentrations are almost identical to maternal serum concentrations. No adverse effects have been attributed to diphenylhydantoin present in breast milk. (See below for teratology.)

Phenobarbital. Phenobarbital may be administered orally, intramuscularly, or intravenously. The usual adult dose is 1 to 5 mg per kg. The total daily dose is usually 60 to 200 mg. Therapeutic phenobarbital blood levels are 15 to 40 μg per ml. Phenobarbital has a relatively long half-life of 4 to 5 days. During pregnancy phenobarbital clearance is increased and dosages may need adjustment. Postpartum observation for toxicity is important. Phenobarbital crosses the placenta readily and is excreted in breast milk. No adverse effects have been attributed to phenobarbital in breast milk.

Diazepam. Oral diazepam is not effective as an anticonvulsant. This drug readily crosses the placenta and accumulates in the fetus. Metabolism in the neonate is slow. Regular use of diazepam during pregnancy or lactation is not recommended. Intravenous diazepam is very effective in the immediate control of seizures and in status epilepticus and has been used by some in eclampsia. It is not recommended as the treatment of choice in eclampsia. As noted it is also not recommended for daily therapy for convulsions.

Other Medications. In Table 1 we have listed other medications which may be encountered by the obstetrician in caring for patients with convulsive disorders. Since the presence of epilepsy per se may be associated with an increased incidence of congenital malformations, almost all medications listed have cautionary warnings.

MANAGEMENT OF STATUS EPILEPTICUS

According to the International League Against Epilepsy the term status epilepticus "is used whenever a seizure persists for a sufficient length of time or is repeated frequently enough to produce a fixed and enduring epileptic condition." Status epilepticus with generalized seizures is a medical emergency with significant maternal and fetal risk. It requires prompt medical management, and hospitalization in an intensive care unit. Treatment includes the following.

1. Establishment of an airway and oxygenation is the first step. In some patients this may require endotracheal intubation. If hypoglycemia is suspected, after a blood sugar is drawn, 25 to 50 grams of a 50 per cent glucose solution should be given. A blood sample for serum anticonvulsant level should be obtained.

2. Intravenous administration of anticonvulsants is necessary. The initial intravenous choice of 10 mg of diazepam is effective. Diazepam has a short duration of action (30 minutes); therefore, this dose can be repeated three times at 20 minute intervals. This may be followed by an infusion of 100 mg of diazepam in 500 ml of saline solution adjusted to deliver 20 to 40 mg per hour, until the seizures are controlled. Then the diazepam dosage is slowly decreased.

After the initial intravenous dose of 10 mg of diazepam, maintenance doses of a longer acting anticonvulsant should be administered (even if diazepam has been effective). An initial intravenous dose of 250 mg of diphenylhydantoin is usually effective. Maintenance dose of diphenylhydantoin may be administered at intravenous infusion rates that should not exceed 0.05 gram per minute up to a total dose of 0.5 gram in patients who have been taking the drug, and up to 1.0 gram in previously untreated patients. Monitoring the patient's blood pressure and electrocardiogram is essential.

Intravenous administration of sodium phenobarbital is also effective in stopping status epilepticus seizures and in preventing recurrence. A slow intravenous infusion at a rate of 0.05 gram per minute to a total dose of 7 mg per kg may be given. An initial intravenous infusion of 100 mg of sodium phenobarbital may be given over a two minute interval and this may be repeated 2 or 3 times at 20 to 30 minute intervals.

3. If seizures continue, slow administration of 4 to 6 ml of intravenous paraldehyde or a slow administration of 500 mg of sodium amytal may be effective for control of status epilepticus.

4. General anesthesia for control of seizures should be used as a last resort and is rarely necessary.

5. Maintenance anticonvulsant therapy after control of status epilepticus depends on the patient's previous treatment history. Usually diphenylhydantoin or phenobarbital is used, with serum concentrations documented as a guideline for appropriate dosages.

6. Although therapeutic levels of medications must be used, the clinician should be aware that the depressant effects of these drugs may cause coma with respiratory depression and hypotension.

EFFECTS OF SEIZURE DISORDERS AND THEIR TREATMENT ON THE FETUS, NEONATE AND CHILD

1. The idiopathic seizure disorders pose a risk of hereditary transmission to the fetus. In a pregnancy with no family history of a seizure disorder, the offspring has a 1 in 200 chance of having a seizure disorder. A woman with an

"idiopathic" seizure disorder has a 1 in 40 risk of having a child with a seizure disorder. Therefore, patients with seizure disorders should receive genetic counselling.

2. The incidence of congenital malformations in the offspring is increased in patients with seizure disorders. Most of this increased risk is for congenital heart disease and orofacial defects. The total risk of congenital malformations is approximately double the rate of malformation in the general population. An increased risk for congenital malformations seems to be more closely linked with the presence of maternal seizure disorders regardless of drug regimens. It is not clear if part of the increase in malformations reported in this group of patients may also be attributed to diphenylhydantoin or other medications.

3. Some newborn infants that were exposed to phenobarbital in utero may exhibit withdrawal symptoms including hyperexcitability, jitteriness, tremor, high-pitched cry, and feeding problems which may start as long as one week after birth.

4. Infants exposed to diphenylhydantoin or phenobarbital may have depressed clotting factors and sometimes neonatal hemorrhage. These defects respond to administration of vitamin K.

The *American Academy of Pediatrics Committee on Drugs* in collaboration with the *American College of Obstetrics and Gynecology Committee on Obstetrics: Maternal and Fetal Medicine* issued a statement relating to anticonvulsant medications and pregnancy in January, 1979. Their recommendations are:

1. No women should receive anticonvulsant medication unnecessarily. When possible, a woman who has been seizure free for many years should be withdrawn from her medication prior to pregnancy. When a woman who has epilepsy and requires medication asks about pregnancy, she should be advised that she has a 90 per cent chance of having a normal child, but that the risk of congenital malformations and mental retardation is two to three times greater than average because of her disease or its treatment. Women who seek advice later than the first trimester of pregnancy should be reassured with the foregoing figures rather than routinely urged to consider abortion. For these women, drug therapy should be continued throughout pregnancy because major anatomical malformations most likely would have taken place already, and the malformations associated with the hydantoin syndrome rarely have significant effect on the well-being of the child.

2. There is no reason at present to advise a woman to switch from phenytoin or phenobarbital to other anticonvulsants about which even less is known. Discontinuation of medication in a woman whose epilepsy is controlled by medicine may cause seizures, and prolonged seizures could cause serious sequelae to her and the fetus.

3. Physicians are often asked for recommendation about breastfeeding for mothers on anticonvulsant medications. A review of published literature shows that most anticonvulsants present in therapeutic levels in the mother also are present in breast milk. However, their concentration is low enough that there is little likelihood of any demonstrable effects on the infant. Thus, there is no evidence at the present time to suggest that a woman requiring anticonvulsants should either stop taking medication or avoid nursing.

TREATMENT OF FEMALE GENITAL TUBERCULOSIS

DAVID L. HEMSELL, M.D.

Tuberculosis of the female genital tract is an uncommon infection that is almost always secondary to infection elsewhere—lungs, kidneys, or bones and joints. It is suspected that involvement is by hematogenous spread, as bacillemia may persist for weeks. It is also possible for pelvic organs to become infected through the lymphatics from peritoneal implants or by direct extension. This protean disease may well exist without signs or symptoms (11 per cent) and may recur long after apparently successful antituberculous therapy. It is diagnosed in two age groups, a younger group of recent immigrants from less well developed countries and an older age group (usually also immigrants) who have been established in the United States for some time.

Percentages of pelvic organ involvement are: fallopian tubes, 90 to 100 per cent; uterus, 50 to 90 per cent; ovary, 20 to 30 per cent; cervix, 1 to 15 per cent; and vagina and vulva, 1 per cent. Incidences of presenting complaints are: menstrual aberrations, either menometrorrhagia or amenorrhea, 10 to 40 per cent; pelvic pain, 25 to 50 per cent; and sterility, 45 to 55 per cent.

The diagnosis of this disease is time consuming and expensive. Exact diagnosis can be made only by inoculation of laboratory animals. A presumptive diagnosis may be made, however, utilizing the following information:

1. Family and past history. A family history is positive for the disease in 20 per cent of cases, and a patient will give a history of previous diagnosis of tuberculosis in 40 per cent of cases.

2. Chest x-ray showing healed lesions (found in 50 per cent of cases, but a normal examination does not rule this out).

3. KUB showing calcified abdominal or pelvic lymph nodes.

4. Positive tuberculin skin test (found in the majority of cases, but a negative test does not rule out genital tuberculosis).

5. Hysterosalpingogram showing fistulas, multiple constrictions along the tube, obstruction of the zone between the isthmus and ampulla, lymphatic or venous intravasation, and/or multiple endometrial adhesions without a history compatible with Asherman's syndrome.

6. Histologic endometrial or surgical specimen showing caseation, calcification, ulceration, fibrosis, hyalinization, and/or tubercles.

The best specimen for diagnosis is endometrium obtained several days before a menses. The greatest concentration of histologic abnormalities will be obtained from cornual regions. A portion of tissue should be submitted both for culture (to confirm the diagnosis) and for sensitivity testing. Two days of menstrual blood may be collected in a cervical cap and cultured in a similar fashion, but with less predictable results. Closed laparoscopy is probably contraindicated if tuberculosis is suspected, owing to the adhesive nature of this disease. A mini-laparotomy or open laparoscopy would be safer and wiser if this is the preoperative diagnosis.

Introduction of more effective antituberculous drugs with fewer side effects has significantly modified therapy for this disease. Original therapy, consisting of long sanatorium stays, bed rest, sunlight, ultraviolet radiation, pelvic diathermy, diets, and vitamin supplementation was associated with a significant requirement for surgical therapy. Postoperative complications such as fistulas and even death were not uncommon. Surgery is almost never required with current therapy. Although there have been great advances in tubal reconstructive surgery, the success rate has been extremely low in patients with previous tuberculosis.

Whereas hospitalization was the rule in the past, it is now infrequently required. Every effort must be made initially to rule out active extrapelvic disease. This can be done with chest x-ray examination, aerosol-induced sputum examination and culture, and culturing and analysis of several first-voided urine specimens. Any treatment regimen still includes adequate rest and nutrition, diet supplements, and appropriate hygiene, as well as identification of reservoirs of active disease in the family and social setting. As is always the case, appropriate patient education is mandatory. Although the gynecologist should consult an infectious disease specialist when pelvic tuberculosis is diagnosed, it is paramount that continued therapy be provided by the gynecologist.

The extent of genital lesions and presenting symptoms serve as indicators for initial therapy. A woman who is asymptomatic with the possible exception of involuntary infertility is usually adequately treated with 5 to 10 mg per kg per day of isoniazid and 15 mg per kg per day of ethambutol as a single dose. After 6 to 12 months of therapy, an endometrial biopsy specimen should be obtained for culture and sensitivity as well as histopathologic examination. A test for cure done in a similar fashion should be performed after 18 to 24 months of therapy. Some stop ethambutol after one year if evaluation then is negative. Women should be followed at 6 month intervals after therapy is completed for one year, and then yearly with endometrial samples obtained for study at each visit. Clinical exacerbations have occurred up to 8 years after active disease was apparently successfully treated. If a biopsy specimen becomes positive after 6 months of therapy or if tubo-ovarian or pelvic masses develop during therapy, rifampin should be added and a laparotomy performed in several weeks with plans for removing the uterus, tubes, and ovaries. With current therapy, however, this is very infrequently necessary.

Should a woman's disease be associated with palpable masses initially, recommended therapy is isoniazid, 10 mg per kg per day, and ethambutol, 25 mg per kg per day, for 60 days, then reduced to 15 mg per kg per day combined with rifampin. Rifampin is given at a dose of 450 mg per day to those weighing up to 50 kg. If a woman weighs over 50 kg, then the dose should be 600 mg per day. This woman should be examined at monthly intervals for the first 3 months and then every 3 months until the end of therapy. Test of cure histologically and bacteriologically as well as evaluation of lungs and urine are indicated at the completion of therapy, 18 to 24 months later. Should masses persist or increase after 3 to 4 months of therapy, the uterus, tubes, and ovaries should be removed irrespective of the patient's age. Ethambutol therapy should be continued for 3 to 6 months postoperatively, and isoniazid for approximately 1 year.

There may be some instances in which the initial diagnosis is made at the time of operation in a patient who is undergoing infertility evaluation or a laparotomy or laparoscopy for other reasons. In general, if foci of disease are 1 cm in size or less, oral antituberculous therapy will prove effective. The disease is usually too widespread to allow complete surgical removal of the multiple implants. Isoniazid and ethambutol at the initial doses (asymptomatic patient) should be given for 18 to 24 months in cases in which there are no masses. If disease is extensive, triple therapy should be utilized.

Surgical therapy is currently recommended only under the following conditions:

1. Persistence or increase in pelvic masses *after* a course of antituberculous therapy;
2. Recurrence of positive culture or histology after 6 months of antituberculous therapy;
3. Persistence of pelvic symptoms after long-term antituberculous therapy;
4. Fistulas that fail to heal;
5. Patients who will not take long-term therapy or return for follow-up.

One should not operate suspecting tuberculosis unless the patient has received at least two weeks of preoperative antituberculosis therapy. Preoperative chemotherapy facilitates surgery and affords a quicker cure than is seen with medical therapy alone. Most of the current failures are due to interruption of self-medication, although inappropriate regimens may be responsible in some instances. Drug resistance is a definite possibility and for that reason it is mandatory to perform susceptibility testing where possible.

Antituberculous drugs are not without risks. Isoniazid may be associated with hepatotoxicity which seems to be related to age and preexisting disease. It is usually reversible and appears 4 to 8 weeks after initiation of therapy. Neurotoxicity has been reported and is ameliorated by pyridoxine. It occurs in 17 per cent of persons reserving 6 mg per kg per day. Dilantin toxicity is potentiated by this tuberculocidal agent.

Ethambutol has been associated with various neuropathies if greater than 50 mg per kg per day of this tuberculostatic antimicrobial are administered. Decreased visual fields and acuity as well as color vision aberrations have been reported. For this reason, pretreatment evaluation by an opthhalmologist is recommended. Ocular symptoms should be sought, and acuity and color perception testing done at 4 to 6 week intervals. Hyperuricemia may also occur.

Rifampin may be associated with hepatotoxicity that is apparently potentiated by isoniazid, heralded by increasing SGOT levels, and is reversible. Patients receiving rifampin should have liver function studies monitored. Decreased effectiveness of coumarin anticoagulants and oral contraceptives has also been reported.

A clinical cure is assumed if clinical symptoms disappear, examination of the pelvis remains or becomes normal, and there is no longer histologic or bacteriologic evidence of *Mycobacterium tuberculosis*. Experience with current modalities of medical therapy indicates that menometrorrhagia, pelvic pain, and amenorrhea will be almost completely cured by even short-course therapy. It is recommended that minimal therapy be continued for 18 to 24 months, however.

There is greater flexibility in current therapy, which is always multi-drug in nature. The goals are the highest safe and tolerated dose for a prolonged period of time. Rifampin and isoniazid appear to be as effective as any previous three drug combination for cavitary pulmonary disease. This treatment undoubtedly may well shorten treatment time, but is investigational at the present time.

If one suspects tuberculous pelvic disease that does not seem to respond to current first-line antituberculous therapy, consideration should be given to nontuberculous mycobacterial infection. This disease is less common than tuberculosis and requires therapy not only with antituberculous drugs but also with conventional antimicrobial therapy such as aminoglycosides, erythromycin, and/or tetracycline. Pathogens include photochromogens, scotochromogens, nonchromogens, and the rapid growers.

PULMONARY TUBERCULOSIS IN PREGNANCY

F. GARY CUNNINGHAM, M.D.,
and GERARD E. BALSLEY, Jr., M.D.

Tuberculosis is a chronic granulomatous infection caused by *Mycobacterium tuberculosis*, *M. bovis*, or so-called atypical mycobacteria. It is characterized by spontaneous remissions and reactivation; the intricate balance maintained between host and parasite is not fully elucidated. Tubercle bacilli are obligate aerobes with a slow division time and whose unique lipid cell-wall components impart characteristic resistance to acids and alkalis, as well as the ability to induce tubercle formation and caseation necrosis. The most common mode of transmission is via aerosolized droplets usually spread by coughing, and the infectiousness of a person with tuberculosis is related to the concentration of bacilli in pulmonary secretions.

From an epidemiological standpoint, *infec-*

tion is defined as a positive tuberculin skin test. This increases with time, and by age 30 approximately 5 per cent of adults have evidence of infection. Clinically apparent infections are termed *new active cases* and are usually due to reactivation, but may represent primary tuberculous pneumonia. In the United States, reactivation tuberculosis is more common among older men, especially those of lower socioeconomic groups. This latter observation is important, since race-susceptibility to tuberculosis is frequently cited; however, it is difficult to separate racial factors from poor hygiene and overcrowded conditions associated with lower socioeconomic factors among some ethnic groups. Symptomatic disease usually develops many years after infection, and events that cause reactivation after a long stable period in some persons remain unknown. Reactivation is generally slowly progressive with caseation and transbronchial spread.

PREGNANCY AND TUBERCULOSIS

Historically, there has been a wide spectrum of medical opinion concerning the advisability of pregnancy when a woman had tuberculosis. Hippocrates advised prompt child-bearing to ameliorate the disease, but in the nineteenth century, tuberculosis was a common indication for abortion. There is no scientific evidence to indicate that pregnancy predisposes to acquisition of primary tuberculosis or to reactivation of latent disease. Current studies show no differences in the short-term and long-term courses of tuberculosis in pregnant women compared to controls matched for age, race, and social and economic status. Changes in pulmonary physiology associated with pregnancy, that is, decreased residual and expiratory reserve volumes, as well as decreased total lung capacity, do not increase susceptibility to infection. However, these changes may decrease the size of a primary lesion and thus make it more difficult to visualize radiographically.

Similarly, current evidence indicates that tuberculosis has minimal effects on pregnancy. Cases of congenital tuberculosis are quite rare, and there is no evidence that infection predisposes to abortions, premature delivery, or increased perinatal mortality. These latter observations undoubtedly are related to early diagnosis and therapy for active tuberculosis with salutary effects on maternal health.

TREATMENT

The significant decrease of active tuberculosis in the United States has resulted from public health preventive measures rather than active therapy for disease. However, chemotherapy markedly alters the outcome in individual patients. Since in any large population of *M. tuberculosis*, a small number of antibiotic-resistant bacilli are selected by therapy with any single drug, a major tenet of chemotherapy is the multiple drug regimen. Thus, the resistant fraction of the bacilli is reduced by exposure to several drugs, each with a different mode of action. Other factors in selection of therapy include a history of prior antitubercular therapy, results of in vitro susceptibility tests, and the relative risk of adverse drug reactions.

Pharmacology of First-Line Antituberculosis Drugs

Isoniazid. *Isoniazid* is an intermediary compound discovered in the synthesis of antitubercular drugs around 1950. It was found to have excellent tuberculostatic properties and remains the mainstay of therapy. Its mechanism of action has not been completely elucidated, but it may block nucleic acid synthesis since it has widespread effects on many enzyme by-products. The standard adult dose is 300 to 400 mg daily and its most common side-effects are neurologic, ranging from peripheral neuritis to encephalopathy. These side-effects are dose related, and are somewhat prevented by pyridoxine, 50 to 100 mg daily. Almost 10 per cent of patients have transient elevations of hepatocellular enzymes with initiation of therapy, but less than 1 per cent develop a picture clinically indistinguishable from viral hepatitis. The latter is uncommon before age 35, and is neither a toxic effect, nor dose-related, and is probably a hypersensitivity reaction. Pregnancy per se is not a contraindication to isoniazid therapy. For example, hepatic function is not impaired, and extensive surveillance has failed to demonstrate fetal anomalies associated with isoniazid.

Ethambutol. *Ethambutol* was introduced in the late 1960s. It is the most tuberculostatic congener of ethylenediamine and has replaced para-aminosalicylic acid as the most commonly used adjuvant to isoniazid. The dose is 15 to 25 mg per kg daily, and infrequent side-effects are usually ocular, manifested by decreased visual acuity and impaired perception of green color. Surveillance of offspring of pregnant women given ethambutol have shown no ocular deficits within the sensitivity of available tests. Moreover, there was no increase in the malformation rate.

Rifampin. *Rifampin* was introduced in 1971. It blocks bacterial RNA transcriptase but human cells are resistant. The customary daily dose is 600 mg and main side-effects are hepatic. When given with isoniazid, there is an uncommon syndrome of hepatocellular necrosis seen almost exclusively in alcoholics. In a retrospective study of pregnant women given rifampin, usually in conjunction with other drugs, the rate of fetuses with anomalies was higher than expected. The most common of these were limb reductions at 8 per 1000; however, there was no control population. These data have been interpreted to contraindicate rifampin during pregnancy except for life-threatening infection. Denying such an effective antitubercular drug on the basis of uncontrolled data and small numbers seems unwarranted, and if indicated, the drug should be given.

Streptomycin. *Streptomycin* was the first antibiotic for therapy of tuberculosis and it still is useful as an adjuvant to isoniazid. Its mechanism of action is by attachment to the 30S ribosomes, which blocks elongation of polypeptide chains. Although largely replaced by rifampin, it is included for life-threatening infection. When given to pregnant women, as many as 15 to 20 per cent of their offspring have detectable eighth nerve damage. Moreover, cochlear and vestibular damage may occur at any stage of fetal development. Although many of these effects were due to dihydrostreptomycin, neither drug currently is recommended for routine use during pregnancy.

Active Infection

For women with less extensive disease, e.g., pulmonary infiltrates without cavitation, isoniazid is given in combination with either ethambutol or rifampin. The latter regimen appears to be more effective as measured by rapid sputum conversion as well as minimal relapse rate. More recently, triple therapy with isoniazid, ethambutol, and rifampin given as initial therapy for minimal tuberculosis has produced cures in 9 months rather than the 18 months required with two-drug regimens. Another advantage is the lesser chance of drug-resistance emerging. For women with cavitary disease, or evidence of dissemination, triple-drug therapy is mandatory, and streptomycin is given initially to the very ill patient.

Tuberculous patients become non-infective within days of initiation of therapy, and even though sputa may contain acid-fast organisms, these mycobacteria will neither grow in culture nor infect others. Hence, prolonged isolation of tuberculous mothers from their infants is neither scientifically warranted nor conducive to compliance with therapy. The uniformly good results from BCG vaccination of offspring born to tuberculous mothers should encourage its use.

Chemoprophylaxis

Isoniazid, 300 to 400 mg daily for 9 to 12 months, is given alone to prevent primary infection or to prevent reactivation. The American Thoracic Society recommends isoniazid chemoprophylaxis in descending priority: (1) household members and other close contacts of patients with recently diagnosed active tuberculosis; (2) tuberculin-positive reactors with a chest radiograph demonstrating nonprogressive lesions; (3) "recent converters," i.e., tuberculin reaction becoming positive within two years; (4) tuberculin reactors undergoing medical treatment known to increase reactivation, e.g., glucocorticoid therapy, immunosuppression, and so forth; and (5) any positive tuberculin reactor under the age of 35.

The decision to include pregnant women in these groups receiving chemoprophylaxis is based on minimal adverse maternal and fetal effects of isoniazid. Since there is no evidence for increased susceptibility of maternal hepatic dysfunction, and since no adverse perinatal outcomes have been attributed to the drug, it seems wise to apply the same health standards to pregnant women as are recommended for the general population. For example, if the decision is made to test women for tuberculin reaction as routine prenatal care, then one should be prepared to administer isoniazid chemoprophylaxis for those with positive tests.

COLLAGEN DISEASES IN PREGNANCY

JACK M. SCHNEIDER, M.D.

As greater understanding regarding the collagen vascular diseases has accumulated, it has become increasingly clear that these disorders reflect various clinical presentations of immunologic dysfunction having the common pathologic finding of inflammatory and degenerative changes in the connective tissues. The connective tissue diseases herein addressed—rheumatoid arthritis, systemic lupus erythematosus, scleroderma, systemic sclerosis, and mixed connective tissue disease—have many features in common, including multisystem involvement; a familial occurrence of some expression of a connective tissue disease; a predilection for women; an increased incidence in the reproductive age group; and episodic exacerbations or remissions. There is also a trend toward improvement of symptoms during pregnancy with a relative worsening or return to pre-pregnancy status after delivery. As with many medical illnesses complicating pregnancy, the selection of approach to management is guided by the necessity to minimize risks for the fetus while optimizing comfort and minimizing morbidity for the mother. In general, then, the "simpler" therapies with long track records and known fetal risks are favored over the more complex and oftentimes risky use of multiple and/or new drugs.

RHEUMATOID ARTHRITIS

It is generally recognized that pregnancy tends to have an ameliorating effect on this multi-organ connective tissue disorder with predominant involvement of the peripheral synovial joints, presumably because of the increased level of free cortisol (plasma), with physiologic alterations in immune responses in pregnancy perhaps playing a role. Relapse, often with apparent exacerbation, frequently follows completion of the pregnancy.

Aspirin is the main anti-inflammatory drug used for this disorder, with doses of 4 to 6 grams per day in divided doses generally sufficient to achieve therapeutic blood levels of 15 to 25 mg per dl. Gastrointestinal side-effects may be avoided by ingestion with food, buffering, or enteric coating. Bowel bleeding may occur by direct effects of the salicylate on mucosa and/or decreased platelet aggregation. Since neonatal bleeding can follow altered platelet aggregation, an attempt to stop aspirin for 10 days or more prior to delivery is an ideal goal. A corticosteroid may be substituted during this period if symptoms require continued therapy. Although the effect of aspirin on prostaglandin synthesis has been implicated as predisposing to prolonged pregnancy and perhaps premature ductus arteriosus closure, this does not pose a significant problem in clinical management requiring alteration of the treatment of the woman.

Phenylbutazone, indomethacin, and other nonsteroidal anti-inflammatory drugs are best avoided in pregnancy because of potential undesirable fetal side-effects.

Antimalarial drugs such as chloroquine may produce an irreversible decrease in visual acuity in both mother and fetus because of retinal damage. Chromosomal damage has also been suggested.

While the gold salts do not appear to cross the placenta because of protein binding, a broad range of adverse effects in the mother limits their usefulness. The same can be said of D-penicillamine with respect to maternal toxicity.

Immunosuppressant agents should be reserved for the life-threatening situation, as in the nonpregnant woman. Cyclophosphamide should not be used in pregnancy.

SYSTEMIC LUPUS ERYTHEMATOSUS (SLE)

This disorder is also a multi-organ chronic inflammatory disease with the prognosis for mother and fetus during pregnancy directly correlated with the severity of renal involvement if present. Women with known lupus nephritis should be counselled *before* pregnancy regarding the increased risks of abortion, stillbirth, intrauterine growth retardation, fetal cardiac lesions (particularly congenital heart block), and preterm delivery.

If SLE is first manifest during pregnancy, the alternate and more common initial diagnosis is preeclampsia. Notation of fever, arthritis, rash, high urinary protein losses ($\geq$ 5 grams per day), thrombocytopenia, dermatologic lesions, and/or neuropsychiatric dysfunction should prompt a laboratory assessment for antinuclear antibody to confirm the diagnosis.

In contrast to the treatment for rheumatoid arthritis, corticosteroids constitute the primary drug therapy for SLE, with aspirin being utilized for symptoms of fever, arthritis, or pleuritis. The benefit of continued steroid therapy throughout pregnancy to prevent exacerbations remains controversial and will probably remain so because of the highly variable clinical course of this disease complicating relatively few pregnancies. Long-term therapy of SLE with corticosteroids in the nonpregnant woman, however, does not appear to alter prognosis. An alternative approach to continuous therapy is the initiation of corticosteroid therapy based upon significant deviation in the levels of C_3, total hemolytic complement, and anti-DNA antibodies discovered during frequent serial assessments. Exacerbations of lupus are typically managed with 60 to 80 mg of prednisone per day in two or three divided doses. Maintenance doses of 10 to 20 mg of prednisone on alternate days are commonly employed. While increased daily dosage of prednisone or the use of 100 mg of intravenous hydrocortisone every 8 hours is recommended if long-term corticosteroid therapy has preceded parturition, appropriate postpartum drug management is unclear since exacerbation of glomerulonephritis in nonpregnant women seems unaltered by prophylactic administration of corticosteroids. Because of the apparent increase in the initial diagnosis of lupus erythematosus or the worsening of lupus nephritis in the early weeks postdelivery, prednisone dosage should probably be continued at the maintenance dosage for 6 weeks postpartum.

Antimalarial drugs pose the same risks and complications as noted in the discussion of the treatment of rheumatoid arthritis. While immunosuppressant agents should be reserved for the life-threatening situation, the cytotoxic antimetabolite azathioprine has been used through the entire pregnancy with possible polydactyly as the only reported teratologic risk. Hemodialysis has been successfully employed during pregnancy in cases of renal failure.

Plasmapheresis has shown such good effect on severe, fulminant expressions of SLE that a national multicenter trial is being undertaken in 1982 to determine long-term benefit, if any. As pheresis has been done in pregnancy without significant complication, this therapy probably constitutes the treatment of choice when severe disease threatens maternal and fetal life. Further, the rare instances of short-term manifestations of lupus in the infant may be preventable by pheresis.

SCLERODERMA

This disease presents either as a localized disorder involving mainly the skin of the fingers and face, or as a systemic expression of the sclerosis (systemic sclerosis) which in turn may be progressive (progressive systemic sclerosis). The localized expression of the disease generally has a benign clinical course.

Progressive systemic sclerosis portends grave risk for maternal and/or perinatal mortality. Treatment is symptomatic and supportive in addressing polyarthritis and fibromyositis (aspirin/corticosteroids), Raynaud's phenomenon and hypertension (vasodilating drugs), and reflux esophagitis (antacids). With lung involvement, prevention and early treatment of infection is critical, as pneumonia is a common complication preceding maternal mortality. Because of the risk of pneumonia, general anesthesia should *not* be employed in women with systemic sclerosis.

SYSTEMIC VASCULITIS

Necrotizing inflammatory lesions of small and medium-sized arteries characterize the pathology of this disorder. The prognosis in pregnancy is unclear because usually only the fulminant cases with cardiac and renal failure are defined in pregnancy, commonly following an initial misdiagnosis of severe preeclampsia. Intervention with prednisone, 60 to 80 mg per day, before cardiac or renal failure occurs may result in sufficient amelioration to allow successful completion of the pregnancy.

MIXED CONNECTIVE TISSUE DISEASE

Whether representing a complex variable expression of SLE or a distinct disorder, the diagnosis of mixed connective tissue disease is utilized in the clinical situation that does not fit rheumatoid arthritis, SLE, scleroderma, or polymyositis, but expresses features of several of these defined connective tissue diseases.

Methotrexate has been employed in this disorder in doses of 25 mg intramuscularly every week. This drug is an abortifacient and teratogen in the first half of pregnancy, but when used in the last half of pregnancy it seems to pose no short-term risk for the infant.

COUNSELING AND CONTRACEPTION

Evident from the above presentation is the need to counsel patients prior to pregnancy in the less life-threatening expressions of the connective tissue diseases (e.g., rheumatoid arthritis and SLE without nephritis) regarding potential risks of needed drug therapy to the fetus. Appropriate contraception counseling and follow-through by the couple are essential to avoid complications of pregnancy or alteration of essential maternal drug therapy in progressive disorders, as in some cases of systemic sclerosis, lupus nephritis, and mixed connective tissue disease. Contraception is a critical consideration when immunosuppressant therapy is being employed, in order to avoid the issue of drug effects on embryogenesis. Since hormonal variations seem to be associated with exacerbation of some of these diseases, oral contraceptives are not the preferred contraceptive method.

ANEMIAS

JOHN C. MORRISON, M.D.,
and STAVROS G. DOUVAS, M.D.

Anemia is one of the most frequent complications diagnosed by the obstetrician and gynecologist. During pregnancy, anemia is especially common, with over 55 per cent of patients having a hemoglobin (Hb) concentration less than 11 grams per dl. Patients with mild anemias demonstrate few overt effects, although malaise and susceptibility to infection are common. Severe sequelae are infrequent in obstetric patients with mild to moderate anemias, although lower birth weights, postpartum hemorrhage, and placental abnormalities have been associated with hemoglobin levels less than 10 grams per dl. In contrast, when the hemoglobin values are less than 6 grams per dl, high-output congestive heart failure and decreased oxygenation of many organ systems is common in all patients. An acute anemia denotes a true decrease in red cell mass and involves (1) diminished erythrocyte production, (2) increased erythrocyte destruction, or (3) erythrocyte loss. The anemia may be due to many factors and frequently there is a combination or mixed pattern which makes accepted diagnostic tests less useful (Fig. 1).

The history and physical examination are seldom helpful except in severe or longstanding anemias. The routine laboratory assessment of an anemia is less reliable in the pregnant patient. Table 1 demonstrates that a packed cell volume (PCV) of less than 35 per cent and a hemoglobin level less than 13 grams per dl are the most commonly used standards for anemia. Because of the hormonal changes during early pregnancy, the relative hydremia results in dilutional or "relative" anemia. Nevertheless, during gestation a PCV <30 and hemoglobin values <10 grams per dl usually denote a true or an absolute anemia.

Iron deficiency anemia accounts for 75 per cent of all anemias diagnosed in the female patient. Iron as well as other necessary elements may be lost at accelerated rates, not absorbed, or be poorly incorporated into the new red blood cell (RBC). No measurable effects of iron deficiency anemia are evident until storage iron is depleted. When iron is then not available for incorporation into new red cells, overt signs of anemia appear. Many disorders and drugs can cause a decreased absorption of iron from the small intestine. Oxalates, carbonates, lack of hydrochloric acid, and mucosal disease states such as lymphoma and regional ileitis are good examples. In patients with chronic infection, cancer, hemochromatosis, or thalassemia, iron may actually be present in excess but cannot be incorporated into newly formed blood cells. In iron deficiency anemia, as with other trace element deficiencies, the diet is usually lacking if the patient is clinically anemic. Poor dietary habits combined with adolescence, normal pregnancy, or chronic blood loss require supplemental iron. In megaloblastic anemias, the production of all cell lines is diminished, with a paucity of white cells and platelets as well as red blood cells. Rare inborn errors of metabolism such as lack of orotic acid can cause megaloblastic anemia. However, 98 per cent of the reported cases are due to folate or vitamin B_{12} deficiency. In the United States megaloblastic anemias and iron deficiency anemia encompass approximately 95 per cent of all anemias diagnosed in women. In short, most of the anemias suspected by the obstetrician/gynecologist can be diagnosed by simple tests which can be performed on an ambulatory basis (Table 1), albeit less reliably in pregnancy.

On the other hand, if severe hematologic disease involving increased destruction of red cells is suspected, active consultation with a hematologist is necessary. These disorders include the hereditary states such as sickle cell hemoglobinopathies, porphyria, spherocytosis and glucose-6-phosphate dehydrogenase deficiency as well as problems with sepsis, toxic agents, immune diseases, and many vascular problems (Fig. 1). Fortunately, these disorders are rare in the patients usually seen by the obstetrician or gynecologist. Finally, there are disorders involving blood loss. In gynecologic patients, polyps, leiomyomata, cancer of the genital tract, and dysfunctional uterine bleeding are common causes for acute and chronic blood loss. Likewise, lacerations or obstetric complications such as abortion, ectopic pregnancy, or third trimester bleeding may lead to acute blood loss (Fig. 1). Chronic blood loss such as that occurring from intestinal lesions or parasites is rare in this country.

Just as more than 90 per cent of the anemias can be diagnosed by the obstetrician or gynecologist on an ambulatory basis, the treatment for most anemias can be similarly rendered. Indeed, the anemic woman, particularly during pregnancy, or when the cause of the anemia is most likely iron deficiency anemia or folic acid deficiency, may be treated with replacement of these elements as a diagnostic/therapeutic test. The treatment of an obvious blood loss is usually best accomplished by eliminating the cause and administering transfusions only if necessary. For the rare hematologic disease such as those involving erythrocyte destruction or the hereditary anemias involving decreased production of erythrocytes, patients should be referred to the hematologist for treatment, as they are for diagnosis. Nevertheless, the obstetrician and gynecologist should be familiar with the rare forms of these anemias, since the management of these patients on a follow-up basis, once the diagnosis is made and the treatment instituted, is within our service. In most of these hematologic diseases therapy is aimed at curing the disease if possible or instituting therapy to prevent exacerbations if removal of the cause is not feasible.

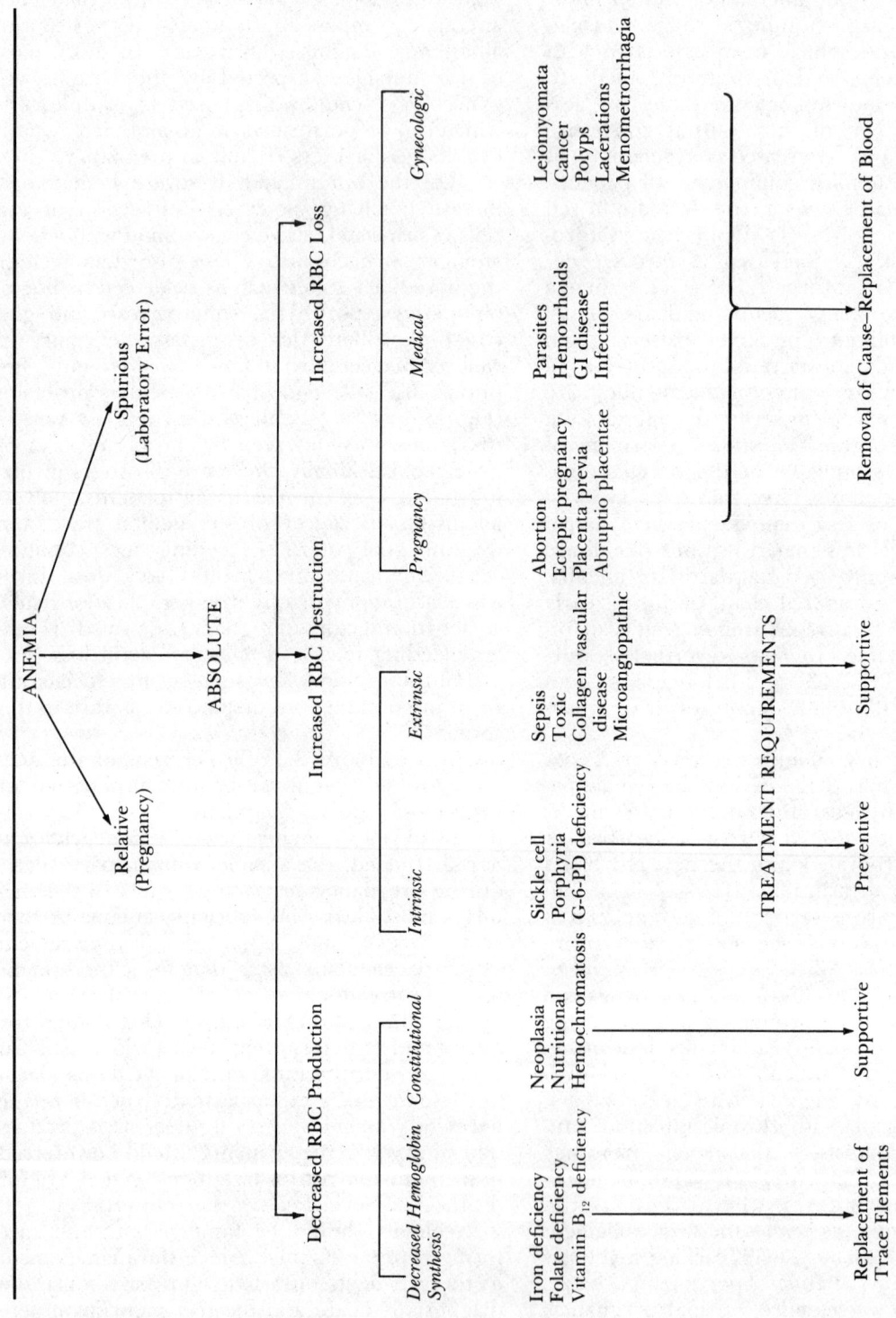

Figure 1. Causes and treatment of anemias.

TABLE 1. Useful Laboratory Tests in the Anemic Patient

	NORMAL NONPREGNANT	NORMAL PREGNANT	ANEMIC
General Screening Assays			
Hemoglobin	12–16 gm/dl	10–13 gm/dl	<10 gm/dl
Packed cell volume	37–45%	30–39%	<30%
Red blood cell count	4.2–5.4 million per cu mm	3.8–4.4 million/cu mm	<3.6 million/cu mm
Mean corpuscular volume	80–100 cu µ/cell	70–90 cu µ/cell	<70 cu µ/cell
Mean corpuscular hemoglobin	27–34 pg/cell	23–31 pg/cell	<20 pg/cell
Mean corpuscular concentration	32–35 gm/dl/RBC	Unchanged	<30 gm/dl/RBC
Reticulocyte count	0.5–1.0%	1.0–2.0%	<0.5–2.0%
Specific Diagnostic Tests			
Serum iron	50–110 µg/dl	30–100 µg/dl	<20 µg/dl
Unsaturated iron binding capacity	250–300 µg/dl	280–400 µg/dl	>400 µg/dl
Transferrin saturation	25–35%	15–30%	<10%
Iron stores (bone marrow)	Adequate ferratin	Unchanged	Decreased
Serum folate	4–16 µ/ml	2–10 µg/ml	<2 µg/ml
Serum vitamin B_{12}	70–85 ng/dl	70–100 ng/dl	<70 ng/dl

Fortunately, more than 95 per cent of the patients with anemia respond to simple trace element replacement. Treatment of iron deficiency anemia should be by oral, elemental iron supplementation, although changes in dietary habits are also crucial. There are many iron preparations but none of them are preferable to simple ferrous sulfate, which is least expensive. Most of these agents contain 200 to 300 mg of iron complex, which yields 40 to 60 mg of elemental iron. Divided administration (three times per day) is preferable because of the absorptive characteristics of the intestinal mucosa. Enteric-coated capsules should be avoided since the iron is released low in the small intestine and cannot be absorbed. Gastrointestinal problems such as diarrhea and constipation may complicate up to 15 per cent of those taking iron. Liquid ferrous sulfate (40 mg per ml) may be substituted in these patients, although dilution of the syrup in 8 to 10 ounces of water or juice is necessary to prevent staining of the teeth. The use of parenteral iron is rarely helpful unless the patient has a gastrointestinal defect which makes the absorption of oral iron impossible, or the patient is noncompliant. Hypersensitivity leads to minor adverse reactions such as a rash and pruritus in 8 to 10 per cent. Major side-effects occur in 0.15 per cent of patients treated with parenteral iron compounds. Likewise, the management of folic acid or vitamin B_{12} deficiency involves simple replacement. Folic acid (0.5 mg) administered twice daily and/or vitamin B_{12} as weekly injections of 7.5 mcg per dose is recommended, and both should be continued for 6 weeks.

Transfusion therapy is necessary for a variety of reasons. Exchange transfusion may be required for the hereditary anemias such as sickle hemoglobinopathies, or thalassemia may require exchange transfusions. This modality is particularly useful during pregnancy, for sickle cell crisis, or prior to a surgical procedure in these patients. Transfusions also may be used preoperatively in any patient prior to major surgery when the hemoglobin is less than 10 mg per dl or in anemic patients with real or potential infection. In those with erythrocyte loss, if the cause of the anemia can be removed and the patient is asymptomatic, transfusions are usually not necessary. For example, postpartum or after minor surgery in asymptomatic healthy women, infusion of red blood cells may not be required even with a hemoglobin as low as 8 gm per dl. Although advances in blood banking and the use of all volunteer donors have made transfusions less dangerous than in the past, the risks of hepatitis and transfusion reactions with subsequent alloimmunization are very real considerations.

Another issue involving transfusion therapy involves the finite resources of blood in this country. Since there are very few communities with adequate stores of blood, transfusions should be given only when required and the appropriate use of component therapy should be emphasized. In most cases the use of packed cells and crystalloid solutions will suffice. If disseminated intravascular coagulation is present, many have recommended whole "fresh" blood to replace clotting factors and platelets. However, this advantage is lost if the blood is more than 6 to 12 hours old, a common occurrence. The use of packed red cells and intravenous solutions is commonly sufficient, particularly if the cause of the disseminated intravascular coagulation is removed. In the event that clotting factors are needed, fresh frozen plasma can be used. In addition cryoprecipitate may be employed if a very small volume of fluid is indicated. In patients with diminished platelet counts infusions of to avoid this problem. However, if at all possible, a pediatrician should be present at the delivery, and naloxone, a specific narcotic antagonist, should be available to reverse respiratory depression in the infant (0.01 mg per kg). Finally, the nursery should be made aware of the potential for infant withdrawal symptoms. Cord blood samples should be sent for drug screening and for hepatitis-associated antigen (HAA) and e-antigen determination in infants of HAA-positive mothers, in order to determine eligibility for hyperimmune globulin prophylaxis.

TREATMENT

Central to all the treatment techniques detailed below is the need for a coordinated medical, social, nutritional, and psychiatric approach with extensive, long-term follow-up. Serial drug screening should be performed. Efforts should be made to remove the patient from her environment and to treat her partner to reduce recidivism.

Abstinence-Oriented Treatment. Depending upon the specific drug(s) of abuse, outpatient or inpatient abstinence oriented treatment, with or without tapering, may be indicated in accordance with the following guidelines:

Outpatient abstinence *without tapering* or maintenance is safe and feasible for users of marijuana, phencyclidine (PCP), psychedelic drugs, amyl nitrate, nitrous oxide, volatile agents, and for occasional users of cocaine.

Inpatient abstinence *without tapering* or maintenance is recommended for regular users of amphetamines and cocaine. Withdrawal of these agents is associated with physical and mental exhaustion, agitated depression, suicidal tendencies, and persistent sleep and appetite disturbances. Serial fetal monitoring should be performed during withdrawal in the third trimester. Although the severity of the psychic changes may be reduced by tapering the dose of amphetamines, the prolongation of fetal exposure is considered undesirable in the absence of marked physiological withdrawal.

Inpatient tapered withdrawal, using phenobarbital, is recommended for users of barbiturates, benzodiazepines, and meprobamate. Withdrawal is associated with gastrointestinal symptoms and, more ominously, with hypotension, seizures, coma, and death. This method is based on a system of substituting an equivalent dosage of phenobarbital for the presumed dosage of the drug of abuse. Although other drugs may be employed for the purpose, we recommend that phenobarbital be substituted for other agents, because it is effective in preventing withdrawal, has a wide margin of safety and has a long half-life, reducing the likelihood of uneven levels and withdrawal episodes. Moreover, it has been used in pregnancy with sufficient frequency that its major risks and effects are familiar to most obstetricians and pediatricians.

Table 4 shows daily doses of common drugs considered equivalent to 30 mg total daily dose of phenobarbital. Starting dosages should be calculated from these equivalents. The appearance of withdrawal symptoms of hypotension, anxiety, or tremor should be covered with an additional 200 mg of short-acting pentobarbital administered hourly until sedation occurs. The basal dose should be re-estimated accordingly. Once a steady state has been reached, levels should be maintained for two days for most drugs; the phenobarbital should then be reduced by no more than 10 per cent or 30 mg daily. Appearance of withdrawal symptoms should be met with a 25 per cent increase in the dose the following day and resumption of tapering, with two specific caveats. First, because withdrawal from benzodiazepines may not occur for up to 10 days, the steady state should be maintained for a week prior to tapering dosage. Second, although barbiturate users of less than 200 mg of phenobarbital (equivalent) daily will generally tolerate withdrawal well, the level at which the fetus experiences withdrawal effects is unknown; therefore, tapering is advised in these patients.

Maintenance. Abstinence from opiates is not feasible for most users and the possibility of occult fetal withdrawal makes even gradual tapering problematic. Also, the use of clonidine, an alpha-agonist currently prescribed in some withdrawal programs, is not recommended during pregnancy. Therefore, methadone maintenance is generally recommended for opiate abusers during pregnancy. Because methadone has

TABLE 4. **Phenobarbital Equivalents of Drugs Which May Be Abused**

	TOTAL DAILY DOSE (MG)*
Amobarbital	100
Butabarbital	60
Chloral hydrate	500
Chlorazepate	50
Chlordiazepoxide	100
Diazepam	50
Flurazepam	60
Glutethimide	250
Meprobamate	500
Methaqualone	300
Oxazepam	100
Pentobarbital	100
Secobarbital	100

*The listed milligrams are considered equivalent to 30 mg of phenobarbital.

TABLE 1. **Useful Laboratory Tests in the Anemic Patient**

	NORMAL NONPREGNANT	NORMAL PREGNANT	ANEMIC
General Screening Assays			
Hemoglobin	12–16 gm/dl	10–13 gm/dl	<10 gm/dl
Packed cell volume	37–45%	30–39%	<30%
Red blood cell count	4.2–5.4 million per cu mm	3.8–4.4 million/cu mm	<3.6 million/cu mm
Mean corpuscular volume	80–100 cu μ/cell	70–90 cu μ/cell	<70 cu μ/cell
Mean corpuscular hemoglobin	27–34 pg/cell	23–31 pg/cell	<20 pg/cell
Mean corpuscular concentration	32–35 gm/dl/RBC	Unchanged	<30 gm/dl/RBC
Reticulocyte count	0.5–1.0%	1.0–2.0%	<0.5–2.0%
Specific Diagnostic Tests			
Serum iron	50–110 μg/dl	30–100 μg/dl	<20 μg/dl
Unsaturated iron binding capacity	250–300 μg/dl	280–400 μg/dl	>400 μg/dl
Transferrin saturation	25–35%	15–30%	<10%
Iron stores (bone marrow)	Adequate ferratin	Unchanged	Decreased
Serum folate	4–16 μ/ml	2–10 μg/ml	<2 μg/ml
Serum vitamin B_{12}	70–85 ng/dl	70–100 ng/dl	<70 ng/dl

Fortunately, more than 95 per cent of the patients with anemia respond to simple trace element replacement. Treatment of iron deficiency anemia should be by oral, elemental iron supplementation, although changes in dietary habits are also crucial. There are many iron preparations but none of them are preferable to simple ferrous sulfate, which is least expensive. Most of these agents contain 200 to 300 mg of iron complex, which yields 40 to 60 mg of elemental iron. Divided administration (three times per day) is preferable because of the absorptive characteristics of the intestinal mucosa. Enteric-coated capsules should be avoided since the iron is released low in the small intestine and cannot be absorbed. Gastrointestinal problems such as diarrhea and constipation may complicate up to 15 per cent of those taking iron. Liquid ferrous sulfate (40 mg per ml) may be substituted in these patients, although dilution of the syrup in 8 to 10 ounces of water or juice is necessary to prevent staining of the teeth. The use of parenteral iron is rarely helpful unless the patient has a gastrointestinal defect which makes the absorption of oral iron impossible, or the patient is noncompliant. Hypersensitivity leads to minor adverse reactions such as a rash and pruritus in 8 to 10 per cent. Major side-effects occur in 0.15 per cent of patients treated with parenteral iron compounds. Likewise, the management of folic acid or vitamin B_{12} deficiency involves simple replacement. Folic acid (0.5 mg) administered twice daily and/or vitamin B_{12} as weekly injections of 7.5 mcg per dose is recommended, and both should be continued for 6 weeks.

Transfusion therapy is necessary for a variety of reasons. Exchange transfusion may be required for the hereditary anemias such as sickle hemoglobinopathies, or thalassemia may require exchange transfusions. This modality is particularly useful during pregnancy, for sickle cell crisis, or prior to a surgical procedure in these patients. Transfusions also may be used preoperatively in any patient prior to major surgery when the hemoglobin is less than 10 mg per dl or in anemic patients with real or potential infection. In those with erythrocyte loss, if the cause of the anemia can be removed and the patient is asymptomatic, transfusions are usually not necessary. For example, postpartum or after minor surgery in asymptomatic healthy women, infusion of red blood cells may not be required even with a hemoglobin as low as 8 gm per dl. Although advances in blood banking and the use of all volunteer donors have made transfusions less dangerous than in the past, the risks of hepatitis and transfusion reactions with subsequent alloimmunization are very real considerations.

Another issue involving transfusion therapy involves the finite resources of blood in this country. Since there are very few communities with adequate stores of blood, transfusions should be given only when required and the appropriate use of component therapy should be emphasized. In most cases the use of packed cells and crystalloid solutions will suffice. If disseminated intravascular coagulation is present, many have recommended whole "fresh" blood to replace clotting factors and platelets. However, this advantage is lost if the blood is more than 6 to 12 hours old, a common occurrence. The use of packed red cells and intravenous solutions is commonly sufficient, particularly if the cause of the disseminated intravascular coagulation is removed. In the event that clotting factors are needed, fresh frozen plasma can be used. In addition cryoprecipitate may be employed if a very small volume of fluid is indicated. In patients with diminished platelet counts infusions of "platelet buttons" can be used as replacement. Fibrinogen which is obtained from pooled serum is no longer commercially available because of the large incidence of hepatitis.

DRUG ABUSE IN PREGNANCY*

NANCY E. JUDGE, M.D.,
and ROBERT J. SOKOL, M.D.

The magnitude of the problem of drug abuse during pregnancy is difficult to estimate because of (1) difficulty in obtaining an accurate history from patients engaged in illegal activities to obtain illicit substances, (2) regional and social differences in patterns of abuse, (3) the failure of addicts to seek prenatal care, and (4) the confounding effects of multiple substance use, including alcohol, cigarettes, and caffeine, on pregnancy outcome. Nonetheless, drug abuse during pregnancy is not rare—over 20 per cent of gravidas at our hospital admit to marijuana use, and at least 2 per cent abuse opiates. Further, drugs of abuse, including amphetamines, cocaine, hallucinogens, marijuana, benzodiazepines, barbiturates, and opiates present a broad and variable spectrum of maternal and fetal risks. In this chapter, as a guide to management, we will first focus on the maternal/fetal/infant complications which may be experienced by drug abusers and of which the clinician should be aware. Management strategies specifically for the assessment and treatment of drug abuse will then be considered. Alcohol abuse is discussed in another article.

MEDICAL/OBSTETRICAL COMPLICATIONS

Maternal Complications. Maternal complications are related to both the drug used and the lifestyle of the user. Most available information is derived from patients addicted primarily to opiates. It appears that when controlled for lack of prenatal care, smoking, and alcohol use, drug users may not be at increased statistical risk for most obstetrical complications; nor do they appear to be more likely than nonpregnant addicts to suffer drug-related problems. In practice, however, these patients do in fact have higher rates of preeclampsia, abruptio placentae, premature rupture of the membranes, and low-birth-weight infants than do non-addicts. Their pregnancies may be complicated by venereal disease, urinary tract infection, hepatitis, subacute bacterial endocarditis, and anemia.

Complications of Fetus and Infant. The consequences of maternal drug use for the offspring are dependent upon the agent and period of exposure. The *teratogenic potential* of most of the drugs of abuse is not well-established; nonetheless, patients should certainly be advised of the suspected associations shown in Table 1. Drug abuse should not in and of itself be considered an indication for therapeutic abortion, but within the framework of these patients' overall life situations, it is at least reasonable to offer the option of pregnancy interruption.

Infants of heroin and barbiturate users are at increased risk for *perinatal morbidity and mortality*. An overdose may expose the fetus to the consequences of maternal hypoxia and metabolic derangement; maternal infections may also include the fetus. Moreover, abuse of these drugs is associated with preterm delivery, intrauterine growth retardation, respiratory depression and hypotonia at birth, and a frequency of meconium staining, with its attendant risk for meconium aspiration, of up to 33 per cent. Adverse neonatal effects have been reported in infants exposed to amphetamines, as well as in those of narcotic and barbiturate users. These effects include hyperactivity, tachypnea, decreased ability to orient to stimuli, and disrupted rapid eye movement (REM) sleep. Infants of opiate users, however, have less respiratory distress syndrome and neonatal jaundice than expected. Further, in pregnancies complicated by opiate abuse, the use of methadone and improved prenatal care appear to increase both infant birth-

TABLE 1. Teratogenic Potential of Drugs of Abuse as Reported in Animal and Human Studies

Amphetamines	Embryotoxic and teratogenic in animal models; transposition of great vessels and cleft palate reported in humans
Barbiturates	Cleft palate reported in conjunction with other agents
Benzodiazepines	Cleft palate, cardiac defects
Cocaine	No known effect
Lysergic acid diethylamide	Chromosomal breakage, increased abortion rate
Marijuana	No definite effect, but possibly increased frequency of anomalies
Methaqualone	Skeletal deformities in rats
Opiates	Effect not well established; possibly increased chromosomal breakage
Phencyclidine	Craniofacial/skeletal syndrome postulated

---

*The authors acknowledge the support of DISCUS, and a grant from the Raleigh Hill Foundation.

undesirable fetal effects, high dose blocking therapy is considered less desirable than establishing maintenance levels. An initial dose of 10 to 20 mg of methadone will prevent withdrawal in the majority of patients and may be given intramuscularly if the patient is in labor or vomiting. Sedation at this dosage suggests a lack of physiological addiction. Virtually all addicts can be maintained at 40 mg daily or less and a gradual tapering of higher doses, at a rate of 5 per cent weekly to reach this level, is advised. If the patient presents in acute withdrawal, an initial dose of meperidine, 50 to 75 mg, may be administered intravenously, since methadone may require up to 60 minutes for onset of action.

Overdose. Cooperative management with a physician expert in drug abuse is highly recommended in caring for the gravid overdose victim. The obstetrician should aid in excluding entities, such as eclampsia, amniotic fluid embolus, and occult abruptio placentae, as well as renal and diabetic conditions, which may be confused with overdose. The obstetrician will also be expected to supervise the assessment of fetal status and to approve agents used in maternal therapy. Although fetal monitoring should be performed, stabilizing maternal condition is the first priority. Moreover, it should be recalled that reversal of maternal hypoxia combined with maternal drug metabolism and elimination may improve an ominous fetal heart rate tracing. In broad general outline, the following steps are appropriate:

1. Assure airway; give oxygen; use cuffed endotracheal tube for comatose or obtunded patients.
2. Monitor mother and fetus; avoid hypoxia, acidosis and alkalosis.
3. Obtain drug screen and chest x-ray.
4. If the mother is apneic, administer naloxone, 0.4 mg intravenously every 6 minutes for three doses as needed.
5. Give glucose, 50 gm intravenous push.
6. Use pressor support, antihypertensives, and anti-arrhythmics, as indicated by the clinical situation.
7. For pulmonary edema, use diuretics and positive pressure ventilation.
8. Encourage emesis, especially for overdose with glutethimide, which has delayed gastric clearance.

Specific agents: (1) Use butyrophenones (e.g., haloperidol 2.5 to 5 mg intramuscularly) for agitation from amphetamines, phencyclidine, or cocaine; diazepam, 5 to 15 mg intravenously, may be used to control seizures. (2) A fluid push of D_5W with potassium chloride, 20 to 60 mEq per liter, followed by alkalinization of the urine using D_5W and sodium bicarbonate, (1 to 2 mEq per kg per liter) and the use of activated charcoal orally will increase barbiturate clearance in severe overdose. (3) To acidify the urine in order to increase phencyclidine and amphetamine clearance, ascorbic acid (500 mg to 2 gm per liter) may be given orally or with an intravenous fluid push of D_5W.

Maternal withdrawal may rapidly follow successful management of an overdose and should be controlled by the techniques previously discussed.

Postpartum. Drug-related risks to both mother and infant persist after birth and should be considered. (1) Most agents are transmitted in breast milk; if infant sedation appears, breast feeding should be discontinued. (2) Infants of drug-abusing mothers are at increased risk for neglect, abuse, learning disabilities, and retarded growth and motor development; placement outside the home is appropriate in some cases. (3) Contraception can also present difficulties—liver disease or poor compliance may reduce the utility of oral contraceptives; the likelihood of venereal disease in association with prostitution increases the risks of the intrauterine contraceptive device. Permanent sterilization may be the only alternative to barrier methods and frequent abortions as contraceptive techniques.

The drug-dependent mother can be and often is a frustrating and difficult patient to manage. A multidisciplinary approach which continues long after delivery currently appears to offer the best chance for improved maternal and infant outcome.

ALCOHOL ABUSE IN PREGNANCY*

ROBERT J. SOKOL, M.D.,
and NANCY E. JUDGE, M.D.

ALCOHOL—A MATERNOFETAL RISK

It has been estimated that approximately 10 million Americans have significant alcohol problems. Although alcoholism was previously thought to be almost entirely limited to men, it is now recognized that problem drinking is not rare among women, particularly among those in the reproductive age range. Thus, for example, among pregnant women on the authors' service, over 10 per cent score positively on the Michigan Alcoholism Screening Test (MAST), a widely

---

*The authors acknowledge the support of DISCUS, and a grant from the Raleigh Hill Foundation.

used and well validated instrument for the detection of alcohol problems. Moreover, some data indicate that women may develop severe medical sequelae, e.g., cirrhosis, more rapidly than men. Therefore, alcohol abuse should be considered an important maternal risk.

Since antiquity, alcohol use during pregnancy has been suspected of having adverse effects on the offspring. Although research findings during the late nineteenth and first half of the twentieth centuries tended to support this suspicion, it was not until 1973 that the term "fetal alcohol syndrome" was coined to denote the following constellation of findings:

1. Growth retardation, both prenatal and postnatal; often these individuals remain small during childhood;

2. Central nervous system involvement, often marked in the neonate by microcephaly; may be manifested by hyperactivity and mental retardation during childhood;

3. Abnormal facies, particularly mid-facial hypoplasia, including short upturned nose, thin upper lip, strabismus, and possibly small palpebral fissures.

Recognition of this syndrome has led to a flood of papers concerning alcohol as a fetal risk—over 800 in the past decade. Based on in vitro and in vivo animal studies, it is clear that in high doses, alcohol (ethanol) and its metabolites are embryotoxic and teratogenic. In humans, approximately 450 cases of fetal alcohol syndrome have now been reported. It appears that the full syndrome probably occurs only in fetuses of chronic alcoholic women who drink heavily during pregnancy.

Full fetal alcohol syndrome occurs in about 2.5 per cent of the pregnancies complicated by abusive drinking or, calculated for all patients, at a rate of about 1 in 1000 births. Were fetal alcohol syndrome the extent of the problem, maternal alcohol ingestion would not be considered an important fetal risk. However, from available studies of human pregnancy, it is clear that fetal alcohol syndrome represents only the tip of the iceberg and that abusive drinking, which may occur in 3 to 5 per cent of pregnancies, is associated with a range of adverse outcomes. These "possible fetal alcohol effects," which may occur in the absence of the full syndrome, are summarized in Table 1. Among very heavy or frequent drinkers, the risk for spontaneous abortion is increased about twofold. Congenital anomalies associated with heavy alcohol intake include cardiac anomalies, particularly septal defects, and genitourinary abnormalities, such as hypospadias. When one examines the overall pregnancy outcomes of patients with significant

TABLE 1. **Risks for Abnormal Pregnancy Outcome in Alcohol-Abusing Gravidas**

	RISK INCREASED	RATE (%)
Spontaneous abortion	2X	30
Perinatal mortality	?Slight	—
Fetal alcohol syndrome	—	2.5
Congenital anomalies—e.g., facial, cardiac, genitourinary and other minor anomalies	4X	40
Intrauterine growth retardation	2.5X	25
Neonatal depression	1.5X	20
Abnormal neurobehavioral development—in children without full fetal alcohol syndrome	Probably	—

alcohol problems, 50 to 70 per cent of the offspring appear to demonstrate some effects.

The documented fetomaternal risks indicate that alcohol abuse during pregnancy should be considered a major public health concern and that appropriate detection and treatment of abusive drinking during pregnancy warrant the attention of the practitioner.

DETECTING THE RISK

The first step in managing alcohol abuse in pregnancy is detecting the problem. Unfortunately, most obstetricians and gynecologists have had no training in obtaining this history. Indeed, our experience is that many clinicians have never detected an alcohol problem among their patients. In addition to the absence of training, another reason for failure to detect this problem is that many clinicians believe that their patients will become angry if asked about alcohol use. This is not the case. If the clinician asks his or her patient, "You don't drink, do you?," one can be sure that the answer will be negative. Denial is a major symptom of alcoholism. The patient does not wish to tell the doctor about her alcohol problem, and when the doctors ask the question in this way, they send the message that they really do not want to know.

To obtain a history of alcohol abuse successfully, some general guidelines should be kept in mind.

1. The clinician must be alert to clues, such as psychosocial disruption. Our experience indicates that women going through a divorce are at greatly increased risk for alcohol abuse.

2. The clinician must transmit a nonjudgmental attitude to the patient. Acceptance by the physician is an important component of the doctor-patient relationship. If the patient perceives

a threat to her relationship to the physician, she is unlikely to discuss her problem.

3. A history of alcohol problems should be obtained as a routine part of the obstetric/gynecologic history, in the same way as other health-related habits are sought.

One series of questions which we have found effective in obtaining a history of alcohol abuse is shown in Table 2. There are, of course, other approaches with which individual clinicians may be more comfortable. We begin with the family history. Although it is true that alcohol problems do tend to be familial, the answer to this question is not crucial. Its purpose is to establish the fact that the physician considers alcohol use a health issue. Alcohol use is next questioned in the review of systems portion of the history, generally immediately after asking about smoking. If the patient smokes and/or has a history of illicit drug use, the chance of alcohol abuse is increased. If she responds that she never takes a drink, then no further questions are necessary. If the patient states she does sometimes use alcoholic beverages, then further questioning is warranted.

Asking the patient directly how much she drinks is unlikely to yield a valid estimate, because of denial. Rather, the clinician should focus on eliciting a history of *tolerance*. Women who have high alcohol intakes may report being able to "hold" a six-pack or one or two bottles of wine without feeling "high." Finally, the question concerning amount of drinking should not be left open-ended. Rather, the clinician should suggest a high amount to transmit the message to the patient that it is "okay" to admit to this level of alcohol intake. Thus, for example, if the patient is a beer drinker, one might ask "How much do you usually drink? Two or three six packs?" Normal drinkers will laugh and answer, "Oh, not that much—just two or three cans." However, some patients will report amounts which may seem truly prodigious to the clinician, leaving little question as to the diagnosis.

MANAGEMENT

Initial Steps

During pregnancy women are motivated to improve their health practices. *Just asking patients about their alcohol use is itself therapeutic.* Many women, including very heavy drinkers, become abstinent during pregnancy. If the physician indicates his/her concern about drinking, this tendency can be maximized. Many women who abuse alcohol have reported to us that it is easier for them to decrease or stop their drinking than it is for them to decrease or stop smoking.

Based on available data from the literature, it appears to be warranted to tell patients that if they can decrease their drinking, they can help themselves have a healthier baby. This statement appears to be true in the case of women who drink very heavily. With respect to women who are moderate drinkers or who occasionally have a drink, data are not available to indicate significant risk to the fetus and, in the opinion of the authors, patients who report that they had an occasional drink early in pregnancy or that they have an occasional glass of wine, for example, on the weekend, should be reassured that it is unlikely to have any adverse effect on the fetus. Finally, the fact that risks of heavy alcohol use have been discussed with the patient should be documented in the medical record.

Further Antepartum Management

Some authors have suggested that women with chronic alcohol problems who continue to drink heavily during early pregnancy have a high enough rate of abnormal outcomes to warrant therapeutic abortion. Review of Table 1 indicates, however, that even among very heavy drinking women, only a limited proportion have infants with the full fetal alcohol syndrome.

TABLE 2. **Flow of Questions Seeking Alcohol Abuse in Routine Obstetric/Gynecologic Examination**

QUESTION	COMMENTS
Family History	
Anybody in your family with alcohol problems?	Establishes that a doctor considers alcohol a health issue
Review of Systems—Habits	
Do you ever take a drink? ↓	If never, no further questions necessary
Beer, wine or liquor? ↓	Preferred beverage
When—weekends, after work, etc.? ↓	Timing
How much does it take to make you feel tipsy or high? ↓	KEY QUESTION—TOLERANCE
How much do you usually drink?	Suggest high amount

Clearly, therapeutic abortion is not warranted in every case. On the other hand, in view of the psychosocial disruption often experienced by these patients, the option of abortion should not be withheld.

Through the antepartum period, it is crucial that the clinician maintain contact with the patient. Laboratory assessment of liver function and repeated drug screens should be obtained. Also, at each antenatal visit the clinician should inquire as to how the patient is doing in controlling her drinking. Repeated encouragement to maintain abstinence or, at least, to minimize drinking episodes, is most helpful. If heavy drinking continues, consultation with an alcohol rehabilitation unit and sometimes referral to Alcoholics Anonymous may be beneficial. Our experience, however, has been that it is difficult to motivate obstetrical patients to see health care professionals other than the obstetrician, so that major responsibility remains with the primary physician.

Specific Alcohol-Related Problems

Both intoxication and withdrawal (abstinence) syndromes may occur during and complicate pregnancy. Some general guidelines may be helpful before proceeding to management of specific problems.

1. Alcohol abuse is associated with poor nutrition. Both alcohol abuse and poor nutrition increase the risk for intrauterine growth retardation, which is, in turn, associated with increased perinatal morbidity and mortality. Nutritional consultation and vitamin supplementation, including thiamine, are appropriate for alcohol abusing gravidas during the antepartum period.

2. Occasional women with chronic alcohol problems may be on disulfiram (Antabuse) when they enter pregnancy. Also, beginning a patient on disulfiram (Antabuse) may be recommended by a consultant. This drug should, however, be avoided during pregnancy, inasmuch as there are convincing data that disulfiram is, in and of itself, teratogenic.

3. Both intoxication and withdrawal problems, which might be treated on an outpatient basis in the nonpregnant state, warrant hospitalization during pregnancy. Alcohol freely crosses the placenta and, based on acute animal studies, appears to be associated with fetal acidosis. Further, although there does not appear to be a fetal withdrawal syndrome of significance for alcohol, as there appears to be for opiates, it is reasonable to suggest hospitalization for fetal surveillance. Electronic and biochemical fetal monitoring are warranted. It should also be noted that alcohol-abusing patients often sign out of the hospital against medical advice. Indeed, hospital sign-out against advice should be considered an indicator for possible alcohol or drug abuse problems, and these problems should be sought if a patient does sign out.

4. The obstetrician will not, in general, be expert in the management of specific alcohol problems. Hence, *consultation* with a clinician expert in this area, often an internist or psychiatrist, is highly recommended. The obstetrician's role should be that of supporting choices for specific medications, in terms of their effects on pregnancy and the fetus, providing appropriate fetal surveillance and maintaining a close doctor-patient relationship.

Intoxication. Alcohol intoxication may be divided into three levels of severity—acute, "pathological," and coma. The characteristics and appropriate treatment of each during pregnancy are shown in Table 3. In pregnancy, intoxication severe enough to bring the patient to the hospital warrants hospitalization. The fact that women who abuse alcohol are at considerably increased likelihood to abuse other drugs as well, is indication for obtaining a "drug screen" for all such patients (see the article *"Drug Abuse in Pregnancy"*). "Pathological" intoxication and

TABLE 3. **Alcohol Intoxication Phenomena and Treatment**

TYPE	CHARACTERISTICS	TREATMENT
Acute	Excitement, followed by lethargy Blood alcohol 0.1 to 0.4 per cent	None specific Obtain "drug screen"
"Pathological"	Aggressive behavior Disorientation Occasionally suicidal Later amnesia	Diazepam, 5 to 10 mg slow IV *or* Sodium luminol, 120 mg IM Protect patient from injury
Coma	Medical emergency Depressed respiration Shock	Airway and respiratory support Prevent aspiration Obtain blood glucose and electrolyte levels and drug screen Give 50 grams glucose IV Evaluate for trauma—chest and skull X rays Start IV—avoid overhydration Gastric lavage, because of possibility of other drugs

coma are very rare. Coma should not, of course, be attributed automatically to alcohol even in known alcohol abusing patients, because of the possibilities of other drug use, trauma, and other causes. This is a medical emergency and consultation should be obtained immediately.

Withdrawal (Abstinence) Syndromes. The complexity of alcohol withdrawal phenomena is frequently underestimated by clinicians unfamiliar with this problem. Indeed, there is a major disagreement, even among experts, as to the most appropriate way to characterize and classify these problems. One classification synthesized from several authoritative sources is shown, along with the characteristics of each stage, in Table 4. Delirium tremens should be viewed as the most severe stage of withdrawal and is associated with significant mortality. Withdrawal symptoms are seen in pregnancy, but the severest stage, delirium tremens, is very rare—only a few cases have been reported in the literature. Many drugs used for nonpregnant patients should be avoided during pregnancy. These include beta blockers and lithium. Specific recommendations for treatment of each stage during pregnancy are shown in Table 5. These recommendations are based on selection of appropriate options for therapy, taking pregnancy into consideration.

Tremulousness is the mildest and most common form of withdrawal symptom. To replace the "missing sedative," some authorities suggest the use of decreasing doses of alcohol for treatment. On the other hand, the effects of barbiturates in pregnancy are well known and they may be used sparingly in this situation. It is crucial, however, to avoid heavily medicating these patients, since there is a risk of substituting dependence upon barbiturates for dependence on alcohol.

Hallucinosis may occur in association with alcoholism even in the absence of withdrawal. Haloperidol is a major tranquilizer related to the phenothiazines. It is an excellent anti-hallucinatory drug, and hypotension is rarer than with phenothiazines, an advantage for use during pregnancy. Although it is considered the drug of choice for hallucinosis, its use in the first trimester should be avoided, since it has been reported to be teratogenic, having been associated with phocomelia.

Seizures during pregnancy constitute an important fetal risk because of hypoxia. Seizures secondary to alcohol withdrawal should be dif-

TABLE 4. **Alcohol Withdrawal (Abstinence) Phenomena**

TYPE	SYNONYM	CHARACTERISTICS
Tremulousness	"The shakes"	Neuromuscular hyperexcitability and autonomic hyperactivity: tremor, nausea, vomiting, restlessness, sleeplessness, tachycardia, sweating
		Acute anxiety
		Severe for 24 to 48 hours
		May last 1 to 2 weeks
Hallucinosis		Hallucinations: almost always threatening; usually auditory, but may be visual or tactile
		Agitation but relatively clear sensorium
		Risk for suicide
		Sometimes seen without withdrawal
Seizures	"Rum fits"	Onset 12 to 48 hours after last drink
		Grand mal
		Often clusters of 2 to 6
		Abnormal electroencephalogram
		About one fourth may proceed to DT's
Delerium tremens	"DT's"	Life-threatening to 5 to 10 per cent of those withdrawing
		Above features, plus increasing blood pressure (sometimes > 180/110), respiratory rate, body temperature, may develop bronchopneumonia, adrenal exhaustion
		About 20 per cent mortality

TABLE 5. **Alcohol Withdrawal Treatment Guidelines for Use During Pregnancy**

TYPE	TREATMENT
Tremulousness	Psychological support
	Mild sedation for sleep—barbiturate
	Avoid dependence on another drug
Hallucinosis	Haloperidol, 5 mg IM q 2 hours initially, then po tid
Seizures	Oxygen by nasal prongs
	Electronic fetal monitoring
	Diazepam, 10 mg slow IV push
	Magnesium sulfate can be considered
Delerium tremens	Quiet, well-lighted surroundings
	Avoid overhydration
	Watch for electrolyte imbalance and hypoglycemia
	Neuroleptics and anticonvulsants, as above
	Thiamine 100 mg IM, plus other B vitamins
	IV corticosteroids for cardiovascular collapse

ferentiated from eclampsia, based on concomitant clinical features and laboratory parameters. In the clinical setting, however, treatment may be required before a decision as to etiology can be made. Currently, diazepam by slow intravenous push should be considered the acute treatment of choice. It is of interest, nonetheless, that seizures related to alcohol withdrawal have been associated in the literature with hypomagnesemia and that magnesium therapy is recommended. Although so far unreported, it may be speculated that treatment with magnesium sulfate in the usual therapeutic anticonvulsant doses might well be an appropriate choice during pregnancy.

Treatment of *delirium tremens* can be expected to require neuroleptics and anticonvulsants, as described above. There is marked disagreement in the literature as to the most appropriate fluid management for these patients. Although some may be overhydrated, vomiting and perspiration may lead to dehydration. Therefore, therapy should be individualized, based upon serum electrolyte levels, blood urea nitrogen, and creatinine clearance.

The Intrapartum Period

Little has been published concerning problems of alcohol abuse as related to labor and delivery. Based on a large study from our Center, it appears that risk for premature rupture of the membranes may be slightly increased and that risks for amnionitis and neonatal infection are distinctly increased. The same data indicated that uterine hypercontractility and fetal distress, with abnormal fetal heart rate tracings, evidence of fetal acidosis, and lowered Apgar scores, are also increased in pregnancies complicated by alcohol abuse. Intrapartum fetal monitoring is indicated. Finally, significant intoxication is sometimes seen upon admission in labor, apparently based on heavy maternal drinking as an analgesic early in labor. Guard against maternal aspiration.

The pediatrician should be informed about alcohol-abusing patients. Neonatal alcohol withdrawal of significance is relatively rare, but does occur. These newborns tend to be jittery, but neonatal seizures, such as those associated with maternal barbiturate abuse, should not be anticipated. However, as shown in Table 1, these infants are at risk for fetal alcohol syndrome, as well as congenital anomalies, growth retardation, and long-term neurobehavioral abnormality. Thus, a long-term plan for infant follow-up should be implemented.

Puerperal Management

Stress reduction is viewed as important in the pathogenesis of abusive drinking. The birth of a new baby and its demands on the mother certainly constitute a major life stress, even for the healthy woman. Thus, maternal drinking may increase during the postpartum period. Further, infants of alcohol abusing mothers have been reported to have sleep state disturbances and decreased ability to habituate to stimuli. An infant with these problems would be expected to be particularly difficult to care for. Thus, alcohol abusing mothers require significant psychological support and the obstetrician should attempt to bring his or her alcohol-abusing patients to long-term therapy for their alcohol problems.

Finally, maternal alcohol abuse may constitute a risk to the infant in terms of failure to thrive and child battering. Consideration, in severe cases of abusive drinking, of infant placement is warranted and may necessitate the involvement of appropriate social service agencies.

AMNIONITIS

DAVID J. NOCHIMSON, M.D.,
and DANIEL CLEMENT, M.D.

Amnionitis usually occurs in association with premature rupture of the membranes or prolonged labor, although it may occur in the absence of both. The most frequent route of infection is transcervical, but transplacental contamination can occur, especially with viral disease and maternal bacteremia.

Many predisposing factors have been elicited, namely parity, malnutrition, coitus (especially in the latter half of pregnancy), vaginal infections, numerous vaginal examinations during labor, and a latent period of approximately 24 hours between rupture of the membranes and the onset of labor. The clinical signs include maternal fever, fetal tachycardia, uterine tenderness, and a purulent (sometimes foul-smelling) discharge from the cervix. Suggestive laboratory findings may include a more accentuated maternal leukocytosis with a possible shift to the left, and white blood cells or bacteria on examination of the amniotic fluid.

Premature rupture of the membranes is the major associated cause of amnionitis and remains one of the more controversial management problems in obstetrics today. If rupture of the membranes occurs at term (greater than 36 weeks), 80 per cent of the patients will be in spontaneous labor within 24 hours. With prudent management of labor, including infrequent pelvic examinations, and with prompt labor and delivery, amnionitis usually is not a major factor. Some authorities recommend a latent period of 6 to 18 hours before instituting oxytocin therapy in the term patient. Others feel that immediate oxytocin therapy should be instituted using a constant infusion pump, with continuous fetal heart rate and uterine activity monitoring, preferably utilizing internal monitoring systems. Controversy exists regarding the use of antibiotic treatment because of inadequate data relating to fetal antibiotic concentrations. Some institutions have noted higher incidences of amnionitis and tend to favor earlier induction of labor with oxytocin and the use of antibiotic coverage.

With rupture of the membranes in the preterm fetus greater than 33 weeks' gestational age, many authorities favor the induction of labor to avoid the serious consequences of amnionitis, feeling that the neonatologist can better treat mild respiratory distress syndrome than a severely infected fetus.

Considerable controversy exists regarding management of premature rupture of the membranes in the preterm pregnancy of less than 33 weeks' gestation. A division of opinion exists regarding the aggressive invasive diagnostic detection of potential chorioamnionitis in order to identify the group of fetuses which require immediate delivery, thus allowing the non-infected group to remain in utero for additional fetal growth. A second group favors initiation of delivery in all premature fetuses with rupture of the membranes in order to avoid chorioamnionitis and an infected fetus. Most all authorities favor prompt delivery of the fetus with signs of developing amnionitis. The use of prophylactic antibiotics in the preterm fetus (less than 33 weeks) with rupture of membranes remains controversial.

The value of prophylactic antibiotic therapy to prevent amnionitis remains controversial. If amnionitis is documented, antibiotics can be started during labor, although some authorities favor prompt delivery, withholding antibiotics until the cord is clamped except with serious maternal septicemia, in which case maternal considerations outweigh neonatal considerations. Ampicillin is used in recommended doses of 500 to 2000 mg intravenously every 6 hours. Some authorities feel that antibiotics should be given during delivery following clamping of the cord (in order to obtain untreated neonatal cultures). After delivery, an aminoglycoside (kanamycin, 500 mg every 6 hours, or gentamicin, 60 to 80 mg every 12 hours) is used, particularly if there is severe infection. Placenta, amnion, and amniotic fluid should be cultured following delivery. At the time of cesarean section, the amniotic membranes and endometrial cavity are preferred culture sites for identification of the organism. If anaerobic pathogens are identified by culture, one may elect to add clindamycin (150 to 300 mg every 6 hours). Others may readily initiate triple antibiotic treatment in the immediate postpartum period as soon as the diagnosis of amnionitis or endometritis is entertained.

The timing and mode of delivery and antibiotic treatment are important and should be individualized following basic management guidelines. Prevention and early detection of amnionitis remains the best treatment. Further studies in the areas of amniotic fluid collection (amniocentesis), culture, Gram stain, and analysis for fetal maturity in the presence of premature rupture of the membranes are needed to improve both the diagnosis and management of amnionitis.

ANESTHESIA FOR LABOR AND DELIVERY

GERARD M. BASSELL, M.D.

The provision of safe methods of pain relief for labor and delivery is an important component of modern obstetric care. Well-chosen analgesia not only enhances the parturient woman's ability to experience the birth process but, by alleviating pain, fear, and apprehension, can produce important physiologic benefits for both gravida and fetus. In this regard, prevention of excessive maternal hyperventilation, mitigation of the parturient's propensity to produce lactic acid during painful labor, and reduction of the catecholamine response to physical and psychological stress are of immense importance to maternal and fetal well-being, particularly in those labors which have been identified as "high risk."

Apart from assuring the effectiveness and safety of the type of analgesia chosen for childbirth, the obstetrician must consider the effect on maternal awareness. Women are increasingly concerned about the passive and often sedated role they have been forced to accept in labor suites in the past, and some have begun to feel that their only alternatives are to refuse all medication during parturition or to seek alternate locations where they could deliver their offspring "naturally." It is unfortunate that such alienation from the medical mainstream has occurred but the lesson is clear: women must be informed, active participants in parturition and, should analgesia be required, only those methods with the largest margin of maternal and fetal safety and minimal effect on the mother's level of consciousness should be considered. Thus, in the paragraphs that follow, emphasis will be given to those types of pain relief which attempt to satisfy the abovementioned guidelines.

ANALGESIA FOR THE FIRST STAGE OF LABOR

Narcotics and Tranquilizers. Narcotics and tranquilizers are the most commonly used means of relieving labor pain. They are usually administered once active labor has begun and, provided that the dosages used are not excessive, should not affect uterine activity or the progress of labor. Meperidine is the narcotic most often employed, as it is believed that less maternal and neonatal depression occurs with it than with other narcotic analgesics such as morphine.

Notwithstanding the apparent advantages of one narcotic over another, there are some guidelines to their use in labor. First, the gravida must realize that the pain relief provided by *safe* doses of drug will be incomplete or, in some women, minimal. Thus, if substantial analgesia is not achieved with the usual intravenous doses of meperidine, 25 to 50 mg, further amounts should not be given. Second, the addition of small doses of tranquilizers, such as hydroxyzine, 25 to 50 mg, can improve the quality of analgesia achieved without a significant increase in the risk of neonatal respiratory depression. Third, the likelihood of adverse effects on the newborn is heightened when narcotics are given to the laboring woman within 3 hours of delivery. Fourth, the availability of the pure narcotic antagonist naloxone allows rapid and effective reversal of neonatal respiratory depression resulting from administration of a narcotic to the mother. Since naloxone exerts its effect almost immediately, there is nothing to be gained by administering it to the parturient immediately before delivery. In fact, such speculative therapy has the disadvantage of reversing any residual analgesia which the gravida may possess at a time when she is most in need of adequate pain relief. It is rational, then, to assess the newborn's level of consciousness and respiratory effort and to administer naloxone (0.01 mg per kg) only if necessary. The preferred route of administration is intramuscular, as naloxone's length of action is shorter than that of the narcotics and renarcotization is a possibility when the newborn receives the drug intravenously. Finally, the inherent limitations of narcotics should be realized. Unlike conduction methods of analgesia which effectively block specific spinal segments without affecting the parturient's level of consciousness, systemically administered analgesics are nonspecific in their action and can produce significant central nervous system depression as an accompaniment of pain relief. Thus, maternal awareness and ability to cooperate can be affected adversely. This is an extremely important consideration and should be weighed against the major advantage of using narcotics during labor, namely, that they do not require the presence of an anesthesiologist.

Epidural Analgesia. Although the administration and management of epidural block requires a significant degree of skill, knowledge, and time commitment on the part of the anesthesiologist or obstetrician, the advantages of the technique to both the laboring woman and the obstetric care team make the amount of involvement worthwhile. During the first stage of labor, pain is perceived at the tenth thoracic through first lumbar spinal segments, so sensory block at these levels by a lumbar epidural technique is usually extremely effective, does not affect the progress of labor adversely, and provides an excellent margin of safety for both mother and fetus. In addition, the laboring woman retains full use of her faculties and can play an active and appropriate role in her own labor and parturition.

Apart from possessing the requisite technical skills, the person providing epidural analgesia must be adept at treating the possible complications. In the vast majority of cases, careful institution and management of the block will prevent complications, but the proper drugs and equipment must always be at hand should untoward events occur. Thus, suction, oxygen, endotracheal tubes, laryngoscopes, and a self-inflating resuscitator must be immediately available in the labor room or on the epidural cart, and thiopental sodium and ephedrine must be prepared and drawn into syringes.

The major complications of epidural block occur either as a side-effect of the block itself or as a result of insertion of the needle or catheter. The latter include accidental perforation of the dura mater or blood vessels in the epidural space and can lead to inadvertent subarachnoid or intravenous injection of local anesthetic if the mishap is not recognized. The epidural block itself can produce hypotension, particularly when the laboring woman has not been adequately hydrated before induction of the anesthetic or if she has been allowed to assume the supine position.

Although each of the complications mentioned above must be explained in detail to the gravida before she can give consent for the procedure, serious consequences of epidural analgesia are, for the most part, avoidable by strict attention to the following guidelines: First, acute intravenous hydration with a minimum of 750 ml of balanced salt solution must precede the initial injection of local anesthetic into the epidural space. The volume of fluid infused will need to be increased if a more extensive block is required, since more sympathetic segments will be involved and the likelihood of hypotension will be increased. Second, gentle aspiration through the epidural needle or catheter should demonstrate subarachnoid or intravascular placement. Negative aspiration does not, however, exclude malposition. Third, even when no cerebrospinal fluid or blood has returned, test doses of local anesthetic should be administered. The initial volume of 2 ml of local anesthetic is given to exclude subarachnoid placement. If it is injected into the cerebrospinal fluid, symptoms and signs of a spinal block should appear within 2 to 3 minutes. If no such events occur, the second test dose is administered. Here, 4 to 5 ml of drug is given to exclude intravascular placement. This amount of local anesthetic should be sufficient to produce symptoms if intravenous injection does, in fact, take place. Thus, the woman should be questioned about such symptoms as sudden drowsiness, unusual tastes, or auditory phenomena. In most gravidas, provided they have been positioned properly, the two test doses will be sufficient to produce segmental analgesia of the tenth thoracic through first lumbar dermatomes. Occasionally, 1 to 2 ml more may be required to include segments missed by the initial administration.

Finally, the importance of position cannot be overemphasized. At no time during labor should the parturient be allowed to lie supine. Aortocaval compression prejudices placental perfusion and, in the presence of epidural block, makes severe hypotension more likely. Even if marked falls in maternal blood pressure do not occur, the apparent cardiovascular stability may be the result of widespread compensatory peripheral vasoconstriction and the uteroplacental circulation may be involved in the phenomenon.

Strict attention to the above points will avoid most of the serious complications related to epidural anesthesia during labor. If side-effects do occur, however, they must be treated rapidly and appropriately. Significant falls in maternal blood pressure must be reversed quickly if fetal well-being is to be unaffected. Thus, frequent measurement of brachial blood pressure after institution of the epidural block will identify any trend toward hypotension, and the rate of intravenous infusion can be increased. Should the blood pressure fall to dangerous levels (less than 100 torr or more than a 20 per cent drop) despite adequate uterine displacement and rapid intravenous infusion, administration of ephedrine is indicated. The initial dose should be 5 mg intravenously and this can be repeated if there has been no upward movement of the blood pressure within 2 minutes of injection.

Accidental injection of local anesthetic intended for the epidural space into the cerebrospinal fluid will produce a more extensive block than intended. Proper attention to test doses and administration of large volumes of drug (say for cesarean section) in intermittent, 4 to 5 ml aliquots will prevent total spinal anesthesia but should it occur, the airway must be maintained (with endotracheal intubation, if necessary), any hypotension should be treated as described above, and the parturient should be told what is happening. This is a situation in which a short-acting anesthetic such as 2-chloroprocaine has a distinct advantage in that the block will be predictably short lived.

Intravascular injection of local anesthetic can present a bolus of drug to the brain and heart sufficient to cause convulsions and even cardiac arrest. Again, these complications should be preventable by adherence to good technique and are less likely to occur when an ester drug with a large margin of safety, such as 2-chloroprocaine, is used. If convulsions do occur, however, the maternal airway must be maintained and oxygen administered, until they subside. Prolonged seizures may occur when longer-acting amide drugs such as bupivacaine are used and may require the intravenous injection of 25 to 50 mg of thiopental sodium to suppress them.

ANALGESIA FOR THE SECOND STAGE OF LABOR

Inhalation Analgesia. It is important to distinguish between the terms "analgesia" and "anesthesia" when describing inhalational methods of pain relief for the second stage of labor. Whereas the former term describes a safe and effective technique by which subanesthetic concentrations of anesthetic gases or vapors are administered to a conscious parturient by mask, the latter refers to production of a state of unconsciousness. There is no place for inhalation *anesthesia* in the conduct of uncomplicated vaginal deliveries. The risks to the mother and her infant far outweigh any perceived benefit. Likewise, administration to term-pregnant women of anesthetic gases and vapors by mask remains safe only as long as subanesthetic amounts are used.

Inhalation *analgesia,* on the other hand, can play an important role in vaginal delivery by producing effective pain relief and relaxation while, at the same time, the parturient retains her ability to cooperate during the expulsion phase. Relatively low inspired concentrations of nitrous oxide (40 to 50 per cent), methoxyflurane (0.2 to 0.4 per cent) or, more recently, enflurane (0.25 to 1.25 per cent) have been shown to be suitable analgesics for the second stage of labor, particularly when combined with bilateral blockade of the pudendal nerves. The small amounts of anesthetic used do not produce loss of maternal protective reflexes, and the high concentrations of oxygen administered aid in the preservation of fetal well-being during the stresses of passage through the birth canal.

Intravenous Analgesia. In situations in which a rapid onset of intense analgesia is required for performance of complicated vaginal deliveries, very low doses of intravenous ketamine are safe and effective. The amounts used are far lower than those required for the induction of general anesthesia; usually 5 to 10 mg are given initially and repeated as required up to a total dose of 25 to 30 mg. In contrast, when employed for induction of anesthesia, 1 to 2 mg per kg is the usual intravenous dose. These small amounts preserve maternal consciousness and protective reflexes, produce their effect rapidly, and are not associated with newborn depression. In addition, the dysphoric side-effects common with larger doses are avoided.

Pudendal Nerve Block. Blockade of the pudendal nerves is a widely used means of providing pain relief for the second stage of labor. The analgesia produced is sufficient for low forceps deliveries and for episiotomy repair. The degree of maternal satisfaction with the technique is enhanced when it is administered in combination with either the inhalation or the intravenous methods outlined above. The major risk associated with pudendal nerve block is intravascular injection of local anesthetic, but precautionary measures such as aspiration before injection, use of the minimum effective dose (10 ml of 2 per cent 2-chloroprocaine or 1 per cent lidocaine per side), and slow injection should prevent serious maternal consequences. Local anesthetics that have been shown to have a prolonged half-life in the newborn (e.g., mepivacaine) should be avoided, as the fetus is exposed to relatively high concentrations of drug owing to the proximity of the injection site to maternal blood vessels.

Subarachnoid (Saddle) Block. Saddle block consists of injecting a very low dose of hyperbaric local anesthetic (tetracaine, 2 to 4 mg, or lidocaine, 20 to 40 mg) into the cerebrospinal fluid with the parturient in the sitting position. The extent of analgesia is limited both by the small amount of drug used and by maintaining the sitting position for 4 to 5 minutes after injection. The ideal block involves only the sacral roots, preserves abdominal muscle tone, and relaxes the pelvic floor.

The complications are those related to sympathetic blockade and perforation of the dura mater. Thus, maternal hypotension is a possibility, as is post–lumbar puncture headache. A significant fall in blood pressure should be preventable by acute intravenous hydration before injection of the local anesthetic (at least 1000 ml of a balanced salt solution). In addition, the limited extent of blockade decreases the likelihood of hypotension. Performance of the lumbar puncture with a 25- or 26-gauge spinal needle reduces the incidence of post–lumbar puncture headache to around 1 per cent.

Saddle block has a number of advantages. First, the technique is simple to perform and, unlike epidural analgesia, there is an easily recognizable end-point, cerebrospinal fluid. Second, the quality of sensory block and perineal muscle relaxation is intense and allows the performance of forceps deliveries and other operative maneuvers comfortably. Third, retention of abdominal muscle tone preserves the parturient's ability to bear down effectively. Finally, the tiny doses of local anesthetic used and their site of injection preclude significant placental transfer of drug.

Epidural Block. Modification of an epidural block that has been used for the first stage of labor to provide pain relief for delivery is a simple matter. Ten to 12 ml of 2-chloroprocaine (3 per cent) is injected through the epidural catheter with the woman in the semi-sitting position to restrict the analgesia to the sacral segments. The same precautions as outlined for induction of the block must be taken to prevent complications. Use of 2-chloroprocaine has the advantage of rapidity of onset, and the 3 per cent concentration produces profound analgesia and perineal muscle relaxation. Like saddle block, this type of analgesia is well suited to most operative vaginal obstetrics.

ANESTHESIA FOR CESAREAN SECTION

The desire of the majority of women to retain consciousness during childbirth extends to cesarean section. Except in very few situations, abdominal delivery can be performed safely under spinal or epidural block. There are, however, contraindications to the use of regional anesthesia. Obvious or suspected hemorrhage, inability to augment blood volume acutely, and patient refusal are the most common circumstances under which conduction block should not be performed.

Regional Techniques. Should regional anesthesia be chosen, the extent of sympathetic blockade will be more widespread, since the required level of loss of sensation extends from the fourth thoracic dermatome. Thus, hypotension is more likely unless acute intravenous hydration has been adequate. For epidural block, at least 1 liter of balanced salt solution should be infused before induction, and for spinal anesthesia, at least 1½ liters. Frequent monitoring of brachial blood pressure should continue until the block has taken effect and the blood pressure has stabilized. At this stage the frequency of measurements can be reduced to every 4 to 5 minutes. Again, adequate uterine displacement is of paramount importance in the prevention of maternal hypotension.

The anesthesiologist must at all times be prepared to administer a general anesthetic should the regional block be inadequate. To this end, all women undergoing cesarean section should receive prophylactic antacid. Likewise, the same precautions against complications should be taken as have been outlined previously.

Systemic Anesthesia. Over the years, the safety of general anesthesia for cesarean section has been improved. Attention has been paid to preventing the common causes of maternal mortality and morbidity associated with anesthesia: inability to intubate the trachea, pulmonary aspiration of gastric contents, and profound hypotension. In addition, more careful attention to maternal position, avoidance of hyperventilation, and development of techniques utilizing lighter levels of anesthesia have contributed to improved neonatal condition.

Preparation for general anesthesia begins with the administration of 30 ml of antacid approximately 30 minutes before induction. When emergency section is necessary, milk of magnesia can be effective in buffering gastric contents within 10 minutes. After assuring adequate uterine displacement, oxygen is administered by tight-fitting mask. Now monitors can be placed, baseline measurements of heart rate and blood pressure recorded, and preparation of the operative field begun.

Induction of anesthesia is commenced once the sterile draping has been completed and all personnel and instruments are ready. A rapid-sequence intravenous technique is performed with thiopental sodium alone (3 to 4 mg per kg) or a ketamine/thiopental sodium sequence (0.5 to 0.7 mg per kg and 2 mg per kg, respectively). Succinylcholine is used to produce relaxation for endotracheal intubation. For the period from injection of thiopental to the point at which correct placement of the endotracheal tube has been verified and the cuff inflated, cricoid pressure is maintained to prevent passive regurgitation of gastric contents. Until the umbilical cord is clamped, anesthesia is maintained with nitrous oxide (40 per cent) in oxygen. Once delivery is complete, the anesthetic is continued with nitrous oxide (60 per cent) and intravenous narcotics.

The maternal advantages of this technique are that regurgitation and aspiration of gastric contents are avoided, oxygenation is maintained, hypotension is prevented, and adequate surgical anesthesia is produced. From the fetal point of view, the drugs used are given in amounts shown to have little or no adverse effect. Overall, this method addresses the known complications of general anesthesia in obstetrics. It is still not risk free, however, and should be reserved for cesarean sections and other emergencies such as disimpaction of a shoulder dystocia or midforceps delivery for fetal distress.

POSTPARTUM HEMORRHAGE

PAMELA J. TROPPER, M.D.,
and ROY H. PETRIE, M.D.

Postpartum hemorrhage occurs in 4 per cent of all deliveries. It accounts for substantial morbidity and approximately 8 per cent of all maternal deaths. The awareness of this potential problem, the identification of patients at risk for this complication, and rapid and effective management can decrease the magnitude of its sequelae.

By definition postpartum hemorrhage is the loss of greater than 500 ml of blood in the postpartum period. It is further categorized into *early* (within 24 hours of delivery) and *delayed* (late, occurring greater than 24 hours but prior to 6 weeks postpartum). There is recognized obvious difficulty with a quantitative definition of significant hemorrhage, as it has been repeatedly demonstrated—at least in the primipara—that the average blood loss is 450 ml—and that visual judgments of blood loss underestimate the true loss almost half the time.

TREATMENT OF EARLY POSTPARTUM HEMORRHAGE

Primary treatment of postpartum hemorrhage requires awareness of the potential in any patient and routine measures which necessitate quick emergency responses, specifically, a large-bore intravenous line and availability of a blood specimen for type and crossmatch. In the presence of heavy bleeding, initial management requires stabilization of the patient and the avoidance of or treatment of shock. Adequate intravenous access must be established using a large-bore intravenous and a central venous pressure line if necessary. Vital signs and urine output must be carefully monitored. Blood should be crossmatched for the patient, anticipating the use of large quantities; Ringer's lactate, colloids, and blood expanders are used until blood is available. A coagulation screen is drawn. In the delivery room, observation of a blood specimen tube for clotting and clot stability will yield faster results than the laboratory and should be done in all instances of postpartum hemorrhage. Fresh frozen plasma should be administered as needed to maintain adequate blood pressure and urine output.

Management of vaginal and cervical lacerations includes adequate assistance for visualization and repair. If a hematoma is present, it is necessary to evacuate the blood clots, identify and ligate any large bleeding vessels, and then further control bleeding by compression, e.g., a vaginal pack or sandbags to the vulva. Embolization techniques using arteriographic localization have been effectively used to control hematoma formation from vulvar and vaginal bleeding sites.

In the presence of uterine atony, uterine massage should be instituted immediately. The operator's hand is introduced into the vagina and the opposite hand is used to massage the fundus through the abdominal wall. Oxytocic agents should be administered. Oxytocin is best administered by adding 20 to 60 units to a liter of intravenous electrolyte solution. Direct bolus intravenous injection may result in hypotension and should be avoided. An electrolyte solution is used to minimize the possibility of water intoxication which may occur after the use of oxytocin with large quantities of fluid. Even small quantities of oxytocin may have an antidiuretic effect. If oxytocin is inadequate to achieve uterine contraction, ergotrate, 0.2 mg, may be administered intramuscularly. Ergotrate may induce marked hypertension and should be used cautiously in patients with a history of hypertension or other cardiovascular disease.

If heavy bleeding persists as a result of uterine atony, the uterus should be manually explored for evidence of retained products of conception and uterine rupture. If products of conception are present they should be removed. If neither of these complications is present, the newer pharmacologic agents to induce uterine contractility should be tried. Prostaglandin $F_2\alpha$ injected through the abdominal wall directly into the uterine musculature in doses of 0.5 to 1 mg will often rapidly produce a tetanic uterine contraction with immediate decrease in blood loss. Prostaglandin E vaginal suppositories may be used as well. It is recommended that these agents be available in the labor and delivery suite for the early management of marked uterine atony prior to the use of surgical intervention.

Other methods of controlling hemorrhage from uterine atony include uterine lavage with hot saline and uterine packing. Both have been successful when traditional oxytocic drugs have failed. Risks of uterine lavage include introduction of infection, and damage to the uterus or external genitalia by the use of an excessively hot solution. Uterine packing alone may decrease hemorrhage but is felt to be unphysiologic by many who argue it distends the uterine cavity and in fact interferes with contractility. If a uterine pack is placed, the patient must be watched carefully for signs of infection and rebleeding, and the patient should not be repacked repeatedly in futile attempts to control bleeding. The uterine pack may be useful to decrease blood loss while preparations for surgical intervention are made.

If all the mentioned techniques fail, surgical intervention is necessary. When other methods have failed one must act rapidly rather than further complicate the situation, potentiating the problems of shock and disseminated intravascular coagulation.

At exploration, bilateral uterine artery ligation alone should be attempted. If bleeding cannot be controlled with adequate uterine artery ligation, one may wish to proceed to hysterectomy. This may be a supracervical or a complete hysterectomy depending on the stability of the patient. Hysterectomy may be preferable to hypogastric artery ligation, for although the latter is effective in reducing pulse pressure in the bleeding vessels, bleeding may persist owing to the presence of collateral circulation.

TREATMENT OF DELAYED (LATE) POSTPARTUM HEMORRHAGE

The treatment of late postpartum hemorrhage is essentially the same as for the early postpartum hemorrhage. Treatment or avoidance of shock is initiated. In the presence of atony, uterine massage and oxytocic agents should be administered. Prostaglandin injection or suppositories should be tried. The absence of intrauterine contents on ultrasonography is reassuring. Evidence of echoes in the uterus does not help in the discrimination of decidual and blood clots versus placental tissue. The presence of fever makes retained products of conception more likely. In the presence of possible endometritis, the use of antibiotics should be considered.

Only if the patient does not respond to oxytocin and ergotrate, or in the presence of persistent fever despite antibiotics, should careful dilatation and curettage be performed. A large blunt or suction curette should be used. Curettage should be done simply to remove any retained products of conception, and care should be taken not to proceed overly vigorously with denudation of the endometrium and removal of portions of the myometrium. Some authorities recommend the use of estrogen after curettage in order to help in the re-establishment of a normal endometrium and avoidance of adhesion formation.

Any coagulation defects should be appropriately treated with fresh frozen plasma or cryoprecipitate and the etiology of the coagulopathy further defined. If all else fails, operative intervention as described for early postpartum hemorrhage will be necessary.

The later or delayed sequelae of massive hemorrhage and its treatment must be remembered. Transfusion may result in decreased platelets, hypocalcemia, renal and pulmonary complications, and later, hepatitis. Prolonged periods of hypotension also predispose the patient to adult respiratory distress syndrome and acute tubular necrosis. The possibility of development of Sheehan's syndrome should be kept in mind. Asherman's syndrome may be a late complication of postpartum infection and curettage.

IMMUNE THROMBOCYTOPENIC PURPURA

ROBERT RESNIK, M.D.

Although many reports demonstrate a mild decrease in the platelet count during pregnancy, it does not fall below 150,000 per cu mm except in the presence of disease states. The diagnosis of immune thrombocytopenic purpura (ITP) is generally considered after a laboratory report reveals a low platelet count, or following the evaluation of petechiae and purpura. The latter are due to bleeding from small vessels in the skin or mucous membranes. Such bleeding usually does not occur unless the platelet count falls to below 20,000 to 30,000 per cu mm, but may be observed at higher levels.

Thrombocytopenia may result from two basic mechanisms. The first involves the failure of the bone marrow to generate megakaryocytes, as observed in drug suppression, viral or bacterial infections, tumor invasion, or vitamin deficiency states (folic acid and vitamin B_{12}). Alternately, thrombocytopenia may be caused by increased sequestration and destruction of platelets and their removal from the circulation by the reticuloendothelial system. Disseminated intravascular coagulation and ITP are examples of the latter mechanisms. Patients with ITP have a bone marrow which is normal or demonstrates increased numbers of megakaryocytes, and a spleen which is rarely palpable; the pathophysiology underlying the disorder is the presence of antiplatelet antibodies-7S immunoglobulin G (IgG), which coat platelets which are then destroyed within the spleen.

IMMUNE THROMBOCYTOPENIC PURPURA DURING PREGNANCY

There is no evidence that ITP is influenced by pregnancy. However, pregnancy may be adversely affected owing to excessive bleeding at the time of delivery, and because the associated 7S immunoglobulin may cross the placenta and produce neonatal thrombocytopenia. Major hemorrhage from mucous membranes, particularly the gastrointestinal tract, may occur throughout gestation with low extremes of platelet counts. Although maternal mortality is very low, perinatal mortality ranges from 10 to 22 per cent in various reports. Most of this fetal wastage is due to abortions and stillbirths. However, since between 50 and 75 per cent of neonates have varying degrees of thrombocytopenia, intracranial hemorrhage is occasionally observed and is considered a significant risk. Some authorities have suggested that cesarean section be performed in all patients with ITP to prevent this serious neonatal complication. However, there is not universal agreement on this point, and abdominal delivery in the presence of profound thrombocytopenia carries significant maternal risk.

TREATMENT

Therapy should be reserved for patients with evidence of bleeding, or platelet counts less than 50,000 per cu mm. Prednisone, 60 to 80 mg daily, is administered, with higher doses occasionally required. A response to corticosteroids is usually observed in approximately 2 weeks, with about one third of patients undergoing complete remission, and some improvement noted in 20 to 30 per cent of patients without complete remission. Corticosteroid dosage may be tapered once the platelet count has reached greater than 100,000 per cu mm.

An alternate form of therapy is splenectomy, which results in remission in 80 per cent of patients treated. Splenectomy should be considered for patients who do not respond to corticosteroids, and has been combined successfully with cesarean section in patients near term with dangerously low platelet counts. In such cases, surgery provides treatment of ITP and an atraumatic delivery for the infant. Ideally, splenectomy should be delayed until the postpartum period, assuming that medical therapy is reasonably effective.

The role of platelet transfusions, particularly around the time of delivery, is controversial because the platelets are removed so rapidly from the circulation. Despite their very brief half-life, such transfusions are commonly used.

MODE OF DELIVERY

This remains a source of considerable controversy. As stated earlier, the principal concern regarding a vaginal delivery is the risk of intracranial hemorrhage in the infant. It should be emphasized that neonatal thrombocytopenia is very common, and may be observed in the post-splenectomy patient who is in remission, because immunoglobulin G is still present. Although some authorities recommend abdominal delivery if the maternal platelet count is less than 100,000 per cu mm, the data to support this type of clinical management are scanty. Recent efforts to evaluate the platelet status of the fetus utilizing scalp blood sampling techniques during labor show promise, since they correlate fairly well with umbilical cord platelet counts. It is possible that the final determination regarding mode of delivery may rest on demonstration of serious thrombocytopenia in the fetus.

CONDYLOMA ACUMINATUM

RAYMOND H. KAUFMAN, M.D.

Condyloma acuminatum is caused by a papovavirus and flourishes during pregnancy. Not uncommonly, small isolated condylomas may multiply during pregnancy and cover large areas of the vulva, vagina, and cervix. Treatment of condylomas will depend upon their location, extent, and size.

1. Important to the eradication of condyloma acuminatum is the eradication of associated vaginal infections, such as trichomoniasis, candidiasis, and *Gardnerella vaginalis* vaginitis. In addition to laboratory studies to identify these infections, cultures should be taken from the cervix, urethra, and anus to exclude the possibility of gonorrhea.

2. Small, isolated condylomas can be treated with 20 per cent podophyllum in tincture of benzoin. This is applied to the isolated condylomas and allowed to dry. The patient should be instructed to wash the area thoroughly in 4 to 6 hours. Extensive use of podophyllum should be avoided, especially during pregnancy, since the medication can be absorbed and has been reported to be associated with intrauterine fetal demise.

3. If the treatment just described is not effective in eradicating the condylomas, trichloroacetic acid (Nevatol) or bichloracetic acid can be applied to the isolated condylomas with wooden applicators. The surface of the warts will turn white, and within several days they will begin to slough off. If necessary, this treatment can be repeated in 1 week.

4. Isolated conylomas can also be treated by cryocautery. A straight probe is applied to the condyloma, and the wart is completely frozen down to its base. The CO_2 laser is even more effective in removing such lesions.

5. Large condylomas involving extensive areas of the vulva and vagina are best treated by surgical excision performed in the hospital. Secondary infection should be treated by the utilization of hot sitz baths and systemic antibiotics, after the depths of the crevices between condylomas have been cultured and sensitivity studies have been performed. With the patient under anesthesia, large vulvar condylomas can be electrodesiccated down to their base, then curetted off with the use of a scalpel or a cutting electric loop. Large vaginal condylomas can be treated in a similar manner. This operative procedure is best performed during the second trimester of pregnancy.

6. If extensive condylomas that fill the vagina, cover the vulva, or appear in both places are present near term, the patient is best delivered by cesarean section rather than being allowed to deliver vaginally with the potential hazards of hemorrhage and infection.

TWIN GESTATION

JOSEPH V. COLLEA, M.D.

Women with twin gestations account for only 1 per cent of all deliveries in any institution, but experience a perinatal mortality which is four (Twin A) and five (Twin B) times that of singleton gestations. Contributing significantly to this excessive mortality are five factors: prematurity (birth weight less than 2500 grams), pregnancy-induced hypertension, intrauterine growth retardation (IUGR), abnormal presentations, and congenital malformations.

Forty-five per cent of first and 55 per cent of second twins are of low birth weight. Twenty-five per cent of women with twin gestations experience hypertensive complications during pregnancy. Twenty-five per cent of first twin and 40 per cent of second twin fetuses are in breech presentations during labor, and as many as 50 per cent of all twin gestations in some series are not diagnosed until the intrapartum period. Consequently, many premature or dysmature second twin fetuses, often in abnormal presentations, are totally unexpected and hastily delivered without the benefit of immediately available neonatal support, which further contributes to twin neonatal morbidity and mortality. Compounding this picture is a congenital malformation rate that is two to three times that observed in singleton pregnancies.

In order to reduce the excessive perinatal mortality associated with twin gestations, obstetricians must:

1. diagnose twin gestations early in pregnancy;
2. prevent the onset of premature labor;
3. diagnose and treat intrauterine growth retardation in one or both twins;
4. manage appropriately the twin fetus in abnormal presentation during the intrapartum period; and
5. maintain a constant vigilance for the development of pregnancy-induced hypertension.

THE DIAGNOSIS OF TWIN GESTATION

The diagnosis of twin gestation can accurately be made by examining the maternal pelvis ultrasonographically late in the first or early in the second trimester of pregnancy. An ultrasound examination to diagnose twin gestations is especially important for women who have previously delivered twins, who have a family history of dizygotic twins, or who have a uterine size-date discrepancy in which the uterus is larger than expected by menstrual dates. In addition, women who have received ovulation-inducing drugs, such as clomiphene citrate, must be screened by ultrasound to rule out the occurrence of multiple gestation.

An ultrasound examination to diagnose twins should also be performed whenever more than one fetal heart rate is auscultated, whenever multiple fetal parts are palpated during the performance of Leopold's maneuver, or whenever the presenting part in the maternal pelvis appears smaller than expected for uterine size or gestational age.

PREVENTION OF PREMATURE LABOR

Patients with known twin gestations should be placed on bed rest at home from 26 to 36 weeks of gestational age in an attempt to prevent premature labor as well as to improve fetal weight gain.

Women with twin gestations who present in early labor (less than 4 cm of cervical dilatation) with intact membranes are candidates for suppression of uterine contractions by tocolytic agents such as magnesium sulfate or ritodrine.

Patients with premature rupture of membranes should be managed according to the obstetric protocols established for singleton gestations.

DIAGNOSIS AND MANAGEMENT OF INTRAUTERINE GROWTH RETARDATION

Once the diagnosis of twin gestation is made, serial ultrasonographic examinations should be performed at 3 to 4 week intervals to verify continued symmetric growth of both fetuses. During the ultrasonographic examination, the fetal biparietal diameter (BPD), head circumference, abdominal circumference, femur length, and estimation of amniotic fluid volume should be recorded for each fetus. The four major ultrasonographic findings that suggest intrauterine growth retardation in one or both of the fetuses are:

1. Oligohydramnios of one or both fetal sacs.
2. Discordant fetal growth: ≥ 0.5 cm difference in biparietal diameter between twins.
3. Asymmetric growth rate of head and body of either twin.
4. Placental infarctions.

If intrauterine growth retardation is suspected or diagnosed by ultrasonographic examination, the patient must be thoroughly evaluated for the cause, and treated appropriately. An integral part of any treatment for intrauterine growth retardation is bed rest. The patient should be placed at bed rest at home or the hospital, as appropriate, and monitored closely for continued fetal growth by serial ultrasonography. Bed rest may be continued throughout pregnancy to ensure adequate fetal growth.

ANTENATAL SURVEILLANCE OF FETAL WELL-BEING

For the patient without evidence of intrauterine growth retardation during twin gestation, routine nonstress tests on each fetus should be performed on a weekly basis beginning at 36 weeks of gestational age. The nonstress test in conjunction with the serial ultrasound data should provide ample surveillance of the twin fetus without intauterine growth retardation.

For women with suspected or diagnosed intrauterine growth retardation, the nonstress test is begun earlier in gestation, as early as 26 weeks depending on maternal-fetal conditions, and repeated twice weekly until delivery. If the nonstress tests are reactive and the growth-retarded fetus demonstrates improved intrauterine growth with treatment, the pregnancy is allowed to continue. If the nonstress tests are nonreactive, a lecithin/sphingomyelin (L/S) ratio for lung maturation is deteriminated on the dysmature fetus. If the lungs are mature, the pregnancy is terminated to prevent fetal wastage.

INTRAPARTUM MANAGEMENT OF TWIN GESTATION

Women who present in advanced labor with premature twin gestations of 26 to 34 weeks' gestation, or with evidence of intrauterine growth retardation of either or both twins, should be delivered by cesarean section.

Women who present in labor at more than 34 weeks' gestational age are managed according to the first twin's presentation: shoulder: cesarean; vertex: vaginal; breech: cesarean.

Patients in labor with twin gestations should have both fetuses monitored for fetal heart rate and uterine contractions in order to diagnose fetal distress. If labor progresses satisfactorily, the first twin in cephalic presentation is delivered spontaneously or by elective low forceps. If labor progression is unsatisfactory, or if a mid forceps procedure is considered necessary for delivery of the first twin, the patient should be delivered by cesarean section.

For patients allowed to labor with twin gestation, a continuous epidural anesthetic may be given for pain relief. Following vaginal delivery of the first twin, the patient may continue in labor provided there is no evidence of significant maternal bleeding or irremediable fetal distress (recurrent late deceleration or severe variable decelerations of the fetal heart rate). Whenever possible, a fetal scalp electrode should be attached to the presenting part of the second twin. The second twin in vertex presentation is delivered either spontaneously or by elective low forceps. If the second twin is in breech presentation, a partial breech extraction may be carried out with application of Piper forceps to the aftercoming head. The induction of general anesthesia with halothane may be required for adequate uterine relaxation during the delivery of the aftercoming head.

The second twin in transverse lie may convert to a breech or cephalic presentation following delivery of the first twin. If conversion to a longitudinal lie does not occur, delivery may be accomplished by internal version and total breech extraction under general halothane anesthesia. If adequate uterine relaxation is not achieved for this manuever, the second twin should be delivered by immediate cesarean section.

FETAL HYDROCEPHALY

FRANK C. MILLER, M.D.,
and MARC R. LEBED, M.D.

Hydrocephalus is the result of an excessive accumulation of cerebrospinal fluid within the brain. The excessive accumulation of CSF can be due to its overproduction by a papilloma of the choroid plexus or, more commonly in the fetus and newborn, to an obstruction to its flow.

Congenitally acquired hydrocephaly occurs in approximately 1 in 2000 live births and recurs in about 3 per cent of patients. The incidence of isolated hydrocephalus, that is without neural tube defect, varies from 0.39 to 0.87 per 1000 live births. Hydrocephaly can occur as an X-linked recessive trait with a 50 per cent recurrence rate in male fetuses. The true incidence of this type of hydrocephaly is unknown although it is estimated to comprise 2 per cent of all cases of isolated hydrocephalus in the newborn.

Evaluation of a pregnant mother with a previously affected infant should include:

1. Serologic evaluation for infectious teratogens;
2. Sonography before the twentieth week to determine the size of the fetal lateral ventricles and cerebral hemisphere and to explore the fetal spine for defects;

TABLE 1. **Etiology of Fetal Hydrocephalus***

Genetic Factors
1. Failure of any part of the CSF pathway to develop. Example, Dandy-Walker syndrome.
2. Stenosis of the aqueduct of Sylvius
3. Cerebellar agenesis
4. Spina bifida cystica
5. Chromosome abnormality such as trisomy 13

Nongenetic Factors
1. Obstructing tumor
2. Postinflammatory fibrosis secondary to viral infection and encephalitis (rubella, cytomegalovirus, possibly mumps) or protozoal infection

*Adapted from Habib, Z.: Obstet. Gynecol. Surv., 36:529, 1981.

3. Amniocentesis for alpha-fetoprotein and chromosome analysis; and

4. Parental karyotyping

Hydrocephaly during the second trimester is usually diagnosed coincidentally with genetic counselling and the associated ultrasound and amniocentesis. It is important to remember that prior to 24 weeks' gestation ventricular enlargement can occur before an increase in the biparietal diameter.

The range of normal variation in ventricular size and ventricular to cortical ratios is quite large during the second trimester. In cases in which questionable abnormalities exist, especially in relation to ventricular dilatation, serial ultrasound examinations and additional consultation should be obtained before a dignosis is established. The diagnosis of mild hydrocephaly does not necessarily result in a severely handicapped infant. The determination of management must involve the typing of the disorder, the extent of anatomic involvement and the experience of the neonatal unit which will care for the infant.

Diagnosis of hydrocephaly becomes easier as gestation advances. One must always be cautious in making the diagnosis in a large fetus because the biparietal diameter or head circumference may be the upper limit of normal for a large normal infant and not due to hydrocephaly. Generally the diagnosis is obvious from widely dilated ventricles or other intracranial abormalities. A word of caution about ultrasound equipment and imaging is needed. Ultrasound images from some of the older equipment will appear dark (because the brain is homogeneous) and may be mistaken for large fluid-filled areas. If there is any question about the diagnosis, obtain consultation from an expert in fetal ultrasound.

The management of a pregnancy with a hydrocephalic fetus is changing almost daily because of the rapidly expanding experience with ventricular shunting (currently some fetuses are shunted in utero). One of the most widely accepted prognostic criteria for hydrocephaly has been the thickness of the cortex at the time of ultrasound scan. An established guideline has been that a 1 cm rim of cortex would justify atraumatic delivery for fetal salvage, provided there are no additional central nervous system lesions. Unfortunately these criteria have failed to consistently predict long-term outcome. The decision on management is best made in consultation with a neurosurgeon and a neonatologist. Their experience and expertise in dealing with these infants will strongly influence the obstetric management.

Atraumatic delivery of a hydrocephalic fetus is probably associated with considerably less intrapartum and neonatal intracranial hemorrhage and thus a better outcome. This is the preferred route of delivery of an infant who is a candidate for shunting. The decision to decompress the fetal head in cases of severe hydrocepahlus or in cases with associated central nervous system lesions is always a difficult one. Technically the insertion of a large bore needle into a dilated ventricle is not difficult. If done vaginally, it is best done under direct vision via an endoscope. The cerebrospinal fluid can be either allowed to drain off or can be aspirated. Transabdominal and vaginal insertion can be aided by visualization with ultrasound to guide the needle to the correct position.

The emotional impact to the parents is often quite staggering, whether the diagnosis is made in mid pregnancy or at term. Parents must be fully counseled regarding the eventual prognosis of the fetus, plans for management during labor, method of delivery, and plans for the newborn, and allowed to fully participate in the decisions that will affect their child.

At this writing there are no acceptable antepartum criteria for the prediction of long-term prognosis except in the grossly affected fetus. Until such a formula is determined, the management of the fetus must be individualized on the basis of (1) the typing of anomaly/abnormality, (2) the extent of anatomic involvement (including thalamic and brain stem involvement), (3) neonatal support available during the immediate neonatal period, and (4) parental input.

POSTPARTUM PELVIC HEMATOMAS

WILLIAM N.P. HERBERT, M.D., and ROBERT C. CEFALO, M.D., Ph.D.

Submucosal bleeding with an intact overlying epithelium (hematoma) occurs in the genital tract in about 1 in 1000 deliveries. More commonly, pelvic hematomas occur after operative vaginal deliveries, but they may follow spontaneous birth. Marked vascularity and congestion of the pelvic tissue appear to predispose to hematoma formation. Disorders of hemostasis, which may include recent maternal ingestion of aspirin, and pudendal block are rare causes of hematoma. Deep cervical lacerations, incomplete rupture of the uterus, and spontaneous rupture of a varicosity in the broad ligament may be associated with a supravaginal hematoma.

Postpartum hematomas of the genital tract can divided into: (1) vulvar type—with bleeding limited to the vulva; (2) vulvovaginal type—involving the vulva, paravaginal tissue, and at times, extending into the ischiorectal fossa; (3) vaginal; and (4) supravaginal—bleeding above the pelvic fascia, possibly retroperitoneal or intraligamentous. Bleeding is often concealed in the vaginal and supravaginal types.

In the immediate puerperium vulvar hematomas are the type most commonly encountered. Hematomas 4 to 5 cm or less in diameter may be managed expectantly, if there is no progression in size. Otherwise, active treatment is required. If the hematoma is adjacent to the episiotomy site, the sutures should be removed, specific bleeding sites ligated, and the cavity obliterated and drained before the perineum and vagina are reapproximated. Frequently, hematomas are opposite the episiotomy site, apparently resulting from tearing of a deep vessel by overdistention of the vaginal outlet. Management is the same. A perineal pad and cold compresses may prevent further bleeding and discomfort.

Vaginal hematomas are less frequently noted, but are more difficult to treat. They may achieve considerable size and compress the urethra, bladder, and rectum, leading to difficulty with voiding and defecation. The surgical approach is the same—incision, ligation of bleeding sites if identified, drainage, and obliteration of the hematoma cavity. Adequate visualization is mandatory and surgical assistance is therefore required. Packing of the vagina for 12 to 24 hours may help prevent a recurrence, but also may interfere with lochia discharge. Packs should be removed by 24 hours.

Supravaginal hematomas may be evident in the immediate or late postpartum period, are least common, and are the most difficult to treat. Blood loss may be substantial, since branches of the hypogastric artery are commonly involved. The patient may describe "bladder pressure" or urgency. Lower abdominal and "deeper" pelvic pain, along with palpation of a mass in the adnexa or lower abdomen, are suggestive of a hematoma. If the mass does not increase in size and the pulse, hematocrit, and blood pressure remain stable, the patient may be treated expectantly. With progression in size or with vaginal bleeding, a complete vaginal examination should be performed to identify particular bleeding sites. Unless the bleeding can be promptly stopped by this approach, abdominal exploration should be performed. Broad ligament hematomas are approached by dividing the leaves of the broad ligament, evacuating the hematoma, ligating the bleeding sites, and reapproximating the anterior and posterior leaves of the ligament. Since the bleeding is frequently arterial rather than venous, topical coagulants such as thrombin or gelatin sponges are usually not helpful. The anatomy is almost always distorted. Great care must be exercised to avoid the ureters, since they may course through the site of hematoma formation. Ureteral catheter placement may be necessary. If bleeding sites are not identifiable, hysterectomy or hypogastric artery ligation may be necessary to achieve hemostasis. Retroperitoneal hematomas may, of course, extend posteriorly to the level of the kidneys.

Regardless of the site of hematoma, close attention must be paid to infusion of crystalloids and blood and its components. As with many surgical situations, assessed blood loss may be markedly underestimated.

Many hematomas discovered in the puerperium occur spontaneously during the descent of the presenting part in normal labor. Early recognition of a hematoma is essential. Inspection of the perineum immediately prior to sending the patient to the postpartum ward, along with immediate vaginal and abdominal examination in all patients complaining of undue perineal or abdominal pain in the postpartum period, will assist in early diagnosis and treatment.

PREGNANCY IN THE PATIENT WITH CHRONIC RENAL DISEASE, ON HEMODIALYSIS, OR FOLLOWING RENAL TRANSPLANT

PAUL R. MEIER, M.D.,
and EDGAR L. MAKOWSKI, M.D.

The coexistence of chronic renal disease and pregnancy places both the gravida and the fetus at increased risk for multiple problems. For the gravida there is an increased risk of induced hypertension (preeclampsia) and perhaps further deterioration of her compromised renal function. For the fetus there is an increased risk of spontaneous abortion, intrauterine growth retardation, prematurity, intrapartum distress, and death. In the past, many patients with known renal disease were advised to avoid pregnancy or to terminate their pregnancy. Currently the techniques for diagnosis and evaluation of renal disease as well as improved medical management justify a more optimistic outlook for pregnancy complicated by a chronic renal disorder.

Although chronic renal disease has many etiologies, it can be divided into three broad categories: glomerular, tubointerstitial, and collecting system diseases. Table 1 subdivides each of the above categories into the more traditional histopathologic or etiologic diagnoses. While each broad category of renal disease may initially present with a different clinical picture, the end result of all three is renal insufficiency manifested by one or more of the following: hypertension, proteinuria, hematuria, or azotemia.

Interpretation of the literature regarding the outcome of pregnancy complicated by chronic renal disease is difficult and often confusing. Many studies are deficient because they fail to establish the exact nature of the renal disorder or the degree of abnormal renal function before, during, and after pregnancy. Other studies date from an era marked by pessimism and active intervention to terminate pregnancies in patients with chronic renal disease. More recently observers have adopted a more optimistic outlook regarding pregnancy associated with renal disease. Although much controversy remains, there is a general consensus that the outcome of pregnancy depends largely on the degree of renal compromise present at the time of the pregnancy and cannot be predicted solely on the basis of specific histopathologic or etiologic diagnoses. Patients with severe renal insufficiency (serum creatinine ≥ 2 mg per dl) are known to have decreased fertility and increased pregnancy wastage. However, normal or near normal renal function augers well for a good pregnancy outcome. Hypertension, if present at the time of conception, significantly worsens the overall prognosis for both the mother with chronic renal disease and her fetus. All patients with chronic renal disease have an increased risk of developing pregnancy-induced hypertension. Finally, pregnancy per se does not appear to adversely affect coexistent renal disease if renal function is normal or only mildly affected and there is no complicating hypertension. Approximate potential risks to the gravida with chronic renal disease and her fetus are listed in Table 2.

The physiologic effects of pregnancy on renal function are multiple. Renal blood flow and glomerular filtration increase 30 and 50 per cent respectively during the course of pregnancy. Ureteral dilation and increased urine stasis are present from early in pregnancy and they cannot be accounted for solely on the basis of uterine compression of the ureters at the pelvic brim. As a result of these dramatic changes in physiologic renal function during pregnancy, there are significant changes in most of the laboratory parameters used to assess renal function. Table 3 compares the normal laboratory values of commonly used renal function tests in pregnant and nonpregnant patients. It is apparent that the laboratory values which are considered to be "normal" in the nonpregnant state are abnormal in a pregnant patient. One of the first indications of unsuspected renal disease may, in fact, be the failure for renal function studies to change during pregnancy.

Ideally, any patient with suspected or known renal disease should be fully evaluated prior to pregnancy. After a careful evaluation of her renal status, a frank discussion regarding the risks of pregnancy for both patient and fetus is possible without the additional stress of a current pregnancy. Unfortunately, this ideal is seldom achieved and the clinician is usually confronted with a pregnant patient who has already developed evidence of renal dysfunction.

The management of suspected chronic renal disease during pregnancy begins with an at-

TABLE 1. **Causes of Chronic Renal Disease**

Glomerular Disorders
  Chronic glomerulonephritis
  Lupus nephritis
  Diabetic nephritis
  Nephrotic syndrome
  Hereditary nephritis

Tubointerstitial Disorders
  Chronic pyelonephritis
  Interstitial nephritis
    Drug-related
    Analgesic
    Radiation

Collecting System
  Nephrolithiasis
  Renal deformity

TABLE 2. **Risks Associated with Chronic Renal Disease and Pregnancy**

A. Patients with Serum Creatinine < 1.5 mg per dl	
Proteinuria	1:2
Hypertension	1:3–4
Transient Worsening of Renal Function	1:6
Permanent Worsening of Renal Function	No definite evidence of permanent deterioration related to pregnancy
B. Fetus	
Prematurity (includes medically indicated and spontaneously premature)	Increased 2 to 3 times
Small for Gestational Age	Increased 4 times
Fetal Mortality	Increased 2 to 3 times
Perinatal Mortality	Increased 4 to 5 times

TABLE 3. **Commonly Used Renal Function Tests**

	NON-PREGNANT	PREGNANT
Serum creatinine	<1.2 mg/dl	<0.8 mg/dl
BUN	<20 mg/dl	<10 mg/dl
Uric acid	<4.5 mg/dl	<3.5 mg/dl
Creatinine clearance	>100 ml/min	>105 ml/min
Urinary protein excretion	<150 mg	<250 mg
Urinalysis		
Specific Gravity	>1.026	>1.026
pH	5–7	5–7

tempt to establish the exact nature of the disease and to evaluate current renal function. A careful history is mandatory and should include specific questions regarding drug (prescription and non-prescription) ingestion and previous episodes of glycosuria, proteinuria, hypertension, or hematuria. Previous medical records should be reviewed for evidence of renal disease or previous renal function studies. A family history may demonstrate the presence of genetic or hereditary renal disease. Physical examination, while complete, should focus on the cardiovascular and genitourinary systems. Measurement of blood pressure in the standing, sitting, and lateral decubitus positions is especially important. In addition, various laboratory studies should be performed, including a complete urinalysis, urine culture, complete blood count, BUN, serum creatinine, and a 24 hour urine collection for creatinine clearance and total protein excretion. In the nonpregnant patient, such additional studies as intravenous pyelography, computed renal tomography, or a renal biopsy should be considered. Occasionally it may be necessary to perform intravenous pyelography or computed renal tomography during pregnancy because of rapid deterioration in renal function.

Based on the information obtained from the initial evaluation, it is usually possible to determine if the patient has any significant renal disease and to appropriately counsel her regarding the remainder of the pregnancy. If the patient is not hypertensive, has no urinary tract infection, has no abnormalities in urinary excretion, and can attain "normal" pregnancy values for her renal function studies, it is unlikely that she has significant renal disease. On the other hand, if renal disease is diagnosed or suspected, it is necessary to institute a careful plan of pregnancy management.

The goals of pregnancy management in patients with chronic renal disease include the detection and treatment of any condition which may jeopardize the gravida's health or her remaining renal function and regular assessment for potential fetal growth retardation or distress.

During the antepartum period, patients with renal disease should be seen biweekly until the last month of pregnancy and then on a weekly basis. At each visit the blood pressure and body weight are to be noted and recorded. A urine sample should be checked for protein and sugar at each visit. Uterine growth is serially evaluated and later in pregnancy fetal movement and amniotic fluid volume are assessed on a clinical basis. Renal function should be assessed with BUN, serum creatinine, and 24 hour urine collection for creatinine clearance and total protein during each trimester of pregnancy. These values should be compared to those obtained at the patient's initial examination; any deterioration in renal function is cause for further assessment and evaluation.

While asymptomatic bacteriuria should be treated in any pregnant patient, treatment is absolutely mandatory in patients with pre-existing renal disease. At least once a trimester a patient's urine should be screened for significant bacteriuria (>100,000 colonies per ml). In the event an infection is detected, the urine should be sterilized and the patient screened for recurrence at least once a month for the duration of her pregnancy. If pyelonephritis develops, the patient should be vigorously treated with intravenous antibiotics and fluids. Following resolution of the acute phase, the patient should be placed on chronic urinary suppressive antibiotic therapy to prevent further infection.

After 24 weeks of gestation, patients with chronic renal disease have about a one in three chance of developing preeclampsia superimposed on their renal disease. Such an event is a diagnostic challenge as to whether the diagnosis is preeclampsia or an exacerbation of renal disease. In fact, it is not always possible to differentiate between the two. If pregnancy is near term, delivery as expeditiously as possible will resolve the problem. Prior to 27 weeks of gestation, severe deterioration in maternal renal status, in the absence of a reversible cause, may necessitate termination of the pregnancy.

It is in the range of 27 to 37 weeks where the conundrum exists. If the mother's condition can be stabilized by bed rest, hospitalization, and frequent evaluations, it is often possible to achieve sufficient fetal maturity to afford an excellent chance of neonatal survival. Should maternal renal function continue to progressively worsen, pregnancy must be terminated. While antihypertensive medications are clearly appropriate for treating chronic pre-existing hypertension, they should be avoided except on a very short-term basis if superimposed preeclampsia is suspected.

The fetus of a mother with renal disease is at risk for many problems. Pregnancy associated with severe renal insufficiency (serum creatinine ≥ 1.5 to 2.0 mg per dl) can be expected to terminate spontaneously in perhaps 50 per cent of the cases. When renal function is less severely affected the pregnancy wastage is reduced, but it is still increased over the normal pregnancy loss rate because of prematurity. The incidence of fetal intrauterine growth retardation (IUGR) is increased and may occur in 25 per cent of pregnancies complicated by chronic renal disease. In the event a fetus is suspected to have IUGR on the basis of clinical assessment, ultrasonography can help to establish the diagnosis. Fetuses with IUGR are at a much higher risk for intrapartum distress and should be monitored appropriately during labor. During the antepartum period, all fetuses of mothers with renal disease should be monitored by daily fetal movement records and weekly fetal heart rate nonstress test from 32 weeks until delivery. If maternal hypertension develops, the fetal environment becomes even more dangerous and necessitates even closer monitoring with premature delivery a distinct possibility. Finally, preterm delivery occurs 2 to 3 times as frequently as in normal pregnancies, but this includes indicated as well as spontaneous deliveries. Unnecessary iatrogenic premature delivery in patients in whom there is no deterioration of renal function or an indicated medical condition is to be condemned. Utilization of readily available tests to establish fetal pulmonary maturity is recommended to prevent needless morbidity secondary to immature lung function.

Nephrolithiasis in pregnancy is rather rare (incidence of renal calculi 0.4 per cent and ureteral stones 0.08 per cent). The management of this problem is similar to that in the nonpregnant patient. Surgery is indicated only after more conservative measures have failed. Patients with renal calculi are prone to persistent urinary tract infections and may require chronic urinary suppressive antibiotic therapy to prevent overt infection. Any pregnant patient with nephrolithiasis should also be evaluated for coexistent hyperparathyroidism.

PREGNANCY IN PATIENTS ON CHRONIC RENAL DIALYSIS AND FOLLOWING RENAL TRANSPLANTATION

Pregnancy rarely occurs in patients on maintenance hemodialysis. Sexual dysfunction, including amenorrhea, anovulatory bleeding, and decreased libido, is common. Nevertheless, women of reproductive age on hemodialysis should be advised that pregnancy is possible, especially if menses return. Appropriate contraceptive measures should be utilized to avoid an unexpected or unwanted pregnancy.

While the likelihood of a pregnancy resulting in the delivery of a full-term infant is less than 25 per cent, a handful of successful pregnancies have been reported in patients on chronic hemodialysis. For the fetus, the major problems are prematurity and intrauterine growth retardation. Assuming that the fetus survives the pregnancy, there is no clear evidence that the associated abnormal maternal metabolic environment causes permanent damage to the fetus. Standard techniques for fetal assessment allow the growth of the fetus and its well-being to be carefully monitored during the last trimester of pregnancy. Pregnant patients on dialysis are confronted with several potential problems. Maintenance of maternal electrolyte balance including normal serum calcium levels as well as the prevention of severe anemia are necessary. This requires adequate dietary calcium intake and frequent serum calcium determinations. The judicious use of transfusions to maintain a stable maternal hematocrit above 25 per cent is indicated. Most successful pregnancies in patients on hemodialysis have been associated with a BUN level of less than 40 mg per dl. It may be expected that total dialysis time required will need to be increased in order to maintain this BUN level since the maternal system is exposed to an increased load of nitrogen excretion from the growing fetus.

Other problems reported in patients on hemodialysis include clotting of the dialysis shunt during the postpartum period and cholestatic jaundice. Whether these problems are related to dialysis or are coincidental is unknown. Several authors report uterine irritability in the third trimester following dialysis. Again the cause and effect relationship is unknown but the occurrence is troublesome and requires that patients be observed closely following dialysis treatments for evidence of premature labor.

Of interest is the finding that even in the face of severe chronic renal disease and the need for hemodialysis, the patient's own renal function may improve during pregnancy and then return to lower values in the postpartum period. Experience with pregnancy occurring during hemodialysis is limited, but it seems appropriate that if pregnancy does occur, every attempt should be made to provide a stable metabolic environment for the fetus. Maternal hypertension, if present, should be treated, and adequate maternal nutrition to nourish both mother and fetus should be provided.

Pregnancy following renal transplantation is a more common event than pregnancy occurring during hemodialysis. Following transplantation, menstruation reappears, on the average, within 6 months. It is appropriate to advise patients to use contraception for 1 to 2 years after transplantation, given the vagaries of life expectancy and adequacy of continuing renal function. After this time period, pregnancy may be allowed in patients who are doing well and who understand the increased risks associated with pregnancy.

Once pregnancy is suspected in a patient with a renal graft, the patient should be followed as a high-risk patient by both an obstetrician and a nephrologist. Immunosuppressive therapy has theoretical risks for the fetus but, in fact, it has been difficult to demonstrate any clear evidence of teratogenicity related to immunosuppressive drugs. Immunosuppressive therapy should therefore be continued as indicated by maternal need and should not be altered for the theoretical fetal risks. These patients should be followed on a biweekly basis until the last month of pregnancy and then on a weekly basis. The patient should be evaluated with frequent serial renal function tests, urine chemistries and sediment, and urine culture. Patients have about a one in four chance of developing pregnancy-induced hypertension, especially if there is any degree of preexisting hypertension. Prematurity complicates the pregnancy in about one in two patients with a renal graft. Additional problems include neonatal adrenal cortical insufficiency and an increased susceptibility to infection in infants whose mothers are receiving steroids for immunosuppression. Finally, in immunosuppressed patients there is an increased chance of cervical malignancy. Patients on immunosuppression should be carefully evaluated for the presence of cervical malignancy during their pregnancy. Labor and delivery are allowed to proceed normally with cesarean delivery reserved for obstetric indications. During the labor and delivery period, the transplant patient should receive supplementary intravenous corticosteroids.

Although a majority of pregnancies following renal transplantation are associated with a good outcome, pregnancy does carry increased risks to the mother and fetus. These risks must be carefully considered and only then should pregnancy be undertaken. Limited experience in patients with renal transplantation indicates that in most cases pregnancy is not associated with a deterioration of renal function.

TREATMENT OF GASTROINTESTINAL DISORDERS DURING PREGNANCY

JOHN W. DOBBINS, M.D.,
and HOWARD M. SPIRO, M.D.

Pregnancy has widespread direct effects on the gastrointestinal tract and, in addition, may make the recognition of gastrointestinal disease more difficult. For example, nausea and vomiting are common in early pregnancy, yet nausea and vomiting are also common complaints of many gastrointestinal disorders, especially those of the pancreas and the biliary tract. The enlarging uterus can also produce changes in the usual manifestations of gastrointestinal disease. Acute appendicitis in the pregnant woman, for example, may lead to pain and tenderness located in the right upper quadrant rather than in the more usual right lower quadrant. Thus, the effect of pregnancy on the gut must be kept in mind in evaluating such women. It is very difficult, indeed, to evaluate acute or chronic abdominal pain in the woman who is pregnant.

REFLUX ESOPHAGITIS

Reflux esophagitis is inflammation of the distal esophagus from the reflux of acid gastric juice; its usual manifestation is heartburn, a burning or painful substernal sensation typically occurring after meals, on lying down or bending over, or on lifting heavy objects. Orange juice will frequently reproduce heartburn in susceptible persons and, conversely, antacids frequently relieve heartburn. Water brash, or regurgitation of gastric contents into the mouth, may accompany heartburn.

A frequent complication of pregnancy, heartburn is especially common in the third trimester; about 40 per cent of pregnant women have such complaints. Present evidence indicates that the heartburn of pregnancy is due primarily to (1) a decrease in lower esophageal sphincter pressure; (2) an increase in intra-abdominal pressure secondary to the enlarging uterus; and (3) decreased responsiveness of the lower esophageal sphincter to increased abdominal pressure. Delayed gastric emptying may play a role but has not been evaluated.

Diagnosis. Reflux esophagitis can be recognized during pregnancy from the symptoms that it engenders, and treatment should be undertaken purely on the basis of symptoms, not diagnostic endeavors. Radiologic studies are unnecessary and should be avoided because of potential risk to the fetus. The use of endoscopy, the Bernstein acid perfusion study, or pH monitoring need be undertaken only if it is unclear that the woman is suffering from reflux esophagitis and only if her physician will alter therapy if something else is discovered, such as a peptic ulcer.

Treatment. The treatment of reflux esophagitis during pregnancy should include the following: (1) elevation of the head of the bed 4 to 6 inches with bed blocks; (2) avoidance of large meals, and especially snacks just before bed; and (3) liquid antacids for symptomatic relief. The H_2 receptor antagonist cimetidine and the dopamine antagonist metoclopramide have proven effective in the treatment of reflux esophagitis, but should be avoided in the pregnant woman.

Cimetidine is effective in reflux esophagitis, presumably because it is a potent inhibitor of both basal and stimulated acid secretion. Teratogenic studies with cimetidine have so far revealed no adverse effects. However, there is no reported experience with this agent during pregnancy, and since it crosses the placental barrier, cimetidine should be avoided. Cimetidine is known to have anti-androgenic effects and has been reported to retard sexual development in fetal rats when given during pregnancy.

Metoclopramide is useful in the treatment of reflux esophagitis because it increases lower esophageal sphincter pressure and stimulates gastric emptying. It also is an anti-emetic and thus may provide an additional benefit to the pregnant woman. Although metoclopramide has now been approved for use in reflux esophagitis in the United States, it should be avoided in the pregnant woman until more is known about its potential effects on the fetus. Moreover, metoclopramide has a high incidence of neurologic side-effects which limit its usefulness.

BILIARY TRACT DISEASE

Gallstones can cause biliary colic, cholecystitis, cholangitis, and pancreatitis; however, they may go undetected throughout life. Biliary colic caused by transient obstruction of the cystic duct or common bile duct results in steady right upper quadrant or epigastric pain of short duration, usually less than 2 to 3 hours. Classically, it occurs an hour or two after a heavy meal and radiates through to the angle of the scapula. When a common duct stone is present, pain tends to be more epigastric and to radiate directly between the shoulder blades. Nausea and vomiting may accompany biliary colic. Although vomiting usually does not relieve biliary tract pain, it is usually not protracted in the absence of pancreatitis or common duct obstruction. When cholecystitis or cholangitis occurs, evidence of inflammation and infection, such as fever, leukocytosis, right upper quadrant tenderness with guarding and rebound, is also present. Cholangitis, of course, can be a severe life-threatening condition, with septic shock, diffuse intravascular coagulation, and so forth.

Fortunately, acute cholecystitis and other complications of gallstones requiring surgical intervention are rare in pregnancy. This is in no small part due to the fact that most women become pregnant in their 20s and early 30s, whereas gallstones usually do not cause symptoms until their bearers are in their late 30s and beyond. Gallbladder contraction is impaired during pregnancy, and so it seems reasonable to postulate that such impaired contractility leads to a lesser frequency of stones obstructing the cystic duct. Of interest in this regard are the many reports of biliary colic occurring after delivery and a seemingly high incidence of cholecystectomy in the year after delivery. Moreover, acute cholecystitis requiring operation during pregnancy is most common during the first trimester when gallbladder contraction is still active.

It is beyond the scope of this article to review the pathophysiology of gallstone formation in detail, but a brief survey of the current state of knowledge is in order. There is considerable evidence that estrogens and progestins, whether endogenous or exogenous (contraceptives), increase the risk of gallstone formation largely by increasing biliary cholesterol saturation. This increased cholesterol saturation is due to a decreased bile acid pool size and especially to a decrease in the size of the chenodeoxycholic acid pool, since chenodeoxycholic acid inhibits cholesterol synthesis.

Diagnosis. The best way to recognize gallstones in the pregnant woman suspected of having biliary colic, cholecystitis or other complication of gallstones is with ultrasonography, since this technique is quite accurate and poses no known risk to the fetus. In skilled hands, ultrasonography is also quite accurate at distinguishing extrahepatic from intrahepatic biliary obstruction in the jaundiced patient, but only rarely will ultrasonography show stones in the common bile duct. As already noted, however, the physician must be aware that as pregnancy progresses, the appendix is displaced toward the right upper quadrant, and in late pregnancy it may be difficult to distinguish between acute appendicitis and acute cholecystitis or pancreatitis. Abnormal pancreatic or liver enzymes along with ultrasonography can be helpful in distinguishing these conditions. Thus, a combination of liver chemistries, pancreatic enzymes, and ultrasonography should clarify what is occurring in most pregnant women who develop right upper quadrant pain with tenderness and guarding, nausea, vomiting, fever and leukocytosis. It must be kept in mind that pancreatitis in pregnancy is usually due to gallstones. If the diagnosis cannot be established with these relatively safe techniques, other diagnostic procedures which require radioisotopes (IDA scan) or x-ray, which pose a threat to the fetus, will depend upon the state of the patient. Keeping in mind that cholangitis may be a life-threatening disorder, the physician will use what diagnostic procedures appear appropriate whenever the situation dictates.

Treatment. Asymptomatic gallstones found incidentally during pregnancy by ultrasound can be ignored on the supposition that they will cause no trouble, particularly as a sluggish gallbladder is less likely to propel them into the cystic duct. Prophylactic cholecystectomy is in order after delivery, we believe, in the woman who is planning on having more children. Clearly, the pregnant woman who develops *only* biliary colic should be treated symptomatically, since the attack usually subsides within a few hours and it is not unreasonable to treat subsequent attacks during pregnancy medically as long as they are infrequent and of no great severity. The woman in whom biliary colic develops during pregnancy, however, should undergo cholecystectomy after delivery. Acute cholecystitis during pregnancy should also be treated medically, at least initially, since it frequently responds to nasogastric suction and antibiotics. Such women should also undergo cholecystectomy after delivery. If acute cholecystitis does not resolve with medical management, or if other complications such as cholangitis or pancreatitis arise, operation should be performed without delay. Indeed, in the presence of cholangitis or pancreatitis from gallstones, operation should be performed as soon as possible as delay is associated with increased mortality for the mother and fetus. Fetal mortality is less than 5 per cent after cholecystectomy, especially in the second and third trimester, but approaches 60 per cent when pancreatitis secondary to biliary tract disease is left untreated.

INFLAMMATORY BOWEL DISEASE

Idiopathic inflammatory bowel disease is classified either as ulcerative colitis or Crohn's disease, although sometimes the distinction is difficult. These diseases frequently involve other organs such as the liver, skin, and eyes, but a description of all their manifestations is beyond the scope of this article. Suffice it to say that ulcerative colitis usually presents with crampy lower abdominal pain, diarrhea, which is frequently bloody, and when rectal involvement is sufficient, there is tenesmus and urgency. Crohn's disease, which can involve any part of the gastrointestinal tract, can resemble ulcerative colitis when it involves the colon, but rectal sparing is usually present. When Crohn's disease involves the terminal ileum, right lower quadrant pain, cramps, and diarrhea are the usual problems, and if small bowel obstruction is present, nausea, vomiting, and abdominal distention will also occur. Both Crohn's disease and ulcerative colitis have exacerbations and remissions with a chronic course, and during exacerbations, fever, leukocytosis, and abdominal tenderness over the involved bowel are present.

It was previously thought that inflammatory bowel disease adversely affected pregnancy, and conversely, that pregnancy might worsen inflammatory bowel disease. More recent experience has suggested a benign interaction between these two processes. Present evidence suggests that ulcerative colitis has no adverse effect on fertility, although Crohn's disease does bring with it an increased risk of infertility, at least during periods of activity. Women with Crohn's disease seem able to conceive when their disease is in remission. It had also been suggested that women with inflammatory bowel disease had an increased rate of spontaneous abortions, but there is no conclusive evidence that the abortion rate in such women is greater than in the normal population. Another misconception has been that pregnancy results in exacerbation of inflammatory bowel disease, but appropriate studies utilizing control populations of nonpregnant women have shown that the exacerbation rate is the same in the nonpregnant patients as in their pregnant counterparts. To be sure, there is about a 40 per cent relapse rate of Crohn's disease in the postpartum period, possibly as a result of a rapid fall in serum cortisol level that occurs during the postpartum period. This hypothesis has not been proven, however, and furthermore, the relapse rate of Crohn's disease in the postpartum period is no greater than in nonpregnant patients and no more severe. Thus, we conclude that pregnancy has no deleterious effects on inflammatory bowel disease and vice versa.

Diagnosis. Diagnostic procedures which pose a risk to the fetus, such as ionizing radiation, should be avoided during pregnancy unless absolutely necessary. In the patient with known inflammatory bowel disease who develops an uncomplicated exacerbation, no diagnostic procedures are necessary and one can simply treat the exacerbation. For example, if a patient with ulcerative colitis in remission develops crampy lower abdominal pain and bloody diarrhea, similar to previous episodes, then she can simply be treated without further diagnostic studies.

In the patient with symptoms suggestive of a complication that may require surgical intervention such as small bowel obstruction or abscess formation, radiologic studies may be necessary. Ultrasonography should be utilized to full advantage in these situations, and although ultrasonography is not good for visualizing the bowel as such, it is good for localizing abscesses. Intestinal obstruction can be detected with the aid of a plain film of the abdomen; although such a plain film involves some radiation, it is estimated that only 300 millirad is delivered to the fetus, certainly a small dose. Present evidence suggests that if the fetus receives less than 25 rads from the fourteenth day until term, no birth defects, retardation, or growth or other abnormalities can be detected.

The patient in whom inflammatory bowel disease develops for the first time during pregnancy may need a more extensive diagnostic workup. Endoscopy, both upper and lower, should be utilized to the greatest extent possible in these situations, since it provides no known risk to the fetus. Endoscopy, however, provides visualization only of the esophagus, stomach, proximal duodenum, and colon, and cannot be counted upon for the diagnosis of small bowel disease unless the terminal ileum is involved. Thus, a small bowel series may have to be performed. However, the radiation involved with this procedure has been estimated at less than 1000 millirad delivered to the fetus. Thus, judicious use of ionizing radiation, and especially not exceeding 2 rads if possible (some believe 10 rads cause no problem), should not result in any harm to the fetus.

Treatment. The treatment of inflammatory bowel disease in pregnancy does not differ from that in nonpregnant persons. Although corticosteroids cross the placenta and can induce fetal abnormality in animals, prednisone and prednisolone, drugs commonly used in the treatment of inflammatory bowel disease, cross the fetal circulation poorly, which helps to explain the low incidence of fetal side-effects when steroids are administered to the mother, and the rarity of fetal putuitary-adrenal suppression. Most data and literature suggest that steroid treatment during pregnancy does not result in an increased frequency of abortion or congenital abnormalities; however, low birth weight has been reported in some studies. Thus, despite experimental observations in animals, administration of corticosteroids during human pregnancy does not appear to be associated with increased risk of fetal malformations, abortions, stillbirths, premature deliveries, or adrenocortical insufficiency. Breast feeding after delivery also appears to be safe; the amount of steroids the nursing infant receives appears to be negligible. More data, however, are needed in this area. Thus, the use of steroids in women during pregnancy or in the postpartum period appears to be safe for the fetus or baby.

There is a theoretical risk associated with the use of sulfasalazine during pregnancy, since sulfonamides can cross the placenta and displace bilirubin from albumin to cause kernicterus. Although sulfasalazine and its metabolites cross the placenta, their ability to displace bilirubin from albumin is small, and an increased incidence of kernicterus in mothers receiving sulfasalazine has not been reported. Sulfasalazine has not been reported to result in an increased incidence of congenital abnormalities, spontaneous abortions, or neonatal jaundice. Sulfasalazine is probably also safe during breast feeding but more studies are needed in this area. We conclude that the usual agents used in the treatment of inflammatory bowel disease, that is, sulfasalazine and steroids, can be used safely during pregnancy.

CONSTIPATION

Constipation is a frequent complaint during pregnancy. By constipation we mean discomfort because the stools are difficult to pass or too hard such that their passage produces pain, incomplete evacuation, or infrequent evacuation. There have been very few good studies of constipation; little is known of the pathophysiology in the general population, and even less in pregnant women. It seems likely that progesterone, a smooth muscle relaxant which has an inhibitory effect on human colonic musculature, plays a role. It has also been postulated that the pressure of the fetus on the distal colon also plays a role, but there are no studies to confirm this hypothesis.

Diagnosis. The diagnosis of constipation can be made by history alone. If there is rectal pain, then hemorrhoids and rectal fissure should be excluded by sigmoidoscopy or anoscopy. Rarely the physician may want to rule out hypercalcemia and hypothyroidism, which can produce constipation. The physician should inquire about the use of aluminum and calcium-containing antacids for heartburn, as these agents often produce constipation.

Treatment. Assuming that no other disorder such as a rectal fissure is present, the primary treatment of uncomplicated constipation is aimed at increasing the bulk and water content of the stool. This is done by increasing dietary fiber and fluid intake, a combination which will increase stool weight and decrease colonic transit time. Dietary fiber can be increased by increasing the intake of fruits, vegetables, and bran. We usually instruct our patients to eat at least three servings of fruits and vegetables per day, and drink 8 to 10 glasses of water. If this is not effective, then bulk agents such as Metamucil, can be added. Starting with 1 or 2 teaspoons per day, the dose is increased until constipation is relieved. Three to 4 tablespoons daily may be required.

Increasing dietary fiber and fluid intake should be tried for at least 6 weeks before being considered ineffective. A few patients will require laxatives or enemas. Milk of magnesia, magnesium citrate, or dioctyl sodium sulfosuccinate (Colace) can be used if the high fiber diet is ineffective. Likewise, a tap water enema may prove helpful. Laxatives and enemas should not be used on a regular basis for constipation, but only sporadically to relieve severe constipation.

PANCREATITIS IN PREGNANCY

WATSON A. BOWES, Jr., M.D.

Pancreatitis is a disorder of unknown cause which is associated with symptoms of abdominal pain, nausea, and vomiting. The reported prevalence of acute pancreatitis in pregnancy varies from 1 in 1000 to 1 in 10,000 deliveries. The higher frequency of the disease undoubtedly is related to a higher index of diagnostic suspicion and the more frequent use of serum and urinary amylase determinations when nonspecific gastrointestinal symptoms arise during pregnancy. The more serious and more complicated cases are more likely to be recognized and, therefore, account for the somewhat biased reporting of extraordinarily high maternal mortality (37 per cent) and perinatal mortality (38 per cent). More recent reports confirming a higher prevalence of the disease as a result of improved biochemical surveillance demonstrate that in 90 per cent or more of the cases the disease is self-limiting and maternal deaths are rare. Perinatal loss is uncommon if the condition is recognized early and treated properly.

It is difficult to determine whether the disease is more or less common during pregnancy than in nonpregnant women of the same age and parity. However, there is some evidence that pregnancy may predispose women to the development of acute pancreatitis. Among women under 30 in whom the diagnosis of acute pancreatitis is made, 50 per cent of the cases occur in association with pregnancy. Several conditions commonly associated with acute pancreatitis, including cholelithiasis, hyperlipidemia, hypoproteinemia, and hyperemesis, are also known to occur with a relatively higher frequency in pregnancy. As many as 75 per cent or more of women in whom acute pancreatitis develops during pregnancy also have cholelithiasis. This association might be even higher if all patients with pancreatitis were diligently investigated for the presence of gallstones. Some of the more unusual and possibly etiologically related conditions which have been reported in cases of pancreatitis during pregnancy are acute and chronic alcoholism, acute fatty liver secondary to tetracycline therapy, chlorothiazide use, acute bacterial and viral infections, carcinoma of the pancreas, and hyperparathyroidism.

Complications of acute pancreatitis in pregnancy include pancreatic abscess, pseudocyst formation, hypocalcemia, hyperglycemia, diabetic ketoacidosis, thrombophlebitis, pulmonary embolism, bronchopneumonia, gastric bleeding, common bile duct obstruction, pancreatic infarction and retroperitoneal hematoma formation, shock, and renal failure. The most serious threats to the fetus are premature labor during the acute phase of the disease, hyperpyrexia, and fetal death due to maternal hypotension.

MANAGEMENT OF PATIENTS SUSPECTED OF HAVING PANCREATITIS DURING PREGNANCY

An increased maternal and perinatal mortality has been associated with one or more of the following laboratory findings: leukocytosis in excess of 20,000; hemoglobin concentration less than 11 gm per dl; serum calcium less than 7.0 mg per dl and hyperglycemia. Consequently, these laboratory tests should be ordered when the diagnosis is established. Interestingly, the level of serum amylase while the most helpful test in establishing the diagnosis, is apparently not related to maternal or perinatal mortality.

Nasogastric suction, which prevents gastric contents from reaching the duodenum and stimulating pancreatic enzyme secretion, usually accomplishes the first objective of management, which is to decrease pancreatic activity.

Intravenous fluids (crystalloids) must be used to replace all nasogastric aspirate and insensible water loss. Patients who are in shock or seriously dehydrated upon admission should be treated with colloids or whole blood for prompt restoration of adequate fluid and blood volume. This is of paramount importance to the well-being of both the fetus and the mother. Nothing will be more dangerous to the fetus than prolonged uteroplacental hypoperfusion secondary to maternal hypovolemia. Daily (or more frequent) serum electrolyte determinations should be checked as long as the patient is on nasogastric suction and replacement intravenous therapy to insure proper electrolyte balance. Special attention must be given to maintaining normal serum potassium and calcium concentrations.

Analgesics given parentally are invariably required because of the intensity of the pain. Meperidine is theoretically less likely than morphine to cause contraction of the biliary ducts.

Anticholinergics such as propantheline (15 to 30 mg every 6 to 8 hours) are not of proven benefit but may help decrease gastric secretion in some cases. Patients find the side-effects of therapeutic doses of anticholinergics very annoying (mouth dryness and blurred vision).

Antibiotics have been advocated by some to prevent the infectious complications of the disease, but most current authorities agree that there is no proven advantage to routine antibiotic therapy in most cases of acute pancreatitis.

Leg exercises, surgical stockings, or special pneumatic hose may help prevent thrombophlebitis, which occurs with increased frequency in association with pancreatitis.

Following resolution of the acute phase of the illness (usually 2 to 4 days), oral feedings and normal ambulation may be resumed. At this time sonographic examination of the gallbladder is in order to determine if cholelithiasis is present. If this is normal or nondiagnostic a cholecystogram performed after the patient has delivered is probably in order. The patient should also be instructed in a high-protein, low-fat diet, served in small frequent meals, as the best protection against recurrence of the disease.

Surgical consultation should be obtained in patients who do not appear to be responding to conservative therapy. Indications for surgical intervention include acute biliary obstruction, a rapidly enlarging abscess, pseudocyst or retroperitoneal hematoma, intestinal obstruction or perforation, or uncontrolled gastrointestinal bleeding. When acute pancreatitis occurs in association with cholelithiasis in early pregnancy, cholecystectomy should be performed 6 to 8 weeks following resolution of the pancreatitis. This will significantly reduce the risk of recurrence. If, however, pancreatitis and cholelithiasis are diagnosed in the second half of pregnancy and resolve with conservative therapy, the cholecystectomy should be performed after the patient delivers.

MYASTHENIA GRAVIS AND MULTIPLE SCLEROSIS IN PREGNANCY

STANLEY van den NOORT, M.D.

MULTIPLE SCLEROSIS

This is a disease of the central nervous system characterized by patches of demyelination which are scattered in time and in anatomical space. It affects at least 1 of every 2000 people. The disease favors young adult women and has an approximate prevalence of 1 of every 1000 women of child-bearing age. The illness is notoriously difficult to identify. Once identified its course is difficult to predict. While the onset may be dramatic, with loss of vision in one eye, ataxia, or paraparesis, it is commonly subtle with vague sensory and motor symptoms, including lower abdominal discomfort, band-like sensations about the pelvis, urgency of urination, a propensity to giggle, electrical sensations on neck flexion, clumsiness, and vertigo. These may lead to erroneous diagnosis of hysteria. In a majority of patients, the disease begins with attacks of neurological deficit which increase over about a week, stabilize, and then begin to improve after several weeks. Attacks may occur once or twice a year at first, with less frequent relapses in later years. Some patients present a slowly progressive course with no clear attacks or remissions. The diagnosis is clinical, with no absolute laboratory test. Laboratory tests are helpful, but least helpful in subtle, early cases. Characteristic laboratory findings include elevated gamma globulin contact and oligoclonal bands of globulin in the cerebrospinal fluid, slowed evoked responses from visual, auditory, and somatosensory stimuli, and white matter lesions on computed tomography.

Treatment of multiple sclerosis is presently ineffective. Acute attacks may respond to prednisone or similar agents, but there is no clear effect on the long-term course of the illness. Many agents are advocated to modify the course, but none to date have survived a well-designed clinical trial. Supportive therapy, physical medicine, and symptomatic approaches help significantly. The overall prognosis is better than is commonly believed by physicians. Including the mild cases with unproven diagnoses, it is probable that the average patient with multiple sclerosis can live a productive life for a normal lifespan.

The pathogenesis of multiple sclerosis is obscure. Genetic predisposition, presumed exposure to a viral agent in the second decade, and a disordered immune system are factors. Suppressor T-lymphocytes disappear in attacks.

The interaction of multiple sclerosis and pregnancy is also overestimated by medical professionals. There is no clear statistical evidence that multiple sclerosis is influenced by pregnancy. Attacks or even first diagnoses appear in pregnancy but not a few patients feel better. It is commonly held by neurologists that exacerbations for first attacks are more commonly seen in the first several months postpartum. This does not have unequivocal statistical support. While postpartum relapse is also seen with suspicious frequency in other "autoimmune" disorders, it may reflect postpartum overwork and fatigue as much as hormonal effects on immune function.

Management of pregnancy in the patient with multiple sclerosis should observe the following guidelines:

1. A decision to interrupt pregnancy is not indicated by the diagnosis of multiple sclerosis. Personal choice in relation to possible increase in risk for multiple sclerosis and concern for capacity to care for children must be balanced with desire to have children and lack of convincing evidence that pregnancy is harmful. There is no evidence that multiple sclerosis influences the outcome of pregnancy. Risk of multiple sclerosis in offspring is statistically increased but trivial for individual families.

2. Management of pregnancy is normal. Unproven treatments for multiple sclerosis should be avoided to reduce risk to the fetus. Attacks or progression of multiple sclerosis in pregnancy may be helped by judicious transient use of prednisone usually as a single dose (40 to 80 mg) once every other day. In severe attacks, daily prednisone may be required for a short period.

3. Physical impairments such as paraparesis with spasticity may alter symptoms of labor and pose problems in delivery requiring spinal anesthetic to reduce adductor spasticity. Constipation is also a stubborn problem requiring enemas, Ducolax, Pericolace, and similar agents. Urgency, incontinence and attendant urinary tract infection require careful management. Bladder spasmolytics may help or may lead to retention. Except for the special management of spasticity, spinal anesthesia should be avoided if possible.

4. Postpartum management may be more relevant to multiple sclerosis than prenatal care. Increased rest and supportive help for several months are desirable. Relapses may benefit from vigorous short-term (4 to 8 weeks) treatment with prednisone (100 mg) in single daily doses for 5 days, then 100 mg in a single dose every other day with decrementing doses as improvement ensues.

MYASTHENIA GRAVIS

Myasthenia gravis is an uncommon disorder of neuromuscular transmission. It affects 1 out of every 20,000 people, but is more common than this in women of child-bearing age. Myasthenia is a highly unpredictable disease which may be mild or severe with dramatic relapses and equally dramatic remissions. Patients requiring respirator care for months may abruptly recover spontaneously and remain well for years on no treatment. Characteristic symptoms include rapid fatigue of eye movements (including opening), facial movements, chewing, swallowing, voice, proximal limb movements, and respiration. Drooping eyelids, flat face, and nasal voice with rapid fatigue and weakness of shoulders and thighs suggest the diagnosis. However, mild cases may be recognized only with difficulty. The diagnosis is established if 10 mg of intravenous edrophonium (Tensilon) provides dramatic if fleeting improvement in strength. A vast majority of patients have thymic hyperplasia and circulating antibodies to acetylcholine receptor proteins. A significant proportion of patients have clinical or subclinical evidence of other disorders of the immune system, such as lupus, rheumatoid arthritis, and thyroiditis.

The pathogenesis of myasthenia is in some way determined by genetic predisposition and development of antibodies to closely related thymic and muscle antigens, with particular elaboration of antibodies to acetylcholine receptor proteins. While the titer of these antibodies is not closely correlated to clinical activity, plasmapheresis produces improvement in some patients suggesting the presence of a circulating factor which determines muscular weakness.

Present treatment of myasthenia varies with age and severity. In a few mild cases, no treatment is needed; in other mild forms, we rely on oral neostigmine (15 to 30 mg every 3 hours) or pyridostigmine (Mestinon) (30 to 60 mg every 6 hours) as agents which enhance cholinergic effects by agonist action and by blocking cholinesterase. Sustained large doses of anticholinesterase drugs damage the neuromuscular junction. In more severe forms, prednisone (20 to 60 mg daily) is instituted in hospital since prednisone may initially worsen symptoms; potassium supplements may modify this initial effect. After a few days, improvement is usual and can often be sustained with prednisone (20 to 60 mg) in a single dose every other day. In young patients with moderate disease, it is usual to recommend thymectomy as an alternative to long-term prednisone treatment. Thymectomy may help a majority of young women with myasthenia; some patients do not improve for many months after surgery. Plasmapheresis on a weekly, fortnightly, or monthly basis has a beneficial effect on some patients who fail to improve with other treatment. Various combinations of these regimens are used. One must often accept some symptoms on any treatment schedule. In a few cases, general immunosuppressants such as cyclophosphamide and azathioprine have been tried with varying effect.

Myasthenics may enter crisis at any time, often without warning. This is a particular problem in the puerperium (perhaps due because of loss of intrinsic immunosuppression by alpha-fetoprotein). It is necessary to decide then whether the crisis is due to: (1) refractoriness to anticholinesterase medication, (2) insufficient dosage of anticholinesterase, or (3) overdosage of anticholinesterase medication. Dramatic fleeting improvement from intravenous edrophonium (10 mg) will identify patients in the second group for continuing treatment with increased levels of neostigmine or pyridostigmine. In the other forms of crisis, anticholinesterase should be reduced or stopped while mechanical support of ventilation is introduced. Hypokalemia should be avoided. A number of drugs adversely affect the course of myasthenia. Myasthenics are notoriously sensitive to curare-like anesthetics; these should be avoided. Parenteral magnesium promotes neuromuscular blockade. A number of aminoglycoside antibiotics can initiate myasthenia—neomycin, streptomycin, gentamicin, kanamycin, polymixin, colistin, tetracycline, and vancomycin. Safer antibiotics include penicillin, erythromycin, and chloramphenicol. Myasthenics are also intolerant of quinine and quinidine.

Most myasthenic patients handle pregnancy without difficulty. Fertility and the probability of normal live birth are normal. Myasthenia may remit, remain unchanged, relapse, or begin during pregnancy. The knowledge that pregnancy can produce remission has caused a few pregnancies. The treatment of myasthenia during pregnancy is unsettled and may vary with severity. Neostigmine and pyridostigmine precipitate early labor and the incidence of prematurity in myasthenia is increased, perhaps for this reason. Single dose, every other day prednisone in modest doses, may be safe. Thymectomy to promote remission before pregnancy should be considered. Plasmapheresis may prove to be a useful means of treatment during pregnancy to avoid high dosage prednisone or pyridostigmine.

A few infants with arthrogryposis (congenital contracture) have been born to myasthenic mothers. Very high titers of antibody and/or decreased fetal activity may dictate vigorous treatment of myasthenia with plasmapheresis to help the fetus.

The incidence of preeclampsia in myasthenia gravis is increased, perhaps in relation to disordered immune mechanisms. Magnesium should be avoided.

During labor, voluntary effort may be reduced. Regional anesthesia is preferred. Chloroprocaine hydrochloride and tetracaine, which are degraded by plasma cholinesterase, should be avoided. Close observation of maternal ventilation is required, and neostigmine 1.5 mg every 2 hours, may be helpful. Neostigmine and pyridostigmine may produce fetal bradycardia presumably without harm.

During the puerperium, the mother has an increased risk of relapse and requires careful observation especially directed to ventilatory adequacy.

About 20 per cent of children from myasthenic mothers develop neonatal myasthenia. This often appears after a day or so, perhaps delayed by persisting levels of maternal alpha-fetoprotein. The myasthenia is presumably due to fetal transfer of anti-acetylcholine receptor antibody from the mother. After diagnosis with edrophonium (1 mg intravenously), treatment with plasmapheresis or neostigmine (.025 mg per kg intramuscularly every 6 hours) will usually produce rapid improvement. After 3 to 4 weeks, treatment can usually be discontinued.

THE MANAGEMENT OF ASTHMA AND RHINITIS DURING PREGNANCY

MICHAEL SCHATZ, M.D.,
RICHARD P. PORRECO, M.D.,
and ROBERT S. ZEIGER, M.D., Ph.D.

GENERAL CONSIDERATIONS

Rhinitis

Chronic rhinitis during pregnancy may have many causes, and optimal therapy requires a correct diagnosis. This can usually be made on the basis of a careful history, a limited physical examination, and the nasal scraping. Sinus films (usually Waters and Caldwell views suffice) with appropriate pelvic and abdominal shielding may occasionally be necessary to identify sinusitis in patients with equivocal clinical findings or to confirm recalcitrant sinusitis in patients not responding to medical therapy. The use of allergy skin testing during pregnancy is discussed below.

Asthma

Asthma occurs in approximately 1 per cent of pregnancies and has been associated with increased perinatal mortality. In addition, severe asthma during pregnancy may be a cause of maternal morbidity and mortality. Although the precise factors responsible for the increased fetal risk remain unidentified, optimal prospective treatment of asthma during pregnancy has been associated with an excellent perinatal outcome.

Pregnancy may also affect the course of asthma in the majority of women. In one study, 24 per cent of women improved during pregnancy while 37 per cent worsened. Although those women with moderate or severe asthma prior to pregnancy are most likely to worsen during pregnancy, even patients with relatively mild asthma may have severe exacerbations during pregnancy. All pregnant women with asthma should be monitored closely for a change in their clinical status so that the therapeutic regimen can be adjusted accordingly. Frequent, regular medical visits during which historical, auscultatory, and spirometric data is evaluated by a physician skilled in managing asthma are essential to achieve successful and safe asthma therapy during pregnancy.

NONPHARMACOLOGIC THERAPY

Pregnancy represents a time of psychological vulnerability and increased stress for virtually all women. In pregnant women with asthma or rhinitis, these stresses may be especially important. First, in women whose symptoms worsen with stress, the stress of normal pregnancy may lead to an exacerbation of symptoms. Conversely, the morbidity associated with asthma or nasal symptoms, especially if the symptoms interfere with sleep, may add substantially to the stress of normal pregnancy. Thus, management during pregnancy must include (1) education of the patient regarding asthma and rhinitis in general and the interrelationships between asthma, rhinitis, and pregnancy; (2) adequate opportunity for the patient to express her concerns; (3) support in the form of regular visits and easy accessibility for unanticipated problems; and (4) reassurance that the internist or allergist, obstetrician, and patient will work as a team to maximize the well-being of mother and fetus.

The first tenet of *immunologic* therapy is avoidance, and this is particularly important during pregnancy since avoidance procedures increase the likelihood of physical well-being without pharmacologic intervention. Information on avoidance of relevant antigens (pollen, mold, dust, dander) and irritants (especially cigarette smoke) should be given to the patient. The patient should be convinced that a decision to trade symptoms and medication for adverse exposure is extremely unwise during pregnancy.

Allergen immunotherapy is utilized for patients with substantial allergic symptoms inadequately controlled by avoidance and medications. Abortions associated with systemic reactions following antigen immunotherapy have been reported. Aside from systemic reactions, allergen immunotherapy appears safe during pregnancy. Based on this information, we recommend that allergen immunotherapy be carefully continued during pregnancy in patients already receiving immunotherapy who appear to be deriving benefit and who are not experiencing systemic reactions. We believe that benefit/risk considerations do not favor *beginning* immunotherapy during pregnancy for most women, since patients just beginning immunotherapy (1) have an undefined propensity for systemic reactions, (2) may be more likely to experience systemic reactions with the frequent dosage increases which occur during initiation of immunotherapy, (3) will derive an unpredictable amount of benefit, and (4) may require long-term treatment before clinical efficacy can be substantiated.

Because skin testing with potent antigens may also be associated with systemic reactions, we recommend that skin tests be performed during pregnancy only if the results will have substantial therapeutic impact. In our experience, this is only rarely necessary since historical information will usually identify dust, mold, dander, or pollen sensitivity for which avoidance instructions may be given empirically.

PHARMACOLOGIC MANAGEMENT

In evaluating a specific medication for use in treating asthma or rhinitis during pregnancy, one must consider (1) human data on the use of that drug during pregnancy, (2) the results and applicability of animal teratogenicity studies, (3) the efficacy and necessity of the medication, (4) its route of administration (topical versus systemic), and (5) the time the drug has been in clinical use.

Rhinitis

Many women will be able to tolerate their nasal symptoms during pregnancy with no pharmacologic therapy. Although this is desirable, especially during the first trimester, troublesome symptoms warrant treatment. Initial pharmacologic therapy, when necessary, depends on the diagnosis, the most troublesome symptoms, and the frequency of symptoms.

Nasal saline may be useful for the nasal dryness, nasal bleeding, and vascular congestion associated with pregnancy. A buffered saline spray (Salinex, Ocean Spray) or saline lavage using the Water-Pik and the Grossan nasal irrigator may be used. The latter is especially useful for patients with prominent postnasal drip during pregnancy.

For intermittent substantial nasal obstruction, oxymetazoline hydrochloride (Afrin) drops or spray may suffice. The patient should be carefully informed of the potential for development of rebound congestion and rhinitis medicamentosa. For more continuous nasal obstruction or for intermittent obstruction inadequately controlled by topical therapy, pseudoephedrine should be used. For intermittent symptoms, 30 to 60 mg as needed may be considered; for more continuous symptoms, 60 mg, three or four times daily or 120 mg slow-release preparations twice daily are useful.

For patients with troublesome allergic or eosinophilic nonallergic rhinitis associated with prominent sneezing and runny nose, antihistamine therapy may be needed. We recommend tripelennamine (PBZ), 25 to 50 mg as needed, for intermittent substantial symptoms, and 50 to 100 mg of the long-acting preparations twice daily for more continuous symptoms. Many patients with eosinophilic rhinitis will respond better to a combination of tripelennamine and pseudephedrine than to either drug alone. For patients who do not respond to tripelennamine or who develop tachyphylaxis, other antihistamines may be considered. For patients with severe eosinophilic rhinitis not responding to oral antihistamine-decongestant therapy, intranasal beclomethasone should be initiated at a dose of two sprays in each nostril twice daily, and tapered to the lowest effective dose.

Although some patients with nasal polyps during pregnancy will require no treatment and others will be adequately controlled by oral antihistamine-decongestant therapy, those with more troublesome manifestations will require intranasal beclomethasone. For patients with severe nasal polyps inadequately controlled by intranasal beclomethasone and adequate treatment of secondary or complicating infection, individual considerations will determine whether oral corticosteroids or nasal polypectomy with local anesthesia is the best choice.

The treatment of bacterial rhinosinusitis during pregnancy involves antibiotics and relief of nasal and sinus obstruction. Various factors contribute to lower serum levels of antibiotics during pregnancy compared to levels after the same dose in the nonpregnant state. Because of this, 500 mg doses (generally three times daily) of amoxicillin, ampicillin, cefaclor, or erythromycin should be used for the treatment of bacterial rhinosinusitis during pregnancy for a 2 to 3 week course. Short-term oxymetazoline nose spray or drops and oral pseudoephedrine (occasionally supplemented by tripelennamine) are useful for control of nasal and sinus congestion associated with bacterial rhinosinusitis. In addition, therapeutic sinus irrigation and drainage may be required for recalcitrant gestational sinusitis.

Rhinitis medicamentosa during pregnancy may be extremely difficult to treat. Although discontinuation of the topical vasoconstrictor is the most important treatment, intolerable congestion frequently results. Several approaches may be useful to control this. First, the patient may be advised to discontinue the topical decongestant initially on one side only. After 1 to 2 weeks, the nostril which is no longer receiving topical decongestant should be relatively normal, and the topical decongestant in the other nostril can be discontinued. Secondly, the substitution of oral antihistamine-decongestant therapy will allow comfortable discontinuation of topical decongestants in some patients. Third, intranasal corticosteroids are quite effective for rhinitis medicamentosa in the nonpregnant state, and may be similarly effective during pregnancy. Systemic corticosteriods are not appropriate for rhinitis medicamentosa during pregnancy; in recalcitrant cases, the least amount of topical decongestant necessary should be used until it can be more easily discontinued post partum.

Asthma

Patients with intermittent mild symptoms who require medication are usually adequately controlled on intermittent inhaled beta$_2$ bronchodilators (isoetharine, metaproterenol, albuterol) or short-acting theophylline preparations. At this time, we consider chronic theophylline therapy the initial treatment of choice for most pregnant women with more continuous mild to moderate symptoms. We generally recommend slow-release anhydrous preparations, beginning with 375 to 500 mg per day in two or three divided doses, increasing as necessary and as tolerated while carefully monitoring clinical response and serum theophylline levels. When the patient is well controlled, the dosage should then be tapered carefully to the lowest effective dose.

Ephedrine is the oldest oral bronchodilator

in clinical use today and appears safe during pregnancy. However, it is generally not effective enough or tolerated well enough when used chronically to be considered a first line bronchodilator drug during pregnancy. Ephedrine may be useful, though, for short-term therapy in a patient already on maximal theophylline doses for a mild to moderate exacerbation such as may be associated with an upper respiratory infection. There are no first trimester human data on the newer beta$_2$-adrenergic agents (metaproterenol, terbutaline, albuterol), and animal studies have not been reassuring with metaproterenol and albuterol. In addition, all three of these drugs have been shown to have substantial inhibitory effects on uterine contractility. For these reasons, we try to avoid oral beta$_2$ sympathomimetics during pregnancy. Although full-dose regular inhalational therapy provides less of a systemic dose, the possibility of adverse effects from this regular, smaller but not necessarily insignificant dose cannot be excluded on the basis of available data. Consequently, long-term high-dose inhalational sympathomimetic therapy during pregnancy is not recommended at this time.

Although cromolyn and beclomethasone are relatively new drugs, their inhalational route and the information available regarding their use during pregnancy suggest probable safety. Moreover, their use seems preferable to the alternatives in patients with moderate symptoms who are poorly controlled on full dose oral theophylline. We recommend that cromolyn be considered first. Further, the use of an inhaled sympathomimetic bronchodilator immediately preceding the administration of cromolyn or beclomethasone, may promote better bronchial penetration and efficacy. As the patient improves, the preceding inhaled bronchodilator may be discontinued.

Current benefit/risk considerations dictate that corticosteroids should be used when clearly indicated for the management of moderate to severe asthma during pregnancy which is unresponsive to the previously cited regimens. Moderate to severe chronic symptoms should be cleared with 30 to 40 mg of prednisone daily for approximately 5 to 7 days. The dose may be tapered over the next 5 days. The regimen that will then be necessary to control the asthma will vary from no medication to, occasionally, regular daily corticosteroids, depending on individual circumstances. For patients who are corticosteroid-dependent prior to pregnancy, corticosteroids should be continued at the lowest effective dose.

Our suggested protocol for the management of acute asthma during pregnancy is shown in Table 1. Epinephrine or terbutaline is used when injectable sympathomimetics are necessary for acute asthma. Epinephrine has been associated with animal and human congenital malformations and decreased uteroplacental blood flow in animals. There are no first trimester human teratogenicity data for terbutaline, and terbutaline may inhibit term labor. For these reasons, our protocol for the treatment of acute asthma during pregnancy tries to minimize the use of injectable sympathomimetics. However, in certain patients with severe acute asthma not responding to other therapy, the benefits of injectable sympathomimetics may still outweigh the potential risks. Although terbutaline is a newer drug, animal teratogenicity studies have been negative, and terbutaline has been shown to preserve or increase uterine blood flow in human beings. Thus, when injectable sympathomimetics are required for the treatment of acute asthma during pregnancy, terbutaline may be a better choice than epinephrine at this time.

Guaifenesin and oral fluids may be useful as expectorants in the supportive treatment of complicating respiratory infections during pregnancy; iodides are contraindicated. Ampicillin, amoxicillin, cefalosporins, and erythromycin are useful and safe for the treatment of bacterial

TABLE 1. **A Suggested Protocol for the Pharmacologic Management of Acute Asthma During Pregnancy**

I. Oxygen
II. Glucose-containing fluids
III. Inhaled beta-2-sympathomimetic by mechanical nebulizer (up to 3 times, 20–30 minutes apart)
IV. For patients not responding to the above, intravenous aminophylline
   A. For patients *not* on oral theophylline, 5.6 mg/kg over 20–30 minutes
   B. For patients on oral theophylline, individual considerations (including time and amount of the last oral theophylline dose, duration and amount of the maintenance oral program, and known prior theophylline levels) will determine whether a half-loading dose (2.8 mg/kg over 20–30 minutes) should precede continuous intravenous administration or not
   C. If continuous aminophylline is indicated, administration by IVAC infusion pump at a dose of 0.4 mg/kg/hour is initially recommended. Subsequent dose adjustments should be made on the basis of frequent theophylline measurements
V. Subcutaneous terbutaline once or twice should be considered for patients not tolerating inhaled bronchodilators and not responding to aminophylline or for patients in impending respiratory failure in spite of the above therapy
VI. For patients responding slowly to the above therapy within the first few hours or those initially severely ill, intravenous methylprednisolone should be given; the dose would usually be 40–125 mg every 4–6 hours

bronchitis complicating asthma during pregnancy (500 mg three times daily for 10 days).

Obstetric management during labor of the controlled asthmatic women is not different from the nonasthmatic patient. Should general anesthesia be necessary, halogenated agents are desirable since they have broncholytic activity. Although exacerbations of asthma during labor are uncommon in prospectively managed asthmatic women, we recommend that patients on oral theophylline or inhaled cromolyn or beclomethasone continue this therapy during labor. Patients on oral theophylline who require surgical intervention may receive intravenous aminophylline.

Steroid-dependent asthmatics should receive supplemental steroids for the stress of labor, delivery, and the puerperium. The following regimen has been recommended: 100 mg of hydrocortisone intramuscularly upon admission to labor and delivery and then every 8 hours for 24 hours, or until the absence of puerperal complications is established. Adrenal insufficiency has been reported only rarely in infants of mothers receiving corticosteroids during pregnancy. Although such infants should be carefully observed for any evidence of adrenal hypofunction, prophylactic treatment is not warranted.

RUBELLA

JOHN W. LARSEN, Jr., M.D.,
and JOHN L. SEVER, M.D., Ph.D.

Rubella virus infection (German measles, three-day measles) is a significant cause of congenital malformations. In order to produce fetal damage, infection of the developing embryo must occur during the period of organogenesis. Since there is no technique which can be used antepartum to tell with certainty if a developing embryo has become infected, management of rubella depends on detection of susceptibility by serologic testing of women and protection of susceptibles by immunization.

DIAGNOSIS

In a child or adult, rubella may be suspected in a patient who has had a maculopapular rash, fever, malaise, arthralgia, and lymphadenopathy behind the ears, occiput, and along the posterior cervical chain. Diagnosis based on clinical evidence alone is inexact. Signs and symptoms may be variable to nonexistent. It has been estimated that one-third of rubella infections of adults are asymptomatic.

When a pregnant woman who may be susceptible to rubella is exposed to the disease, serologic tests for rubella antibodies should be performed. One of the most useful tests for this purpose is the hemagglutination-inhibition test (HI). Serologic tests which give results similar to those obtained with the hemagglutination-inhibition method include indirect hemagglutination (IHA), radioimmunoassay (RIA), latex agglutination (LA), fluorescence (FA), and enzyme-linked immunosorbent assay (ELISA). A pregnant woman who has a positive test for rubella antibody at the time of exposure is protected from rubella viremia and thus the fetus is also protected. A susceptible woman who has been exposed should be retested in 3 to 4 weeks. If the time of exposure cannot be determined with certainty, it should be remembered that the incubation period for rubella is approximately 2 weeks, after which an additional few days are required for the development of a significant level of antibody. The diagnosis of acute rubella infection is made when serology converts from negative to positive. If the patient was first seen after the onset of symptoms, it would still be possible to demonstrate a significant rise in antibodies in some cases, since peak antibody titers are not reached until 10 to 14 days after the onset of the rash. In such cases, it may be helpful to supplement the routine antibody test by also measuring rubella IgM antibodies. These antibodies appear a few days after the rash and remain present for about 1 month.

For the hemagglutination-inhibition tests, the physician should remember that, for proper comparison of serologic antibodies measured by dilution techniques, both serum specimens should be assayed simultaneously. Under such circumstances, a fourfold or greater increase in antibody titer is considered significant. In order to accomplish such testing, there are two practical considerations: (1) it is necessary for either the physician initiating care or the laboratory that receives the first specimen to save a frozen aliquot until the second specimen can be obtained; and (2) it is necessary for the physician initiating care to send both specimens to the same laboratory.

Surveys of pregnant women infected with rubella have shown that the incidence of fetal infection is variable. The incidence of major malformations such as microcephaly, cataracts, deafness, and cardiovascular defects may be as great as 50 to 60 per cent when infection occurs during the first 2 months of pregnancy. The malformation rate subsequently declines toward zero as the period of fetal organ formation has been completed. After the fifth month of gestation, there is no evidence of damage.

Fetal morbidity related to rubella is not limited to major malformations. Persistence of virus has been demonstrated in every organ system, causing the "expanded rubella syndrome" which includes: anemia, encephalitis, hepatitis, myocarditis, nephritis, osteomyelitis, pancreatitis, pneumonitis, and thrombocytopenia. Virus may persist in the central nervous system for more than 10 years before causing a fatal progressive panencephalitis. The risk of disease due to very long viral persistence has not been quantitated, but there may be some risk regardless of the stage of pregnancy during which the infection occurred.

MANAGEMENT OF THE PREGNANT WOMAN INFECTED WITH RUBELLA

The physician who takes care of pregnant women has the following responsibilities with respect to rubella:

1. At the initial visit, whether or not there has been known rubella exposure, a pregnant woman should have her rubella antibody status measured by the hemagglutination-inhibition test or other antibody test that is sensitive and suitable for screening.

2. HI-negative patients should be warned of the risk of rubella infection and be advised to avoid contact with persons known to be infected.

3. HI-positive patients should be advised that they are protected from rubella provided their positive antibody status was not the result of recent infection and seroconversion while pregnant. In practice, it is best to know that a patient was HI-positive *prior* to conception. In particular, it is wise to screen for rubella antibody at the outset of an infertility work-up and management program.

4. Patients diagnosed as having rubella while pregnant should be given a full explanation of the possible unfavorable effects of the virus on the fetus. Abortion is now widely available for women who are less than 24 weeks pregnant. A pregnant woman, especially if she developed rubella very early in pregnancy, might wish to have her pregnancy aborted rather than risk giving birth to an infant with congenital rubella. It should be emphasized that the physician's proper role in such instances in to convey information related to the diagnosis, risks of disease, and risks of treatment. We believe that it is not proper for the physician to actively advocate whether or not the patient should be aborted. Difficult as it may be, that decision should remain with the patient, provided her physician has given her sufficient information upon which she can rely.

TREATMENT OF CONGENITAL RUBELLA

Newborn infants with congenital rubella should be isolated to prevent spread of the virus throughout the nursery and obstetric service. The oropharyngeal secretions, urine, and feces of congenital rubella patients are usually noninfectious by age 6 months. However, in some cases, virus shedding persists for as long as 1 year.

Since there is no specific therapy for the rubella virus, treatment of congenital disease is directed at correcting or relieving organ dysfunction. Major eye, ear, and cardiovascular defects require prompt specialty consultation. It is quite important that the initially asymptomatic newborn *not* be lost to follow-up. Delayed manifestations of disease, such as partial hearing loss, vestibular dysfunction, psychomotor retardation, and seizures may not become evident for several years. Particularly close surveillance should be maintained to detect deficient hearing. A central hearing defect may be the only manifestation of disease. It may not be present or obvious in the newborn period; however, if the primary defect is properly diagnosed and the patient is treated with hearing aids and special education, secondary defects of speech and learning can be minimized.

TREATMENT OF ACQUIRED RUBELLA IN CHILDREN AND ADULTS

For the infected child or adult, the course of rubella is usually benign. No therapy is required other than minor pain relievers, such as aspirin or acetaminophen, and bed rest for a few days. The illness may be complicated by thrombocytopenia, arthralgia, and arthritis, which are particularly likely to occur in women of childbearing age. Rarely, encephalitis occurs. Complications usually resolve without treatment.

Should the infected patient be hospitalized for any reason, strict isolation should be enforced. The usual mode of transmission is by nasopharyngeal secretions which can be infectious from up to one week before clinical illness and until two weeks after clinical remission. Blood, urine, and feces from rubella patients may be infectious, also.

PREVENTION OF RUBELLA

The obstetrician-gynecologist may best prevent rubella by routinely screening for rubella antibody in women of childbearing age and conducting appropriate immunization. A vaccine of live attenuated virus is available and has proven to be effective. The vaccine should be given to any woman or girl who is sero-negative and *not* pregnant, and 3 months should elapse before any immunized woman attempts to conceive. The vaccine virus can be transmitted to the products of conception and, on that basis, abortions have been performed for women inadvertently immunized while pregnant, even though the magnitude of risk of fetal malformation from such infection is probably very small.

AMNIOCENTESIS FOR THE ANTENATAL DIAGNOSIS OF GENETIC DEFECTS

ALBERT B. GERBIE, M.D., and SHERMAN ELIAS, M.D.

One of the most exciting advances in the history of obstetrics is the development of techniques to monitor for genetic disorders in the fetus. Before this, genetic counseling could only provide probabilities based upon family history, and couples at risk for having offspring with such disorders could never have a child without taking the chance that it might be affected. Now it is possible to provide a definite answer. If the fetus is determined to be affected, the couple has the choice of terminating the abnormal pregnancy. Fortunately, in most circumstances the physician can reassure the couple that the abnormality in question is not present. Thus, rather than choosing sterilization or nonselective abortion of all pregnancies, these couples may now proceed in having children with greater confidence of a normal outcome.

Detection of many genetic disorders requires analysis either of amniotic fluid or amniotic fluid cells which can be obtained only by amniocentesis. It is the obstetrician who has the responsibility to review the medical and family history of the couple to determine whether or not antenatal diagnosis should be offered. Mandatory requirements to provide safe and reliable antenatal studies are as follows:

1. Appropriate genetic counseling;
2. Performance of the amniocentesis by an obstetrician experienced in this procedure;
3. Availability of ultrasonography;
4. An experienced laboratory with expertise in culturing amniotic fluid cells and performing the necessary cytogenetic and biochemical analyses.

INDICATIONS

The following conditions are now clearly accepted as indications for offering genetic amniocentesis:

Advanced Parental Age. The most common indication for antenatal diagnosis is advanced maternal age. The mean maternal age (the age of the mother when the affected child is born) in trisomy 21 is approximately 35 years, whereas the mean maternal age in the population is about 27 years. A woman aged 35 at the birth of her child has a 1 in 365 risk of having a child with Down syndrome; at age 39 the risk is 1 in 139; at age 45 the risk is 1 in 32 (Table 1). How-

TABLE 1. **Risk of Having a Liveborn Child with Down Syndrome or Other Chromosomal Abnormality by 1 Year Maternal Age Intervals from Ages 20 to 49 Years***

MATERNAL AGE	RISK OF DOWN SYNDROME	TOTAL RISK FOR ALL CHROMOSOME ABNORMALITIES
20	1/1923	1/526
21	1/1695	1/526
22	1/1538	1/500
23	1/1408	1/500
24	1/1299	1/476
25	1/1205	1/476
26	1/1124	1/476
27	1/1053	1/455
28	1/990	1/435
29	1/935	1/417
30	1/885	1/384
31	1/826	1/384
32	1/725	1/322
33	1/592	1/285
34	1/465	1/243
35	1/365	1/178
36	1/287	1/149
37	1/225	1/123
38	1/177	1/105
39	1/139	1/80
40	1/109	1/63
41	1/85	1/48
42	1/67	1/39
43	1/53	1/31
44	1/41	1/24
45	1/32	1/18
46	1/25	1/15
47	1/20	1/11
48	1/16	1/8
49	1/12	1/7

*Modified from Hook, E. B., and Chambers, G. M., Birth Defects Original Article Series, Vol. 13, No. 3A, New York, Liss, 1977, pp. 123–141; and Hook, E. B.: Obstet. Gynecol. 58:282–285, 1981, with permission.

ever, trisomy 21 is not the only chromosomal abnormality that increases with maternal age. Other autosomal trisomies (most commonly trisomy 18 and 13) and some X-chromosome polysomies (e.g., 47,XXX and 47,XXY) also increase with maternal age (Table 1). Accordingly, couples should be informed about the risk of all chromosome disorders (not just Down syndrome) at a given maternal age in order to make an informed decision. Finally, the risk of fathering a child with Down syndrome appears to approximately double that of the maternal age risk when the paternal age is past 55.

Previous Child with a Chromosomal Abnormality. It is reasonable to offer antenatal studies to all couples who have had a previous child (or stillborn, or aborted fetus) with either autosomal trisomy or sex chromosome polysomy. However, it should be recognized that the risk of recurrence may not be as high as sometimes stated. Specifically, above the age of 25 the recurrence risk for Down syndrome is probably no greater than that for maternal age risk alone. On the other hand, women who gave birth to a child with Down syndrome under age 25 have a recurrence risk in the range of 1 per cent. Although data are limited, the recurrence risk following the birth of a child with a chromosomal aberration other than trisomy 21 is in the range of 1.5 to 2 per cent for either the same or for a different chromosomal abnormality.

Parental Chromosomal Translocation or Other Chromosomal Abnormality. A less common indication for antenatal diagnosis which may carry a relatively high risk for abnormal offspring is the presence of either a balanced chromosomal translocation or inversion in a parent. Usually such a parent would be identified after the birth of a child with an unbalanced complement, or as part of an evaluation for repetitive spontaneous abortions. For example, 2 to 3 per cent of individuals with Down syndrome have a translocation, usually between chromosomes 14(D) and 21(G). About 25 per cent of these occur *de novo* with no apparent increased risk for subsequent siblings with Down syndrome beyond that of the general population risk. However, if the mother is a balanced 14/21 carrier, the empirical recurrence risk is about 10 per cent. If the father carries the same translocation, the empirical risks are much lower, perhaps in the range of 1 to 3 per cent. Other translocations or structural chromosomal rearrangements (e.g., inversions) do not necessarily carry the same recurrence risk. Counseling in such cases is usually complex and best provided by experienced geneticists.

Antenatal Sex Determination. Women at risk for X-linked recessive disorders that are not amenable to accurate diagnosis in the male fetus (e.g., Duchenne muscular dystrophy, X-linked hydrocephalus) may elect amniocentesis for antenatal sex determination. Couples with male fetuses know there is a 50 per cent risk of its being affected. On the other hand, couples with female fetuses could be reassured that (with rare exceptions) their child will be unaffected.

Mendelian Disorders. Mendelian disorders result from mutations at single gene loci. The locus may be on an autosome or on a sex chromosome, and it may be dominant or recessive in nature. Depending upon the mode of inheritance, the risk of an affected offspring ranges from 25 to 50 per cent.

Inborn errors of metabolism are inherited in Mendelian fashion. Any disorder in which a biochemical defect is demonstrable in fibroblasts is potentially detectable in cells cultured from the amniotic fluid. These disorders are usually autosomal recessive diseases necessitating that both parents be carriers to have an affected child. One in 4 of their children would then be so affected. These diseases are characterized by failure to thrive, mental retardation, and death in infancy.

In certain Mendelian disorders, linkage analysis can prove useful in prenatal diagnosis, since it may be possible to make a diagnosis on the basis of closely linked genes which tend to be transmitted together. Among the close linkage relationships that have been informative are myotonic dystrophy and ABH secretor locus, hemophilia A and glucose-6-phosphate dehydrogenase deficiency, and 21-hydroxylase deficiency and HLA.

Recent advances employing restriction endonucleases that cleave DNA within specific base-sequence recognition sites promise to greatly expand diagnostic capabilities of Mendelian disorders utilizing amniotic fluid cells. Disorders in which such techniques have already proved useful in antenatal diagnosis include sickle cell anemia, hemoglobin H disease, some variants of beta-thalassemia and alpha-thalassemia.

Neural Tube Defects. Failure of embryonic neural tube closure leads to anencephaly or spina bifida or meningocele. Such disorders are inherited in polygenic/multifactorial fashion. After the birth of one child with a neural tube defect, the recurrence risk is 2 to 5 per cent. Such couples should be offered amniocentesis for determination of alpha-fetoprotein levels. Experiences with amniotic fluid alpha-fetoprotein assays for the prenatal diagnosis of neural tube defects reveals a detection rate for anencephaly of 98.3 per cent and for spina bifida 84.6 per cent. False-positive values occur, although most experienced laboratories report a true false-positive rarely (0.1 to 0.2 per cent). A common cause of falsely elevated alpha-fetoprotein levels is contamination of the amniotic fluid with fetal blood. Measurement of amniotic fluid cholinesterase is useful in differentiating a true elevation of alpha-fetoprotein from a falsely positive level owing to fetal blood contamination. Other causes of falsely elevated alpha-fetoprotein include a dead fetus, multiple pregnancy, omphalocele, gastroschisis, open skin defect, and teratomas. Ultrasonographic evaluation of the fetal head and vertebral column should be utilized as an adjunctive technique in antenatally diagnosing neural tube defects.

AMNIOCENTESIS PROCEDURE

The couple must receive appropriate genetic counseling and understand the reliability and limitations of prenatal diagnosis. In addition, they must be informed regarding the potential risks of amniocentesis which include abortion, fetal injury, maternal hemorrhage, infection, blood group sensitization, failure to obtain amniotic fluid, and failure to grow amniotic fluid cells. In our genetic counseling unit we tell couples that the risk of abortion as a result of the procedure itself is about 1 in 200. The couple should be told when the results can realistically be expected, usually 3 to 5 weeks.

Genetic amniocentesis is optimally performed at about the sixteenth week of pregnancy (i.e., from the first missed menses). Ultrasonographic examination prior to amniocentesis is important to verify fetal life and gestational age, locate the placenta, diagnose multiple gestation, detect gross fetal malformations, exclude hydatid mole, and delineate uterine or adnexal abnormalities. The patient should void prior to the amniocentesis.

The actual procedure is performed under strict aseptic conditions. A local anesthetic is injected into the selected insertion site and a 20 or 22-gauge 3½ inch spinal needle with stylet is inserted transabdominally into the amniotic cavity. The stylet is removed and several milliliters of amniotic fluid are withdrawn and discarded to minimize the possibility of maternal contamination. If a bloody sample is obtained, the fluid can usually be cleared by aspiration into additional syringes. Twenty to 30 ml of amniotic fluid is then aspirated, and transferred to either sterile siliconized glass or plastic tubes, properly labeled, and transported at ambient temperature to the laboratory. Immediate preparation of the fluid is preferred, although samples have been safely transported over long distances. Following the procedure, the patient should be observed and instructed to report any bleeding, loss of fluid, pain, or fever. All Rh-negative unsensitized women pregnant by a Rh-positive male should receive anti-D globulin (Rhogam). Finally, all aborted fetuses and all newborn infants should be evaluated for disorders.

By using the outlined technique and the expertise of an experienced laboratory, complications of genetic amniocentesis have been exceedingly few and errors extremely rare. Finally, because of the vital consequences of the results, only an experienced team of obstetricians, geneticists, and laboratory personnel should undertake responsibility for amniocentesis and amniotic fluid analyses for intrauterine genetic diagnosis.

Section 2
THE NEWBORN

IMMEDIATE RESUSCITATION OF THE NEWBORN INFANT

WALTER L. MILLAR, M.D.

Immediate resuscitation of the newborn actually begins prior to birth. The obstetrician should ensure the availability of adequate equipment and personnel as part of the preparation for delivery. The presence of additional medical personnel is helpful when there is evidence of meconium staining, fetal distress, or significant pre-existent maternal or fetal illness.

Under the conditions of modern obstetric care, most babies are born fully capable of making the metamorphosis from intra-abdominal parasite to semi-independent air-breather without medical intervention. Care of the newborn consists of providing simple supportive measures for this majority, while promptly resuscitating those few babies whose transition is compromised.

Diagnosis and therapy are conducted concurrently. The overriding urgency of establishing respiratory exchange via the lungs makes a rather simple approach appropriate for this complex situation. The resuscitator must accomplish five tasks no matter whether the newborn is perfectly healthy or severely depressed:

1. Establish a patent airway;
2. Minimize thermal stress;
3. Perform a limited, efficient physical examination, which is repeated as necessary;
4. Ensure that the lungs are being ventilated;
5. Ensure adequate cardiovascular function.

AIRWAY PATENCY

Establishing a patent airway is the first priority of resuscitation. The oropharynx should be expeditiously suctioned as soon as the head is delivered. Ideally, this suctioning takes place while the thorax is still compressed inside the birth canal, so that passive thoracic reexpansion serves to facilitate initial aeration of the lungs.

In the presence of meconium staining, this initial suctioning is the single most important step in preventing meconium pneumonitis. One may attempt to aspirate the stomach as well as the pharynx with a catheter attached to a de Lee suction trap. The color and consistency of the aspirate serve as a guide to further therapy.

Following pharyngeal aspiration, the delivery is completed. It is common practice to clamp and cut the umbilical cord while holding the infant at or below the level of the placenta. The infant is next transferred to a neutral thermal environment and wiped dry. An open-sided resuscitation table with overhead controlled radiant heat is an ideal site to carry out the succeeding measures. If thick meconium has been noted in the amniotic fluid or pharyngeal aspirate, it is important to remove any meconium lying in the trachea, if possible before the first breath has spread it peripherally in the lungs.

Thick meconium requires the largest-bore suction catheter possible. By definition, this is an endotracheal tube of appropriate size (Table 1). The trachea is intubated by direct laryngoscopy, and the resuscitator applies direct suction by mouth to the endotracheal tube connector as the tube is withdrawn. Leaving the laryngoscope in place during this process facilitates reintubation and permits differention between tracheal and pharyngeal aspirate. The aspirate is inspected when the tube is cleared by blowing, and the trachea is reintubated.

Tracheal suction is repeated until the aspirate is negligible. The tube is then reinserted to an appropriate depth (Table 1) and the lungs are ventilated with 100 per cent oxygen. Even if the pharyngeal aspirate shows relatively thin meconium, but the baby "looks bad" (see below), tracheal aspiration, intubation, and intermittent positive pressure ventilation are likewise indicated. Once the infant "looks good," a catheter may safely be passed via nose or mouth to empty the stomach of any residual meconium.

If adequate deep suctioning was performed with the head on the perineum, thin meconium in the baby who "looks good" presents little risk of severe pneumonitis. The potential hazards of laryngoscopy and intubation, of breath-holding, laryngospasm, bradycardia, hypoxemia, and reversion to fetal circulation may well constitute a greater risk.

In the absence of meconium, a patent airway is best maintained in a slightly head-down, lateral decubitus position. The resuscitator should resist the temptation to repeatedly suction the airway. Deep nasopharyngeal suction before the onset of regular breathing may cause severe bradycardia and breath-holding.

TABLE 1. **Tracheal Suction of the Newborn**

	ESTIMATED WEIGHT OF NEWBORN (KG)		
	1	2	≥3
Endotracheal tube size (mm inner diameter)	2.5	3.0	3.5
Depth of insertion (cm from tip to lip)	7	8	9

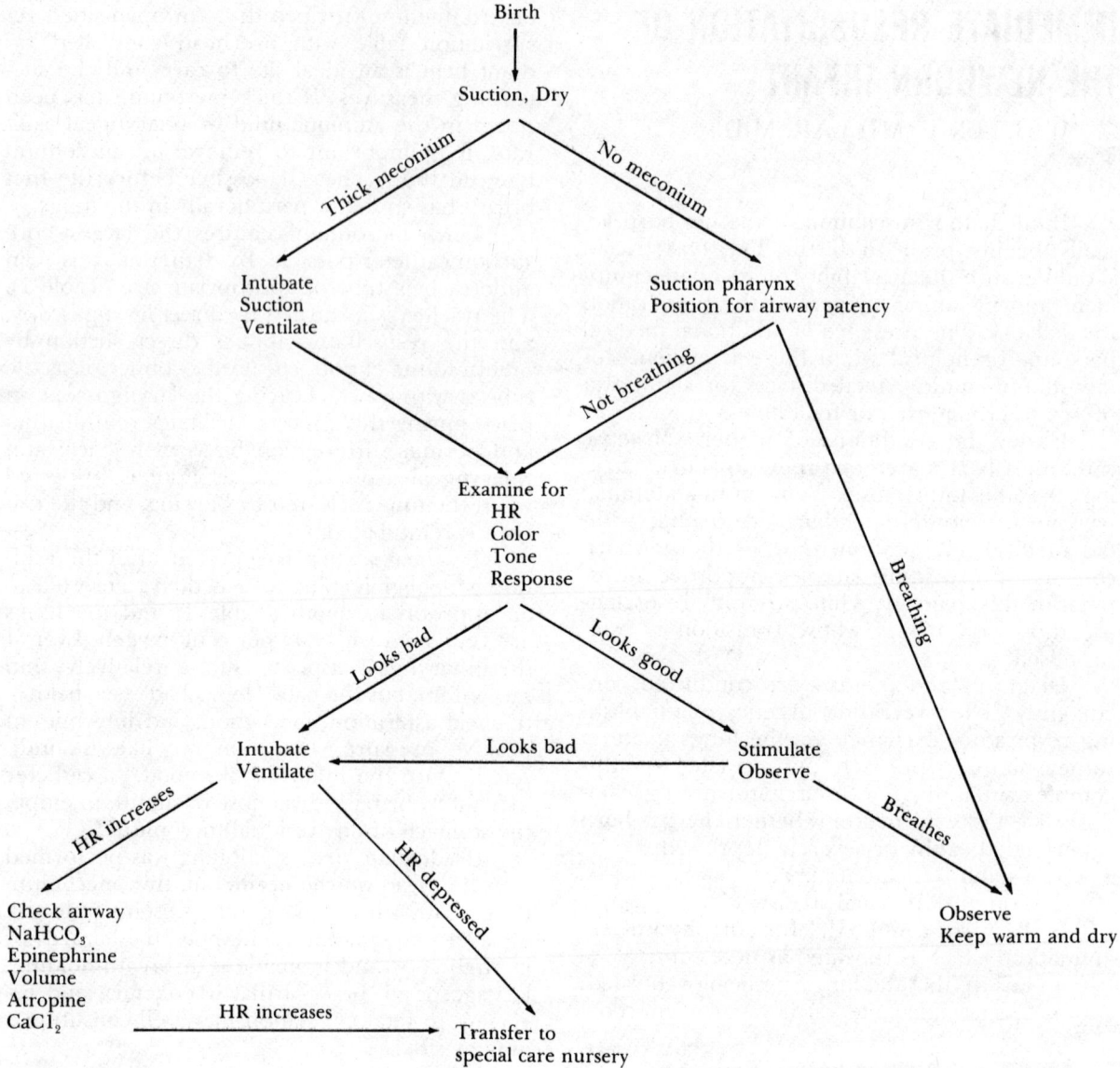

Figure 1. Resuscitation of the newborn.

VENTILATION

The resuscitator must next differentiate between those babies who require immediate artificial ventilation and those who can—and should—be allowed to initiate ventilation on their own. A brief cardiovascular and neuromuscular examination is immediately performed and is repeated at a minimum of 1 and 5 minutes. The Apgar score summarizes the result of this examination but is *not* the criterion for decision-making.

The initial examination is done while the infant is being dried and positioned for airway patency. Respiratory effort is observed. Skin color and capillary filling are inspected. Heart rate is monitored by auscultation of the precordium or palpation of the umbilical stump. The extremities are assessed for flexor tone or active motion. Any response of the muscles of face, extremities, or diaphragm is observed during the stimulation of suctioning and drying.

The majority of healthy babies initiate ventilation in the first minute of life. In the absence of any complicating factors or medical misintervention, ventilation becomes progressively regular and sustained. The immediately vigorous infant needs only to be kept dry, warm, and properly positioned while being observed in the first minutes of life.

Infants who are not breathing are differentiated at the initial examination into two groups: those unable to breathe unassisted, and those who have the ability to breathe but do not.

The apneic baby who "looks good" has a normal cardiovascular and neuromuscular examination. That is, the skin is well perfused (blue rather than pale, rapid capillary refill), heart rate is greater than 80 and regular, extremities are actively flexed, and stimulation produces a grimace, movement, or gasp. The respiratory center may be depressed by narcotics given the mother during labor, or by a reflex response to airway obstruction ("primary apnea") unique to the newborn.

The drug-depressed newborn may initiate regular respiration as its arterial CO_2 rises, but if apnea persists too long, hypoxia will supervene and produce further respiratory and cardiovascular depression. This infant, who now "looks bad," requires ventilation, stimulation, and reversal of narcotics with naloxone. "Adult" strength naloxone (Narcan, 0.4 mg per ml) should be injected intramuscularly in a dose of 10 to 20 μg per kg.

The infant with reflex breath-holding will usually begin to gasp within a minute; if the airway is clear and the resuscitator does not stimulate the airway, gasping will soon give way to regular ventilation. So long as the heart rate remains above 80 and the muscle tone is good, the resuscitator should resist the temptation to instrument the airway, slap the baby's skin, or administer analeptic drugs.

The infant who exhibits skin pallor, poor capillary refill, cardiac rhythm either below 80 beats per minute or irregular, flaccid extremities, or no response to stimulation "looks bad." Asphyxia has progressed to the point where it may no longer stimulate ventilation because it has begun to depress the respiratory center as well as every other cellular function.

Such an infant is in extremis and requires immediate ventilation. Ventilation by bag and mask may be briefly attempted before endotracheal intubation is performed. Once a tube of appropriate size has been inserted to the proper depth, 100 per cent oxygen is administered via a resuscitation bag, the lungs are auscultated, and the epigastrium is inspected for movement. However, neither breath sounds nor diaphragmatic movement is a completely reliable sign of proper tube placement. If ventilation has not produced a rising heart rate within 30 seconds, the tube should be checked against esophageal or endobronchial placement by laryngoscopy.

CARDIOVASCULAR FUNCTION

The majority of infants depressed at birth respond to ventilation with 100 per cent oxygen with gratifying rapidity. The infant suffering from acute birth asphyxia who immediately "pinks up," increases cardiac rate, and initiates spontaneous ventilation may usually be extubated in the delivery room in the absence of prematurity, sepsis, or other complicating factor. If any doubt exists, it is safer to leave the tube in place.

In the rare situation in which ventilation of the lungs does not initiate an immediate improvement in cardiac response, closed-chest cardiac massage is initiated at a rate of 80 to 100 per minute by depression of the mid-sternum by 1 to 2 cm. Spontaneous improvement in cardiac rate usually results in less than a minute.

In the exceedingly rare case in which these measures are ineffective, the position of the endotracheal tube must be verified again before pharmacologic therapy is initiated. Epinephrine, 10 μg per kg; sodium bicarbonate, 1 to 2 mEq per kg diluted to a 4.2 per cent solution; and Ringer's lactate, 10 ml per kg may be infused via an ordinary butterfly or short plastic IV-cannula inserted percutaneously into the dilated umbilical vein; flushing of the dark color of the vein verifies intravascular placement. Additional therapy may include calcium chloride, 10–20 mg per kg, or atropine, 0.02 mg per kg. As soon as a stable cardiac rhythm is established, an umbilical artery catheter should be placed for arterial pressure monitoring and blood gas sampling.

RESPIRATORY DISTRESS SYNDROME

MICHAEL F. EPSTEIN, M.D.

Respiratory distress syndrome, or hyaline membrane disease, continues to be the major cause of morbidity and mortality in the premature newborn. When delivery occurs before the fetal lung has developed, the capacity to produce adequate amounts of surface active material (primarily the phospholipid, disaturated phosphatidylcholine, SPC, or lecithin, and to a lesser degree phosphatidylglycerol, PG), the newborn's lungs tend to collapse with each breath out. Widespread atelectasis leads to hypoventilation and mismatched ventilation and perfusion in the lung. The hypoxemia, hypercarbia, and acidemia that result further compromise the metabolic function of the lung as well as contribute to systemic shock and collapse. The newborn with severe respiratory failure presents with intercostal and subcostal retractions and flaring of the nasal alae as he exerts increased inspiratory pressure to open his collapsed lungs with each breath. He breathes rapidly (> 60 breaths/min) in an attempt to increase minute ventilation, and he makes a grunting noise on expiration as he tries to maintain some degree of end expiratory pressure. Cyanosis in room air indicates a failure of these compensatory mechanisms. Without respiratory support the outcome is usually fatal, and even with mechanical ventilation and sophisticated metabolic, fluid, and pharmacologic support, the mortality for respiratory distress syndrome remains 10 to 15 per cent. Morbidity in terms of intraventricular hemorrhage, chronic lung disease, and retrolental fibroplasia further add to the toll of this disease.

The diagnosis of respiratory distress syndrome is a clinical one based on finding the above mentioned signs of respiratory distress accompanying the classic radiographic appearance of the lungs—homogeneously distributed, granular, ground glass densities in all lobes with air bronchograms and decreased lung volumes. Although the chest x-ray of group B streptococcal pneumonia may be indistinguishable from that of respiratory distress syndrome, other newborn lung diseases such as transient tachypnea or retained fetal lung liquid, aspiration of meconium, blood, or amniotic fluid, and congestive heart failure with pulmonary edema should be easily distinguishable. The presence of negative blood cultures, immature phospholipid indices in amniotic fluid obtained at or before delivery (SPC< 500 µg per dl, L/S < 2:1), a beneficial response to continuous positive airway pressure (CPAP), and a classic course of worsening disease for 2 to 3 days followed by improvement over 2 to 3 days and resolution by one week of age are all supportive evidence for the diagnosis of respiratory distress syndrome. Additional epidemiologic clues are the increased incidence of respiratory distress syndrome in multiple gestations, males, infants of diabetic mothers and Rh-sensitized women, asphyxiated babies, infants delivered by cesarean section without labor, and the markedly increased incidence with shorter periods of gestation (~ 70 per cent at 28 weeks to 5 per cent at 36 weeks).

The treatment of the infant with respiratory distress syndrome can range from simple supportive measures in the most mildly affected infants to the limit of sophisticated, technical care for severely affected babies in a newborn intensive care unit. There are, however, several general areas of therapy that apply to all babies with respiratory distress syndrome, and involve maximizing the potential of each baby to adequately adapt to extrauterine life. The ability of the baby's lungs to produce surfactant is determined both by developmental maturation as well as by postnatal events. Among the latter, several can compromise the lung's ability to make surfactant and support adequate ventilation including: hypothermia (< 96.7°F), hypoglycemia (blood glucose < 20–30 mg/dl), asphyxia (pH < 7.25, Pco_2 > 45 torr), hypoxia (arterial Pao_2 < 50 torr), and hypotension (systolic blood pressure <30 mm Hg at 28 weeks, <50 mm Hg at term) and anemia (Hct <45 per cent). Therefore, careful monitoring of vital signs (including blood pressure) and obtaining blood from either a radial artery puncture or puncture of a warmed heel for a rapid determination of blood glucose, hematocrit, and blood gases is the first step in assessment and treatment.

One of the most important goals of this initial assessment is the determination of how sick the baby is likely to become. This step is critical for physicians in community hospitals faced with the decision whether or not to transfer a baby to an intensive care nursery. It is also important in Level II and Level III nurseries in deciding the appropriate level of intervention and support.

A critical part of this determination of severity of illness is the ability to predict whether the baby will develop respiratory distress syndrome. The newborn infant's stomach, within the first 30 minutes after delivery, contains primarily fetal pulmonary fluid swallowed in utero. Therefore, gastric fluid phospholipids reflect the status of fetal lung maturity. Tanswell has described a single-step gastric aspirate shake test as follows: 0.5 ml gastric fluid, 0.5 ml saline, and 1.0 ml 95 per cent ethanol; shake vigorously for 15 seconds and let the tube rest undisturbed for 15 minutes. The presence of a rim of stable bubbles covering two-thirds of the air-fluid interface is a reliable indicator that the risk of developing respiratory distress syndrome is very small (< 5 per cent). In contrast, the absence of bubbles is associated with a 67 per cent risk.

Another simple test which is useful for predicting the risk of respiratory distress syndrome is cord blood total protein concentration. If these are < 4.6 gm per dl, there is a greater likelihood of respiratory distress syndrome. This measurement can be made in minutes with a refractometer on serum from a hematocrit determination.

The chest x-ray is frequently difficult to interpret in the first 1 to 2 hours after delivery; however, uniformly diminished aeration indicates that a baby is likely to show progressive respiratory failure. In addition, an early chest x-ray helps to rule out other treatable causes of respiratory distress such as pneumothorax or diaphragmatic hernia.

Careful and continuous attention should be paid to maintaining the baby in a neutral thermal environment to reduce metabolic demands for oxygen consumption for temperature regulation. Radiant warming tables, heating lights, and incubators are alternative methods. If the blood glucose is below 20 to 30 mg per dl and the baby is in respiratory distress, glucose should be administered intravenously over 2 minutes in a dose of 200 mg per kg as 10 per cent dextrose in water. Continuous intravenous administration of 10 per cent dextrose in water at a rate of 100 ml per kg per day will usually suffice to maintain an adequate blood glucose level. Intravenous access can usually be achieved with a 25 to 27 gauge butterfly needle in a small vein on the dorsum of the hand or foot or in a scalp vein. If peripheral venous access is impossible to achieve, a 3.5 or 5 French catheter can be inserted 2 to 3 cm into the umbilical vein after dividing the cord 1 to 2 cm from the abdominal wall. Care should be taken not to advance the catheter into the portal vein, an hepatic vein, or the heart, across the foramen ovale, or into a pulmonary vein. An x-ray of the abdomen and chest can quickly identify the catheter's position.

If the blood pressure is low and there is evidence of poor peripheral perfusion (tachycardia, weak pulses, slow capillary refilling, metabolic acidosis) volume expanders should be administered. If anemia coexists, packed red blood cells or whole blood would be the expander of choice. Otherwise, 5 per cent albumin, fresh frozen plasma, or if neither were available, isotonic sodium chloride or sodium bicarbonate solutions would suffice.

The evaluation of respiratory status, however, finally depends on the measurement of pH and the partial pressures of oxygen (Pao_2) and carbon dioxide ($Paco_2$) in arterial blood. Blood for these measurements can be obtained from an indwelling arterial catheter (in an umbilical, radial, ulnar or posterior tibial artery), from a peripheral artery puncture, or by heel puncture to obtain arterialized capillary blood from a pre-warmed heel. A new instrument that measures arterial Po_2 transcutaneously ($TcPo_2$) has provided a noninvasive means of continuously monitoring Po_2 but provides no information about $Paco_2$ or pH.

If an infant needs ventilatory support from the time of delivery, we proceed directly to insertion of an umbilical artery catheter. When an infant is not as critically ill from the onset, we use a combination of radial artery blood sampling, arterialized capillary blood sampling and transcutaneous Po_2 measurement for initial assessment.

Once the general condition is assessed, decisions as to transport and further treatment can be made. Since there is no specific "cure" for respiratory distress syndrome, the goal of treatment is to insure optimal condition of the baby in terms of maintaining tissue oxygenation and avoiding acidosis, i.e., the maintenance of normal respiratory function. A number of alternative methods are available to attain this goal; however, much critical knowledge of respiratory, circulatory, and metabolic pathophysiology in small premature infants with respiratory distress syndrome remains undefined. Therefore, many aspects of routine management are based on personal and institutional experience.

The maintenance of tissue oxygenation and prevention of respiratory acidosis depends primarily on the balance between the exchange of gases in the lungs and the metabolic demands of the tissues. The latter can be minimized by: (1) maintenance of the baby in a neutral thermal environment; (2) provision of adequate calories to meet basal needs; and (3) efficient organization of medical and nursing handling to minimize stress. If careful attention is paid to these details, the need for ventilatory and circulatory support may be lessened.

Respiratory support varies from providing additional oxygen by raising the fraction of inspired oxygen concentration (FIo_2) the baby is spontaneously breathing to total mechanical ventilatory support. Respiratory support is provided in order to maintain the arterial blood gases in the following range: Pao_2 50 to 70 torr, $Paco_2$, 40 to 45 torr, and pH 7.30 to 7.35. Perhaps the most critical is the Pao_2 since hypoxemia leads to compromise of tissue function. Hypoxemia may be associated with intraventricular hemorrhage in the brain, necrotizing enterocolitis, asphyxial myocardial failure and elevated pulmonary artery pressure with the attendant risk of persistence of right-to-left fetal circulatory shunts (persistent fetal circulation). Hyperoxemia ($Pao_2 > 100$ torr) is also dangerous since elevated Pao_2 increases the risk of retrolental fibroplasia, posing a major threat of blindness to the small premature infant treated with oxygen.

The desired Pao_2 is often reached in babies with mild respiratory distress syndrome by simply adding oxygen to the infant's inspired air.

Oxygen should be warmed and humidified. Careful attention must be paid to the temperature of the nebulizer heater since unwarmed oxygen flowing into a head box can lead to hypothermia, and overheated oxygen can lead to hyperthermia. Both conditions can significantly increase oxygen consumption in the baby. The FIO_2 in the incubator or head box should be checked at least hourly to assure that it remains at the desired concentration.

If an $FIO_2 > 0.50$ is needed to maintain the Pao_2 between 50 and 70 torr, we institute continuous positive airway pressure (CPAP) via a nasopharyngeal tube. There is some evidence that early use of CPAP shortens the length of time a baby with respiratory distress syndrome needs oxygen supplementation or mechanical ventilation. Although some methods to determine the optimal CPAP have been described, we empirically begin at 4 to 5 cm H_2O. A good response to CPAP is a 15 to 20 torr rise in Pao_2, and CPAP is gradually increased from 4 to 10 cm H_2O until either this increase in Pao_2 is achieved or CO_2 retention occurs. Occasionally CPAP may result in a decline in Pao_2 owing to overdistention of the lung or impeded venous return and decreased cardiac output.

If nasopharyngeal CPAP results in little or no improvement, there may be inefficient transmission of the pressure from nasopharynx to trachea because of the baby's crying or open mouth. The tube then is advanced into the trachea for a further trial of CPAP. Care is taken during intubation not to advance the tube beyond the carina, and a chest x-ray is obtained immediately to ensure correct tube position.

If, despite 8 to 10 cm H_2O CPAP delivered by endotracheal tube, an $FIO_2 > 0.70$ to 0.80 is needed to maintain $Pao_2 > 50$ torr, we proceed to mechanical ventilation, using a time-cycled, pressure-driven ventilator. In addition to hypoxemia despite $FIO_2 > 0.70$ to 0.80 other indications for mechanical ventilation are: (1) multiple prolonged apnea spells leading to bradycardia; (2) a $Paco_2$ that increases to > 60 torr in the first 24 hours; (3) a $Paco_2$ that results in a severe respiratory acidosis (< 7.20).

Ventilation settings of inspiratory and end expiratory pressure, rate and FIO_2 are adjusted to maintain the Pao_2, $Paco_2$, and in the desired ranges.

The goal of ventilator treatment is optimal condition of the baby with minimal respiratory support. The usual course of respiratory distress syndrome is gradual worsening for 48 to 72 hours followed by gradual improvement. In the absence of complications, babies ventilated for severe respiratory distress syndrome usually can be removed from respiratory support by 5 to 7 days after birth.

Two additional aspects of respiratory support deserve attention. First, some babies are very difficult to ventilate adequately. These are usually larger babies (> 2.0 kg) who breathe vigorously but inefficiently and who do not synchronize with the ventilator. We have found that achieving paralysis with the neuromuscular blocker pancuronium (Pavulon, 0.05 to 0.1 mg per kg intravenously, repeated as needed) allows more efficient ventilation at lower settings of FIO_2 and pressure. Also, our impression is that paralysis reduces the risk of pneumothorax. Pancuronium has had no discernible effect on blood pressure, but seems to result in an increase in peripheral edema, probably owing to the elimination of muscle activity and venous stasis. Pancuronium is continued until a significant improvement in lung compliance is noted, as judged by a decrease in the required inspiratory pressure, usually 24 to 48 hours after the medication is begun.

Second, chest physiotherapy is a routine part of ventilator management. Every 2 to 4 hours the baby receives chest vibration and percussion following instillation of 0.5 ml 0.9 per cent sodium chloride into the endotracheal tube. The tube is then suctioned, taking care to insert the suction catheter gently and not beyond 1 to 2 cm past the carina. The lungs are then gently hyperinflated manually with an anesthesia bag at the current FIO_2.

Other important areas of management of the baby with respiratory distress syndrome include the following: (1) circulatory support with volume and when needed cardiotonic drugs such as isoproterenol or dopamine; (2) metabolic support to maintain normal glucose and electrolyte values and to avoid the opposite extremes of fluid overload (and the risk of a patent ductus arteriosus, congestive heart failure and bronchopulmonary dysplasia) and dehydration (and the risk of ischemic damage to organs such as the bowel with necrotizing enterocolitis; (3) nutrition, initially parenteral using amino acids and fat emulsions given intravenously and eventually enteral using special premature formulas or supplemented breast milk; (4) antibiotics (usually a penicillin/aminoglycoside combination) which are instituted intravenously in all babies with respiratory distress until blood, gastric aspirate, and tracheal cultures indicate the absence of bacterial infection.

The careful attention to these areas of initial assessment and respiratory, circulatory, and metabolic support have been largely responsible for the significant improvement in birth weight specific survival in babies with respiratory distress syndrome.

HYPOGLYCEMIA, HYPOCALCEMIA, AND HYPOMAGNESEMIA IN THE NEWBORN

SHELDON B. KORONES, M.D.

HYPOGLYCEMIA

Pathophysiology. Storage of energy-yielding substrate throughout gestation, particularly during the last trimester, is probably directed toward sustaining the neonate during the first postnatal days because caloric needs after birth must be supplied from external sources, and it may be days before glycogen stores are significantly replenished. After delivery, the baby's glycogen stores are depleted abruptly; in normal term infants, approximately 90 per cent of hepatic glycogen is consumed by the end of the third postnatal hour. It rises gradually thereafter to attain adult concentrations by the end of the third week. As carbohydrate stores are consumed, fat becomes a significant source of energy. An "energy crunch" is therefore created when the maternal supply line is cut while a sudden need for increased energy is created by the asphyxia of normal birth, the work of establishing respiration, a massive loss of body heat, and the initiation of muscle activity. While these events are ordinarily well managed by normal term neonates, infants who are stressed are likely to fare poorly for want of glucose.

Within 2 hours after birth, the normal neonate's blood glucose declines from a cord level of 70 to 80 mg per dl to 50 mg per dl. The earliest defense against a declining blood glucose concentration is the acceleration of glycogen breakdown (glycogenolysis); the secretion of glucagon is increased and the secretion of insulin decreased. Activation of certain hepatic intracellular enzymes inhibits glycogen formation from glucose, thus also contributing to restoration of blood glucose levels. Release of hepatic glucose is further enhanced by the onset of gluconeogenesis. In sheep, gluconeogenesis begins within 3 minutes after birth; it seems quite likely that in human neonates the process also begins very soon after delivery. The "energy crunch" of the immediate postnatal period is thus transiently alleviated by the release of hepatic glucose and by the use of free fatty acids (lipolysis) as an additional fuel.

The limited capacity of certain high risk infants to cope with the perinatal "energy crunch" is in sharp contrast to normal term infants who adjust without difficulty. Premature infants are more vulnerable to hypoglycemia because of their smaller stores of energy substrates. The malnourished fetus who could not accumulate adequate stores of substrate is similarly vulnerable. During asphyxic episodes in utero, glycogen stores are rapidly depleted; asphyxiated infants are therefore likely to become hypoglycemic. Thus, in several clinically identifiable circumstances, diminished glycogen and fat storage often result in neonatal hypoglycemia. The most frequently encountered situations are prematurity, intrauterine malnutrition, asphyxia, and postnatal cold stress.

Hypoglycemia also occurs in the presence of adequate stores of fat and glycogen when there is excessive insulin secretion. Infants of diabetic mothers are archetypical examples of hypoglycemia resulting from hyperinsulinism. Neonates with severe hemolytic disease of the newborn (Rh disease) may be similarly affected. Protracted hypoglycemia caused by hyperinsulinism is associated with maternal administration of chlorpropamide, which stimulates both maternal and fetal islet (beta) cell activity. Maternal administration of propranolol and beta-mimetic tocolytics have also been reported in association with neonatal hypoglycemia.

BIOCHEMICAL CRITERIA AND CLINICAL SIGNS

Hypoglycemia may be symptomatic or asymptomatic; in either event it is defined by serum or whole blood glucose levels. In low birth weight or preterm infants, hypoglycemia is present when whole blood glucose is less than 20 mg per dl (serum glucose less than 25 mg per dl). In term infants during the first 72 hours of life, hypoglycemia is defined by a whole blood glucose level below 30 mg per dl (serum below 35 mg per dl). After 72 hours of age, whole blood and serum values below 40 and 45 mg per dl, respectively, are hypoglycemic.

Clinical signs are clearly identifiable, but they are not specific for hypoglycemia. The signs of hypoglycemia also occur in the presence of central nervous system disorders, septicemia, hypocalcemia, hypomagnesemia, cardiorespiratory disorders, and several others in which blood glucose levels may be low or normal (Table 1). The signs of hypoglycemia include apnea, cyanosis, rapid and irregular respirations, tachyp-

TABLE 1. **Clinical States Associated with Hypoglycemia in the Newborn**

Intrauterine malnutrition
Fetal asphyxia
Cold stress
Central nervous system hemorrhage
Central nervous system malformation
Adrenal hemorrhage, insufficiency
Infants of diabetic mothers
Erythroblastotic infants (Rh)
Maternal tolbutamide, chlorpropamide, and propranolol
Abrupt stop of intravenous glucose, ≥ 10 per cent
Cyanotic congenital heart disease with congestive failure
Septicemia

nea, tremors, jitters, twitches, convulsions, lethargy, coma, pallor, sweating, upward rolling of eyes, weak or high pitched cry, and refusal to feed. The relationship of these signs to hypoglycemia is credible only if they clear a short time after the administration of intravenous glucose.

Intrauterine Malnutrition. Hypoglycemia occurs in approximately 20 per cent of infants who are malnourished in utero. Males are affected twice as frequently as females; hypoglycemia occurs more often in the smaller of twins, particularly with a weight discrepancy in excess of 25 per cent. Symptoms have been reported in 50 per cent to 90 per cent of these hypoglycemic infants. In small-for-dates babies, hepatic glycogen stores are reduced and the capacity for gluconeogenesis is diminished. Hepatic weight is diminished, but the brain is less affected by growth retardation. Thus, in normally grown fetuses at term, the liver is approximately one-third the weight of the brain; in malnourished fetuses, hepatic weight is one-seventh of the brain. The glucose requirement of a normal sized brain cannot be satisfied by a diminutive liver. Fat depots are also considerably reduced; and the provision of free fatty acid is thereby restricted.

Screening for blood glucose levels should be performed with a chemical reagent strip (Dextrostix) at least every 4 hours for the first 3 to 5 days of life. If low levels are indicated on the strip, laboratory determinations are essential.

Infants of Diabetic Mothers. In the infant of a diabetic mother, fetal hyperinsulinism enhances the decline in blood glucose to hypoglycemic concentrations which usually occur between 2 and 4 hours after birth. This is followed by a spontaneous rise to normal levels between 4 and 6 hours of age. Approximately half the infants of insulin-dependent mothers will develop glucose levels below 30 mg per dl in whole blood. In gestational diabetes, approximately 20 per cent are affected. Occasionally hypoglycemia is protracted; rarely it may appear as late as 12 to 24 hours of age.

Adequate screening of these infants can be accomplished by use of reagent strips (Dextrostix) at 1, 2, 4, and 6 hours of age. Laboratory determinations of blood glucose levels are necessary if the Dextrostix reads below 45 mg per dl.

Erythroblastosis Fetalis (Rh). Low blood glucose levels occur in almost a third of moderately or severely affected infants, and in 5 per cent of all erythroblastotic babies regardless of severity. The incidence of hypoglycemia is highest when the cord hemoglobin concentration is less than 10 gm per dl. Blood sugar levels may fall transiently before or after exchange transfusion, most often during the first day of life but occasionally later. Blood glucose levels should be monitored every 2 to 4 hours during the first day of life, and regularly every 6 to 8 hours thereafter for the ensuing 3 days.

Premature (Very Low Birth Weight) Infants. Hypoglycemia is common in infants whose birth weight is less than 1500 grams. It may occur very soon after birth or several days later. Hepatic glycogen stores are presumably low in these immature infants, and the increased metabolic demands imposed by extrauterine life often deplete supplies rapidly. This is accentuated by cold stress, asphyxia, and respiratory difficulty, all of which are frequent in these small infants. Blood sugar levels should be monitored with reagent strips at least every 4 hours for the first few days of life.

TREATMENT

With an awareness of the clinical circumstances described above, hypoglycemia can usually be prevented by early administration of intravenous fluid calculated to deliver an appropriate quantity of glucose continuously. Therapy should maintain blood glucose at physiologic levels while avoiding hyperglycemia, which often stimulates excessive insulin secretion. The normal neonatal liver at term generates glucose at an approximate rate of 5 to 8 mg per kg per minute. Vulnerable infants who are not yet hypoglycemic should therefore receive a solution that is calculated to deliver 5 to 8 mg of glucose per kg per minute.

Most neonatologists agree that when hypoglycemia occurs, intravenous glucose is indicated whether or not clinical signs are evident. Some advocate a push dose of 20 or 25 per cent dextrose, 2 to 4 ml per kg of body weight. Others contend that such a bolus stimulates excessive islet (beta) cell activity with resultant wide fluctuations in blood glucose levels. If bolus administration is utilized, it is followed by continuous infusion of glucose at a rate that delivers 6 to 8 mg per kg per minutes, occasionally more. If only a continuous infusion is used, glucose should be administered at a rate between 8 and 10 mg per kg per minute.

Prevention and treatment of hypoglycemia are most effective when the volume and concentration of an infused dextrose solution are determined by the amount of glucose that must be administered. The appropriate volume and concentration of a solution can be readily calculated using conversion factors as follows:

1. For 10% dextrose: ml/kg/24 hours = mg/kg/min of glucose × 15
2. For 15% dextrose: ml/kg/24 hours = mg/kg/min of glucose × 10
3. For 20% dextrose: ml/kg/24 hours = mg/kg/min of glucose × 8

Examples of calculations are shown in Table 2. The daily fluid volumes in the table may occasionally vary from actual calculations by only a few ml/24 hours.

If blood glucose levels remain low after one hour of intravenous glucose therapy, a steroid should be added. The need for steroid therapy is infrequent. One may utilize hydrocortisone, 5 mg per kg per day (intramuscular), in divided doses every 12 hours, or prednisone, 2 mg per kg per day (oral), given in two divided doses every 12 hours. Steroid therapy is usually continued for 2 to 3 days, then terminated abruptly.

HYPOCALCEMIA

Hypocalcemia (serum calcium less than 7.0 mg per dl) usually occurs within the first 48 hours of life. Early hypocalcemia is thought to be related to transient neonatal hypoparathyroidism. Serum calcium is low, phosphorus may be high, and magnesium is sometimes diminished. Low serum calcium levels are related to gestational age rather than birth weight; the shorter the gestation the lower the calcium. The small-for-dates infant is therefore not more vulnerable to hypocalcemia. Hypocalcemia is most likely to occur with perinatal asphyxia, in small premature infants, and in infants of diabetic mothers. A history of abruptio placentae or placenta previa is not unusual. The symptoms of early hypocalcemia, if any are discernible, are not often neuromuscular. Rather, they include apnea, cyanotic episodes, edema, high-pitched cry, and abdominal distention. Even these manifestations, however, have not been proved to be of specific hypocalcemic origin.

Therapy may be oral or intravenous. Ten per cent calcium gluconate is preferred. Whether given orally or intravenously, 75 mg of elemental calcium per kg per day should be administered. For oral therapy, four divided doses may be used. Intravenous therapy should provide continuous infusion. Intravenous administration of calcium must be monitored closely; infiltration in the subcutaneous tissue causes severe skin sloughing. Furthermore, inadvertent overdosage may cause profound bradycardia. Calcium therapy is contraindicated in infants who are receiving digitalis preparations.

HYPOMAGNESEMIA

The normal serum magnesium level in the neonate is 1.2 to 1.8 mg per dl. Hypomagnesemia rarely occurs as an isolated phenomenon; it most often accompanies hypocalcemia. It is encountered most frequently in infants of diabetic mothers. It is occasionally encountered during or after exchange transfusions. Laboratory determinations of serum magnesium are essential for proper evaluation of infants with signs of neuromuscular excitability. This is particularly important in hypocalcemic infants who do not respond to calcium therapy. If clinical signs are attributable to magnesium deficiency, they disappear promptly after appropriate therapy. An intramuscular dose of 50 per cent magnesium sulfate (0.2 ml per kg of body weight) is given every 4 hours for the first day. The need for subsequent therapy is determined by serial serum magnesium determinations. Magnesium sulfate may also be administered by slow intravenous infusion, utilizing the same dosage as for intramuscular administration.

HYPERBILIRUBINEMIA OF THE NEONATE

LEO STERN, M.D.

Neonatal jaundice, a condition visibly affecting 30 per cent of all newborn infants, refers to the unconjugated (indirect-acting) hyperbiliru-

TABLE 2.

SOLUTION	GLUCOSE (mg/kg/min)	FACTOR	INFUSED FLUID (ml/kg/24 hours)
10% Dextrose:	10	x 15 =	150
10% Dextrose:	8	x 15 =	120
15% Dextrose:	12	x 10 =	120
15% Dextrose:	8	x 10 =	80
20% Dextrose:	12	x 8 =	96

binemia resulting from the inability of the immature neonatal liver to handle the presenting bilirubin load. Because of the normally suffused polycythemic appearance of the newborn infant's skin, jaundice is rarely visible below 5 mg per dl so that by adult standards of normality (> 2 mg per dl), excessive jaundice would be considered to be present in an even greater number of newborns than the above quoted figure.

The hepatic immaturity for bilirubin metabolism affects all three aspects of liver function (uptake, conjugation, and excretion), although the rate-limiting step is thought to be a delay in the conjugation of bilirubin with UDP glucuronic acid enzymatically mediated by a glucuronyl transferase to its mono and then diglucuronide forms. Physiologically, this converts the bilirubin from a lipid-soluble to a water-soluble form (indirect-acting to direct-acting with the Erlich aldehyde reagent), thereby enabling its excretion into the bile ducts and the gastrointestinal tract.

In physiologic terms, such hyperbilirubinemia depends on the balance between the load presented, ranging from the normal breakdown of neonatal red blood cells, to the excessive rates of production of bilirubin in the various forms of hemolytic disease of the newborn, and the capacity of the liver to handle what is presented to it. This hepatic capacity has an equally marked variable ability related to heredity and genetic factors, the presence or absence of enzyme inhibitors (cf breast milk factor, etc.), and an equally important individual variation in the rate at which hepatic function matures, principally in the first 5 to 10 days of life. Thus whether or not an individual infant becomes jaundiced and the degree to which this occurs will depend on both factors. In these circumstances an infant with an immature liver may become exceedingly jaundiced in the presence of only the normal neonatal breakdown of red blood cells, augmented dramatically by only mild hemolysis, placental transfusion which provides additional hemoglobin, or resorption of relatively small amounts of extravasated blood from tissue bruising or cephalhematomas. In contrast a severely affected infant with hemolytic disease of the newborn may show little or no jaundice even in the face of severe and progressive anemia in the presence of a relatively mature hepatic conjugating mechanism.

SIGNIFICANCE OF HYPERBILIRUBINEMIA

The rationale for therapy is based on the avoidance of and protection against bilirubin encephalopathy (kernicterus) in which there is deposition of unconjugated (water-insoluble) bilirubin in the central nervous system. Bilirubin which is conjugated (direct-acting) and is thus made water-soluble will not precipitate out of plasma (essentially a water solution) and, therefore, poses no danger for entry to the central nervous system *irrespective of its level*. The unconjugated fraction is, however, insoluble in water and relatively soluble in lipids, so that it will tend to come out of solution in plasma and enter lipid-rich areas such as the skin and brain unless it is bound to albumin, which serves not only as its carrier in plasma, but also makes the resultant molecule (bilirubin-albumin complex) too large to diffuse outward from the vascular system. The normal-term infant has an albumin level of about 3 grams. On a 1:1 basis this permits the binding of 8.3 to 8.7 mg per dl bilirubin per gram of albumin (the precise amount is pH dependent), accounting for a normal full-term binding ability of approximately 24 to 27 mg per dl. It is from this calculation that the clinically recognized level of 20 mg per dl as being a useful dividing line between "safe" and "at risk" levels is derived and which provides the biochemical substantiation for the clinical observation. It must be noted, however, that the small premature infant has closer to 2 grams of albumin, reducing the normal amount capable of being bound to a figure of 16 to 18 mg per dl and that a variety of other factors may conspire to further lower the binding ability in specific individual instances.

The term "physiologic" jaundice is a misleading one and should be abandoned. There is no qualitative difference in the bilirubin itself at any level, and the factors which operate to promote its egress from plasma and entry into the central nervous system may be present at extremely low levels particularly in the sick, small premature infant. A lower level (< 12 mg per dl) should not be considered as physiologic simply because it is less dangerous than a higher one.

Factors that promote dissociation of the bilirubin-albumin complex include acidosis, hypothermia, sepsis, and asphyxia. In addition, a number of drugs are capable of displacing bilirubin from its albumin bond by a competitive binding mechanism. These include sulfisoxazole (Gantrisin), salicylates, and sodium benzoate, the latter being a commonly used stabilizer and preservative vehicle for a number of parenteral drug preparations (e.g., caffeine sodium benzoate, diazepam). It must be remembered that such agents may not only be administered directly to the infant but can also be transported to some extent across the placenta and are additionally able to reach the infant via the breast milk of a nursing mother. In addition, some endogenous substances (free fatty acids, hematin) are capable of similar competitive displacement. Free fatty acids may be increased secondary to hypothermia, hypoglycemia, and excessive use of heparin, as well as from skin reabsorption of soaps (a mixture of long and short-chain fatty acids) used as a substitute for the now discredited hexachlorophene preparations. The capacity of heme to displace bilirubin from albumin likely accounts for the greater risk of kernicterus in the presence of hemolytic disease and does not reflect any toxic differences in the properties of the bilirubin produced from hemolytic as opposed to nonhemolytic causes. It is also thought that carboxyhemoglobin produced in the excessive breakdown of red blood cells may have a similar displacing action.

Finally, it should be noted that whatever blood-brain barrier exists to the transport of bilirubin from the circulation to the central nervous system does not show any evidence of maturation with time. This assumption is an inaccurate inversion of the fact that even under severe circumstances the infant's serum bilirubin level, which normally reaches its zenith between the fourth and fifth day of life, almost invariably declines after the first week of life as a result of hepatic maturation. However, under conditions of permanent hepatic dysfunction (Crigler-Najjar syndrome) or delayed forms of hemolytic disease (glucose-6-phosphate dehydrogenase deficiency when the child is placed in clothing preserved in mothballs after the first week of life), kernicterus will occur beyond that period of time if the level goes high enough. What prevents kernicterus from usually occurring in adults is not a more "mature" blood-brain barrier but a more mature liver. Thus the adult liver can handle seven times more bilirubin on a per diem basis than is normally presented to it from the daily degradation of hemoglobin, and, therefore, adults with severe hemolysis will become only mildly, if at all, jaundiced. Even massive hepatic destruction (e.g., acute fulminating hepatitis or toxic liver destruction) will cause death from liver failure before a high enough level to produce kernicterus occurs.

TREATMENT

While a bilirubin level of 20 mg per dl seems safe in an otherwise well full-term infant, this relationship does not hold for the small premature infant who is otherwise ill or for the full-term infant in whom the factors associated with facilitative bilirubin-albumin dissociation or displacement are present. Moreover, the standard Evelyn and Malloy technique for the determination of serum bilirubin is accurate on repeat determinations only at best at a 5 to 10 per cent level, leaving the possibility that at this level (20 mg per dl) there is a ± 2 mg per dl margin of error associated with the technique itself. For these reasons some method of determining the presence or absence of the potential for bilirubin-albumin affinity designated as bilirubin-binding capacity or saturation potential is desirable.

There are now in excess of a dozen such techniques which can be used for these determinations. Of these, Sephadex G-25 separation of free (unbound) bilirubin from the heavier bilirubin-albumin complex by virtue of their different ability to pass through the Gel Column represents a simple and easily available method to establish and use. The presence of free bilirubin in any significant amount will turn the Gel from white to yellow. The addition of an Ictotest tablet to the supernatant will result in the formation of a purple ring in the column as a result of the presence therein of free bilirubin, which can also be estimated quantitatively by washing the columns followed by spectrophotometric determination of the bilirubin present in the effluent.

The use of such methods yields a more accurate index of risk in any individual infant at any given time thereby allowing for better individualization of a "safe" and/or "risky" level of serum bilirubin. In addition it can avoid unnecessary exchange transfusions in infants who, despite adverse circumstances, demonstrate adequate binding capacities and who might otherwise be empirically considered as candidates for therapeutic intervention at lower levels of serum bilirubin.

Exchange Transfusion. Exchange transfusion is the only certain way of lowering serum bilirubin. It is a washout technique and is not, therefore, specific for bilirubin but is the standard against which the efficacy of all other methods of lowering serum bilirubin should be compared. The exchange procedure is usually performed via the umbilical vein which remains patent and can under the usual circumstances readily be entered up to 7 days of age. One can also use an umbilical artery, particularly if there is already an arterial catheter in place for purposes of blood gas monitoring. De novo entry into the artery can usually be accomplished up to 72 hours of age but is difficult after then. In the event that an initial procedure is required after the first week of life, a cut-down through the skin above the umbilicus at a higher level into the umbilical vein will usually be successful.

Fresh blood, no older than 5 days but preferably less than 3 days old, should be used. It should be typed and crossmatched for both major and minor group incompatibility. In severe emergencies the mother's own blood may be used without the necessity for crossmatch. The blood is commonly anticoagulated and preserved as either ACD (acid citrate dextrose) or CPD (citrate phosphate dextrose) with the latter having the advantage of preservation of 2,3 DPG in the donor blood and its resultant easier unloading of oxygen from the red blood cell. Citrate, however, confers a low pH on the donor blood (citric acid) and is also responsible for the consumption of ionized calcium by formation of a calcium citrate complex. Heparin, which avoids both the acidosis and calcium consumption, may be used as an anticoagulant in its place; but although its anticoagulant properties are excellent, it has no preservative capability and heparinized blood must be utilized within 36 hours unless converted to a citrated preservative pack by 24 hours of age.

The standard single volume exchange transfusion (the newborn has a blood volume ranging from approximately 80 to 120 ml per kg) will usually result in a reduction of the serum bilirubin level to approximately 50 to 60 per cent of its pre-exchange value. Because of the increasing ratio of donor to recipient blood removed as the procedure continues, the efficacy of the transfusion with respect to bilirubin removal falls off along a parabolic curve; and the greatest proportion of bilirubin is thus usually removed with the *first 100 ml exchanged*. The so-called double-volume exchange transfusion will only remove an additional 20 per cent of the bilirubin and may not be justified in the event that the infant's clinical condition is perilous or the transfusion procedure is being poorly tolerated. In isoimmune hemolytic disease (Rh, ABO) the exchange procedure, in addition to removal of bilirubin, may also remove large amounts of antibody and its earlier performance may thereby reduce the subsequent level of hyperbilirubinemia, and thereby the necessity for repeat procedures.

Complications of the procedure include infection, thrombosis, sepsis, perforation, and air embolism. Hyperkalemia from old blood and bleeding secondary to thrombocytopenia (platelets are rapidly lost in donor blood) may also occur. Hypocalcemia may occur secondary to the calcium ion-citrate complexing even though the total serum calcium will be normal or even high. Calcium should, therefore, be added in the form of calcium gluconate periodically during the exchange procedure (1 cc every 50 to 100 ml). As the glucose content of both ACD- and CPD-preserved blood is high (approximately 300 mg per dl), there is a reactive insulin response to the exchange transfusion. With the sudden removal of the glucose load at the conclusion of the procedure, the remaining insulin levels may result in a post-exchange hypoglycemia which can be both symptomatic and severe, especially in instances (e.g., severe Rh incompatibility) in which the blood glucose is low or marginal to begin with.

Long-term complications include both hepatic cirrhosis and hepatosplenic arteriovenous malformations, in addition to which there is a possiblity of serum hepatitis which, although rare, carries both high morbidity and significant mortality in this age group.

Phototherapy. Phototherapy, clinically practiced as exposure of jaundiced infants to a variety of light sources, has in the last decade become a common and accepted method for decreasing the serum bilirubin. In vitro, photoirradiation of bilirubin solutions results in an energy-induced oscillation of the bilirubin molecule with the resultant loss of two hydrogen atoms (photo-oxidation). The use of blue light has been advocated as being superior because of its greater concentration in the activating wavelength (450 mm). Recent evidence, however, suggests that the in vivo effect (which occurs not in plasma but in the skin) is not the result of any significant photo-oxidation but is rather due to an internal isomerization of the bilirubin molecule which converts the water-insoluble unconjugated (indirect-acting) bilirubin into a water-soluble molecule by rupture of its internal linking triple hydrogen bonds, thereby permitting the passage of unconjugated bilirubin through the liver into the gastrointestinal tract. This mechanism may in addition reduce the reabsorption of bilirubin from the gastrointestinal tract (see below).

Clinically, the delineation of this mechanism would serve to explain the failure to demonstrate any in vivo toxicity of phototherapy as would be expected in a photo-oxidative reaction (there is no reason why bilirubin would be the only molecule selectively destroyed from this intensity of photo-irradiation). Moreover, since the isomerization reaction requires only about 1/100 the amount of light energy needed for photo-oxidation, it would explain why a great variety of white, cool, and day lights seem to be equally effective in producing a serum bilirubin reduction.

Complications of phototherapy include the danger of burns and evaporative water loss, with the latter increasing in severity in smaller more immature infants as a result of their greater surface area to body weight ratio. Moreover, in cases where significant hemolysis (from any cause) is present, the reduction of bilirubin alone, without the removal of antibody or correction of anemia, may result in a progressive anemia which might otherwise have been avoided if exchange transfusion or a modification thereof had been used. Because of this, its use as a primary method of approach to hyperbilirubinemia resulting from hemolytic causes is not recommended. If it is utilized, extreme care must be taken to carefully ascertain and correct the presence of an underlying anemia.

Paradoxically, the relative ease with which phototherapy can be administered also constitutes one of its clinical shortcomings. Its very simplicity and ease of usage results in a temptation to simply treat hyperbilirubinemia as a disease without investigating its cause. Moreover, infants who might otherwise have been transferred to regionalized more highly staffed and equipped centers for investigation and treatment are now more likely to be retained in primary care type units with occasional unfortunate negative outcomes resulting.

The bronzed baby syndrome results from photoirradiation of infants with an elevated direct-acting (conjugated) bilirubin level. The coloration is due to the presence of a series of dipyrroles from the photodecomposition of the glucuronidated bilirubin. It is self limiting and is not associated with any hepatic toxicity other than that which may have caused the elevated direct-acting fraction initially. The syndrome will not occur in the absence of an elevated direct-acting component whose presence should be viewed as a contraindication to such therapy. Indeed, other than in the presence of extreme hemolysis, where the elevated direct fraction represents an imbalance between conjugation and excretion of bilirubin, the presence of an elevated direct acting fraction *demands* investigation as to cause and not attempts to simply lower the level.

Hepatic Enzyme Induction. Hepatic enzyme induction widely utilized in Europe and some other countries may be effectively used to both prevent the rise of and hasten the reduction of the serum bilirubin after birth. This can be accomplished either by treatment of the mother in the latter weeks of gestation or of the infant postnatally. The agent in greatest use clinically is phenobarbital, of which a postnatal dose of 3 to 8 mg per kg per day orally appears to be effective, although, in view of the delay in metabolism of phenobarbital by the neonatal liver, it is not surprising that a single parenteral injection given in the first 24 hours of life appears to be equally effective.

As with most other enzyme induction phenomena, the effect is an "all-or-none" turn-on; and once an increase in enzyme activity is obtained, increasing the dosage of the inducing agent does little to enhance the effect. Although all aspects of hepatic metabolism (uptake, conjugation, and excretion) are enhanced by the drug, it seems likely that the major (and rate-limiting) step influenced is the hepatic conjugation of bilirubin mediated by the enzyme UDP glucuronyl transferase. Where successful, the effect takes approximately 48 hours to achieve and the approach should, therefore, not be used where it has been decided that a rapid or immediate lowering of the serum bilirubin is desired. Other agents capable of inducing such an effect include alcohol, diphenylhydantoin (Dilantin), diethylnicotinamide (Coramine), and a variety of organic pesticides, among which dicophane (DDT) has been proven to be effective in clinical trials. However, phenobarbital remains both the original experimental agent and the only one in common clinical usage and, therefore, the agent with which there is most experience to date.

Interference with Enterohepatic Circulatory Reabsorption of Bilirubin from the Gastrointestinal Tract. This method affords an additional mechanism of lowering serum bilirubin. Meconium contains approximately 1 mg bilirubin per gram. Since the average term newborn infant has about 200 grams of meconium in the gastrointestinal tract at birth, there is thus available a pool of 200 mg of bilirubin, a figure which represents approximately 15 to 20 times the endogenous daily production of bilirubin from the normal degradation of heme. In the human adult the presence of bilirubin in the gut would not be considered to be of any real risk, since the bilirubin exists in the water-soluble conjugated diglucuronide form. Unlike the adult situation, however, the fetal and newborn gastrointestinal tract contains large amounts of beta-glucuronidase capable of removing the glucuronide fraction and leaving lipid-soluble bilirubin, which can then be reabsorbed via the enterohepatic circulation into the vascular system. This feature explains the presence of elevated serum *indirect* bilirubin levels in cases of neonatal gastrointestinal obstruction, as well as the bilirubin-lowering effect of early oral feedings. The feedings promote the early expulsion of meconium, thereby reducing the available enteric reabsorptive bilirubin pool rather than, as has been commonly believed, reducing the bilirubin levels by maintaining a better state of hydration.

Previous attempts at binding bilirubin in the gastrointestinal tract by the use of cholestyramine or activated charcoal have been unsuccessful. The use of Agar feedings has, however, resulted both in a significantly reduced bilirubin level in plasma and an increase in the amount of bilirubin excreted in the gut. Agar is both a mild laxative and binder of bilirubin with the resultant bilirubin-Agar complex being too large to be reabsorbed into the circulatory system. The approach, while it is effective, does not yield rapid results and its use is best kept for prophylactic rather than active therapeutic purposes.

BREAST MILK JAUNDICE AND OTHER HEPATIC INHIBITORS

It is commonly accepted that breast-fed infants tend on the average to show higher serum bilirubin levels than their bottle-fed counterparts, an effect which is not due to any relative degree of dehydration in the breast-fed group. It has also been demonstrated that the milk of some women contains one or more aberrant steroids capable of inhibiting the activity of glucuronyl transferase in vitro. Although it has been suggested that the substance is 3α 20β pregnanediol, there is considerable dispute as to the precise characterization of the substance itself, although there is agreement on its presence. The inhibitory factor is not transferred in colostrum, and early jaundice (before the third or fourth day of life) in a breast-fed baby should thus not be ascribed to this possibility. Whether or not an individual infant whose mother's milk contains the inhibitor will or will not become jaundiced, and the extent to which this will occur depends both on the strength of the inhibitor and the degree of immaturity of the liver. Moreover, the rapid increase in hepatic functional maturity after birth may allow an infant to tolerate breast-feeding without a further rise in serum bilirubin, where 1 or 2 days previously the feeding was clearly implicated in a rise in serum bilirubin. Because of this, it is prudent to discontinue breast-feeding in jaundiced newborns for a 24 to 48 hour period, and then reinstitute it. In the vast majority of instances there will be no further effect even though an inhibitor is subsequently demonstrable in the particular breast milk in question.

In the rare case, there is an inhibition so strong involved (together with a slowly maturing hepatic system) that it will result in persistent and repeated re-elevation of indirect-acting serum bilirubin each time breast-feedings are re-commenced. The effect usually resolves by 1 month of age, but on occasion persistent mild recurrent hyperbilirubinemia has been demonstrated up to 6 months and even as long as 1 year of age. Although disconcerting to the parents, such elevations (usually well below 8 to 10 mg per dl) are of no risk, and with careful parental reassurance breast-feeding can be continued despite this occurrence.

There are in addition a number of other substances that appear to be capable of inhibiting hepatic conjugating ability, with resulting unconjugated hyperbilirubinemia. These include novobiocin, the esther proprionate derivative of erythromycin (Ilotycin), and large doses of the phenothiazine derivatives. In addition, there is increasing suspicion that oxytocin and its derivatives used for induction of labor may have a similar effect on the fetal liver, thereby accounting for a difference in bilirubin levels in oxytocin-induced versus non-induced infants.

SEIZURES IN THE NEONATAL PERIOD

FEIZAL WAFFARN, M.D.

Seizures in the neonatal period are of relevance to the obstetrician, as they may be a consequence of maternal disorders or of events related to labor and delivery. Their occurrence serves as an index of perinatal morbidity and as an indicator of those infants at risk for later neurologic deficit or developmental delay.

The clinical manifestations of neonatal seizures differ from those of the older child or adult, because of incomplete maturation and organization of the central nervous system. As a result, they are unlike the clonic seizures seen in adults. The more immature preterm infant will manifest seizures as subtle, nonrhythmic, disorganized movements of the trunk and extremities which may be described as "thrashing" or "swimming" motions. These are accompanied by repetitive movements of the eyes, lips, and tongue. With increasing gestation, the seizures are more rhythmic with tonic and/or clonic movements which spread at random to the other extremities. Sustained tremors or jitteriness may be categorized as "seizure-equivalents," as infants with this movement disorder are also at increased risk for later abnormalities in development. Both full-term and preterm neonates may manifest more than one type of seizure.

The type of seizure is of little value in localizing the anatomic site of the lesion or in establishing the etiology. The majority of neonatal seizures occur as a result of complications associated with pregnancy or labor and delivery, and characteristically manifest in the 72 hours following birth. These infants can therefore be readily identified at birth and monitored for seizures in the observation nursery. Neonates with a diagnosis of seizures or suspected of having seizures should ideally be transferred to a neonatal intensive care unit. The following descriptions apply to clinical situations in which neonatal seizures occur most frequently.

SEIZURES SECONDARY TO PERINATAL ASPHYXIA

Hypoxic-ischemic encephalopathy following perinatal asphyxia is the leading cause of seizures in both the term and preterm infant. The degree of perinatal asphyxia is invariably extreme as documented by ominous fetal heart rate patterns, profound metabolic acidosis in cord blood, 5 minute Apgar score less than 5, or the need for prolonged resuscitation at birth. The onset of seizures is usually 6 to 12 hours following delivery. They increase in frequency by 24 hours of life. Though the primary etiology is cerebral hypoxia-ischemia and edema, other contributory factors such as intracranial hemorrhage, hypoglycemia, and hypocalcemia may be responsible for the persistence of these seizures and their refractoriness to therapy. Repetitive seizures may compromise effective respiration. Diagnosis is by the clinical history, age at onset of seizures, and blood gas determinations to document hypoxia and acidosis. CT scan and cranial ultrasonography are of limited value in documenting hypoxic-ischemic encephalopathy in the immediate postnatal period.

Therapy is directed toward correcting ongoing hypoxia and acidosis by the administration of oxygen, and assisted ventilation if respiration is compromised. Anticonvulsant therapy should be promptly initiated, and intravenous fluids restricted to minimize cerebral edema.

SEIZURES SECONDARY TO INTRACRANIAL HEMORRHAGE

The three types of intracranial hemorrhage that commonly cause neonatal seizures are periventricular-intraventricular hemorrhage, primary subarachnoid hemorrhage, and subdural hemorrhage.

Periventricular-Intraventricular Hemorrhage. This form of hemorrhage is most frequent in preterm infants with birth weights less than 1.5 kg. The initial site of hemorrhage is the periventricular germinal matrix with subsequent rupture into the cerebral ventricles. A frequent neurologic sign that follows intraventricular hemorrhage is seizures, which occur between the second and fourth day of life. These infants also suffer from perinatal asphyxia and respiratory distress syndrome, which increases the risk of hemorrhage. Periventricular-intraventricular hemorrhage can be reliably diagnosed by cranial ultrasonography or CT scan. The current management of intraventricular hemorrhage is supportive and directed toward minimizing its extension and the development of post-hemorrhagic hydrocephalus. Seizures resulting from large intraventricular hemorrhages are at times persistent and may remain refractory to anticonvulsant therapy.

Primary Subarachnoid Hemorrhage. Primary subarachnoid hemorrhage is thought to result from minimal trauma and/or hypoxia sustained at birth. It is equally common in both term and preterm infants. The lesser degrees of these hemorrhages are clinically silent. When associated with seizures, they represent small to moderate hemorrhages over the cerebral convexities. The time of onset of seizures is variable, but is usually within 72 hours of delivery. These infants are otherwise free of neurologic or cardiorespiratory symptoms. Diagnosis is by demonstration of blood-stained cerebrospinal fluid on lumbar puncture or by CT scan. Anticonvulsant therapy is indicated.

Subdural Hemorrhage. Subdural hemorrhage over the cerebral cortex usually follows a difficult forceps or vacuum extraction of a large term infant. Since the hemorrhage is venous in origin, the neurologic signs are gradually progressive and are not usually manifest until 24 to 48 hours following delivery. The infant may present with focal or generalized seizures, and then become progressively unresponsive. Diagnosis of a subdural hemorrhage may be confirmed by a CT scan or a subdural tap. Other indirect supportive evidence includes a serial decrease in hematocrit values or rapid increase in head circumference. Therapy is directed toward the urgent relief of increased intracranial tension by surgical evacuation of the hematoma, minimizing cerebral edema and initiating anticonvulsant therapy. With improved obstetric tehcniques, the incidence of clinical subdural hemorrhage has declined.

SEIZURES SECONDARY TO METABOLIC CAUSES

Hypoglycemia is a common metabolic cause of seizures in the neonatal period. Those at greatest risk are infants of diabetic mothers, low-birth-weight infants, small-for-gestational-age infants, and postmature infants. This same group is also at risk for perinatal asphyxia and, hence, may have more than a single cause of seizures. Signs of hypoglycemia may be (1) neurologic, with seizures, irritability, or lethargy; (2) nonspecific, with apnea, or temperature instability; or (3) completely asymptomatic. These infants need to have their blood sugar levels monitored closely during the first three postnatal days when they are at greatest risk. The method of screening is by chemical reagent strips (Dextrostix), verifying borderline values by blood glucose determinations. A diagnosis of hypoglycemia is made when the blood glucose level is below 30 mg per dl. Initial correction is by an immediate intravenous infusion of a 1 to 2 ml per kg per dose of 25 per cent dextrose. This is immediately followed by a maintenance intravenous infusion of dextrose at the minimum rate of 500 mg per kg per hour. The blood glucose level should be maintained between 45 and 90 mg per dl. Anticonvulsants are indicated if seizures persist.

Hypocalcemia occurring within the first 3 days may be associated with neonatal seizures. However isolated hypocalcemia as a cause of seizures is uncommon. These infants are at risk for seizures because of associated perinatal asphyxia, being infants of diabetic mothers, or being premature. Hypocalcemia and hypomagnesemia may occur together and cause seizures which persist, unless both causes are corrected. These seizures are usually of later onset. The diagnosis is made when the serum calcium level is below 7.5 mg per dl and the serum magnesium level is below 1.5 mg per dl. Hypocalcemia is corrected by an initial intravenous infusion of calcium gluconate, 200 mg per kg per dose, which is continued at a maintenance rate of 500 to 700 mg per kg per day. Magnesium as a single intramuscular injection of 0.2 ml per kg per dose of a 50 per cent magnesium sulfate solution is usually adequate to correct hypomagnesemia. A second dose is rarely needed 12 to 24 hours later.

SEIZURES SECONDARY TO PERINATAL INFECTIONS

Neonatal seizures secondary to bacterial meningitis are more common than those due to the transplacental group of viral infections. The common pathogens are the group B streptococci, *E. coli* and the Klebsiella-Pseudomonas group. The onset of seizures is usually toward the end of the first week of life and is invariably preceded by nonspecific symptoms. If infection is suspected, a blood and cerebrospinal fluid culture should be obtained and antibiotics started immediately. The antibiotic regimen currently recommended is a combination of a penicillin (e.g., ampicillin) and an aminoglycoside (e.g., gentamicin). A positive culture from the cerebrospinal fluid confirms the diagnosis. Therapy includes appropriate antibiotics for 3 weeks and long-term anticonvulsant therapy.

The transplacental infections commonly referred to as the "TORCH" group, and including syphilis, have intracranial involvement to a varying degree. Seizures in the postnatal period are uncommon. When they do occur, there is also evidence of microcephaly, hydrocephaly, intracranial calcifications, meningioencephalitis, or chorioretinitis. Disseminated neonatal herpes infection is an exception where the presenting sign may be seizures followed by a vesicular rash appearing suddenly within the first week of life. Diagnosis is by clinical history, serology, and virus isolation. Besides anticonvulsant therapy, specific therapy for syphilis, herpes, cytomegalovirus, or toxoplasmosis is indicated.

SEIZURES SECONDARY TO DRUGS

Drug Toxicity. Recently a group of neonates with tonic seizures of early onset have been identified whose presenting signs include the need for ventilatory resuscitation at birth, hypotonia, apnea, and bradycardia. The seizures have been directly related to toxic levels of local anesthetic (mepivacaine and lidocaine) in the infant's circulation, secondary to paracervical block, pudendal block, or infiltration analgesia in the mother. These seizures may be distinguished from those secondary to perinatal asphyxia in that they occur within 6 hours of delivery and characteristically subside by 12 to 24 hours when postasphyxic seizures are most frequent. The diagnosis is made from the perinatal history and confirmed by the presence of elevated levels of drug in the infants' blood and urine. Therapy is primarily directed toward increasing diuresis to promote urinary excretion of the drug. Gastric lavage and exchange transfusion are less effective. Short-term anticonvulsant therapy may be indicated.

Drug Withdrawal Secondary to Maternal Addiction. Methadone, alcohol, and short-acting barbiturates are the drugs most likely to cause neonatal seizures as a part of the withdrawal syndrome. Seizures are seldom the presenting sign. Infants with methadone withdrawal present with jitteriness, irritable behavior, increased sweating, sneezing, and diarrhea. Seizures usually occur 1 to 3 days after the onset of these symptoms. Seizures are less common in infants in withdrawal from heroin. In contrast, neonates in withdrawal from short-acting barbituates and alcohol have onset of seizures usually within 24 to 48 hours following delivery. Tremors and jitteriness are other prominent signs.

Diagnosis is by maternal history and by demonstration of the drug in the infant's urine in the first day or two of life. Infants suspected of alcohol withdrawal may also have features of the fetal alcohol syndrome. Therapy is primarily that of treating the withdrawal syndrome. In the presence of seizures, anticonvulsant therapy should also be added.

SEIZURES SECONDARY TO RARE AND MISCELLANEOUS CAUSES

Neonatal seizures are also seen as part of the clinical picture in some rare metabolic disorders, chromosomal anomalies, and congenital malformations of the central nervous system. Pyridoxine (vitamin B_6) dependency may present as seizures refractory to anticonvulsant therapy and show an immediate response to 50 mg of intravenous pyridoxine. Other metabolic causes include disorders of amino acid metabolism and urea-cycle enzyme defects. The characteristic finding in these disorders is that the seizures and other symptoms follow the institution of oral feeding. Diagnosis is by collecting appropriate blood and urine samples while the infant is being fed, and then to exclude the offending substance from the diet.

Infants with trisomy 13 or 18 develop neonatal seizures secondary to abnormal brain development. The infants can be readily identified by their multiple congenital anomalies. Other congenital malformations of the central nervous system associated with neonatal seizures are lissencephaly, schizencephaly, and pachygyria. Diagnosis is confirmed by karyotyping, CT scan, or an autopsy. Parental counseling is indicated.

MANAGEMENT OF NEONATAL SEIZURES

From the above account it should be apparent that more than one cause may be responsible for the onset of seizures in a given neonate. Even when a single cause is readily identifiable, e.g., perinatal asphyxia, other contributory causes including hypoglycemia, hypocalcemia, or infections should be sought. The initial investigations should include (1) blood gas and pH determinations for evidence of hypoxia and acidosis; (2) blood glucose determinations; (3) serum calcium and magnesium analysis; and (4) blood and cerebrospinal fluid culture. These studies should be performed promptly since each of the corresponding disorders warrant immediate therapy. Further diagnostic studies should be based on the clinical history and the results of these initial investigations.

Phenobarbital is the most widely used anticonvulsant and adequately controls neonatal seizures in the majority of instances. If seizures should persist, a second anticonvulsant, phenytoin (Dilantin) is added. The initial loading dose of both drugs is given intravenously to rapidly achieve adequate blood levels. The dosages are given in Table 1. Since individual infants metabolize both drugs at widely varying rates, blood levels should be monitored periodically for maximum therapeutic effect. These infants are sent home on maintenance doses of oral phenobarbital, which they continue for at least 6 to 12 months.

PROGNOSIS

The prognosis depends on the primary etiology of the seizures. Infants with massive intracranial hemorrhages, severe asphyxia, and developmental disorders involving the central nervous system have a high perinatal mortality and significant neurologic deficits. Early identification and prompt treatment of the reversible causes of seizures are usually associated with a better prognosis. As a group, however, infants who have had seizures in the neonatal period are at an increased risk for permanent neurologic and developmental handicaps, even if they appear normal at the time of discharge. Close pediatric follow-up for at least the first year of life is essential.

TABLE 1. **Neonatal Dosage of Anticonvulsant Drugs**

DRUG	TOTAL LOADING DOSE	MAINTENANCE DOSE	THERAPEUTIC SERUM CONCENTRATION
Phenobarbital	10 mg/kg/dose IV; Repeat in 2 hours if seizures persist, for total of 20 mg/kg/24 hours	5 mg/kg/24 hrs divided q 12 hrs IV, IM, PO	15–30 mcg/ml
Phenytoin (Dilantin)	15–20 mg/kg/24 hrs IV	5 mg/kg/24 hrs divided q 12 hrs IV	10–20 mcg/ml

EVALUATION OF THE NEONATE FOR CONGENITAL ABNORMALITIES

SHERMAN ELIAS, M.D., and
ALBERT B. GERBIE, M.D.

Birth defects occur in approximately 3 to 4 per cent of infants. It is their sudden and unexpected appearance that causes the change in the delivery room atmosphere from one of laughter and happiness to sudden silence. A carefully obtained family and prenatal history coupled with the utilization of the new prenatal diagnostic techniques can often avoid the unexpected delivery of an abnormal infant with its emotional trauma for parents, physician, and hospital staff. In addition, the pediatric staff can be alerted and prepared for the necessity of immediate treatment.

The obstetrician must be particularly concerned with obtaining a history with respect to advanced parental age, family members with either congenital birth defects or mental retardation, unexplained stillbirths or multiple spontaneous abortions, and ethnic origin which may indicate an increased risk for a specific abnormality (e.g., Tay-Sachs disease in Ashkenazic Jews). It is necessary to elicit information concerning teratogen exposures. Important teratogens include alcohol, thalidomide, aminophyllin, methyl mercury, phenytoin, trimethadione, warfarin (coumarin), heroin, methadone, diethylstilbestrol, lithium, tetracycline, cigarette smoking, high doses of x-irradiation, hyperthermia, and certain viruses and protozoa (e.g., rubella, cytomegalovirus, herpes, and toxoplasmosis).

Important prenatal findings which may alert the clinician to an abnormal fetus include intrauterine growth retardation, breech presentation, hydramnios, oligohydramnios, premature labor, and fetal arrhythmias. In such cases, ultrasonography or x-ray studies may prove useful in establishing a diagnosis.

PHYSICAL EXAMINATION OF THE NEONATE (OR STILLBORN)

The neonatal examination is essentially the same as the examination of an older child, but certain points require amplification. It is best to start with the head and progress toward the feet.

Head. Head circumference should be carefully measured and evaluated against fetal head circumference standards. Anencephaly, hydrocephaly, microcephaly, and abnormal head shapes are obvious and highly significant. True congenital anomalies must be distinguished from normal obstetrical changes such as caput succedaneum and molding. The number of fontanelles should be noted, and the sutures examined for overriding, separation, and craniostenosis. Abnormal slants of the palpebral fissures, hypertelorism or hypotelorism, and epicanthal folds should alert the clinician to the possible presence of a chromosomal abnormality. The sclera are usually slightly blue; however, a deep blue tinge may indicate osteogenesis imperfecta. Subconjunctival hemorrhages are not uncommon in the normal neonate. Absence of one or both eyes or microophthalmia indicate severe defects which may either be isolated abnormalities or part of a broader syndrome (e.g., trisomy 13). Funduscopic evaluation may reveal either cloudy corneas, or cataracts which should lead to high suspicion of an intrauterine infection (e.g., rubella). Coloboma may be present in multiple malformation syndromes or as an isolated finding.

Ears. The position of the external pinna relative to the rest of the head should be evaluated. Abnormal helices and low-set ears are frequently associated with chromosomal abnormalities, renal abnormalities, and various syndromes.

Nose. Since infants are obligate nose breathers, any difficulty in respiration should alert the physician to the possibility of choanal atresia. This can be excluded by transnasal passage of a soft catheter bilaterally. Midfacial hypoplasia and abnormal nasal development is characteristic of the coumarin syndrome and the Conradi Hünermann syndrome.

Mouth. Cleft lip or palate is readily apparent. Clinically, however, careful examination both visually and digitally should be done. Retention cysts (Epstein's pearls) are frequently found, but are of no clinical significance. Neonatal teeth may be occasionally seen, particularly in American Indians. Microglossia is a common feature in the Pierre-Robin anomaly, and macroglossia is frequent in the Beckwith-Wiedemann syndrome. Protruding, fissured tongue secondary to maxillary hypoplasia and a narrow palate is characteristice of Down syndrome.

Chin. Both prognathism and micrognathia are frequent findings in various syndromes. They also may be normal variants.

Neck. A short neck may indicate the Klippel-Feil anomaly. Branchial and thyroglossal cysts are readily apparent. The thyroid should be palpated for goiter. A low posterior hairline or webbed neck are frequent features of Turner syndrome.

Chest. Careful inspection and palpation of the chest will reveal pectus carinatum, pectus excavatum, fractured ribs, clavicular fractures, widely spaced nipples, hemangiomas, lymphangiomas, and abnormal point of maximum cardiac impulse (e.g., dextrocardia). Auscultation may reveal congenital cardiac defects, pulmonary hypoplasia, or diaphragmatic hernia.

Abdomen. A single umbilical artery is seen in approximately 1 per cent of all live births. It is more common in infants who are chromosomally abnormal or in twins. Also, it is a frequent finding associated with cardiovascular, gastrointestinal, and renal abnormalities. Omphalocele, gastroschisis, umbilical hernia, and "prune belly" syndrome are apparent on inspection. Abdominal distention may indicate polycystic kidneys, organomegaly from blood group sensitization, infection, perforation of a viscus, necrotizing enterocolitis, distended bladder, or intestinal obstruction. Tumors which may appear in the neonatal period may include Wilms' tumor, nephroblastoma, neuroblastoma, and teratoma.

Back. Spina bifida, meningocele, and meningomyelocele are obvious. The entire vertebral column should be palpated for scoliosis.

Genitalia. In the female infant, the labia should be separated to detect imperforate hymen with hydrocolpos or hydrometrocolpos, or vaginal agenesis. A white mucoid discharge is not uncommon and is due to the influences of maternal estrogen. Several days after birth, bleeding may be noted as a result of withdrawal of these estrogens. In the male, hypospadias, with or without chordee, may be present. The testes should be palpated in the scrotum, and the size and consistency noted. If undescended, they may occasionally be brought to the normal position pushing down gently over the inguinal canal. Clitoral hypertrophy and ambiguous genitalia require immediate evaluation. These may be a manifestation of the adrenogenital syndrome which can be life threatening.

Anus. Imperforate anus is obvious upon examination.

Extremities. Constriction deformities (e.g., camptodactyly, popliteal webs) may result from fetal constraint such as with prolonged ruptured membranes with oligohydramnios. Both polydactyly and oligodactyly may be components of multiple malformation syndromes or isolated findings. Congenital dislocation of the hips may be diagnosed by abducting the legs and palpation of a click in the hip region. Abnormalties of the feet may be positional, or may result from a fixed deformity such as talipes equinovarus. Such fixed flexion deformities may be inherited in polygenic/multifactorial fashion with a 2 to 5 per cent recurrence risk in future offspring. Flexion deformities of the legs are not infrequent findings in breech presentations. Either absence or marked decrease in size of the nails may indicate ectodermal dysplasia or teratogenic exposure (e.g., hydantoin). Finally, skeletal dysplasias should be readily apparent.

Skin. The infant's entire skin surface should be inspected for hemangioma, ichthyosis, pigmented nevi, sebaceous cysts, and café-au-lait spots. A minor variant is a blue discoloration sometimes called "mongolian spot." This is frequently seen over the back and buttock and is of no clinical signficance.

Neurological Examination. Infants may be tremulous for a variety of reasons, including (1) metabolic disorders (e.g., hypoglycemia, hypocalcemia, hypomagnesemia); central nervous system disorders (e.g., hemorrhage, hypoxia, hyperviscosity syndrome); and drug withdrawal (e.g., heroin, methadone, barbiturates). Neonatal seizures may be the result of hypoxia, metabolic disorders, hypoglycemia, intracranial hemorrhages, infection, drug withdrawal, electrolyte imbalance, cerebral edema, and hyperviscosity syndrome. Hypotonia is a frequent feature in Down syndrome, the Präder-Willi syndrome, central nervous system injury, infection, intracranial hemorrhage, Werdnig-Hoffmann disease, myasthenia gravis, congenital benign hypotonia, or congenital muscular dystrophy.

SPECIFIC CONGENITAL ANOMALIES

A number of congenital abnormalities are readily apparent either by physical examination or by laboratory investigation. These may be broadly categorized into chromosomal, mendelian, polygenic/multifactorial, and environmental in etiology. It is beyond the scope of this article to review all congenital abnormalities. An excellent resource for additional information is *Birth Defects, Atlas and Compendium* (D. Bergsma, editor, Williams & Wilkins Company, Baltimore, 1979, 2d edition). We shall only consider a select group which we consider particularly important for obstetricians to recognize.

Chromosomal Disorders

Down Syndrome. Down syndrome is by far the most common and best known of the chromosomal disorders (See article entitled "Amniocentesis for Antenatal Diagnosis"). Recent estimates place the frequency rate in the North American population at 1 in 1000. The majority of cases are due to nondisjunction, producing cells with 47 chromosomes including an extra number 21 chromosome. Approximately 3 per cent of the cases involve a chromosomal translocation, usually 14/21. Phenotypic features include hypotonia, flat facies, slanting palpebral fissures, epicanthal folds, speckled iris (Brushfield spots), low bridged nose, broad and protruding tongue, "spade-like" hands, abnormal dermatoglyphics (e.g., 50 per cent of cases with a simian crease), excessive skin over the nape of the neck, congenital heart defects (40 per cent of cases), intestinal abnormality (duodenal atresia being disproportionately represented), intrauterine growth retardation, and wide gap between the first and second toes. Mental retardation (in the range of 25 to 50 I.Q.) is invariably present. Life expectancy is shortened, with about one third dying during the first year; half by age 3 or 4; the remainder living into adulthood. Congenital heart defects may be a major cause of early death; however, many of these defects are now surgically correctable. The incidence of Down syndrome increases with advancing parental age.

Trisomy 18. Trisomy 18 occurs in approximately 1 in 7000 live births in North America. Intrauterine growth retardation is invariably present and the mean survival time is only 2 months, though a few survive into the second decade or more. Approximately 80 per cent of these infants are female. Phenotypic features include generalized hypertonia, head with a prominent occiput, low-set malformed ears, short sternum, limited hip abduction, distally implanted thumb, hypoplastic nails, and prominent calcaneus. A characteristic posture of the fingers is usually present with the second and fifth digits overlapping the third and fourth digits. Severe cardiac malformations and profound mental retardation are present in virtually all cases. As with other autosomal trisomies, trisomy 18 is found with increased frequency in advanced parental age.

Trisomy 13. This rare syndrome occurs in approximately 1 in 20,000 live births in North America. Trisomy 13 is also associated with advanced maternal age. Most cases of translocation trisomy 13 occur de novo, but a few are inherited from phenotypically normal parents who carry a balanced translocation. Phenotypic features include cleft lip and palate, hypotelorism with severe eye anomalies (e.g., microophthalmia or anophthalmia), central nervous system malformations (e.g., arrhinencephaly, holoprosencephaly) severe growth retardation, sloping forehead, malformed low-set ears, postaxial polydactyly, "rocker-bottom" feet, abnormal dermatoglyphics, congenital heart defects, urogenital defects (e.g., cryptorchidism in males, bicornuate uterus and hypoplastic ovaries in females), and polycystic kidneys. All of these infants are severely mentally retarded. Most infants die within the first 3 months of life.

Cri-du-Chat Syndrome (5p- syndrome). This syndrome involves a deletion of part of the short arm of chromosome number 5. The frequency is approximately 1 per 20,000 live births in the North American population. Phenotypic features include severe developmental delay, microcephaly, various somatic abnormalities, and a characteristic high pitched, cat-like cry. Approximately 85 per cent of cases are sporadic, whereas 15 per cent are inherited from a phenotypically normal parent who carries a balanced chromosomal rearrangement, either translocation or inversion. The characteristic cat-like cry disappears in late infancy. Severe mental retardation is characteristic.

45, X Syndrome. 45, X chromosomal complement is associated with the Turner syndrome and occurs with a frequency of approximately 1 in 10,000 females. Physical abnormalities which may be present in the newborn include webbing of the neck, coarctation of the aorta, edema of the dorsum of the hands and feet, and a low nuchal hairline. However, many of these infants remain undiagnosed until later life.

Mendelian Disorders

Diseases produced by single mutant genes whether transmitted in dominant or recessive fashion, or on an autosome or on an X chromosome, are uncommon disorders. Although individually rare, mutant genes cause abnormalities in approximately 1 per cent of liveborn infants and the risk in certain families for an affected offspring is 25 or 50 per cent depending on the particular mode of inheritance.

Inborn Errors of Metabolism. Almost all of the inborn errors of metabolism involve enzyme or peptide-hormone deficiency states. The inborn errors of metabolism may generally be subdivided into several categories: (1) mucopolysaccharidoses; (2) mucolipidoses and other disorders of carbohydrate metabolism; (3) lipidoses; (4) aminoacid disorders; and (5) miscellaneous biochemical disorders. The obstetrician who is not a geneticist cannot be expected to be informed on all aspects of the clinical features of these disorders. However, the obstetrician should obtain appropriate consultation when a question arises concerning an inborn error of metabolism.

Of particular importance in the newborn are the inborn errors of aminoacid metabolism. They frequently present with vomiting, failure to thrive, protein intolerance, hypotonia and/or hypertonia, lethargy, coma, and unusual odor, and may be confused with more common problems such as sepsis. Initiation of diet therapy can be life-saving or can prevent irreversible brain damage.

Neonatal screening for phenylketonuria is mandatory in many states. Further extension of such screening programs may include the aminoacid disorders, galactosemia, and congenital hypothyroidism. Infants with genetic defects of cortisol synthesis often exhibit adrenocortical insufficiency. About half of such infants will be found to have 21-hydroxylase deficiency characterized by virilization, with or without salt loss. Müllerian and gonadal development are unaffected. 21-Hydroxylase deficiency and other forms of congenital adrenal hyperplasia must be excluded when assessing a neonate with genital ambiguity. In the case of 21-hydroxylase deficiency, untreated infants may develop hyponatremia, hyperkalemia, dehydration and possibly death from adrenal insufficiency.

Cystic Fibrosis. Cystic fibrosis is the most common disease caused by a single mutant gene in Caucasian children. The estimated incidence of this autosomal recessive disorder is approximately 1 in 1000 in the American population. Most of the clinical problems are the result of obstruction of organ ducts by abnormally thick secretions. The basic defect is unknown. Cystic fibrosis may present as an acute surgical emergency in the newborn period as a result of meconium ileus. The other clinical features, such as chronic pulmonary disease, steatorrhea, cirrhosis of the liver, cor pulmonale, prolapse of the rectum, glycosuria, massive salt loss and dehydration, coma, and eventual death develop later in childhood.

Skeletal Dysplasias. There are over 40 known conditions which may result in skeletal dysplasias. Achondroplasia is the most common occurring nonlethal condition. Thanatophoric dysplasia and lethal perinatal osteogenesis imperfecta are the most widely occurring lethal skeletal dysplasias. Correct differential diagnosis can be established only through careful clinical and radiologic evaluations.

Polycystic Kidney Disease (Perinatal Type). In this autosomal recessive form of polycystic kidney disease, infants have marked abdominal distention because of huge symmetric renal masses; they die within 6 weeks. In contrast to other forms of polycystic kidney disease, liver involvement is relatively minimal, with little periportal fibrosis. Oligohydramnios may be present in such pregnancies. This may result in an infant with Potter facies (low-set floppy ears, micrognathia, deviated nose) and multiple joint contractures. Ultrasonography may prove useful for antenatal diagnosis in subsequent pregnancies.

Polygenic/Multifactorial Disorders

These disorders result from the cumulative effects of several genes (polygenic) and their interactions with environmental factors (multifactorial). Frequently such disorders involve single organ systems. After the birth of one child with a disorder believed to be inherited in polygenic/multifactorial fashion, the likelihood of recurrence is usually in the range of 2 to 5 per cent.

Neural Tube Defects. The estimated incidence of neural tube defects is approximately 1 to 2 per 1000 births in the United States. Embryologically and genetically, spina bifida and anencephaly appear to be related, the etiology in both being a failure of neural tube closure. Hydrocephalus in the presence of spina bifida should be considered a secondary manifestation of the spinal defect; hydrocephalus without spina bifida is etiologically distinct. Infants with anencephaly will succumb shortly after birth. Infants with either meningocele or meningomyelocele should be evaluated immediately by a neurosurgeon for surgical repair. In subsequent pregnancies the couple should be informed about genetic amniocentesis and prenatal diagnosis (see article entitled "Amniocentesis for Antenatal Diagnosis").

Congenital Diaphragmatic Hernia. There are several types of diaphragmatic hernia, most of which are not life-threatening. Three fourths of these defects are on the left side. In 50 to 75 per cent of infants it exists as an isolated defect. However, pulmonary hypoplasia and the pulmonary vasculature abnormalities may coexist. In large defects the pulmonary hypoplasia may be so pronounced that resuscitation of the neonate is impossible. Usually the infant has relatively minor difficulty breathing initially, but begins to have increasing difficulties in the first few hours of life. The abdomen is scaphoid, and the infant shows the classical triad of symptoms: dyspnea, cyanosis, and apparent dextrocardia (the result of mediastinal displacement). The differential diagnosis must include tension pneumothorax and true cardiovascular abnormalities. Initial management includes endotracheal intubation, nasogastric tube to decompress the stomach, and fluid and electrolyte maintenance. Immediate surgical consultation must be obtained.

Tracheoesophageal Fistula. The incidence of esophageal atresia with or without tracheoesophageal fistula is about 1 in 3000 births. At least 7 different anatomic varieties of tracheoesophageal fistula have been described. About half the infants with tracheoesophageal fistula have other anomalies, with renal, cardiac, and rectal defects being most common. Recently the so-called VATER association (an acronym for vertebral, anal, tracheoesophageal, radial, and renal anomalies) has been recognized. Infants with this disorder frequently have only one umbilical artery, further emphasizing that the umbilical cord should be carefully inspected. Early recognition of the infant at risk should include a search for an obstructive lesion prior to the first feeding to avoid aspiration.

Congenital Heart Defects. There are many forms of congenital heart disease which may present in the neonatal period. Such defects occur in 5 to 8 per 1000 live births. Usually abnormalities of the cardiac system are isolated structural defects; however, they may be part of a multiple system malformation syndrome. The most commonly encountered cardiac abnormality is patent ductus arteriosus with the characteristic feature of a systolic murmur at the second or third left intercostal space and bounding peripheral pulses. Only rarely is the classic "machinery murmur" heard in the neonatal period. Infants with acyanotic heart defects (e.g., atrial and ventricular septal defects, patent ductus arteriosus, coarctation of the aorta) usually remain asymptomatic during the neonatal period. Congenital heart defects that usually present with cyanosis in the neonatal period include tricuspid or pulmonary atresia, truncus arteriosus, transposition of the great vessels, total anomalous pulmonary venous drainage, and hypoplastic left or right heart syndrome. Cyanotic congenital heart disease is a medical emergency which requires immediate consultation with a cardiovascular specialist.

In addition to cyanosis, poor feeding, failure to gain weight, tachypnea, poor peripheral pulses, pulsatile liver, and radiographic evidence of pulmonary parenchymal disease should all alert the physician to the presence of congenital heart disease.

Cleft Lip and Palate. Cleft lip and cleft lip with cleft palate appear to be etiologically related, and in most cases, considered to be inherited in a polygenic/multifactorial fashion. Cleft lip and cleft palate are usually not life-threatening abnormalities; however, there may be difficulties in feeding with resultant aspiration. In addition, these infants may have upper airway obstruction. Immediate therapy includes maintenance of an oral airway and referral for surgical repair. The infant must be carefully evaluated for associated malformations since cleft lip and/or cleft palate may be components of multiple malformation syndromes (e.g., trisomy 13). The risk of recurrence of cleft lip (with or without cleft palate) or cleft palate alone depends upon the particular family history. For example, with one previously affected sibling the recurrence risk ranges from 2 to 4 per cent. If only one parent is affected, the recurrence risk is in the range of 4 to 6 per cent. If both parents are affected, the risks range from 25 to 35 per cent.

Omphalocele and Gastroschisis. An omphalocele is a saccular malformation of the umbilical cord containing various portions of the intestinal tract, with the umbilical ring being widely open. This defect is generally covered by a membranous extension of the peritoneum. Elements of the umbilical cord may be present in the wall of the sac. The umbilical defect may vary in size from 1 to 2 cm, to massive, obliterating most of the abdominal wall. The contents of the omphalocele may be just one loop of bowel or the entire intestinal tract, with liver and spleen being included. This defect occurs in approximately 1 per 6000 live births. Associated abnormalities of the cardiovascular system (16 to 20 per cent), genitourinary system (40 per cent), and central nervous system (4 per cent) may occur. The Beckwith-Wiedemann syndrome, consisting of macroglossia, macrosomia, umbilical defect, and hypoglycemia, should be investigated in the infant with omphalocele.

A gastroschisis is a similar defect, except the umbilical cord is normally inserted. In addition, there is a full-thickness defect of the abdominal wall away from the midline, and the sac is absent. Intestinal malrotation is commonly observed in gastroschisis.

In both omphalocele and gastroschisis, emergency measures are directed toward preventing evaporative heat and water loss from the exposed viscera. This may be accomplished by covering the defect with warm, saline-soaked gauze sponges or loosely wrapping the entire abdomen with warm towels or plastic sheets. The prognosis is usually good once the repair is accomplished and the intestinal function established. Intestinal obstruction due to adhesions may be a problem, particularly in small lesions. It is important not to attempt to reinsert the eviscerated organs into the abdominal cavity prior to transporting the infant to the care of a pediatric surgeon. Nasogastric suction is useful for gastric decompression. Intravenous fluid replacement should be given and feedings withheld.

Intestinal Atresia or Stenosis. Intestinal obstruction in the neonate is clinically manifest by abdominal distention, vomiting, and obstipation. In approximately 25 per cent of cases intestinal atresia is secondary to other intestinal or abdominal defects. Isolated intestinal atresia is usually attributed to interference with mesenteric blood supply. Atresia occurs in the jejunum (50 per cent), the ileum (43 per cent), and in both jejunum and ileum (7 per cent). A high obstruction is often manifest antenatally by the presence of hydramnios. Duodenal atresia is present in about 8 per cent of infants with Down syndrome. Intestinal atresia should be suspected when infants fail to pass meconium within the first 24 hours after birth.

Intestinal stenosis may become clinically apparent later in infancy with constipation or diarrhea (secondary to alterations in intestinal flora).

Management of the neonate suspected of having an intestinal obstruction includes intravenous fluid replacement, withholding feedings, and gastric decompression. Maintenance of electrolyte balance is crucial.

Section 3
GENERAL GYNECOLOGY

INFECTIOUS VAGINITIS

KENNETH L. NOLLER, M.D.

Although infectious vaginitis is one of the most frequent reasons for women to visit a gynecologist, only recently has it been possible to identify, diagnose, and treat many of the specific causes of this malady. In the past, it was recognized that infections with yeast and *Trichomonas vaginalis* organisms were common, but all other causes of vaginitis were classified as "nonspecific." We now know that this large group of patients represents women with infections caused by a number of specific agents. If these agents are correctly identified, and if appropriate treatment is planned, most women will become symptom-free with relative ease. In addition, with treatment of the male sexual partner(s), recurrences are infrequent. Thus, modern management of vaginitis involves the following three principles: (1) identification of the causative organism, (2) appropriate systemic therapy, and (3) treatment of the male sexual partner(s). The term "nonspecific vaginitis" should rarely if ever be used in modern gynecology. Additionally, topical vaginal creams, except for antifungal agents, probably should not be used. In general, such vaginal preparations are ineffective against well-established infections.

The common causes, symptoms, diagnostic criteria, and appropriate treatment in infectious vaginitis are indicated in Table 1.

INFECTIONS DUE TO YEAST AND FUNGI

Although many species of yeast and fungi may live in the human vagina, most symptomatic infections are the result of an overgrowth of *Candida albicans* or *Torulopsis glabrata* organisms. The patient will often complain of a thick, white vaginal discharge, but the main symptom is severe perineal itching. With severe infections, vulvar, perineal, and periurethral excoriations may result in severe burning with voiding.

In most patients, the cause may be easily identified by means of a saline or potassium hydroxide preparation of the vaginal discharge. In some with mild infections, the organism may be difficult to see in clinical preparations, and vaginal culture on an appropriate medium may be necessary.

Two medications that are currently avail-

TABLE 1. **Common Causes of Infectious Vaginitis in the United States**

CAUSATIVE ORGANISM	SYMPTOMS	DIAGNOSIS	TREATMENT*
Yeast, fungus (*Candida albicans, Torulopsis glabrata*)	Perineal itching; thick, white discharge	Saline preparation; KOH preparation; culture	Miconazole; clotrimazole
Gardnerella vaginalis (*Haemophilus vaginalis, Corynebacterium vaginalis*)	Profuse malodorous discharge	"Clue cells" on saline preparation, bacterial culture	Tetracycline, 500 mg four times a day for 10 days; metronidazole, 500 mg three times a day for 5 days; metronidazole 2 grams single dose; (erythromycin, 250 mg four times a day for 10 days)
Trichomonas vaginalis	Profuse malodorous discharge; yellow-green discharge	Saline preparation	Metronidazole, 250 mg three times a day for 7 days; metronidazole, 2 grams, single dose
Chlamydia species (several organisms can cause symptoms)	Thin white discharge; little odor, if any; occasional itching	Culture (? cytology)	Tetracycline, 500 mg four times a day for 7 days; erythromycin, 250 mg four times a day for 7 days
Mycoplasma species (various mycoplasma may cause symptoms)	Thin, usually clear discharge (rarely cause of significant clinical symptoms)	Culture	Tetracycline, 500 mg four times a day for 7 days; erythromycin, 500 mg four times a day for 7 days
Beta-Streptococcus	Severe vaginal burning (infrequent cause of vaginitis)	Culture (bright-red vaginal mucosa)	Penicillin, ampicillin

*Less effective modalities indicated in parentheses.

able will eradicate infections due to these organisms in virtually every case: miconazole and clotrimazole. Either may be used nightly for 5 to 7 days, with nearly universal clearance of symptoms. However, reinfection is *very common* unless the male sexual partner(s) is also treated. Only recently has it been recognized that yeast organisms are present on the foreskin, folds of the skin on the penis, and the ruga of the scrotum. The male should spread the cream on the shaft of the penis and scrotum several times on consecutive days, or medication may be put in the vagina just before intercourse. The second method is preferable because the medication is spread over the surfaces of the vaginal and penile skin by the mechanism of coitus.

INFECTIONS DUE TO *Gardnerella vaginalis*

Many of the infections that were previously identified as "nonspecific vaginitis" are now known to be due to the bacterium *Gardnerella vaginalis*. Unfortunately, the taxonomy of this bacterium is confusing. In the last few years, the same organism has also been known as *Haemophilus vaginalis* and *Corynebacterium vaginalis*. The accepted name is now *Gardnerella vaginalis*.

Infection with this bacterium causes a profuse malodorous vaginal discharge. The odor is characteristic, and the diagnosis can often be suspected at the initiation of pelvic examination. A small amount of vaginal discharge may be examined in saline suspension, and the presence of large numbers of epithelial cells covered with bacteria ("clue cells") is presumptive evidence of infection with this bacterium. Leukocytes are also often present in large numbers. If the diagnosis is in doubt, a general bacterial culture of the vagina may be obtained to confirm the presence of *Gardnerella* organisms.

Many therapies have been suggested for eradication of this bacterium. At the present time, the oral use of tetracycline, 500 mg four times a day for 10 days, or of metronidazole, 500 mg three times a day for 5 to 7 days, appears to be the best choice. In patients sensitive to these drugs, ampicillin or erythromycin may be used as second-line therapy. Recently, the use of a single oral dose containing 2 grams of metronidazole has been supported by some clinicians.

In *Gardnerella* infections, the male sexual partner(s) should be treated with the same course of medication as the female. Reinfection is almost certain unless the male is treated.

When a *Gardnerella* infection occurs during pregnancy, neither tetracycline nor metronidazole should be used. Ampicillin appears to be the best choice in pregnancy. Erythromycin (base or steroid forms only) may be used in penicillin-sensitive patients.

INFECTIONS DUE TO *Trichomonas vaginalis*

Many older textbooks state that *Trichomonas* vaginitis is the second most frequent cause of leukorrhea. Although common, this organism now ranks behind yeast and fungi and behind *Gardnerella* in frequency and may even be seen less frequently than chlamydial infections. Nevertheless, trichomoniasis continues to be a common cause of vaginal symptoms. The patient usually complains of a profuse yellow-green discharge that has an unpleasant odor. The protozoan that causes this infection may be readily identified on a saline preparation of the vaginal discharge.

Although many treatment regimens have been devised, the only acceptable treatment currently (except in pregnancy) is the use of metronidazole. This drug is almost uniformly effective in eradicating the organism from the female genital tract. However, reinfection is very frequent unless the male sexual partner(s) is treated at the same time. Patients using this medication must be cautioned against the intake of alcohol during treatment.

Metronidazole should not be used during pregnancy. Unfortunately, there are no other uniformly effective medications available. The use of povidone-iodine gel and douche may decrease symptoms. However, this treatment rarely completely eradicates the organisms from the female genital tract.

CHLAMYDIAL VAGINITIS

A number of organisms are included in the chlamydial species. Several of these may cause symptoms when present in the lower female genital tract. This group of organisms represents the second most frequent cause of nonspecific vaginitis. These organisms also frequently cause nonspecific urethritis in males. Although the organism may be easily cultured using a special medium, the procedure is costly and not universally available. Presently, studies are under way to determine whether the Papanicolaou smear may be utilized as a sensitive and specific method for identifying chlamydial infections.

Patients with chlamydial vaginitis will often complain of a thin, white, bubbly vaginal discharge with little odor. Occasionally, itching may be present. Treatment with either tetracycline, 500 mg four times a day for 7 days, or erythromycin, 250 mg three times a day for 7 days, is usually effective. In this infection, the male sexual partner(s) also may likely have symptoms. Once again it is most important to treat both sexual partners.

MYCOPLASMAL VAGINITIS

Although one or more *Mycoplasma* species may be cultured from the vagina of many females, this is rarely a cause of significant symptoms. Very rarely no other cause will be found, but cultures for *Mycoplasma* organisms will be positive. The utilization of an appropriate culture technique is virtually the only method to identify this group of organisms. Erythromycin or tetracycline may be used to treat the infection in the same manner as was described for chlamydial infections.

STREPTOCOCCAL VAGINITIS

On rare occasions, beta-streptococcal organisms will be the cause of vaginitis. The patient usually complains of severe vaginal burning and a very "hot" feeling in the perineal area. When examined, the vagina will appear to be fiery red, resembling the pharynx of patients with streptococcal pharyngitis. Culture for beta-streptococcus will be positive in these cases. Penicillin should be used in treatment.

COMBINED INFECTIONS

It is very common for more than one pathogen to be present in the female vaginal tract at any one time. In these patients, an attempt should be made to identify a simple treatment plan that will eradicate all of the organisms. Additionally, endocervical cultures should be performed for the presence of *Neisseria gonorrhoeae* when infectious vaginitis is present.

DYSTROPHY

DONALD WOODRUFF, M.D.

The term dystrophy commonly has been applied to muscular conditions such as "progressive muscular dystrophy," and is a disorder arising from defective or faulty nutrition. In 1966, during the transitionary period between the hoped-for demise of the terms "leukoplakia and kraurosis," dystrophy was applied to various "white vulvar lesions" by Norman Jeffcoate. In 1971, the International Society for the Study of Vulvar Disease made the first attempt to classify the dystrophies into three categories proposed by the organization:
1. Hyperplastic dystrophy
    A. Typical hyperplasia (largely chronic dermatitis and hyperkeratosis)
    B. Atypical hyperplastic dystrophy—mild, moderate and marked
2. Lichen sclerosus (et atrophicus). The modifying term et atrophicus was eliminated because the epithelium as determined by certain studies such as tritiated thymidine and acridine orange fluorescence demonstrated cellular overactivity in the thinned epithelium. No specific atypical variety of lichen sclerosus is described; thus, the occasional transition from lichen sclerosus to cancer is felt to be related to an intervening area of epithelial hyperplasia.
3. Mixed dystrophy is obviously "a combination of lichen sclerosus and hyperplasia".

The classification was devised for two reasons:

1. In order to eliminate ambiguous terms such as leukoplakia which, obviously, means only white patch and is most classically associated with chronic dermatitis and hyperkeratosis; and

2. To offer some predictable evaluation of the specific alteration that may identify the patient at risk and thus demand close follow-up or definite therapy.

Chronic dermatitis is common since the vulva is constantly moist; cracking and splitting of the skin are frequent; and the vulva is constantly exposed to many local irritants such as protective appliances used at the time of the menstrual period, bubble baths and bath oils, local anesthetic agents, colored and perfumed toilet papers, and so forth. Long-term chronic irritation leads to thickening of the epidermis, elongation of the rete pegs (acanthosis) and hyperkeratosis, the latter giving the condition its grayish-white color. These histopathologic features are of those described for "leukoplakia" in the past. Atypical changes are demonstrated by abnormal maturation in the rete tips (pearl formation). There are no specific gross changes to differentiate the typical from the atypical changes. Consequently biopsy is imperative to identify the specific histologic details.

Lichen sclerosus, so named because of its irregular, whitish-gray pattern with accentuation of the skin markings (lichenification), may be found in any age group. Prior to the menarche, the lesions are uncommon and yet often disturbing and misdiagnosed. Of significance in this group of patients is the elimination of other irritants in symptomatic treatment, for example, intravaginal estrogen and local hydrocortisone: Testosterone, commonly used in the postmenopausal patient, is not recommended for the prepubertal child. If the problem cannot be controlled by the above medications, a 2 per cent progesterone preparation in aquaphor base is recommended.

During the menstrual years, vulvar lichen sclerosus is not common. However, because of the underlying collagenization, it often produces constriction and fissure formation at the fourchette. It is imperative to make the appropriate diagnosis by biopsy and then treat the patient symptomatically, often by excision of the fissure, undermining the adjacent vagina and using the vaginal epithelium to recover the defect. In the postmenopausal patient, lichen sclerosus is commonly symptomatic and produces severe irritation and itching. In this age group, testosterone is the appropriate therapy, and in 75 to 80 per cent of cases, applications 2 or 3 times a day for 2 months will thicken the epithelium and improve nutrition. The author prefers a 2 per cent preparation in stearin-lanolin base, although the base may be petrolatum or even Vaseline. Lower percentages have not been successful and stronger preparations have not produced better results. It should be appreciated that testosterone does not relieve itching. Consequently, it is necessary in most instances to use a fluorinated hydrocortisone in association with testosterone. It is not suggested that these agents be mixed, since the former treats the symptom and should be used only as necessary, while testosterone must be used over long periods of time. It is wise to continue topical testosterone therapy in order to maintain good nutrition. One application rubbed in thoroughly once a week is usually adequate. Reversion to the original lichen sclerotic condition may well take place if the medication is discontinued for long periods of time.

Finally, it is important to use biopsy freely if ulceration or marked focal thickening (hyperkeratosis) appears. The latter often demonstrates only benign hyperkeratosis, but it is possible that in such areas, a malignant lesion may develop. It is important to make the patient aware of side-effects that may accrue from testosterone therapy. Clitoral enlargement and increased libido are seen in approximately 20 per cent of the cases. Systemic effects, such as the appearance or increase in facial hair have been reported but must be extremely rare. If any adverse reaction occurs, it is wise to alter the therapy and use progesterone as noted above.

The mixed dystrophies are extremely common. As noted above, lichen sclerosus may, over a period of time, demonstrate focal areas of thickening with hyperkeratosis and acanthosis. These patients should be treated symptomatically, and if the lichen sclerosus is prominent, testosterone is the treatment of choice. Nevertheless, it should be understood that testosterone is not the treatment for the hyperplastic variety of dystrophy.

In the case resistant to topical agents, particularly those falling into the category of chronic dermatitis with hyperkeratosis (typical hyperplastic dystrophy), the subcutaneous injection of fluorinated hydrocortisones may be dramatically successful. The author prefers Triamsynalone (Kenalog), usually 2 cc of the 1 cc = 10 mg preparation, injected in focal areas. The area should be anesthetized first with 1 to 2 per cent lidocaine solution. Relief can be expected for 4 to 6 months in such instances. Since these patients have been chronically symptomatic, the relief is often dramatic. The treatment may be used in focal areas or over the entire external genitalia. The author prefers to initially treat a focal area in order to demonstrate the results or lack thereof. Systemic steroids are not recommended.

The use of subcutaneous alcohol can be effective, but should be used only as a last resort. The blocking of the entire vulva by the injection of 0.1 to 0.2 cc of absolute alcohol at 1 cm intervals from the mons to the perineum will eliminate the itching in a great majority of the cases. The patient should be warned that there is initial swelling and numbness for at least 3 to 4 weeks. In general, the results have been successful if the agent is used correctly, that is, not injected into the deeper tissues or into the epithelium itself. Symptomatic relief lasts for 6 or more months: Vulvectomy should not be performed unless a malignant process is present. Such procedures as denervation are rarely, if ever, necessary, and laser treatment is currently not recommended.

Finally, it should be emphasized and re-emphasized that biopsy plays a major role in the evaluation of such patients and in the effort to eliminate the possibility of malignant disease, and follow-up is mandatory.

VAGINAL ADENOSIS

HUGH R. K. BARBER, M.D.

Diethylstilbestrol (DES) was synthesized in 1938. It was inexpensive, potent orally, and was used for a great number of hormonally associated problems as well as for threatened abortion and pregnant diabetic patients. Cellular or organ changes secondary to the administration of DES were not identified until 1971. At that time, Herbst, Ulfelder and Poskanzer reported a link between DES and cancer of the female reproductive organs. An unusual cancer of the vagina and/or cervix had developed in a number of young women whose mothers had taken DES type drugs during pregnancy.

Since that time, other abnormalities have also been found, including tissue placed abnormally on the cervix or vagina. The tissue is not cancerous and has not been shown to be an approximate precursor of clear cell adenocarcinoma, but has caused a great deal of concern. Adenosis is defined as the abnormal presence of glandular epithelium in the vagina. Glandular structures are always located superficially, closely related to surface epithelium. In about 20 to 25 per cent of patients exposed to diethylstilbestrol in utero, structural changes in the vagina and the cervix have been reported by Stafl. He also found an 87 per cent incidence of vaginal adenosis in the patient exposed to DES. The anterior fornix often appears shortened and is less elastic than usual. A cervical hood which gives the appearance of a coxcomb may be present, and the cervix appears red. There is often red granular mucosa, small cysts, or papillary lesions that may be multicentric in appearance. On palpation there is a sandy irregularity. Reports have suggested that squamous cell lesions would be a major problem among these women, but this has not materialized. At this point in time, it is felt that women exposed to DES appear to be at no greater risk for squamous lesions than their nonexposed counterparts.

The question of whether there is an increased incidence of breast cancer in women who receive DES is under investigation, but there currently are no hard data to confirm this. The other problem raised concerns fertility and the outcome of pregnancy in women exposed in utero to DES. Barnes and her colleagues reported on the fertility and the outcome of pregnancy in women participating in the National Cooperative Diethylstilbestrol Adenosis (DESAD) project. Among DES-exposed women who became pregnant, 81 per cent had had at least one full-term live birth.

MANAGEMENT OF THE DES-EXPOSED PATIENT

All asymptomatic girls who have been exposed in utero to DES should receive a thorough pelvic examination at the time of their first period. They should also be examined if they have not had their period by age 14. Younger girls should be examined if they have abnormal bleeding or discharge has developed. Whenever prenatal exposure is probable and any symptoms are present, further investigation is imperative, regardless of the patient's age. This investigation should not be concluded until it is certain that no lesion is present.

The examination should include inspection, palpation, and Papanicolaou smears of the cervix and vagina which are carried out with a spatula that scrapes the mucosa. Colposcopic examination is carried out after the Papanicolaou scrapings have been obtained. The value of colposcopy is controversial. Colposcopy has never detected an unsuspected clear cell adenocarcinoma. However, in the hands of the experienced colposcopist it does serve to identify proliferating metaplasia, and this is important because often a report is rendered saying that dysplasia is present. Thus, the colposcopic examination can be helpful in identifying this change. However, as a routine screening method, colposcopy has not been shown to be superior to a very careful examination and palpation. After the colposcopic examination has been carried out, Lugol's staining of the cervix and vagina should be done. Lugol's solution is usually unnecessary and inspection and palpation are more important in determining the areas that need biopsy and subsequent examination.

Contraception for the DES-exposed woman should follow the same guidelines as for the non-exposed patient. These patients often have cervical deformities and an inelasticity of the fornices making it difficult for them to use a diaphragm. Kaufman has shown that there are often changes in the uterus that may make the insertion of an intrauterine device difficult. The pill is not contraindicated in these patients and it may help improve the appearance of the cervix and vagina.

The management and follow-up of these patients has progressed from the use of an acid preparation, progesterone suppository, and excision of the fornices with skinning of the cervix to treating the involved areas with cryotherapy, hot therapy, laser therapy and repeated punch biopsies. Currently the plan has changed from an aggressive management to merely following these patients with careful pelvic examinations and Pap smears. Repeat examinations are usually performed approximately every year and if there is any evidence of change either locally or in the Pap smear, the time interval should be shortened. Colposcopic examination is of value initially but does not need to be repeated at every visit. However, if the patient has an abnormal Papanicolaou smear, colposcopy is mandatory.

In a certain number of these patients the adenosis will disappear spontaneously by age 22 or 23. In the experience of the author, the adenosis only needs treatment when it is accompanied by a marked ectopy that gives rise to a significant and annoying discharge. It is imperative that careful follow-up be carried out because many of these patients have an enlarged T-zone. It is in this area that neoplastic changes may occur. Whether there will be an increased incidence of neoplasm when these patients are in their 40s or 50s remains to be seen. Currently they do not seem to be at any greater risk for developing squamous lesions than their non-exposed counterparts.

The DES problem and the complications arising from it are iatrogenic. Yesterday's cure has become today's folly, and the medical profession must take steps to prevent this from ever happening again. We must be prepared to answer the patient's questions on any drug therapy employed. We must guard against overtreatment, and work to change attitudes and provide a better understanding between the provider of medical care and the consumer.

DISORDERS OF PELVIC SUPPORT
RAYMOND A. LEE, M.D.

It is generally agreed that the support of pelvic structures depends on the endopelvic fascia, the uterosacral and cardinal ligaments, and the levator muscle. This intact fascial system with its attachments to the vaginal fornices and the upper two thirds of the lateral vagina provides a well-supported vaginal tube, which in turn is the most important supporting structure for the uterus and vaginal vault. Traumatic (obstetric) stretching, "wear and tear of living," occupational and unusual athletic endeavors, heredity, and postmenopausal attenuation all contribute in varying degrees to development of pelvic relaxation. Additional contributing factors that promote uterine descensus are obesity, asthma, and other chronic lung conditions.

The symptoms of uterovaginal prolapse are rather vague; frequently, the degree of relaxation is inconsistent with the severity of symptoms. The most frequent symptoms are pelvic pressure, a "falling-out sensation," or the feeling of sitting on a ball. Occasionally, something "protruding from the vagina" is associated with standing, walking, or ineffective evacuation of urine or stool.

UTERINE DESCENSUS (UTERINE PROLAPSE OR PROCIDENTIA)

Prolapse of the uterus may result in the descent of the cervix to the introitus (first degree), protrusion of the cervix through the introitus (second degree), or prolapse of the entire uterus (third degree). Rarely, because of severe medical conditions in an elderly patient, a pessary may be indicated; however, the preferred treatment is operation. Although some surgeons may disagree, operations such as the Manchester, Watkins-Wertheim interposition, Spaulding-Richardson, and Le Fort procedures, previously described for correction of pelvic relaxation, are generally considered to be only of historic interest at this time. Modern surgical therapy consists of a vaginal hysterectomy and appropriate anterior and posterior colpoperineorrhaphy. It should be understood that even though the condition may not improve and operation may eventually be required, correction is not necessarily urgent and should be deferred until the patient has sufficient symptoms and is medically prepared. Several techniques for vaginal hysterectomy are acceptable, any one of which will yield satisfactory results when properly accomplished. Nevertheless, the method of providing support after the hysterectomy—not the specific technique of hysterectomy itself—is the crux in correcting pelvic relaxation. An appropriate procedure will result in a safe, effective anatomic support, providing a functional vagina and correction of bladder and bowel dysfunction.

It is not my intention to review the individual steps of vaginal hysterectomy but rather to highlight specific points of importance. My colleagues and I prefer not to catheterize the bladder before operation. The presence of urine in the bladder does not impede the progress of the procedure; if the bladder is accidentally penetrated during the procedure, the immediate gush of urine aids in its recognition. The attenuated, stretched-out uterosacral and cardinal ligament complex must be shortened considerably, the amount depending on the degree of pelvic relaxation. To accomplish this safely, we routinely palpate the ureter between the index finger and the laterally placed Deaver retractor in all vaginal hysterectomies. Occasionally, because of uterine enlargement secondary to uterine fibroids, adenomyosis, or subinvolution, morcellation of the uterine fundus is necessary for delivery of the fundus. If the fundus is left intact, it tends to "milk off" the previously placed ligatures on the uterosacral and cardinal ligaments.

Morcellation can be safely performed with no increased morbidity and minimal blood loss after both uterine vessels have been clamped, cut, and suture ligated.

Uterine prolapse will invariably be associated with some degree of enterocele, which generally increases in size as the degree of prolapse progresses. After excision of the enterocele sac, we customarily place a modified McCall suture, approximating a heavy portion of the vaginal sacral ligament far superior (2 cm) to the vagina and lateral to the wing of the rectum and incorporating the intervening peritoneum. This, in effect, obliterates the posterior cul-de-sac and thus reduces the opportunity for later development of an enterocele or vault prolapse. Ligation of the sac at a high level with a second retroperitonealizing suture is a fundamental principle in the repair of all acquired hernias. This creates a solid block of support under the floor of the cul-de-sac and firmly approximates the fascial supports.

CYSTOCELE

With progressive stretching or attenuation of the cervicopubic fascia, the posterior aspects of the bladder and the urethra descend into the vagina and produce a cystourethrocele. Occasionally, this relaxation is encountered in the nulliparous patient; however, most cases occur in parous women. Obesity, asthma, and other upper respiratory conditions are often associated causes of cystocele. Cystocele alone without uterine descensus rarely produces appreciable symptoms and usually does not necessitate surgical repair. Occasionally, surgical repair of an asymptomatic cystocele leads to urinary incontinence not previously present or a troublesome urinary fistula from the urethra or bladder. The patient should be reassured that even though a cystocele may enlarge over the years, no serious illness will result if surgical correction is delayed. When the cystocele protrudes through the vaginal introitus, or if the patient has pelvic pressure and the sensation of sitting on a ball, surgical repair is justified.

When operation is undertaken, an anterior colporrhaphy (which is only a single facet in the pelvic repair) is the most effective treatment for cystocele. This is accomplished by plication of the endopelvic fascia (bladder capsule) with fine interrupted polyglycolic acid sutures. Overzealous repair of the cystocele or undercorrection of the urethral and bladder neck support should be avoided. Accurate, carefully placed sutures that tighten the tissues through which the urethra passes and firmly support the bladder neck increase resistance to the flow of urine and will result in good urinary control. Careful excision of the redundant anterior vaginal wall and accurate approximation of its edges are necessary for preservation of a functional vagina and avoidance of a retracting scar that may result in dyspareunia or urinary incontinence.

RECTOCELE

Bulging of the posterior vaginal wall and underlying rectum through the rectovaginal fascia results in a rectocele. A mild degree of rectocele (rarely causing symptoms) is present in all multiparous patients. A large rectocele may cause a sense of pelvic pressure, rectal fullness, or incomplete evacuation of stool. Occasionally, a patient may find it necessary to reduce the posterior vaginal wall manually in a backward direction to evacuate stool effectively from the lower rectum. Examination (with the index finger in the vagina and the middle finger in the rectum) reveals a thinned-out septum, which can involve varied lengths of the rectovaginal area. Distinguishing a high rectocele (involving the entire rectovaginal septum) from an enterocele may sometimes be difficult. Generally with the patient straining, a rectovaginal examination will confirm the presence of abdominal contents sliding into the enterocele sac.

When an operation is necessary, a posterior midline incision is extended up to the transverse suture line of the vaginal vault repair. An adequate repair consists of plication of the rectovaginal fascia, approximation of the levator and peroneal muscles, and excision of the redundant vaginal wall. Again, overzealous approximation of levator or peroneal muscles (resulting in a transverse bar) or resection of an excessive portion of the vaginal wall may result in dyspareunia that may be difficult to eliminate.

POSTHYSTERECTOMY VAGINAL VAULT PROLAPSE

Although vaginal inversion occasionally occurs after vaginal hysterectomy, abdominal hysterectomy is responsible for almost an equal number of cases. Unfortunately, some patients with considerable pelvic relaxation are still managed by an abdominal hysterectomy, and vaginal prolapse ensues postoperatively. Occasionally, an abdominal operation is justified (ovarian tumor, invasive carcinoma of the cervix) in a patient with substantial pelvic relaxation. Unless specific measures are taken (excision of a large wedge of the posterior part of the vagina and also the cul-de-sac peritoneum and approximation of uterosacral ligaments), prolapse of the vagina may occur. Other patients seem to be "hernia prone" and have a history of hernias of the groin, umbilicus, or previous abdominal incisions, an indication of a generalized weakness of vaginal tissues.

Some operations (Marshall-Marchetti-Krantz or Burch procedures) that pull the vaginal wall forward encourage a hernia of the posterior cul-de-sac. Even in a patient with a well-performed hysterectomy, years of wear and tear and postmenopausal atrophy may lead to a vault prolapse. The symptoms and indications for repair of posthysterectomy vault prolapse are those already described for pelvic relaxation.

If good long-term support and vaginal functions are to be obtained, the surgeon must be experienced and able to dissect, identify, and properly approximate the appropriate supporting structures. The basic principles of repair consist of (1) excision of the enterocele sac and obliteration of the cul-de-sac, incorporating the principles of McCall, Waters, and Torbin, (2) support of the corners and apex of the vagina to the vaginal sacral (wings of the rectal) ligaments, and (3) complete anterior and posterior colpoperineorrhaphy. At the Mayo Clinic, we prefer a technique that "cones down" and narrows the vagina yet maintains a functional size, because this technique has yielded favorable results. Infrequently, in a young patient who has had several operations and who presents with a shortened, narrowed vagina, the abdominal approach and presacral fixation by means of a sheet of Teflon mesh are necessary. In our experience, this has been the only indication for this approach. Whether the patient has prolapse of the cervical stump, complete uterine procidentia, or posthysterectomy prolapse, the underlying cause, symptoms, and means of surgical correction are essentially the same.

URINARY INCONTINENCE

ALFRED E. BENT, M.D.,
and DONALD R. OSTERGARD, M.D.

The bladder functions to store and expel urine under voluntary control. Urinary incontinence is the demonstrable involuntary loss of urine that is socially or hygienically unacceptable. Occasional urinary incontinence which occurs in normal women does not merit investigation or treatment other than reassurance.

The most significant advance in the management of female urinary incontinence has been the application of more extensive investigative procedures to determine the causes of incontinence and identify patients who will not benefit from surgery.

A systematic evaluation of patients with lower urinary tract symptoms will allow a diagnosis of 90 per cent of patients without in-depth urodynamic studies. The initial step is urinalysis and urine culture. The second phase includes urogynecologic history and physical examination, neurological examination, uroflowmetry with residual urine, urethrocystoscopy, CO_2 cystometry, urethral calibration, and the Q-tip test. Water cystometry is done to rule out false-positive bladder instability found with CO_2 cystometry. The final triage, reserved for approximately 10 per cent of patients, includes multichannel urodynamic recordings, water cystometry, urethral closure pressure profiles, cough profiles, instrumented uroflow to determine voiding mechanism, and vesical contraction inhibition. Other specialized testing may also be included. A classification of urinary incontinence follows:

Genuine stress incontinence (urethral sphincter incompetence);

Unstable bladder (neurogenic bladder, detrusor dyssynergia, bladder hyperreflexia);

Retention of urine with overflow incontinence;

Congenital;

Urinary fistula and diverticula;

Functional disorders.

MANAGEMENT

Genuine Stress Incontinence. The causes of genuine stress incontinence or urethral sphincter incompetence are anatomic, scarred urethra (iatrogenic or traumatic), and urethral denervation.

Anatomic stress incontinence is the involuntary loss of urine through an intact urethra as a result of a sudden increase in intra-abdominal pressure, in the absence of a bladder contraction or other lower urinary tract pathology. During the stress of coughing, the proximal portion of the urethra drops below the pelvic floor. The increase in intra-abdominal pressure induced by coughing transmits to the bladder, but not to the urethra. Since the urethral resistance is overcome by the increased bladder pressure, leakage of urine results. On urodynamic evaluation there is a decreased functional length of the urethra, decreased urethral closure pressure, and abnormal response of the sphincteric mechanism in reaction to stress, assumption of the upright posture, and bladder filling.

The best treatment is a retropubic surgical approach to replace the urethra within the abdominal cavity with minimal urethral fixation or para-urethral dissection so as to avoid adverse effects on the otherwise normal urethral sphincteric mechanism. Suspension is accomplished by placing sutures in the peri-vaginal fascia 2 cm lateral to the urethra. These sutures are then anchored to Cooper's ligament. Intraoperatively, steps are taken to promote scarification of the perivaginal fascia to the pelvic side wall to allow permanent fixation. Vaginal plication of the urethra no longer has a place in the modern treatment of anatomic stress incontinence owing to the potential for scarification, denervation, and devascularization.

The elderly at-risk surgical patient may respond to vaginal estrogen therapy alone, or in combination with an alpha-adrenergic stimulator such as phenylpropanolamine (Propadrine), 25 to 50 mg up to 4 times daily.

At least 10 per cent of patients with a clinical complaint and the physical findings of urinary stress incontinence alone have an unstable bladder. Symptoms of frequency, urgency, and urge incontinence are strong predictors of an unstable bladder.

A urethra scarred from previous surgery or trauma becomes rigid and fixed, and loses its function as a sphincteric unit. This stove-pipe urethra observed and palpated at urethroscopy defies any management other than purposeful obstruction or a neourethra fashioned from bladder wall.

Temporary bladder denervation may be caused by drug therapy (phenothiazines, phenytoin, antihistamines) or infection with *E. coli* which releases an alpha-adrenergic blocking agent. Permanent urethral denervation results from neurologic disease or previous disruption of the nerve supply to the urethra and bladder during radical pelvic surgery. Treatment of this latter condition at present is unsatisfactory.

Unstable Bladder. An unstable bladder is present in 10 to 20 per cent of the female population, though symptoms may be present in many fewer because the urethral sphincteric mechanism maintains continence. The causes may include cerebral atherosclerosis, upper motor neuron lesion, psychosomatic outflow obstruction, and unknown. Diagnosis is by water cystometry, which detects 50 to 85 per cent of abnormalities in the supine position, and detects another 10 to 13 per cent when the test is performed in the standing position with the provocative measures of cough and heel bounce.

Outflow obstruction is relieved by dilatation or external urethrotomy. Other treatment measures are generally unsatisfactory. Anticholinergic therapy such as oxybutynin chloride (Ditropan), 5 mg orally 2 to 4 times daily; dicyclomine hydrochloride (Bentyl), 10 mg 2 to 4 times daily to a maximum of 80 mg per day; imipramine hydrochloride (Tofranil), 25 to 50 mg 2 to 4 times daily; or flavoxate hydrochloride (Urispas), 200 mg 3 times daily to a maximum of 1200 mg daily, may produce improvement in 60 per cent of patients. Those without other neurologic defects may improve with bladder drill, psychotherapy, or biofeedback. Pelvic floor stimulation has produced beneficial results in some patients. The surgical approach to an unstable bladder has proven helpful in up to 60 per cent of selected cases. Denervation of the bladder described by Sundberg may be indicated in those cases of urgency or reduced bladder capacity which are unresponsive to medical therapy and show a good response to unilateral or bilateral anesthesia of the inferior hypogastric plexus. The procedure is a resection of one or both hypogastric nerves performed vaginally.

Urinary Retention with Overflow Incontinence. Urinary retention and overflow resulting from lower motor neuron lesions and autonomic neuropathy, which persists after management of the primary disease, are best managed by intermittent self-catheterization.

Overdistention of the bladder as occurs in the postoperative period is a temporary problem managed by decompression of the bladder with a suprapubic or urethral catheter maintained for 24 to 48 hours to allow the bladder to regain its muscle tone. Careful observation must follow removal of the catheter to prevent recurrence.

A distal obstruction with resulting trabeculation of the bladder is treated by dilatation or external urethrotomy. Ninety per cent of such obstructions are in the distal female urethra.

Congenital Incontinence. Ectopic ureter is diagnosed by intravenous pyelogram and cystoscopic examination. It may be overlooked until later in life, and must not be excluded from suspicion.

Urinary Fistulas and Diverticula. Diagnosis of urinary fistula (urethrovaginal, vesicovaginal, ureterovaginal) is suggested by history and most commonly follows abdominal hysterectomy, radiation therapy for gynecologic cancer, or radical pelvic surgery. Postoperative vesicovaginal fistulas are best repaired vaginally by the Latzko technique. Fistulas associated with tumors and radiation therapy require an abdominal approach with use of an omental patch, or may have to be treated with urinary diversion if very large. Urethrovaginal fistulas are repaired vaginally and may require a Martius flap.

Urethral diverticula are diagnosed by urethroscopic examination, positive pressure urethrography with a Tratner catheter, and urodynamics to determine the relationship of the peak urethral pressure to the location of the diverticulum. A diverticulum distal to peak urethral pressure is treated by the Spence procedure, which is a marsupialization of the urethral vaginal mucosa up to the diverticulum. Diverticula proximal to the peak urethral pressure must be carefully dissected from the para-urethral tissue, excised at the base, and the urethral defect closed with interrupted sutures over a urethral catheter.

Functional Disorders. When extensive urodynamic evaluation has failed to reveal a cause for continuing symptoms, and treatment measures have provided no relief, a psychiatric evaluation is indicated. A few well-timed questions may reveal prolonged life situational stresses, chronic depression, or functional symptoms such as headaches, backaches, and gastrointestinal symptoms. One third of patients will reject therapy, and one third will benefit.

DYSMENORRHEA

ROBERT E. CLEARY, M.D.

Dysmenorrhea is one of the most common gynecologic complaints. It remains the greatest single cause of lost school days among adolescents and the greatest cause of lost work hours among women. Only the common cold has a greater impact on time lost from school or work.

The term dysmenorrhea is derived from several Greek words and means literally difficult monthly flow. On the basis of symptoms and findings elicited from the history and physical examination, dysmenorrhea can be classified as primary or secondary. Primary dysmenorrhea implies that the individual's symptoms are not attributable to any recognizable pelvic pathology. Typically, the symptoms have their onset within twelve months of menarche and are characterized as lower abdominal cramps in the suprapubic region with radiation to the lower back and upper thighs. The pain is most intense on the first three days of menses, usually subsides within 24 to 48 hours, and is frequently associated with nausea, vomiting, diarrhea, or headache. Dysmenorrhea is called secondary if it arises from recognizable pelvic pathology.

The successful treatment of primary dysmenorrhea necessitates excluding painful periods caused by endometriosis, pelvic inflammatory disease, intrauterine devices, adenomyosis, uterine myomas, endometrial polyps, cervical stenosis, and congenital and obstructive abnormalities of the uterus. In the secondary form of dysmenorrhea, treatment is directed at the specific underlying cause.

Treatment should always include careful evaluation of the psychological component of the symptoms. In some cases of mild dysmenorrhea, all that may be necessary is an explanation of the cause of the symptoms and reassurance that there is no serious pelvic pathology after a careful history is taken and pelvic examination is performed.

The excessive and abnormal uterine contractions occurring in women with primary dysmenorrhea are caused by increased amounts of prostaglandins generated in menstrual fluid. The pain of menses in women is thought to arise from three mechanisms: increased uterine contractions, ischemia from reduction of uterine blood flow, and a direct effect of prostaglandin endoperoxides in lowering the pain threshold of nerve terminals in the uterus.

The recent discovery that the nonsteroidal anti-inflammatory drugs (NSAID) relieve menstrual pain by inhibiting prostaglandin synthesis in menstrual fluid has resulted in widespread clinical trials of these compounds in dysmenorrhea. All NSAID studied so far have been shown to suppress prostaglandin synthesis by inhibition of the enzyme cyclo-oxygenase (also known as prostaglandin synthetase). One group of the NSAID, the fenamates, also work as prostaglandin antagonists (Figure 1). The currently available prostaglandin synthetase inhibitors (PSI), their dosage, and some of the toxic side effects are listed in Table 1. These drugs do not need to be given prior to the onset of menstrual flow since their absorption and onset of action has been shown to be rapid.

The major side effects of NSAID occur in the gut and the central nervous system. Nausea, vomiting, diarrhea, and ulcers occur more frequently with aspirin and indomethacin than with the other NSAID. Headache is a common side effect, especially with indomethacin. Less frequently seen are dizziness, confusion, and syncope. Other rare side effects are edema, reversible alteration of liver enzymes, urticaria, angioedema, and bronchospasm in patients with asthma.

Oral contraceptives have always been a very effective form of treatment of dysmenorrhea. The combined pill has been shown to decrease the amount of prostaglandins present in menstrual fluid secondary to endometrial hypoplasia induced by the contraceptive steroids. Unless the patient desires oral contraception, it would be far safer to prescribe one of the nonsteroidal anti-inflammatory agents. There are serious vascular and metabolic side effects associated with the use of oral contraceptives, and it is no longer possible to justify the use of these agents for dys-

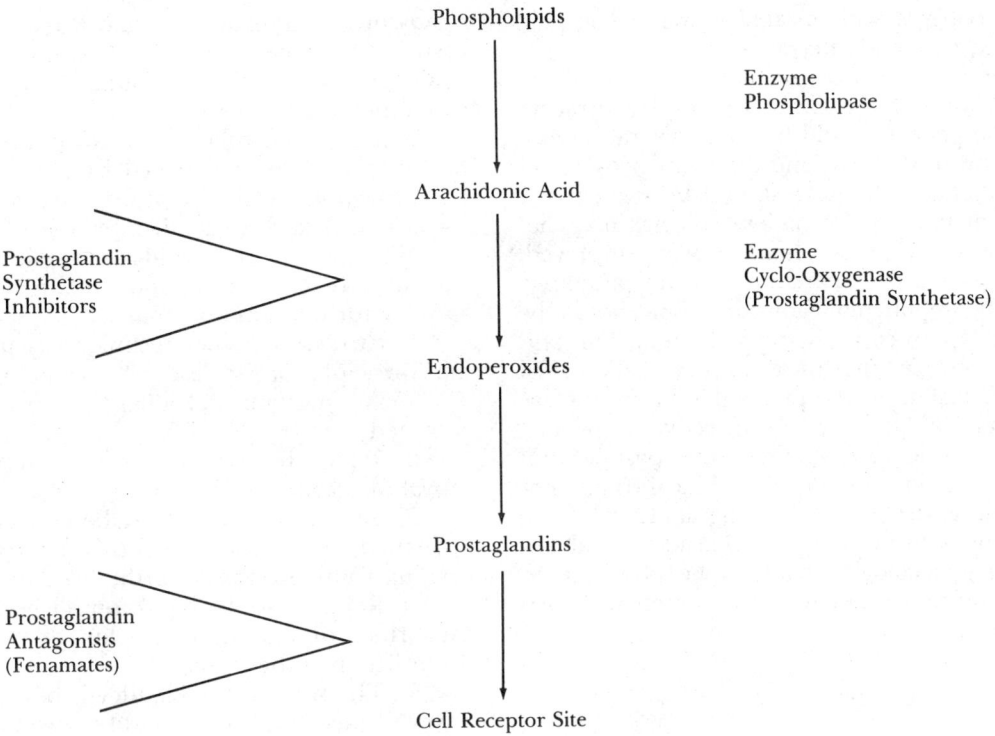

Figure 1. Mode of action of prostaglandin antagonists

menorrhea when the pain of menses seldom persists beyond 48 hours and can be controlled by other drugs. If a patient has painful menses and also desires to continue using her intrauterine device (IUD), the NSAID should be tried. Several of the NSAID have been shown to reduce the cramps and menstrual blood loss associated with the IUD. Obviously the specific treatment of dysmenorrhea will hinge on the choice of contraception by the patient.

Other forms of therapy for dysmenorrhea include the beta-receptor agonists, calcium antagonists, alcohol, and presacral neurectomy. Unfortunately, even the newer beta-mimetic agents are not devoid of B_1 activity and serious cardiovascular side effects can occur. Nifedipine, a calcium antagonist, has been shown to be effective in primary dysmenorrhea, but it also has serious vascular side effects. Two ounces of whisky had been a "time-honored remedy" for menstrual cramps. Unfortunately, the accompanying state of inebriation prevents this agent from being the recipe of choice. Today, presacral neurectomy is limited almost entirely to in-

TABLE 1. **Available Prostaglandin Synthetase Inhibitors (PSI)**

CLASS	DRUG	TRADE NAME	DOSE	PAIN RELIEF	APPROVED	COMMENT
Salicylates	Aspirin		650 mg 4 times/day	Poor	Yes	
Indoles	Indomethacin	Indocin	25 mg 3 times/day	Good	No	Toxic to Gut
	Sulindac	Clinoril	150 mg 2 times/day		No	New Drug
Fenamates	Mefanamic acid	Ponstel	250 mg 4 times/day	Good	Yes	Diarrhea
	Meclofenamate sodium	Meclomen	100 mg 3 times/day		No	New Drug
Propionic Acids	Ibuprofen	Motrin	400 mg 4 times/day	Good	Yes	
	Naproxen	Naprosyn	500 mg initial dose 250 mg 4 times/day	Good	Yes	
	Naproxen sodium	Anaprox	550 mg initial dose 275 mg 4 times/day	Good	Yes	
	Fenoprofen calcium	Nalfon	200 mg 4 times/day		No	New Drug

fertility patients with incapacitating pelvic pain associated with endometriosis.

The dysmenorrhea of most patients will respond to one of the NSAID or oral contraceptives. The patient should be given several months to respond to therapy, and different prostaglandin synthetase inhibitors should be tried if the first agent fails. If the patient still has no relief after the above measures have been employed, a more exhaustive search for pelvic pathology should be reinitiated. Consideration should be given to laparoscopy, hysterosalpingogram, and hysteroscopy in the unresponsive patient. In nearly all instances, the prostaglandin synthetase inhibitors will prove to be effective with relatively few side effects. Over the past several years, the results of controlled clinical trials comparing these drugs with existing analgesics have shown them to be a major pharmaceutical advance in gynecology, enabling the physician to offer significant relief to most women with primary dysmenorrhea.

VESICOVAGINAL FISTULA

THOMAS B. LEBHERZ, M.D.

As Mengart aptly stated, "It is no sin to cut into the bladder, the sin is not to recognize it."

Vesicovaginal fistula in the United States is seen primarily as a complication of gynecologic surgery, occasionally as a complication of radiation and neoplasm, but almost never as an obstetric complication except after cesarean section. In my experience, this problem is most common after abdominal hysterectomy but does occur after vaginal hysterectomy and/or with anterior colporrhaphy. Graber, O'Rourke, and McElrath (1964) indicated that serious injury to the bladder occurs in almost 2 per cent of hysterectomies.

Vesicovaginal fistula is likely to develop as a result of unrecognized or improperly repaired bladder trauma. It may occur as a result of postoperative necrosis secondary to devascularization, as can occur with bladder dissection, or with a suture placed into or immediately adjacent to the bladder lumen.

The presence of unexplained hematuria following an operative procedure should alert the physician, especially if the hematuria lasts longer than 48 hours. If a fistula is recognized or suspected, prolonged catheter drainage is in order since spontaneous healing can be anticipated if no infection coexists. Early diagnostic cystoscopy is most helpful, and if a suture is evident, it can be cut and continuous catheter drainage can correct the fistula. Unfortunately, spontaneous cure is rare.

Timing of fistula repair is important. The use of steroids is controversial but in my hands has proven especially helpful for early repair of fistulas, at 3 to 8 weeks, if infection is not present. Whether or not steroids are used, the fistula site must be pliable and not inflamed prior to surgery for optimal outcome.

Regardless of what technique is used, certain principles of fistula repair are paramount.

1. All infection and inflammation must have subsided.
2. Wide dissection, mobilization, and removal of scar tissue is a must.
3. The fistula area must be converted into a cleaned, fresh wound (controversy exists concerning routine removal of the fistulous tract).
4. Repair should be accomplished so that the orifice of one viscus no longer overlies or underlies the other viscus.
5. The tract in the bladder is best closed by a row of inverting sutures, and a second layer of anatomically strong tissue should be interposed between the two fistulous tracts.

Although the dorsolithotomy position is adequate for most repairs, the knee-chest position is especially useful in repair of fistula sites at the vaginal cuff and use of a headlamp is strongly advised. A suprapubic catheter should be placed at the beginning of the procedure. I prefer a 22 French Silastic type Foley catheter for this purpose since a plugged suprapubic catheter can ruin a perfect repair. Fine dissecting scissors and angulated scissors are often helpful, as is a fine-tipped suction instrument. A pediatric Foley catheter placed through the vaginal side of the fistula into the bladder will allow caudad traction of the fistula and thus allow the operator to make the operative site more available for dissection. Polyglycolic acid or Polyglactic 9–10 sutures, 3–0 and 2–0, are used throughout the repair. Small "peanuts" or cotton pushers, soaked in dilute epinephrine, are helpful in accomplishing tissue mobilization and often improve visibility. If the fistula is adjacent to the ureters, ureteral catheters must be inserted as a precautionary measure.

The vaginal flap technique devised by Raz and Leach at UCLA has been found to give the best results. If the fistula is low at the bladder base or trigone, vaginal flaps are outlined in unscarred areas of the vagina. A large posterior flap is developed with its base near the vaginal apex. This tissue is then dissected toward the fistula until scarred vagina is evident. The scarred vaginal mucosa around the tract is circumscribed and removed up to the tract edges. No attempt is made to remove the fistula tract. A small anterior flap of normal vaginal mucosa is developed between the fistula and the meatus. With the tract in view, 3–0 inverting sutures are placed at either side of the tract; using these for fistula delineation, additional tract-inverting sutures are placed to completely close and invert the fistula tract into the bladder. Nonremoval of the tract prevents iatrogenic enlargement of the defect and prevents the often brisk bleeding seen when the tract is excised. A second layer of inverted 3–0 sutures is placed in the endopelvic fascia in an opposing direction. Approximately 1 cm of the anterior vaginal flap is trimmed away and the posterior flap advanced over the repaired fistula so that the vaginal closure site does not overlie the bladder closure site. When the fistula is high in the vagina a similar procedure is carried out, but in this situation a large anterior vaginal flap is developed and managed in the same manner.

The bladder repair site should be tested before vaginal closure. This is done by instilling 400 cc's of sterile milk or indigo carmine–stained solution. If the fistulous tract is in the trigone, indigo carmine should be injected intravenously and the ureteral orifices observed cystoscopically for egress of stained urine. A urethral Foley catheter is inserted and an antibiotic-soaked vaginal pack is placed for 24 hours. Both catheters are attached to gravity drainage. The Foley catheter is clamped the next day, and if the suprapubic catheter drains well the urethral catheter is removed.

The patient is discharged on the fifth to seventh hospital day. On the tenth to fourteenth postoperative day a cystogram is performed using the suprapubic catheter. If no extravasation of dye is evident on the cystogram and the patient is voiding without significant residual, the suprapubic catheter is removed. Prophylactic antibiotics are routinely used since any infection in the operative site will doom the repair to failure. Twenty-three cases have been managed in this manner at UCLA, with no failures.

PELVIC TUBERCULOSIS AND FEMALE GENITAL TUBERCULOSIS

GEORGE SCHAEFER, M.D.

Pelvic tuberculosis and female genital tuberculosis are different entities. Unfortunately, these conditions have been confused in the past and the terms used interchangeably.

Pelvic tuberculosis occurs when principally the peritoneum is involved, with or without generalized miliary involvement of the serosal surface of both abdominal and pelvic organs and frequently the omentum. This superficial involvement does not impair the reproductive function of the patient. If the miliary deposition of the tubercles is acute, ascitic fluid forms and may be either free in the abdominal cavity or encysted between loops of bowel and dense adhesions. The rapid appearance of large peritoneal effusions in children is strongly suggestive of tuberculous peritonitis. Fluid that forms rapidly in this instance is also frequently bloody. Usually the tubercles which stud the intestine, omentum, bowel, and bladder heal by fibrosis and the fluid is absorbed. However, the tubercles may break down, causing necrosis which results in caseation and the formation of dense, thick adhesions binding pelvic and abdominal viscera together.

The diagnosis of pelvic tuberculosis is usually made at operation or by laparoscopic examination. Pelvic tuberculosis or peritoneal tuberculosis was described in the older literature in which cures were attributed to opening the abdomen and letting air in. Treatment for this condition is with antituberculosis drugs, isoniazid and ethambutol, in doses that will be described below for female genital tuberculosis.

Female genital tuberculosis, on the other hand, implies involvement of the *mucosa* of the fallopian tubes, with or without spread to the uterus and to the ovaries. Peritoneal involvement may or may not be present in this condition.

Coexisting Peritoneal "Pelvic" and Female Genital Tuberculosis. In both conditions the lesions are a result of the same or successive hematogenous seedings. Tuberculous peritonitis, like female genital tuberculosis, is not a primary disease. It results from miliary spread from the lungs (most commonly) or it may arise from a tuberculous focus in the intestine, mesenteric nodes, or bladder. Tuberculous peritonitis is seen in combination with female genital tuberculosis in about 50 per cent of the cases; however, one can occur without the other.

FEMALE GENITAL TUBERCULOSIS

As a result of a recent analysis of data from an extensive pathologic study of female genital tuberculosis by Nogales-Ortiz and his co-workers in Spain, the frequency of involvement of various pelvic organs should be altered from what was previously described.

In over 1400 cases of female genital tuberculosis in the Spanish study, the fallopian tubes were found to be involved in 100 per cent of the cases, the endometrium in 79 per cent of the cases, the myometrium in 20 per cent, the cervix in approximately 25 per cent, and the ovaries in 11 per cent.

The only one of these figures I would take issue with is the degree of involvement of the ovaries. It has been my experience that if the ovary is bisected, involvement of the hilus will be found in a greater percentage of cases. Our figures show involvement of the ovaries in about 25 per cent of the cases.

Age. Earlier surveys showed the peak of genital tuberculosis to be between 20 and 40 years of age. More recent surveys report the mean age to be 42 years with a range from 24 to 80 years. The younger age group had a higher incidence in the immigrant population, whereas disease was more likely to be found in the older age group in the United States and Canada, that is, in countries where the disease was usually recognized early and treated with antituberculosis drugs. I have recently reported six cases of postmenopausal genital tuberculosis; in the past I had not seen this condition frequently in the older age group.

Diagnosis. The diagnosis of female genital tuberculosis will more frequently be made if a high index of suspicion is maintained for this entity. Suspicion should be aroused in (1) patients who give a history of primary infertility (in some infertility clinics this can be as high as 10 per cent or more, although the average cited is 5 per cent); (2) patients who have chronic pelvic pain that persists over a long period of time, is not severe, and is made worse by the menstrual cycle; and (3) patients with a history of poor general health persisting over a period of months associated with weight loss, undue fatigue, low-grade fever, and vague abdominal pains should prompt further investigation for genital tuberculosis, particularly if the "chronic pelvic inflammatory disease" does not respond to the usual antibiotic therapy.

Physical examination may reveal bilateral tubal ovarian masses, or there may be no palpable disease or only slight induration in both adnexal regions.

The presence of female genital tuberculosis can be ruled out if the tuberculin test is negative. However, a positive tuberculin test does not imply a definite diagnosis of female genital tuberculosis, since the tuberculin test does not differentiate genital tuberculosis from pulmonary or extrapulmonary disease. It may sometimes be falsely positive in fever, pregnancy, influenza, brucellosis, or measles.

The most common method of diagnosing genital tuberculosis is by endometrial curettage performed shortly before the menstrual period. Half of the specimen should be sent for histologic examination and the other half for bacteriologic examination for tubercle bacilli.

A hysterosalpingogram done in the course of the workup of an infertile patient may reveal changes that are characteristic of tuberculosis of the uterus and tubes; however, a definitive diagnosis cannot be made from x-ray studies alone and must be confirmed by histologic or bacteriologic examination.

Laparoscopy has been used in the diagnosis of female genital tuberculosis. This is not without danger and cases have been reported of perforation of the bowel or bladder with the laparoscope. Open laparoscopy is a safer procedure. Laparoscopy can not always differentiate between pelvic tuberculosis and female genital tuberculosis, since involvement of the serosa of the tubes does not necessarily mean involvement of the mucosa.

TREATMENT

Treatment of female genital tuberculosis depends on whether the disease is minimal or advanced. Minimal disease is usually asymptomatic, except for sterility, and is diagnosed by finding tuberculous endometritis on curettage or biopsy, or tubercle bacilli on culture of the curettings.

Advanced genital tuberculosis is diagnosed by the presence of palpable tubo-ovarian masses plus histologic or bacteriologic evidence of tuberculosis.

Minimal female genital tuberculosis should be treated with isoniazid, 300 mg daily, plus ethambutol, 20 mg per kg or approximately 1200 mg per day, orally in the morning. This should be continued for at least 18 to 24 months. Six months and 12 months after initiating treatment, endometrial curettings or biopsies should be examined bacteriologically and microscopically. If these are negative, a hysterosalpingogram can be done. On rare occasions, patency of the tubes may be reestablished, but this does not guarantee that conception will occur since the mucosa of the tube has been destroyed or rendered fibrotic and the cilia nonfunctional. Ectopic pregnancy may occur when tubes show some patency.

Treatment of advanced genital tuberculosis starts with isoniazid, 300 mg daily, and ethambutol, 20 mg per kg per day orally. The patient should be examined at monthly intervals for 3 to 4 months. If tubo-ovarian masses are still present after this period of antimicrobial therapy, surgery should be performed. This entails a bilateral salpingectomy and, if the ovaries are bound down and cannot be separated from the tubes, bilateral salpingo-oophorectomy and hysterectomy. In patients over 35 to 40 or in postmenopausal patients, total abdominal hysterectomy and bilateral salpingo-oophorectomy is the treatment of choice after 3 to 4 months of antituberculosis drugs. For several days before operation and for approximately 2 weeks after operation, rifampin, 600 mg daily in the morning, may be used to cover the operative procedure.

At the present I have avoided the use of streptomycin, particularly in elderly patients, because of the danger of impairment to auditory and vestibular function. I do not use both rifampin and isoniazid for a long period of time because of the danger of hepatitis, although the use of rifampin for a short period of time has not resulted in hepatic toxicity. Hepatic toxicity from isoniazid is rare. It may occur in elderly patients, in alcoholics, and in combination with rifampin, or in patients with a history of previous hepatitis. Hepatic toxicity can usually be diagnosed on history alone in approximately 85 per cent of the patients. If clinical symptoms do appear, liver function tests should be done. If these are positive, treatment with rifampin or isoniazid should be discontinued.

Female genital tuberculosis is occasionally first diagnosed in the pathology laboratory after removal of the uterus or tubes. In such instances, the patient should immediately be given antituberculosis drugs, namely isoniazid and ethambutol. Rifampin should be used for 2 to 3 weeks if the disease is advanced. The medication should be continued for approximately 18 months postoperatively, although there is reason to believe that if all the tuberculous tissue is removed, this period of treatment may be shortened to 9 to 12 months.

There are conflicting views as to whether a successful pregnancy may be expected after treatment for female genital tuberculosis. My experience is that a full-term pregnancy rarely occurs in a woman who has had genital tuberculosis, although it may occur in pelvic tuberculosis in which the mucosae of the uterus and tubes have not been involved. It may also occur if female genital tuberculosis is diagnosed and treated early when only one of the tubes has been initially involved. However, tuberculosis is a disease that involves organs bilaterally and the unilateral tuberculous salpingitis is seldom seen.

Tuboplasty operations which have now come into vogue should not be done in patients with female genital tuberculosis. The probability of a full-term pregnancy is extremely unlikely and the risk of miliary spread is present.

PELVIC INFLAMMATORY DISEASE
RONALD S. GIBBS, M.D.

Diagnosed approximately 800,000 times per year in the United States, pelvic inflammatory disease* (PID) has as its presenting symptoms abdominal-pelvic pain, fever, vaginal discharge, and less commonly nausea, vomiting, and urinary symptoms. Pelvic examination usually reveals tenderness, especially of the adnexa, and often a palpable mass. Because the signs and symptoms are nonspecific, additional diagnostic procedures may be indicated. These techniques include culdocentesis, sonography, and laparoscopy. A number of microbes appear to be involved in PID: *Neisseria gonorrhoeae*, *Chlamydia trachomatis*, other anaerobic and aerobic bacteria, and occasionally, genital mycoplasmas. Appropriate work-up includes complete blood count, urinalysis, blood cultures (though these are rarely positive), and cervical culture (for *Neisseria gonorrhoeae* only, on selective media). If peritoneal exudate is obtained by culdocentesis or laparoscopy, the specimen should be cultured for aerobes and anaerobes.

GENERAL PRINCIPLES OF TREATMENT

First, it is vitally important to rule out, with confidence, surgical emergencies such as ectopic pregnancy or acute appendicitis, which may mimic PID. Except in a few circumstances (discussed later), PID is treated with supportive therapy and antibiotics. Because women who wear intrauterine devices are 4 to 9 times more likely to develop PID, removal of the device during an acute attack (after instituting antibiotic therapy) has been recommended by many.

Women with PID may be treated as either inpatients or outpatients, depending upon the severity of the episode. Clear indications for inpatient treatment are: (1) patient toxicity with high fever, marked pain, or peritonitis, (2) vomiting and dehydration, (3) suspected tubo-ovarian abscess, and (4) an uncertain diagnosis when acute surgical emergencies need to be excluded. Some authorities believe that nearly all women with PID should be admitted, since inpatient

---

*In this article, pelvic inflammatory disease will be defined as an acute or chronic infectious process of the upper female genital tract, with its focus of attack being the fallopian tubes. Alternative terms include acute or chronic salpingitis. Postoperative and postpartum pelvic infections are not included.

therapy may avoid later infertility. At present, there are no data to support that belief.

Current recommendations from the Centers for Disease Control (August, 1982) take into consideration recent data on the microbiology of PID. The treatment of choice has not been established. No single agent is active against the entire spectrum of pathogens, and many of the suggested examples of therapy have not been adequately tested in clinical trials.

OUTPATIENT TREATMENT

For women with milder forms of PID, treatment consists of bed rest at home in the semi-Fowler's position, analgesics, and antibiotics. Currently recommended treatment schedules from the Centers for Disease Control are: cefoxitin (Mefoxin), 2.0 grams IM, *or* amoxicillin, 3.0 grams PO, *or* ampicillin, 3.5 grams PO, *or* aqueous procaine penicillin G, 4.8 million units IM—each with probenecid, 1.0 gram PO. Each of these is then to be followed by doxycycline (Vibramycin), 100 mg PO twice daily for 10 to 14 days. Tetracycline hydrochloride, 500 mg PO four times a day, is an alternative but must be given more often and is less active against some anaerobes.

Sexual partners should be examined for sexually transmitted diseases and treated promptly with a regimen effective against uncomplicated gonococcal and chlamydial infection (such as doxycycline, 100 mg PO twice daily for 7 days). All patients should be seen again in 48 to 72 hours, and test of cure culture should be performed.

Removal of the IUD is appropriate, although in many cases cure can be achieved without removal. When there is not a prompt response removal of the IUD becomes mandatory. Because removal of the IUD may lead to transient bacteremia, it seems wise to remove it about an hour after the first dose of antibiotic has been given.

Former treatment schedules using penicillin-ampicillin *or* tetracycline are no longer recommended.

INPATIENT TREATMENT

For women with more serious episodes of PID, inpatient observation and therapy are indicated. Supportive therapy should consist of analgesics and intravenous fluids to correct volume depletion and electrolyte imbalance. The patient should be placed at bed rest in the semi-Fowler's position to promote dependent drainage. There is no standard antibiotic regimen, and in view of the present uncertainty about causative microorganisms, a variety of regimens have been suggested. Recommended are:

1. Doxycycline, 100 mg IV, every 12 hours, *plus* cefoxitin, 2.0 grams IV every 6 hours. Continue IV medications for 4 more days, depending upon clinical course. Oral doxycycline, as above, is recommended after discharge from the hospital to complete 10 to 14 days of therapy. This regimen would not provide optimal coverage against anaerobes and would not be preferred for patients with suspected or proved tubo-ovarian abscess. It does provide excellent coverage for gonococci, including penicillinase-producing varieties, and for *Chlamydia trachomatis*.

2. Clindamycin, 600 mg IV every 6 hours, *plus* gentamicin or tobramycin, 2.0 mg per kg IV, then 1.5 mg per kg IV every 8 hours, for patients with normal renal function. Continue IV medications, as above. The oral medication recommended for continuation of this therapy is clindamycin, 450 mg PO four times a day. In view of the potential for adverse reaction with oral clindamycin and the empiric nature of the treatment, oral doxycycline also seems to be a suitable alternative.

3. Doxycycline, 100 mg IV every 12 hours, *plus* metronidazole, 1.0 gram IV every 12 hours. Continue IV drugs as above. For oral therapy, CDC recommendations are to continue both drugs orally in same dosage.

SURGICAL TREATMENT

As seen in many genital tract infections, surgical intervention is occasionally necessary for PID. Indications may be described as follows:

1. Ruptured tubo-ovarian abscess. This condition is a surgical emergency, requiring prompt drainage, in addition to antibiotic therapy.

2. Failure of antibiotic therapy. Persistent signs and symptoms usually indicate a pelvic abscess. After a reasonable trial of antibiotics, women with persisting findings are also surgical candidates.

3. Persistent mass or pain. After acute symptoms have resolved, some patients have residual masses or severe pain (probably from adhesions). Persisting masses may require surgical intervention, as they may obscure adnexal neoplasia, and persistent incapacitating pain may be best treated surgically. In neither of these instances is there great urgency, and the decision should be made after thorough counseling of the patient.

4. Other conditions. In some other situations, the patient's condition may also be handled best by surgical intervention. An example would be an elderly woman who desires sterilization and who has chronic, recurrent PID.

PROGNOSIS

The outlook for survival is, of course, excellent, although ruptured tubo-ovarian abscess with septic shock does present a serious threat to the patient's life. Unfortunately, the outlook for future fertility is not so bright, as tubal obstruction increases markedly with successive episodes of PID. Furthermore, patients who have had PID are also more likely to develop tubal pregnancy.

SEXUALLY TRANSMITTED DISEASES

DAVID CHARLES, M.D.

GONORRHEA

This disease remains an important health problem although the exact degree of its communicability is generally unknown. Only disseminated gonococcal infection can be diagnosed solely by physical examination. Consequently, all other forms of gonococcal infections require identification of *Neisseria gonorrhoeae* by gram smear and culture.

In women the most common site of gonococcal infection is the endocervix. The majority of women with gonococcal cervicitis are asymptomatic and frequently such individuals will not seek medical attention until the disease has spread to adjacent tissues. Consequently, since such women can be asymptomatic for several months, they constitute the largest reservoir for the gonococcus.

The most serious sequel of untreated gonococcal cervicitis results from the spread of the pathogen to the fallopian tubes. Acute salpingitis occurs in at least 15 per cent of women with gonococcal cervicitis. Extension of the infection most frequently occurs at the time of menstruation and as a result the tubal infection may be associated with pelvic peritonitis and abscess formation. The latter complications constitute the spectrum of pelvic inflammatory disease. The physician must realize that *Neisseria gonorrhoeae* is not the only cause of pelvic inflammatory disease. In fact, in only about 50 per cent of women with adnexitis can the gonococcus be isolated from the endocervix, and in only about 10 per cent can the organism be isolated from cultures of tubal aspirates. Currently, it appears that salpingitis is most frequently a polymicrobial infection associated with a variety of aerobic and anaerobic organisms as well as *Chlamydia trachomatis*. Consequently, the exact role of any single bacterial species in the etiology of adnexitis remains to be delineated. Likewise, there is no unanimity pertaining to the ideal antimicrobial therapy for pelvic inflammatory disease.

In all women with asymptomatic gonococcal cervicitis rectal cultures for *N. gonorrhoeae* should be obtained because about 40 per cent of such patients will have positive cultures in the absence of a history of rectal coitus. Even in patients who are suspected of having gonorrhea, 10 per cent will have positive rectal cultures and negative endocervical cultures. Asymptomatic rectal gonorrhea may persist for many months, and in women symptomatic gonococcal proctitis is still an uncommon infection.

Pharyngeal gonococcal infection occurs in persons who have had oral sex and is usually asymptomatic and not contagious. The rationale for treating this form of gonococcal infection is its association with disseminated gonococcemia. Overall, the pharynx is the commonest site of primary infection in patients with gonococcal septicemia, and disseminated gonococcemia develops in about 25 per cent of patients with pharyngeal infection. Currently, it is impossible to readily predict which strains of the organism have the ability to cause disseminated gonococcal infection and so it is recommended that all patients with pharyngeal infection be treated. In all cases of suspected pharyngeal infection a culture is mandatory as there is no pathognomonic symptom complex, and a Gram stain is of no value as the oropharynx contains other species of *Neisseria* as well as *Branhamella* which are identical in appearance to the gonococcus.

Disseminated gonococcal infection is usually preceded by asymptomatic cervical, rectal, or pharyngeal infection. The strains of *N. gonorrhoeae* isolated from such patients differ from the usual isolates in that they are usually more sensitive to penicillin but are resistant to the bactericidal activity of normal human sera and complement. In normal hosts the relative sensitivity or resistance to bactericidal agents of certain strains of this organism may be a major factor that establishes the invasive potential of the organism. The most characteristic clinical manifestations of disseminated gonococcal infection are tenosynovitis, arthralgias, septic arthritis, and dermatitis. Although the typical skin lesions associated with tenosynovitis or septic arthritis are virtually diagnostic of disseminated gonococcal infection it is important to culture all mucosal sites for the gonococcus.

For over 30 years penicillin has been one of the primary antimicrobial agents used in the single dose treatment of gonorrhea. During this period of time, however, the susceptibility of *N. gonorrhoeae* to this antibiotic has decreased, and as a result larger doses are necessary in order to avoid treatment failures. The increasing resistance of the gonococcus to penicillin led to the following recommendations by the United States Public Health Service for the treatment of uncomplicated gonococcal infections: 4.8 million units of procaine penicillin G intramuscularly after the oral administration of 1.0 gram of probenecid; or for those with proven penicillin allergy, 0.5 gm of tetracycline hydrochloride orally 4 times a day for 5 days. Other recommended forms of therapy for uncomplicated gonococcal infections are listed in Table 1.

The majority of penicillin-resistant strains of *N. gonorrhoeae* do not produce beta-lactamase and are referred to as "intrinsically resistant." The emergence of penicillin resistant beta-lactamase–producing strains of this organism throughout the world has however been reported during the past few years. Consequently, reculturing of patients after therapy is now essential to determine whether the disease has been cured. Strains of *N. gonorrhoeae* reisolated from patients treated with penicillin G or one of its congeners in recommended doses should be assumed to be beta-lactamase producers until proved otherwise. Such patients should receive spectinomycin, 2.0 grams intramuscularly, as beta-lactamase–producing gonococci are usually resistant to tetracycline. Recently the Centers for Disease Control reported the first known case of gonococcal urethritis caused by a spectinomycin-resistant penicillinase-producing strain of *N. gonorrhoeae*.

For uncomplicated anogenital gonorrhea caused by such strains, cefoxitin, 2.0 grams in a single intramuscular injection, preceded by the oral administration of 1.0 gram of probenecid is recommended. An alternative regimen for such infections is a single daily dose of 9 tablets of trimethoprim-sulfamethoxazole for 3 days. This latter regimen should be used for 5 days for the treatment of pharyngeal infection. The reason for prescribing the combination of trimethoprim and sulfamethoxazole for several days is the fact that treatment of males for acute uncomplicated anogenital gonorrhea with single doses of 9 tablets yield cure rates ranging from 70 to 80 per cent. The latter cure rates are significantly lower than those achieved with standard treatment regimens. The sulfamethoxazole-trimethoprim combination should not, however, be prescribed for the treatment of gravid or lactating women with uncomplicated gonococcal infections.

Spectinomycin, cefoxitin, ampicillin, and amoxicillin should not be prescribed for patients with pharyngeal infection because they are associated with a cure rate of less than 50 per cent. Aqueous procaine penicillin G with 1.0 gram of probenecid is, however, about 95 per cent effective in eradicating *N. gonorrhoeae* from the pharynx.

As will be seen from the above discussion, no one ideal safe therapeutic regimen for the treamtment of uncomplicated anogenital and pharyngeal gonococcal infections is available. Even for infections caused by beta-lactamase–

TABLE 1. **Treatment of Uncomplicated Gonococcal Infections**

SITE OF INFECTION	DRUGS OF CHOICE	ALTERNATIVE DRUGS	COMMENTS
Lower genital tract	Aqueous procaine penicillin G, 4.8 million units I.M. in divided doses at two sites, preceded by probenecid, 1.0 gm by mouth, OR oral ampicillin or amoxicillin, 3.5 gm, and probenecid, 1.0 gm, OR tetracycline hydrochloride, 500 mg four times a day for five days.	A single I.M. dose of spectinomycin hydrochloride, 2.0 gm, OR cefoxitin sodium, 2.0 gm I.M., preceded by probenecid 1.0 gm by mouth, OR trimethoprim-sulfamethoxazole, 9 tablets as a single dose daily for three days.	There is an incidence of 0.1 per cent procaine reaction with aqueous procaine penicillin G. For patients who are allergic to both penicillin and tetracycline the drug of choice is spectinomycin. For gravid patients allergic to penicillin, spectinomycin may be used. OR erythromycin, 750 mg 4 times a day for 5 days.
Oropharynx	Aqueous procaine penicillin G or tetracycline in the same dosage as for lower genital tract infections.	Trimethoprim-sulfamethoxazole, 9 tablets as a single dose daily for 5 days.	Ampicillin, amoxicillin or spectinomycin should not be used as they are associated with a failure in excess of 50 per cent. For gravid patients allergic to penicillin, although it is of suboptimal efficacy, erythromycin should be used.

negative strains of *N. gonorrhoeae,* each of the single-dose regimens currently recommended by the United States Public Health Service has drawbacks of toxicity, less efficacy at some anatomic sites, or cost. All single-dose regimens are ineffectual for coexisting infection with *C. trachomatis,* and the new third generation cephalosporins are of no avail. Of the new parenteral cephalosporins, cefotaxime is from drug susceptibility studies the most effective cephalosporin against both beta-lactamase–positive and beta-lactamase–negative strains of *N. gonorrhoeae.*

Hospital admission is advisable for the majority of patients with acute pelvic inflammatory disease. The reason for hospitalization is that the clinical diagnosis may be in error and laparoscopy not infrequently will reveal the presence of such conditions as ectopic pregnancy or acute appendicitis. Likewise, inappropriate antimicrobial therapy in ambulatory patients with acute salpingitis can result in extension of the suppurative process and eventuate in a pelvic or tubo-ovarian abscess as well as infertility. Until recently acute salpingitis was arbitrarily divided into two varieties, namely gonococcal and non-gonococcal solely on the basis of the presence or absence of *N. gonorrhoeae* in the endocervix. Laparoscopic studies indicate that direct culture from the peritoneal cavity or fallopian tube is important not only for determining the microbiologic etiology of acute salpingitis, but for successful therapy. Recent studies have shown that isolates of *N. gonorrhoeae* from the fallopian tubes of patients with acute salpingitis are frequently more resistant to penicillin G, ampicillin, and cefoxitin as compared to isolates of this organism from patients with asymptomatic gonorrhea. Such findings are in accord with the fact that single-dose penicillin, ampicillin or cefoxitin therapy is ineffective in the treatment of acute salpingitis. Appropriate antibiotic therapy for acute and subacute salpingitis is outlined in Table 2. In patients who fail to improve within 48 to 72 hours, additional antimicrobial therapy in the form of clindamycin or metronidazole is indicated. This applies specifically to patients who have delayed seeking treatment and those who have had one or more previous episodes of acute salpingitis. In such patients the salpingitis is due to a polymicrobial infection and the an-

TABLE 2. **Treatment of Acute Salpingitis**

	DRUGS OF CHOICE	ALTERNATIVE DRUGS	COMMENTS
Ambulatory patients	Aqueous procaine penicillin G, 4.8 million units I.M. injected in divided doses at two sites, preceded by probenecid 1.0 gm orally, followed by ampicillin, OR amoxicillin, 500 mg orally four times a day for 10 days, OR ampicillin, 3.5 gm orally, with probenecid, 1.0 gm, followed by ampicillin, 500 mg orally 4 times a day for 10 days, OR tetracycline, 500 mg orally 4 times a day for 10 days.	Spectinomycin, 2.0 gm I.M. daily for 7 days.	Hospital admission is advisable if nausea or vomiting precludes the use of oral medication or if there is failure of patient compliance or the infection is caused by penicillinase-producing strains of *Neisseria gonorrhoeae.*
Hospitalized patients	Aqueous sodium or potassium penicillin G, 20 million units I.V. daily until improvement is observed, followed by ampicillin or amoxicillin, 500 mg orally four times a day until 10 days of therapy has been achieved. OR doxycycline, 200 mg I.V. followed by 100 mg every 12 hours I.V. until improvement is observed, followed by 100 mg orally every 12 hrs. until 7 days of therapy has been achieved.	Cefoxitin sodium, 2.0 gm I.M. or I.V. every 8 hours for 7 days.	If the patient has received prior treatment or has a past history of pelvic inflammatory disease or if no therapeutic response occurs after 72 hr. of treatment, a polymicrobial infection must be considered. For such patients additional therapy in the form of clindamycin phosphate, 600 mg I.V. every 6 hr, or metronidazole, 500 mg I.V. every 8 hrs, plus tobramycin sulfate, 1.5 mg per kg body weight I.V. every 8 hr is required.

aerobic component must be treated. It is essential that the sexual partners of all patients with salpingitis where the gonococcus is implicated be examined for asymptomatic gonorrhea or nongonococcal urethritis.

The treatment regimens for disseminated gonococcal infection are listed in Table 3. Since up to 25 per cent of disseminated gonococcal infections occur in gravid patients it is essential that the obstetrician be conversant with the standard therapy of this syndrome. In all cases of disseminated infection "test of cure" follow-up cultures of specimens from previously infected sites must be obtained, especially if clinical symptoms are slow to resolve. The need for such measures is emphasized by the fact that several cases of disseminated infection are caused by penicillinase-producing strains of *N. gonorrhoeae*. For the treatment of such infections, spectinomycin is the drug of choice.

From this discussion it will be noted that the therapy of gonorrhea to date cannot be standardized because of the emergence of antimicrobial-resistant strains of *N. gonorrhoeae*. There are therefore two prerequisites for improving the treatment of this infection. Firstly, public health authorities should provide detailed information pertaining to the geographic location of all antimicrobial resistant strains of the organism, and secondly, all descriptions of antibiotic trials should detail the antibiotic sensitivity of the strains of *N. gonorrhoeae* prevalent in the populations studied. Recent reports that some strains of the organism produce penicillinase and the emergence of a spectinomycin resistant beta-lactamase–producing strain of *N. gonorrhoeae* underscore the need for such measures.

SYPHILIS

Although syphilis remains the third most common notifiable communicable disease in the United States, its incidence has increased in the past few years. In 1980 there was a 33.4 per cent increase in the number of reported cases of primary and secondary syphilis compared to 1977. The rates per 100,000 population increased by 26.3 per cent, from 9.5 in 1977 to 12.0 in 1980. An important feature in this current trend for the obstetrician is the fact that the rate of primary and secondary syphilis in women from 1977 to 1980 has increased by 17 per cent. This trend among women is reflected by an increased incidence of congenital syphilis. The latter can, however, be decreased by reducing the incidence of syphilis in gravid women, and by adequate treatment and follow-up.

It is important for early diagnosis and treatment that a physician regard all genital sores as syphilitic until proven to be otherwise. Likewise, in the treatment of patients with gonorrhea who are found to have genital sores or papules, or an unidentified rash, a diagnosis of concomitant syphilis must be entertained. Extragenital sites, such as the lips, tongue, and pharynx, can also be involved. One generalization is appropriate in respect to primary syphilis. Any indolent, painless ulcerated lesion, irrespective of location if the erotic areas of the body are involved, should alert the physician to suspect syphilis. Except for location, a chancre, both histologically and in its response to treatment, is the same whatever the anatomic site. Dark field microscopic examination of material scraped from the lesion is the single most accurate way of identi-

TABLE 3. **Treatment of Disseminated Gonococcal Infection**

DRUGS OF CHOICE	ALTERNATIVE DRUGS	COMMENTS
Potassium or sodium penicillin G, 10 million units daily I.V. until improvement is noted, followed by ampicillin or amoxicillin, 500 mg four times a day orally for 7 days._OR_Ampicillin or amoxicillin in an initial oral dose of 3.0 gm, with probenecid, 1.0 gm, followed by ampicillin or amoxicillin, 500 mg orally 4 times a day for 7 days.	Spectinomycin, 2.0 gm I.M. twice daily for 3 days._OR_Tetracycline, 500 mg orally 4 times a day for 7 days._OR_Erythromycin, 500 mg orally 4 times a day for 7 days._OR_Cefoxitin, 2.0 gm I.M. or I.V. every 8 hours for 7 days.	Spectinomycin is the treatment of choice for penicillinase-producing strains of *Neisseria gonorrhoeae*.For gravid patients who are allergic to penicillin, erythromycin, 750 mg orally 4 times a day for 7 days, OR spectinomycin can be used.Hospitalization is indicated for patients with purulent joint effusions or other complications as well as those who fail to comply with the oral dosage regimens.

fying primary syphilis. Unfortunately, darkfield examination of oral lesions may be unreliable since *Treponema pallidum* may be morphologically indistinguishable from *Treponema microdentium*, a normal inhabitant of the mouth. Local application of antibiotic ointment, alcohol, or antiseptic creams should be avoided until a definitive diagnosis has been established. If such measures have been adopted by the patient, the physician must rely on serologic tests to complement clinical judgment.

The function of serologic tests for syphilis is to enable clinicians to diagnose and treat the disease. The incubation period for syphilis varies from 10 to 90 days, but primary syphilis will develop in the majority of patients within 6 weeks of exposure. Consequently, the VDRL, which is a nontreponemal serologic test, is positive in only about 70 per cent of patients with primary syphilis, as it can take as long as 3 months for positive results after exposure. A positive VDRL test is present in essentially all cases of secondary syphilis. The VDRL test may be quantitated and is especially useful for follow-up evaluation of the response to treatment.

In suspected primary syphilis with repeatedly negative dark field microscopy reports, as for example when topical antibiotics have been used, a specific treponemal test is useful. The most commonly used treponemal test is the FTA-ABS, but it should not be used as a routine screening test for the serologic diagnosis of syphilis. In patients with late latent syphilis as well as adolescents and adults with or without evidence of congenital infection, serologic tests are only one aspect of assessment. The final decision to treat a patient depends on clinical judgment.

The recommended treatment for this disease is given in Table 4. The drug of choice for all stages of syphilis is benzathine penicillin G. What is unique about this preparation of penicillin is that it is a repository form which is absorbed so slowly following intramuscular administration that it produces low blood levels of penicillin for several weeks. An injection of 600,000 units of this formulation results in blood levels of 0.03 to 0.2 unit per ml for about 2 weeks in all nongravid patients. The recommended dose of this drug for the treatment of primary and secondary syphilis produces treponemocidal levels for at least 2 weeks in pregnant patients and is highly efficacious for the prevention of congenital syphilis. A time-dosage relationship is crucial in the treatment of syphilis and a continuous blood level above 0.03 unit per ml for 10 days is essential. The bactericidal effect of penicillin on the *T. pallidum* is most effective when the organism is in the process of replication, an activity that occurs about every 30 hours. A major advantage of benzathine penicillin G is that treatment can be accomplished by a single dose which obviates the need for multiple injections of the short-acting penicillins and avoids the hazards of noncompliance when oral

TABLE 4. **Treatment of Syphilis**

STAGE OF DISEASE	DRUGS OF CHOICE	ALTERNATIVE DRUGS	COMMENTS
Primary, secondary or early latent	Benzathine penicillin G, 2.4 million units I.M. as a single dose—one-half the total dose into two separate sites; OR aqueous procaine penicillin G, 600,000 units, I.M. daily for 8 days.	Tetracycline, 500 mg orally four times daily for 15 days; OR erythromycin, 500 mg orally 4 times daily for 15 days.	The alternative drugs should be prescribed for patients who are allergic to penicillin. It should be noted that the treatment of gonococcal infections with procaine penicillin will treat incubating syphilis but not primary disease.
Late latent or latent of undetermined duration	Benzathine penicillin G, 2.4 million units I.M. weekly for 3 weeks.	Tetracycline, 500 mg orally 4 times daily for 30 days; OR erythromycin, 500 mg orally 4 times daily for 30 days.	
During pregnancy	Benzathine penicillin G, 2.4 million units I.M. weekly for 3 weeks.	Erythromycin, 750 mg orally 4 times a day for 20 days.	Although tetracycline cannot be used in pregnancy, those patients who are allergic to both penicillin and erythromycin, doxycycline 200 mg every twelve hours for 15 days has prevented congenital syphilis in the infants.

antimicrobial agents are prescribed. For patients with neurosyphilis, treatment with benzathine penicillin G has not proved efficacious because therapeutic levels of penicillin are not achieved in the cerebrospinal fluid. For neurosyphilis, aqueous penicillin or aqueous procaine penicillin is the drug of choice.

For the nongravid patient with proven or suspected penicillin allergy, tetracycline hydrochloride, 1 hour before or 2 hours after meals in dosages of 500 mg 4 times a day for 15 days, or erythromycin as the base, stearate or ethinylsuccinate in dosages of 500 mg 4 times a day for 15 days can be prescribed.

Gravid patients who are allergic to penicillin should not receive tetracycline because this antimicrobial agent has potential adverse effects upon fetal dentition and bone. Oral erythromycin has been shown to be poorly absorbed in gravid women and the recommended dosage used for the treatment in nongravid patients is associated with low maternal serum levels. Furthermore, there is marked patient to patient variation in maternal serum concentration after the oral administration of erythromycin. Such observations would account for congenital syphilis in the progeny of some mothers who received erythromycin therapy. Unfortunately there is no alternative antimicrobial agent that is entirely free of toxicity to mother and fetus. Consequently, erythromycin should be prescribed in dosage of 750 mg 4 times a day for 20 days to any gravid patient who is allergic to penicillin.

At the time one prescribes treatment to any patient with syphilis, it is prudent to advise the patient of the possibility of a Jarisch-Herxheimer reaction, which occurs in more than 50 per cent of patients with primary or secondary syphilis. The reaction occurs within 12 hours of the initiation of treatment and is characterized by fever, shaking chills, myalgia, headache, lethargy, and tachycardia, and in patients with secondary syphilis recrudescence of the rash. The patient should be reassured that the reaction is of short duration and will respond symptomatically to antipyretics.

HERPES GENITALIS

Genital infection with the herpes simplex viruses (HSV) has a higher prevalence rate than other sexually transmitted diseases. Consequently, genital HSV infections have been a source of increasing concern during the past decade. Much of the concern has emanated from the recognition of the risk of severe neonatal infections in the progeny of infected women, the possible association with cervical cancer and, more recently, squamous cell carcinoma in situ of the vulva as well as the present lack of effective modalities of therapy.

Since there is no national surveillance system for genital herpes infection, no reliable data are available to determine the magnitude of the problem. It is most prevalent, however, in the 15 to 30 year age group, and the rate of infection of the sexual contacts of individuals with genital HSV infection has been estimated to be at about 75 per cent. HSV consists of two antigenically distinct types—HSV 1 and HSV 2—and like all the viruses of the herpes group they are indigenous to man. Thus, after the primary infection the patient has a persistent infection as the viral genome remains in the host. This latter phenomenon accounts for the reactivation of the infection under certain circumstances despite the presence of circulating antibody. The utopian treatment of genital HSV infections would be one directed at the primary infection within a week of its inception so as to prevent latent infection when the virus remains in an inactive and nonreplicating state in the spinal root ganglia.

HSV 2 has been the predominant type associated with genital infections, but as fellatio and cunnilingus have increased in the patient population with genital herpes, more and more HSV 1 infections have been reported. HSV 1 can be isolated from the genital tract lesions in at least 50 per cent of patients with recurrent infection and from about 10 per cent of individuals who after their initial primary infection have no clinical evidence of the disease.

It is not known what precipitates recurrences of genital herpes, although they appear to be more common in men than in women. Recent data suggest that the risk of recurrence is related to the type of virus. Genital HSV 1 infection has been shown to be less likely to recur than HSV 2 infection. Likewise, among patients with primary HSV 2 infection, recurrences are more likely to occur in individuals with high titers of HSV 2 neutralizing antibody in their convalescent-phase serum. It is thus possible that the presence of neutralizing antibody after primary HSV 2 genital infection may be indicative of an increased risk of recurrent infection due to the presence of latent infection. When the quantity of periodic active viral replication attains a certain threshold level, shedding of the infectious virus occurs and recurrent clinical disease may result.

If the primary infection is confined to the cervix or vagina, the diagnosis of HSV infection may be overlooked, as the majority of cases are asymptomatic or subclinical. Only when the vulva is involved do herpetic vesicles and ulcers become symptomatic. Such lesions develop on an erythematous base and are associated with inguinal lymphadenopathy and on occasion constitutional symptoms. Such clinical manifestations of primary herpes genitalis occur anywhere from 2 to 12 days after sexual exposure and can persist for 4 to 6 weeks. Recurrent infections are not usually associated with inguinal lymphadenopathy and the eruption may last for only a few hours. Lesions of recurrent infection due to reactivation of the virus may appear every few weeks or only once or twice a year. The diagnosis of herpes genitalis is made on the clinical appearance of the lesions and is confirmed by the presence of multinuclear giant cells with intranuclear inclusion bodies in smears obtained from the base of the vesicles. Detection of viral antigen in infected cells and isolation of the virus can be used to substantiate the diagnosis. Since herpes genitalis is often associated with other sexually transmitted diseases it is important to screen patients with this infection for syphilis and gonorrhea. After the diagnosis is confirmed it is essential to inform the patient about the etiology of the disease and its recurrent nature. If the patient is conversant with the infectious potential of the active lesions and the high probability of their recurrence, dissemination of the disease to sexual partners may be reduced.

Although there are many claims that particular therapeutic regimens have been efficacious, to date there is no treatment that has been unequivocally shown to arrest genital herpes. The fact that so many different modalities of therapy are claimed to be of value is in itself evidence that none is probably of much value. Treatment of the acute attack is not the same as eradication of the infection and elimination of recurrent infection.

Antiviral drugs of the purine and pyrimidine family such as iododeoxyuridine and adenine arabinoside when systemically administered do reduce replication of HSV but are too toxic for use in patients with uncomplicated genital herpes. Furthermore, they do not eradicate the latent virus. Topical application of these agents is of minimal value as the compounds do not penetrate the skin in sufficient concentrations to inhibit viral replication.

A nucleoside analogue of adenine arabinoside, namely acyclovir (acycloguanosine), has been shown to be highly active both in vitro and in various animal studies against several herpes viruses. It has also been found to be effective for the treatment of human corneal ulcers caused by HSV. Recent studies indicate that intravenous therapy with this antiviral agent can significantly shorten the period of active replication of HSV in mucocutaneous lesions. The absence of toxicity makes acyclovir an attractive drug with which to conduct therapeutic trials in patients who have marked discomfort from HSV genital infections. Like the other antiviral agents it does not however eliminate latent infection, and consequently it does not prevent recrudescence of the infection after cessation of therapy. Formulations for the oral administration of acyclovir are currently being evaluated and it is possible that prolonged oral administration of this compound could prevent recurrent disease and reduce the risk of possible transmission of HSV to sexual contacts.

Another therapeutic approach to the treatment of genital herpes for which no benefit has been demonstrated is the use of smallpox vaccines. Other immunologic approaches involving inactivated HSV vaccines, transfer factor, or levamisole which causes immunomodulation, particularly of the cellular immune response, have been suggested. At this time no large double-blind studies have unequivocally demonstrated the efficacy of any of these agents.

Topical or systemic steroids are contraindicated in patients with genital herpes. Likewise, photodynamic inactivation of HSV with heterocyclic dyes, such as neutral red, proflavine, or methylene blue in the presence of incandescent or fluorescent light, should not be used, not only because of its potential oncogenicity, but because it is of little therapeutic value to patients with recurrent infections.

Many topical preparations have been used for the treatment of this disease including boric acid, ether, ether-alcohol, povidone-iodine, alcohols, and merthiolate. All are of questionable value, although the drying agents such as alcohols and ether, while not curative, at least have the advantage of causing the lesions on the vulva to rapidly dry up.

The primary infection is often extremely painful, particularly during the first week, and sedation with meperidine or oxycodone may be necessary. The nonsteroidal antiinflammatory agent indomethacin in a dosage of 25 mg four times daily for 7 days in conjunction with analgesic agents aids in the amelioration of the symptoms. Indomethacin alone is efficacious for the symptomatic relief of recurrent infections. Tepid sitz baths are beneficial when edema of the vulva is a major clinical feature of the disease.

Since this clinical entity has such a variable course from the point of view of recurrent infection, any new modality of treatment must be subjected to extensive double-blind studies. Eventually more effective prophylactic and therapeutic measures may enable us to control this sexually transmitted disease. In the meantime, however, the most important aspects of management are the relief of pain in primary infections, instruction of patients in hygienic measures, and sexual abstinence as well as tracing any sexual partner who may have been at risk of exposure to the infection.

CHLAMYDIAL INFECTIONS

During the last decade, as the result of the availability of specific culture techniques, the obligatory intracellular parasite *Chlamydia trachomatis* has been shown to be a common sexually transmitted pathogen and the cause of many genital tract infections. In males, it is the causative agent of many cases of epididymitis and at least one third of the cases of nongonococcal urethritis. In fact, in developed countries, urethritis due to this procaryotic organism appears to be the most common sexually transmitted disease.

Although *C. trachomatis* has been frequently isolated from the cervix of female sexual partners of men with chlamydia-positive nongonococcal urethritis, the clinical spectrum of chlamydial infections in women has not been completely established. Among women seeking general gynecologic care the prevalence of chlamydial genital infections has been shown however to exceed that of infections with *N. gonorrhoeae*. This pathogen has a predilection for the endocervix. Chlamydial cervicitis is often asymptomatic, but when symptoms such as a mucopurulent discharge are present they are indistinguishable from those caused by other genital pathogens. In this regard, chlamydial infections resemble those due to the gonococcus. Asymptomatic infections are, however, more common in patients with *C. trachomatis* than in those with *N. gonorrhoeae*.

Physicians need to be aware that concomitant gonococcal infections are frequently present in patients with chlamydial cervicitis. Any mucopurulent endocervicitis in a sexually active patient should be considered due either to the gonococcus or *C. trachomatis,* and if tests for *N. gonorrhoeae* are negative, then the patient should be treated for a presumptive chlamydial infection. Her sexual partner should be evaluated for nongonococcal urethritis and if he has had such an infection in the previous 6 weeks he should be treated.

Most chlamydial infections in women are restricted to the cervix or urethra. There is some evidence to indicate that chlamydial infections in women might be regarded as self-limiting. However, treatment is mandatory in view of the numerous studies which demonstrate the etiologic role of *C. trachomatis* in acute salpingitis, the Fitz-Hugh-Curtis syndrome, the urethral syndrome, neonatal conjunctivitis, and pneumonia, as well as its potential to cause cellular atypia and cervical dysplasia. Furthermore, as asymptomatic infections in women may serve as a reservoir for the dissemination of *C. trachomatis,* therapy might aid in the control of genital infections due to this organism as well as nongonococcal urethritis in their sexual partners.

The incidence of chlamydial infection of the cervix in gravid patients has been variously reported to be between 2 per cent and 18 per cent, and at least 20 per cent of such individuals transmit the infection to their infants during parturition. Chlamydial inclusion conjunctivitis is currently the most common form of infectious conjunctivitis in the neonate. Although chlamydial conjunctivitis, otitis media, and pneumonia in the neonate are unlikely to be life threatening, there are no long-term studies available which would allow one to predict the frequency of long-term ocular, auditory, or pulmonary sequelae. Laboratory improvements in the methodology for the diagnosis of chlamydial infections are essential before screening of patients can be initiated on a large scale and effective control measures instituted.

A diagnosis of chlamydial infection depends on the isolation of *C. trachomatis* by tissue cell culture by the use of irradiated McCoy cells or serologic studies. Both procedures are not readily available to the physician in practice, although most virology laboratories can perform tissue isolation of the organism. The growing interest in chlamydial infections among many medical specialities, health departments, and private laboratories promises to increase the availability and reduce the cost of screening procedures for these infections.

The increased incidence together with the diverse clinical manifestations of chlamydial infections have stimulated microbiologic laboratories to study the in vitro susceptibility of *C. trachomatis* to various antimicrobial agents. Such studies have shown that penicillin, ampicillin, the aminoglycosides, spectinomycin, nalidixic acid, and metronidazole are essentially inactive while tetracycline, doxycycline, and erythromycin are the most active against this organism. Consequently, tetracycline, doxycycline, and erythromycin are the drugs of choice for treating chlamydial infections.

To date no strains of *C. trachomatis* have been shown to be resistant to tetracycline. Treatment failures with tetracycline are indicative of lack of patient compliance or that the diagnosis should be further evaluated because the infection could be due to a pathogen other than *C. trachomatis*. Since there is no avialable effective single dose treatment for chlamydial infections, patient compliance may be difficult, especially as prolonged therapy is essential for the eradication of the organism.

For lower genital tract infections and the urethral syndrome, tetracycline, 500 mg 4 times daily for 10 days, or doxycycline, in an initial oral dosage of 200 mg followed by 100 mg twice daily for 10 days, is the treatment of choice. There is no evidence to indicate that longer courses of treatment are more effective. The sexual partners of such patients should receive the identical therapeutic regimen. In pregnancy, erythromycin is the drug of choice and this antibiotic should be prescribed in an oral dosage of 500 mg 4 times daily for 10 days.

For patients with acute salpingitis due to *C. trachomatis* who do not require hospitalization, oral doxycycline or tetracycline in the same daily dosage as used for lower genital tract infections is effective therapy when administered for 14 to 21 days. The reason for prolonged therapy is that chlamydial salpingitis has a more protracted course than that due to *N. gonorrhoeae*. For patients who require hospitalization treatment should commence with intravenous doxycycline in an initial dosage of 200 mg followed by 100 mg every 12 hours until there is clinical evidence of amelioration of the infection. Oral treatment with doxycycline in the same dosage should then be continued until the patient has received at least 14 days of therapy.

The importance of genital tract infections due to *C. trachomatis* as a medical and public health problem at the present time is obvious. Asymptomatic chlamydial cervicitis contributes in no small measure to the high incidence of nongonococcal urethritis in males. Thus, whether or not the patient is symptomatic, treatment is imperative.

VAGINAL TRICHOMONIASIS

This infection, which is caused by the flagellate protozoon *Trichomonas vaginalis*, has its highest incidence in women during the years of greatest sexual activity, namely those females between 16 and 35 years of age. Women with vaginal trichomoniasis commonly complain of vaginal discharge and pruritus vulvae although approximately one third of such individuals are asymptomatic. Urinary frequency, dysuria, dyspareunia, and lower abdominal discomfort are other symptoms which patients may experience with this infection. The onset of symptoms often coincides with menstruation, when the vaginal pH ranges from 5.5 to 6.5, which is the optimal range for the growth of this organism.

A diagnosis of vaginal trichomoniasis depends on the demonstration of the organism by microscopic examination of the discharge or by growth of the protozoon in a selective culture medium. It is imperative that any specimen obtained be examined microscopically as soon as possible, as the characteristic motility of the organism is essential in substantiating the diagnosis. The protozoon can readily be cultured on Feinberg's medium and after incubation at 37° C for 48 hours. Microscopic examination will reveal the presence of the flagellate. Cultures on this specific medium are valuable for the assessment of cure after treatment. The Papanicolaou smear may also demonstrate the presence of the organism but is less comparable in its diagnostic value to direct microscopy or culture. Since trichomonal vaginitis is frequently associated with gonorrhea, cultures should also be obtained for the gonococcus.

Metronidazole is the drug of choice. Treatment should also be prescribed for the patient's male sexual partners, although the majority are asymptomatic. Because of poor patient compliance with a prolonged course of metronidazole therapy, a dosage regimen of a single oral dose of 2.0 grams or 0.5 gram every 6 hours for 3 days is recommended. Patients should be cautioned to avoid all alcohol during treatment with metronidazole because this drug has a disulfiram-like effect.

Metronidazole induces mutations in bacteria and high doses in laboratory animals have been shown to be teratogenic. Consequently the drug should not be prescribed for gravid patients in the first trimester of pregnancy since its safety for the embryo and fetus has not been established. For such individuals, local therapy with hypotonic saline douches to alleviate the symptoms can be prescribed although such measures rarely eradicate the infection. Likewise, metronidazole therapy should be restricted in later pregnancy and during lactation to patients in whom local measures produce no amelioration of their symptoms.

VAGINAL CANDIDIASIS

This form of vaginitis most often is caused by the yeast-like fungus *Candida albicans* which is a normal constituent of the flora of the mouth, gastrointestinal tract, and vagina. This organism is usually an innocuous saprophyte and can be isolated from the vagina of up to 50 per cent of asymptomatic healthy women and it is therefore not invariably sexually acquired. Pregnancy, diabetes mellitus, hypoparathyroidism, and broad-spectrum antibiotic therapy predispose to vaginal candidiasis. Likewise, women taking steroidal antifertility compounds, corticosteroids, or immunosuppressive agents are more liable to colonization by this organism. The pathogenicity of *C. albicans* can be correlated with its overgrowth. *C. albicans* is frequently cultured from the urethra of male sexual partners of women colonized with this organism. Many of the male partners develop symptomatic urethritis or balanitis. The presenting symptom of vaginal candidiasis is pruritus vulvae which, in severe infections, is associated with edema of the vulva.

The diagnosis is made by the presence of white patches on the vulva, vaginal mucosa and ectocervix and substantiated by microscopic examination of the cottage cheese–like vaginal discharge. A sample of the vaginal discharge can be mixed on a slide with a few drops of a 10 per cent solution of potassium hydroxide, and the dimorphous fungus will be observed on microscopy. Alternatively, a Gram stain of a sample of the vaginal discharge can be performed when the yeast forms appear as gram-positive ovoids and the pseudohyphae as long gram-positive tubes. An increasing number of cases of vaginal candidiasis are caused by *Candida glabrata*. This organism can be differentiated from *C. albicans* only by fermentation reactions following culture on Sabouraud's glucose agar. Although *C. albicans* can readily be cultured on Sabouraud's medium, it is frequently difficult to ascertain whether the woman has a true infection or whether the isolate is a constituent of the normal vaginal flora.

Although a variety of antifungal compounds are available for the treatment of candidal vulvovaginitis, it is clear that the clinical efficacy of such agents may be offset by the failure of many patients to complete the prescribed course of therapy. For many years most antifungal agents for vaginal infections have been routinely prescribed for 14 days or more, but such courses of therapy may be abandoned prematurely by patients who experience rapid symptomatic relief.

A variety of intravaginal medications have been used for the treatment of vaginal candidiasis. Until recently nystatin was the drug of choice. Therapy consisted of the vaginal insertion of a suppository containing 100,000 units of the compound twice daily for 14 days. Because of the long course of treatment, patient compliance was often poor.

During the past few years a new group of antifungal agents, the synthetic imidazole derivatives, have proven highly efficacious in the treatment of vaginal candidiasis. The first of these compounds to be made available was miconazole. A vaginal cream containing 2 per cent of the drug used once daily at bedtime for 7 days appears to be more effective than the 14 day treatment with nystatin. Clotrimazole, a related compound, is available as a vaginal tablet containing 100 mg of the drug and also as a 1 per cent vaginal cream. Either formulation is effective when used daily for 7 days. Both these compounds are approved for use in pregnancy. Since virtually all topical antifungal agents are formulated as creams or pessaries for intravaginal use, they often prove to be cosmetically unacceptable to some patients and as such may contribute to many therapeutic failures. Consequently, in order to overcome this problem and reduce the duration of treatment, miconazole-medicated vaginal tampons inserted twice daily for five days have been made available for clinical trials and found to be very effective. A further imidazole derivative, econazole nitrate, has proved to be highly successful in the treatment of vaginal candidiasis. Studies indicate that the daily insertion of a 150 mg vaginal ovule for three days is more effective than clotrimazole therapy. Further studies are however required to ascertain the relationship between total antifungal dose, duration of therapy, and therapeutic success of the various imidazole derivatives in order to establish optimal conditions for the topical treatment of vaginal candidiasis.

NONSPECIFIC VAGINITIS

Any abnormal vaginal discharge that cannot be attributed to gonorrhea, vaginal trichomoniasis, or candidiasis is usually described as nonspecific vaginitis. This is a common disorder in clinical practice and its incidence appears to have increased during the past several years. Controversy exists as to the cause of this condition, but there is increasing evidence that *Gardnerella vaginalis*, which was formerly known as *Haemophilus vaginalis*, or *Corynebacterium vaginale* is implicated in most cases. This pleomorphic gram-negative coccobacillus is a common vaginal commensal which may have a pathogenic role when present in large numbers. Currently it is considered that *Gardnerella vaginalis* acting synergistically with anaerobes such as *Bacteroides* species and *Peptococcus* species are the cause of most bacterial vaginitides.

Clinically the patient presents with a creamy, malodorous vaginal discharge, a pH value in excess of 5.0, but without extensive evidence of inflammation. A wet saline smear demonstrates the presence of epithelial cells whose surface is stippled by small coccobacilli and referred to as "clue cells." The addition of a drop of 10 per cent potassium hydroxide to the wet-mount specimen causes the release of the "fishy" odor, which is reliable corroborative evidence of this form of vaginitis. A gram-stain of an undiluted specimen of the vaginal discharge will show large numbers of small gram-negative coccobacilli as well as "clue cells," but almost a complete absence of lactobacilli. A definitive diagnosis can be obtained only by culturing a specimen of the undiluted vaginal discharge on Columbia chocolate agar or Casman's blood agar. Routine culturing for bacteria is inadequate for the isolation of *Gardnerella vaginalis*.

The treatment of nonspecific vaginitis has also been controversial. Part of the confusion in the treatment of this entity has been fostered by the fact that *Gardnerella vaginalis* is present in the vaginal microflora of many asymptomatic women. Nonspecific vaginitis is a common and troublesome complaint of many women and the practice of treating this entity empirically with "all-purpose vaginal creams" is to be deplored because such preparations are ineffective. Originally, sulfonamide creams were advocated because of symptomatic improvement but all sensitivity tests demonstrate that *Gardnerella vaginalis* is uniformily resistant to sulfonamides. Oral ampicillin for a week or more was at one time advocated as the treatment of choice but such therapy is often ineffective even when the sexual partner is also treated. Similarly, treatment with doxycycline is not curative.

Metronidazole is now emerging as the treatment of choice for this condition. The efficacy of metronidazole, which is an anaerobic microbicidal agent and moderately active against *Gardnerella vaginalis*, is in accord with the concept that anaerobic bacteria act synergistically with *Gardnerella vaginalis* to cause nonspecific vaginitis. Clinical experience implies that this entity is frequently a sexually transmitted disease and it is essential that the sexual partner be treated. Even treatment with metronidazole does not necessarily eradicate *Gardnerella vaginalis*, but the drug may sufficiently alter the vaginal flora to create an environment that is hostile to its replication. This may be the reason why metronidazole is highly efficacious in the treatment of nonspecific vaginitis. The mechanism of action of metronidazole in the treatment of nonspecific vaginitis warrants further study because it is effective in curing this troublesome form of vaginitis.

BARTHOLIN CYSTS AND ABSCESSES

EDWARD W. SAVAGE, M.D.

Bartholin's cysts are very common. They are caused by obstruction of Bartholin's duct, usually near its orifice. Occlusion of the duct is frequently due to infection but may also result from trauma. Lacerations or mediolateral episiotomy repair may injure or ligate the duct. The contents of cysts vary, depending upon the cause of the obstruction. The normal mucus may appear sanguinous or brown in color if the cyst is caused by trauma, or it may appear cloudy if the cyst is caused by infection.

An abscess is extremely tender and may have a large surrounding area of inflammation. Incision and drainage give immediate relief; but the abscess may recur or a cyst may form because the channel of escape for gland secretions closes when the incision heals.

If the abscess has begun to drain spontaneously, it is frequently necessary to enlarge the opening to allow adequate drainage.

Proper treatment of Bartholin adenitis in the acute stage consists of bed rest, administration of analgesics and systemic antibiotics, and Sitz baths. When abscess formation is evident, incision and drainage are performed. The incision is made along the mucosa that is distended over the abscess. If there is an area of impending rupture through the skin, the incision may be made there. The mucosal site is usually preferred because of less discomfort, less distortion of the vulva, and more satisfactory healing. In addition, if the channel remains open, the mucosal site is more appropriate for discharge than is the skin of the labia.

Marsupialization may be performed under anesthesia and is a common, usually preferred, method of treatment for a Bartholin's cyst or abscess. Since the cyst or abscess wall is composed primarily of the duct of the gland, this procedure may preserve the duct channel and thus the secretory function of the gland for vaginal and vulval lubrication. It is a less involved technical procedure and eliminates many of the complications resulting from excision of the cyst.

Marsupialization may be performed under local, regional, or general anesthesia. A vertical incision is made in the vaginal mucosa over the center of the cyst and outside the hymenal ring. It should be as wide as possible to enhance the patency of the stoma postoperatively. An alternative method is the apposition of elliptical incisions and removal of an oval portion of the mucosa overlying the cyst. After the cyst wall is opened and its contents are drained, the cyst lining is everted and sutured to the vaginal mucosa with interrupted 2-0 chromatic catgut suture. Excision of a portion of the cyst wall does not appear to increase the possibility that the stoma will remain patent. Drains and packs are usually not necessary. Postoperative care includes daily Sitz baths after about the third postoperative day.

Marsupialization is advocated primarily for

Bartholin's cysts but may work satisfactorily if the abscess wall is well formed and the tissue is not excessively friable. However, there is a 10 to 15 per cent recurrence rate that results from closure and secondary fibrosis of the orifice following marsupialization. The use of packs, gauze wicks, or drains has not prevented closure of the stoma. One technique employs a Word catheter placed into the cavity to maintain patency of the orifice while the initial edema is subsiding and healing is taking place. This may prevent reocclusion of the orifice; however, catheter retention is a problem and may produce additional postoperative discomfort.

The decision to excise (rather than marsupialize) a Bartholin's duct cyst should be determined by (1) recurrence following marsupialization and (2) recurrent infection deep in the gland. There should be no attempt to excise significantly infected, inflamed tissue. Furthermore, thickening at the base of the gland may represent a rare neoplasm, and this possibility should be considered in the patient over the age of 40 years.

To remove Bartholin's duct cysts, it is usually best to make an elliptical incision in the mucosa that is distended over the cyst. A mucosal incision is preferable to an incision in the skin. If the incision is made through the skin, it is often difficult to dissect the cyst wall from the more delicate and thin mucosa without incising or tearing it. An opening accidentally made through the mucosa may result in a permanent fenestration in the affected labium. On the other hand, if the incision is made on the mucosal side, usually no difficulty is encountered in dissecting the cyst from the inner surface of the skin. Excising a small ellipse of mucosa with the cyst allows a focus for traction and helps prevent rupture of the cyst.

The inflammation and scarring sometimes associated with Bartholin's cysts make blunt dissection difficult if not impossible. Metzenbaum scissors are helpful in sharp dissection of the cyst from the surrounding tissue. If the cyst is large, it may have extended posteriorly, close to the rectum. Care must be exercised to avoid damage at this point. Complete removal of the gland tissue adherent to the cyst wall is essential, for residual glandular tissue may result in the formation of a tender nodule or recurrent cyst. The noncystic portion of the gland feels indurated in contrast to the surrounding tissue and is easily palpated and dissected.

Beneath the Bartholin's cyst is the vestibular bulb, which is composed of anastomosing venous channels. Care must be exercised to avoid bleeding when the gland is dissected from its attachment to the vascular bulb. The entire cavity must be obliterated by approximating the walls with fine absorbable sutures. The mucosa is finally closed using 2-0 absorbable sutures. Bleeding from the area may result in a postoperative hematoma of the labia, which may dissect up over the mons pubis and onto the abdominal wall beneath Scarpa's fascia. The hematoma usually responds to conservative measures such as bed rest, ice, and pressure packs. Attempts to ligate vessels upon reoperation are usually futile, though sometimes it is necessary to evacuate the hematoma and drain the incision.

Cultures should be obtained from all cysts and abscesses of the Bartholin's duct so that appropriate antibiotic treatment may be instituted when necessary. Precise identification may become especially important in the infrequent instances when serious sequelae, such as *Bacteroides* bacteremia and synergistic gangrene of the surrounding tissue, occur.

UTERINE MYOMAS

JAMES A. MERRILL, M.D.

Myoma (leiomyoma) is a well circumscribed, benign uterine tumor arising from smooth muscle within the myometrium. It is estimated that 20 to 25 per cent of women over the age of 35 have uterine myomas. The tumors occur most frequently during the reproductive years and commonly undergo regression, often complete, following the menopause. Most myomas produce no symptoms. However, it has been estimated that as many as 60 per cent of all pelvic laparotomies in women are done for the indication of myomas. Myomas commonly are multiple, located variously within the uterus and attached to it. Rarely myomas are subject to a variety of degenerative phenomena, usually of no clinical significance. Sarcomatous change occurs in less than 1 per cent.

TREATMENT

Indications. The principal indication for active treatment is *symptoms* which have been thoroughly evaluated and for which no cause other than uterine myomas has been found. In patients without uterine enlargement the finding of normal endometrium and an irregular endometrial cavity is an example of such evidence.

Treatment also may be indicated for patients with asymptomatic tumors if the tumor is unusually *large* (possibly larger than a 3 month pregnancy), *increases in size* during observation, or cannot be distinguished definitely from a solid *ovarian tumor* or other lesion of greater significance. Rapid growth may be defined as a gain of 6 weeks gestational size within an interval of less than 1 year. Ultrasonography may be helpful in establishing a baseline. No controlled clinical trials have demonstrated that women on oral contraceptives are at increased risk for growth of myomas. Low-dose oral contraceptives are not necessarily contraindicated in patients with small myomas.

In carefully selected cases of *infertility* and/or repeated *fetal wastage,* in which all causes have been excluded and the uterus is judged to be of 8 weeks gestational size or less, treatment by myomectomy may be considered.

Methods. *Observation* and reassurance is most frequently the appropriate treatment. This is particularly so if the patient is asymptomatic, has small tumors, or is menopausal. Curettage and progestin therapy, such as medroxyprogesterone acetate (Provera), 10 mg daily, is recommended for the patient with symptomatic myomas who is approaching the menopause. Patients should be examined every 6 months for unusual growth or development of symptoms.

For patients in whom active treatment is indicated, as described above, *surgery* is preferred. Usually this is *total hysterectomy.* If the tumors are small the hysterectomy may be done vaginally, particularly if there is associated pelvic relaxation. The author does not recommend morcellation of myomas and their removal by the vaginal route. Most often the abdominal approach is preferred. Since very large tumors may distort the ureters and make them liable to surgical trauma, the operator should consider the possibility of placing ureteral catheters prior to hysterectomy in selected cases. Hysterectomy should not be done without prior endometrial sampling if the patient complains of abnormal bleeding.

The issue of removal of ovaries at the time of hysterectomy is not related to uterine myomas, and that decision must be based upon factors of age, patient desire for preservation of the ovaries, the gross appearance of the ovaries, and the potential for subsequent ovarian malignancy. Since the risk of any woman developing ovarian cancer during her lifetime is only 1 per cent, the probable benefit of ovariectomy is small. However, ovarian cancer has been reported to occur in 5 to 10 percent of women with prior hysterectomy for benign disease. Commonly a minimum age recommended for prophylactic oophorectomy at the time of hysterectomy is within the fifth decade of life. Oophorectomy prior to this time should be limited to women with specific indications, such as family history of ovarian cancer, previous ovarian neoplasm or, possibly, cancerphobia.

Myomectomy is rarely indicated, and is done only to improve or preserve reproductive function. Myomectomy may be accomplished through the vagina in cases of pedunculated submucous myomas, employing a wire loop and electrocautery. Myomectomy, if indicated, is usually done by the abdominal approach. The indications, as stated above, include selected cases of infertility and repeated pregnancy loss, or when a tumor is in a location likely to interfere with normal delivery. A prior thorough evaluation of fertility is essential. Myomectomy carries a high frequency of postoperative complications of adhesions and bowel obstruction. The literature indicates that 15 per cent of patients undergoing myomectomy had recurrence of tumors and 10 per cent required subsequent treatment. When myomectomy is done to preserve or improve reproductive function, the risks and limited potential for success must be explained to the patient.

The author recommends occlusion of the ovarian and uterine vessels during myomectomy to decrease blood loss. The infundibulopelvic ligaments may be occluded with rubber-shod clamps and the ascending uterine vessels with either a Bonney clamp or a rubber catheter passed through bilateral incisions in the base of the broad ligaments to encircle the lower uterine segment. Optimally, a single vertical midline incision in the *anterior* fundus should be used to remove all of the myomas. This is less likely to cause adhesions than multiple incisions and if they form, those on the anterior wall of the uterus are less likely to involve the oviducts and ovaries. Obviously some myomas will not be accessible through a single or an anterior incision but an attempt should be made to do so. Further, effort should be made to remove the tumors without entrance into the uterine cavity. The uterine incision(s) should be closed with a minimum of suture material. Interrupted sutures of #0 Vicryl are used to approximate the myometrium. A continuous suture of 4-0 Vicryl should be used to imbricate the serosa, thus reducing the raw surface area and the risk of postoperative adhesions. There may be an advantage to uterine suspension when posterior incisions have been necessary.

In the past, *radiation* has been used for the treatment of myomas in some clinics. It is mentioned here only to be condemned, for radiation has no place in the treatment of uterine myomas today.

MYOMAS DURING PREGNANCY

Reports indicate that the incidence of uterine myomas during pregnancy is 0.3 to 7 per cent. Myomas usually precede the pregnancy but may not become apparent until pregnancy occurs. Myomas usually increase in size during pregnancy but this is largely the result of edema or degeneration and probably does not represent true proliferation of the tumors. During the second and third trimesters, increase in size of myomas may produce or increase pressure symptoms.

Degeneration may produce symptoms of gradual or acute pain, usually associated with localized tenderness. Since it may be difficult to distinguish this from other acute intra-abdominal accidents or inflammation, operation is sometimes necessary for this reason. However, in the majority of patients, degeneration does not indicate surgical intervention. Such patients are best treated by bed rest, analgesia, and careful observation. Surgery is rarely necessary, and myomectomy is followed by an increased incidence of abortion and premature labor.

Myomas may produce fetal malpresentation, uterine inertia, or mechanical dystocia. Fortunately, most tumors rise out of the pelvis as pregnancy progresses. However, if cesarean section is necessary, myomectomy is not advised at the same operation. In the majority of cases, successful vaginal delivery can be anticipated. Postpartum hemorrhage is more likely to occur when the uterus contains myomas and should be anticipated.

ENDOMETRIOSIS

ROBERT W. KISTNER, M.D.

Endometriosis is a rather ubiquitous, potentially disabling disease that seems to be increasing in incidence. It is a frequent cause of infertility and has been reported to account for 25 to 30 per cent of fertility problems in the human female. If male factors were excluded, endometriosis would probably be the most common cause of infertility in women over age 25.

Although this disease may have always existed, the term "endometriosis" was first coined by John Sampson in 1922 and since that time has been described, defined, and classified in over 2000 reports. Yet it is still an enigmatic disease. At least a dozen theories attempt to explain the histogenesis of endometriosis, but the most logical, I believe, is still that of Sampson—namely, retrograde menstruation via the oviduct with recurrent peritoneal insult month after month, year after year, in women who unfortunately do not have periods of menstrual cessation. The disease is, therefore, common in the nullipara and uncommon in the multipara.

The most frequently involved areas are the ovaries and the cul-de-sac. This is consistent with the menstrual tubal reflux theory. Predisposing factors are undoubtedly of importance in the development of endometriosis. Recent studies indicate that race per se is not relevant. A familial tendency has been reported, particularly in sisters, but also in mothers and daughters.

Since all women menstruate into their peritoneal cavities simultaneously with vaginal efflux, the important question to be answered is, "Why does the menstrual effluvium attach and grow in some women, but not in others?" Undoubtedly, the former are not protected immunologically, whereas the latter are. Future research should be directed toward determining the cause of this protection, rather than newer methods of treatment.

Specific physical and psychological characteristics have been attributed to patients with endometriosis. These women are tense perfectionists with an insatiable desire to excel. They express demanding and specific goals for their lives, are usually well dressed, and usually have trim figures. In one study, most of the patients were employed in responsible administrative positions or in professions such as law, medicine, and teaching.

It should be noted, however, that these personality traits occur in career women who have elected a prolonged delay in initiating a family; perhaps it is the prolongation of peritoneal insult rather than the somatotype that is etiologic. Of course, when a planned delay has been accomplished with the use of oral contraceptives, the incidence of endometriosis seems to be diminished. Oral contraceptives effectively reduce the quantity and quality of the tubal efflux.

SIGNS AND SYMPTOMS

The classic symptom complex includes dysmenorrhea, deep dyspareunia, and infertility. Only 30 per cent of patients are completely asymptomatic. Because reliable and simple endoscopic procedures are now available, the diagnosis can easily be made visually and/or histologically. Laparoscopy provides an ideal method for determination of the extent and severity of the disease, thus permitting accurate classification prior to therapy. Treatment should not be instituted until precise diagnosis and classification have been established.

Classification in terms of severity or stage of development of the disease has proved to be useful, not only in selection of appropriate therapy, but also in evaluation and reporting of results of treatment. We introduced a classification in 1977, which has been augmented and approved by the American Fertility Society.

ENDOMETRIOSIS AND INFERTILITY

What is the mechanism of infertility in patients who have endometriosis? When endometriosis is extensive, the alteration of tubal and ovarian physiology is ominous, and the relationship to infertility is easily explained. However, in early stages, it is difficult to rationalize a cause and effect.

Prostaglandins may play a role in such patients. It has been suggested that degeneration of ectopic endometrial tissues releases prostaglandin, resulting in local vasospasm, hypoxia, tissue destruction, and uterine contractions. Physiologic levels of prostaglandins have been shown to be necessary for ovum release, normal tubal motility, uterine relaxation and contractility, and steroidogenesis. An increased concentration of prostaglandins in peritoneal fluid may result in alterations in tubal motility, ovum release, and steroidogenesis.

TREATMENT

The objectives of treatment are to secure relief of pain, permit adequate coitus, prevent abnormal bleeding, and, of course, to preserve or increase the possibility of pregnancy. Conservative surgery accomplishes all of this in many patients, but pregnancy itself has been suggested as the optimum in prophylaxis and therapeutics. The signs and symptoms of endometriosis frequently, though not always, regress during the period of gestation and for varying periods of time thereafter.

In 1958 I suggested that this improvement may be due in part to a transformation of the functioning endometriotic tissue into decidua by increased levels of chorionic estrogen and progesterone. This concept led to the combined use of synthetic estrogens and progestins to create a so-called pseudopregnancy.

Subsequently, in 1971, danazol (Danocrine) was introduced; it creates a so-called pseudomenopause.

But what about conservative surgery? That usually means, following preliminary dilatation and curettage and laparoscopy, an exploratory laparotomy, excision and/or fulguration of endometrial implants, resection and plication of the uterosacral ligaments, and uterine suspension. Additional surgery, such as appendectomy or presacral neurectomy, is performed when and as indicated.

Pregnancy rates following conservative surgical procedures depend upon the stage of the disease. We reported a pregnancy rate of 76 per cent in stages I and II in 232 patients and a pregnancy rate of 38 per cent in stages III and IV in 106 patients. Others have reported similar results.

Hormonal therapy is indicated in patients having stage I or IIa disease. A variety of schemes have been devised for the medical management of this illness. The hormonal pseudopregnancy approach yields pregnancy rates of 45 to 55 per cent in Stages I and IIa, and danazol has been reported to be even more effective than that. Some investigators also believe that danazol produces fewer side-effects, but this has not been corroborated in other studies. In doses of 800 mg per day, serious side-effects, such as depression, weight gain, acne, and hirsutism, have caused many patients to discontinue treatment.

An analysis of reported data suggests that at present both danazol in a reduced dose of 400 mg per day and the hormonal pseudopregnancy approach have about the same incidence of side-effects, and the pregnancy rate is essentially the same for both in stages I and IIa.

Danazol may be used preoperatively in a dose of 400 mg per day for 3 months in stages IIb, III and IV. I think it is excellent, and other investigators agree. Preoperative therapy decreases the size and number of endometriotic areas, diminishes vascularity, and theoretically decreases the risk of postoperative adhesions.

SHOCK—A GENERAL PLAN OF MANAGEMENT

DENIS CAVANAGH, M.D.,
and DONALD E. MARSDEN, M.D.

Shock is a condition in which the circulating blood volume is less than the capacity of the vascular bed. This disparity leads to hypotension, reduced perfusion of vital organs, and cellular hypoxia. Anaerobic metabolism is utilized by cells to compensate for hypoxia, but this leads to the accumulation of lactate and pyruvate in the poorly perfused tissues, and the development of a metabolic acidosis. The end result is metabolic dysfunction, autolysis, and cellular death.

Shock is not a disease in itself but the response of the body to a range of life-threatening situations (Table 1). Management involves resuscitative measures to combat and reverse shock before irreparable damage is done to vital organs, and specific therapy to remedy the basic cause. The management of the condition is often made more complex because the basic disease may cause both shock and a coagulopathy which then adds a hemorrhagic element to further aggravate the shock. Examples of this situation are septic shock and abruptio placentae. Blood transfusion given in the treatment of shock may lead to a coagulopathy, through either incorrect crossmatching or failure to recognize the need for coagulation factor replacement when large amounts of stored blood are infused. Thus, throughout the management of the patient in shock one must keep in mind the possibility of secondary conditions developing as the result of the disease or its treatment, because these will compound the already serious situation. The priorities for the management of the shocked patient are represented by the mnemonic "ORDER" (Table 2).

O—Oxygenation involves an adequate supply of oxygen, a clear airway, and a satisfactory tidal volume. In the conscious patient breathing normally, 8 to 10 liters per minute of 100 percent oxygen by mask or nasal catheter is adequate. But if the patient cannot maintain a clear airway or adequate tidal volumes, then intubation, or in some cases tracheostomy, and positive pressure ventilation may be required. Adequate ventilation is confirmed by arterial blood gas determinations, but in the initial phases of management one must be careful not to allow the performance of such tests to interfere with more urgent procedures.

R—Restoration of the circulating blood volume is a vital part of the management of shock. Consideration must be given to the type and number of intravenous lines, the fluids used for replacement, and the monitoring of infusion rates. Large-bore cannulas (14, 16, or 18 gauge) in peripheral veins are ideal but may be hard to place in the patient in shock. Number 16 gauge polyethylene catheters can often be placed easily in the veins of the antecubital fossa even in severe shock. Should these alternatives fail, considera-

TABLE 1. **Classification of Shock**

1. Hypovolemic shock
   A. Hemorrhagic shock. Associated with postpartum or postabortal hemorrhage, ectopic pregnancy, placenta previa, abruptio placentae, rupture of the uterus, dysfunctional uterine bleeding, benign and malignant uterine neoplasms, rupture of ovarian neoplasms, and obstetric and gynecologic surgery.
   B. Fluid loss shock. Associated with excessive vomiting, diarrhea, diuresis, or too rapid removal of ascitic fluid in patients with hepatic cirrhosis.
   C. Supine hypotensive syndrome. Associated with compression of inferior vena cava by pregnant uterus.
   D. Shock associated with disseminated intravascular coagulation. Intrauterine dead fetus syndrome and amniotic fluid infusion.
2. Septic shock (endotoxic shock). Associated typically with infected abortion, chorioamnionitis, pyelonephritis, and postpartum endometritis; may be hypovolemic; has cardiogenic component.
3. Cardiogenic shock
   A. Failure of left ventricular ejection
      1. Cardiac arrest (asystole or ventricular fibrillation)
      2. Myocardial infarction.
   B. Failure of left ventricular filling
      1. Cardiac tamponade. Associated with coagulation defects
      2. Pulmonary embolism. Associated with infusion of air or fat, or with thrombophlebitis associated with pregnancy, use of hormones, extensive pelvic surgery, or sickle-cell disease.
4. Neurogenic shock
   A. Chemical injury. Associated with aspiration of gastrointestinal contents.
   B. Drug-induced. Associated with spinal anesthesia.
   C. Inversion of uterus with vasomoter collapse.
   D. Electrolyte imbalance. Associated with hyponatremia from any cause.

The conditions cited in the list may operate independently or in combination. When a pregnant woman is in shock, the fetus also is in shock.
(From Cavanagh, D., Woods, R. E., O'Connor, T. C. E., and Knuppel, R. A.: Obstetric Emergencies, Harper and Row, Hagerstown, Md., Reproduced with permission. 3rd ed., 1982.

TABLE 2. **The ORDER of Priorities in Managing the Patient in Shock**

O OXYGENATE
   Assure an airway
   8–10 liters/min by closed mask, nasal catheter, or endotracheal tube

R RESTORE CIRCULATING VOLUME
   One or more IV lines
   Initially crystalloids or colloids
   Where possible, blood for blood, but remember clotting factors
   Initial monitoring by central venous pressure

D DRUG THERAPY
   Avoid vasopressors as a general rule
   Digitalize if in cardiac failure
   Specific drugs for condition

E EVALUATE
   Response to therapy
   Basic cause
   Fetal condition if appropriate

R REMEDY THE BASIC PROBLEM
   Surgery if appropriate
   Specific antibiotics if organism identified

tion should be given to performing a surgical "cut-down" on a peripheral vein, preferably in the arm, or placement of a central venous line by either the subclavicular or the supraclavicular route. The latter procedures are fast and usually simple in experienced hands, but one must keep in mind the fact that a complication such as pneumothorax in a patient already in shock may be a terminal event. At the time of insertion of the intravenous line, blood is drawn for a complete blood count with a differential white blood count, platelet count, coagulation profile, and SMA (complete) as well as for blood grouping and crossmatching. It is wise to perform all of these studies at this time in all patients in shock.

One would ideally like to replace fluid lost with a similar fluid: blood with blood, electrolyte solution with electrolyte solution, and so on. However, in the initial phases either crystalloid solutions (sugar and electrolytes) or colloids (plasma proteins) will often be used because crossmatching takes time. It is best to avoid Ringer's lactate solution because the metabolic acidosis is further aggravated by the additional lactate. A solution such as 5 per cent dextrose in normal saline with added bicarbonate is more appropriate. Where hemorrhage is massive and red cells are necessary to allow oxygen transport to the tissues, uncrossmatched blood may be used. This has traditionally been Group O, Rh-negative blood with low titers of anti-A and anti-B, but blood of the patient's own group, if that is accurately known, is equally suitable. Remember that unless blood is drawn within 24 hours of transfusion it is deficient in labile clotting factors and platelets, and this deficiency must be remedied by infusion of fresh frozen plasma and platelets. A reasonable approach is to give two bags of fresh frozen plasma after the first six bags of stored blood, and one pack of fresh frozen plasma for every four subsequent bags of blood. One pooled platelet pack should be given after every six bags of blood. With large volume transfusions, warming of infused blood is also essential to avoid hypothermia.

The volume of fluid infused may be very large and the pulse, blood pressure, and urine output are often not accurate reflections of requirements and response. Central venous pressure (CVP) and pulmonary artery wedge pressure (PAWP) monitoring are useful in the management of fluid replacement. Although the PAWP is more reliable in certain circumstances, the process of insertion is not one that is appropriate in the emergency situation or for inexperienced personnel. It is better in the earlier phases of resuscitation to insert a central venous line, preferably through an antecubital vein, and if at a later stage wedge pressures appear desirable, to remove the central catheter over a guide-wire and then insert a flotation catheter using the same guide-wire.

D—Drug Therapy, though of secondary importance when compared with oxygenation and restoration of circulating volume, must be seriously considered at this stage. Patients with tachycardia and a raised central venous pressure should be digitalized, once it has been ascertained that there is no contraindication. Vasoactive drugs may play a role in the management of shock. In the "warm hypotensive" phase (early stages) of shock, vasopressors such as metaraminol may be used to maintain a blood pressure sufficient to assure a urinary output of at least 30 ml hourly. In the later, "cold hypotensive" phase of shock when vasoconstriction is most pronounced, vasodilators such as chlorpromazine may be used in conjunction with volume replacement. Dopamine, 200 mg in 500 ml of 5 per cent dextrose solution, run at a rate sufficient to maintain blood pressure, is a very useful agent, but because of its potency must be used with great care.

Other drug therapy that should be considered at this stage includes steroids in pharmacologic doses (dexamethasone, 20 mg as an intravenous bolus, and 6 mg per kg daily as a continuous infusion), antibiotics for patients with septic shock, morphine for patients with pain, pulmonary embolus, or myocardial infarction, and heparin for patients with amniotic fluid embolism. Patients in shock from postabortal or postpartum hemorrhage should receive intramuscular Ergotrate and an intravenous infusion of oxytocin.

E—Evaluation of the situation is critical at this stage. Frequently, when one sees a person in shock the resuscitative measures discussed above must be undertaken rapidly and even reflexly. But having established basic therapy for the patient, one should pause to evaluate the response of the patient to the initial therapy, the basic etiology of the shock, and what further investigations and therapy are required. The results of initial laboratory studies are evaluated and further tests ordered as appropriate. Blood gas studies may be repeated, or done for the first time if they have not been done before. This is the time for a more detailed history and physical examination than was possible earlier. This would be the appropriate time to consider whether a Swan-Ganz flotation catheter should be inserted. Although theoretically too late, this may be the first practical opportunity to obtain blood, urine, pus, or secretions for microbiologic study.

And at this stage one must evaluate which treatments are most appropriate to remedy the basic cause of the shock.

R—Remedy the cause if at all possible by specific treatment. This may simply require the removal of a retained placenta or products of conception in postabortal or portpartum hemorrhage. Patients with severe antepartum hemorrhage will require examination with a "double set-up" to ascertain the source of bleeding and to rupture the membranes if vaginal delivery appears feasible. Patients with uterine rupture will need laparotomy, and in most cases, hysterectomy. Intractable postpartum hermorrhage, unresponsive to oxytocic agents, demands uterine exploration. If no remediable cause is found, a laparotomy should be performed with a view to hysterectomy or hypogastric and ovarian artery ligation. Although ligation of these vessels will control hemorrhage in many situations, it is unwise to push conservatism too far, and often hysterectomy will be a more prudent initial course. This is technically the easiest course in most postpartum patients. Severe vaginal bleeding following hysterectomy, or in patients with extensive malignant disease, may often be controlled by hypogastric artery ligation.

In septic shock, the nidus of infection must be removed or adequately drained. Hence, in shock following septic abortion uterine evacuation is performed within 6 hours of obtaining adequate antibiotic coverage. Hysterectomy should be considered if shock persists despite uterine evacuation, if the uterus exceeds 16 weeks in size, if perforation has occurred, if the infecting organism is *Clostridium welchii*, if a toxic or corrosive douche has been used, or if the patient is oliguric.

Finally, it must be emphasized that there are many situations in which adequate control of shock cannot be achieved until surgical intervention has remedied the basic cause, and surgery must proceed despite the presence of shock. The classic example of this situation is ruptured ectopic pregnancy, but there are many other similar situations. Excessive delay may allow irreversible shock to develop before the cause is corrected.

DYSPAREUNIA AND VAGINISMUS

JAMES P. SEMMENS, M.D.

Dyspareunia (pain with intercourse) occurs with sufficient frequency that 40 per cent of women under 40 years of age at the time of a routine gynecological visit (Pap smear, family planning, and so forth) desired to discuss it as a significant personal problem and request an evaluation during examination. Among 200 of 500 patients in an office survey who expressed concern with coital pain and discomfort, 1 in 10 listed dyspareunia as a primary complaint. Two thirds of these patients were menopausal. Dyspareunia was the primary motivation for 60 per cent of the volunteers participating in a study of the effects of menopause on vaginal physiology currently being conducted by the author.

Though women under 40 reported a 40 per cent incidence of dyspareunia, the frequency of the occurrence of pain or discomfort may only occur 4 to 6 times during a given year; 50 per cent of women over 50 had discomfort as often as every third or fourth sexual encounter. The incidence and frequency continues to increase during the 60s and 70s. Our current research indicates that estrogen deprivation plays a significant role by not providing adequate lubrication in both the quiescent and aroused states. Coital frequency may be an additional factor affecting the menopausal age group.

Physical, physiologic and psychological factors may be involved in dyspareunia. Unfortunately, the physical factors are not always detectable because they are related to the congestive changes in the lower third of the vagina in response to sexual arousal, a situation not present during a routine gynecological examination. Also, hymenal tabs, redundant or excessive skin in the region of the posterior fourchette and perianal area, or vaginal scar tissue may serve at one time or another as a triggering mechanism which may not be discernible at the time of examination.

SEXUAL HISTORY

Dyspareunia is considered a sexual dysfunction and unless the gynecologist is willing to at least elicit a sexual history oriented toward the problem, the examination will be more of a disservice then a help to the patient. The examiner needs to elicit the onset of the woman's complaint, her first awareness of vaginal discomfort, be it during coitus or with insertion of a tampon. The physician needs to know what attempts she has made to resolve the discomfort, if the discomfort has become progressively worse or has remained the same, and whether there are times that the patient is free of pain. Another important factor to be aware of is whether or not the sexual partner has been involved in the counseling or treatment and whether any suggestions have been made regarding coital activities, positioning, frequency, or the use of lubricants.

Another area frequently omitted in this type of sexual history is the couple's index of comfort with their method of contraceptive control, as it relates to their coital activities. Frequently, a female partner feels that she has physical problems which would contraindicate the use of oral contraceptives. She finds herself using oral contraceptives at the insistence of her sexual partner and her physician, who is usually a male. The implication is that contraceptive control and sexual opportunity for the male partner is of more concern than her physical well-being, to which she responds negatively with complaints of dyspareunia and vaginismus. Ideally, the physician prescribing contraceptives should be made aware of the couple's coital frequency and sexual needs. Younger couples are quite negative about methods which require prior preparation or taking time out during the coital relationship, such as the application of gels, foam, or creams. The dyspareunia may simply be a message of dissatisfaction with their method of contraception or an effort to achieve an audience for complaints referable to sexual communication as well as contraceptive control.

ORGANIC CAUSES

The differential diagnosis involves a thorough investigation of physical causes to rule out organic lesions which may be primary or secondary as well as superficial at the level of the introitus or deep above the level of the levators.

Superficial Primary Lesions. Patients with superficial primary lesions are difficult to examine owing to hypertrophy of the levators, and spasm of the levators and the adductor muscles of the thighs.

Conditioned plus organic problems may involve vaginismus as a result of faulty sex education, leading to fear or hysteria; usually the problem is aggravated by a clumsy sexual partner. A principal finding is pain and involuntary spasm when attempting to examine the patient and a reported history of pain and inability to attain coital containment of the penis. Many of these women will report discomfort and pain with tampon insertion as well.

Genital trauma, with a history of foreign bodies in the vagina and traumatic experiences with removal during childhood and preadolescence, may also contribute to dyspareunia. Perineal trauma may also have been incurred, as with a bicycle crossbar accident. A third category of patients are those who have experienced sexual assault.

Primary lesions of the vaginal introitus may include a rigid hymen, requiring surgical correction, imperforate hymen, agenesis of the vagina, or a vaginal septum extending the full length of the vaginal tract.

Superficial Secondary Lesions. Local trauma may include burns (including radiation), repairs of lacerations, episiotomy repairs, clitoral circumcision, rectocele, and cystocele repair scars.

Inflammatory lesions (acute and chronic) may be vulvar, including Bartholin cysts, or granulomatous lesions which may involve sinus tracts and scarring as well as vaginal narrowing.

Urethral lesions include caruncles of the urethral meatus, infection of Skene's glands, and urethral diverticuli.

Anal lesions include proctitis, fissures, and fistulas, as well as hemorrhoids, particularly those which are thrombosed.

Redundant or webbed skin between the posterior fourchette and anus or a "dashboard" posterior repair which is traumatized during attempts at intromission acts as a triggering mechanism, especially if the female partner is not lubricated, or if there is little or no lubrication of the perineal area.

Deep Organic Lesions. With deep primary lesions, there may be mild levator spasm but pain is more apt to be elicited above the level of the levators. Vaginal obstruction may be due to hypoplasia of the vagina, Gartner duct cyst, or a vaginal septum. Pelvic tumors may include primary vaginal neoplasms, or vaginal extension of neoplastic disease in the genital urinary tract or rectosigmoid areas.

Deep Secondary Acquired Lesions Include the Following: Vaginal infection, causing induration and tenderness (trichomonal, monilial, and bacterial).

Vaginal irritation from chemical causes; with use of condoms, diaphragms, lubricants, jellies, douches, vaginal medication, feminine hygiene sprays, and so forth;

Vaginal scarring and obstruction as well as lubricative difficulties following irradiation;

Uterosacral tenderness because of deep thrusting by the male partner which is socially and culturally motivated by myth and misinformation;

Endometriosis, especially when uterosacral lesions are present; however, the lesions may involve the adnexae and the cervix as well;

Retrodisplacement of the uterus usually when associated with fixation of the adnexal structures as in endometriosis, inflammatory disease, or previous pelvic surgery, including tubal ligation;

Ovarian prolapse;

Post-hysterectomy vaginal scars resulting in a foreshortened vagina or a scar which includes adnexal structures at the apex or angles in a fixed position;

Ovarian and uterine tumors, especially large cysts and myomata of the pelvis;

Bowel lesions, including hemorrhoids, diverticula, and proctitis; vaginismus and colitis may exist in the same hypertonic type of patient.

Failure to localize lesions causing specific tenderness or duplication of pain as experienced during coitus by the patient may be an indication for an examination under anesthesia or a laparoscopic examination. Frequently, the pain caused by endometriosis is not related to the extent of the lesion (a small powder burn may be more tender than a large endometrioma of the ovary). Also, fine inflammatory adhesions which may follow bowel or pelvic infection or ectopic pregnancy, etc., are usually not palpable. The laparoscope not only permits visualization of these lesions but also may be used to biopsy the lesions or lyse the adhesions.

PSYCHOGENIC ETIOLOGY

When all efforts have been made to rule out a physical cause of the problem, the psychological aspect may be dealt with. The patient needs to be advised of the psychosomatic implications of the diagnosis and approach to therapy. It is important to once more affirm the onset of the difficulty—the conditions under which it occurs and any cause and effect relationship she or her partner may have attached to the problem. A decision needs to be made whether or not the therapy should involve both sexual partners; in most cases, the problem involves the relationship, and will improve only with understanding by both the individuals concerned. If the clinician is uncomfortable with the therapeutic approaches at this level, it is best to refer to a competent sex counselor or sex therapist.

TREATMENT

Any physical abnormalities found (superficial or deep) should be treated appropriately by medical and/or surgical means. Physical problems which cannot be corrected or may be only partially relieved need to be discussed with the patient or couple and options offered. It is not the intent of this review to discuss each clinical entity in depth. How to deal with specific problems caused by lesions of endometriosis or the vaginal lubricative problem of the female diabetic requires that each clinical entity be properly treated and controlled. Then, as part of therapy, it will be necessary to rehabilitate the patient psychologically to relieve the remaining apprehension and anxiety stemming from past experiences of coital pain.

Reassurance may not be enough. Being cured of a physical problem does not necessarily reverse the patient's sexual comfort index. Therefore, additional psychological approaches may be necessary to allow individuals to undergo transitional changes at their own pace. This total treatment should include some instruction in the Kegel vaginal muscle exercises and the liberal use of a good vaginal lubricant as supportive therapy. Once self-confidence is restored, these adjuncts to sexual communication will be retained or rejected on an individual basis by the patient.

One of our most effective tools has been the sexological examination which teaches the dysfunctional female to utilize these muscle structures of the perineum to enhance her sexual pleasure and to assure a more active role during the coital experience. We recommend the foaming sexual lubricant (Transi-lube) developed in our clinic and currently being distributed by Young's Drug Products, Inc. When vaginal dilation is required, we employ the disposable plastic syringe covers (10 cc, 30 cc, and 50 cc) rather than the more expensive rectal dilators used in the past. These can be given to the patient and disposed of after the need for them expires.

A female co-therapist, counselor, or nurse is the most effective professional person to teach the patient to identify the muscular structures in the perineum and to learn to use the vaginal dilators. She should be present at the time of the sexological examination to allow her to establish a dialogue with the patient. This dialogue will allow her to pick up valuable information as she works with her on a one-to-one basis while giving instructions initially and at subsequent visits.

Dyspareunia, vaginismus, and primary and secondary nonorgasmic response represent a continuum in degree of failure and disappointment for both partners. The cause may be physical, physiologic, or psychological. Initially, the problems create high levels of anxiety, and in the chronic stage, severe depression. In therapy, both the emotional and the physical aspects of the problem need to be treated. Patients should be treated with the full resources of an empathetic physician. The problems of the menopausal patient are unique in that estrogen deprivation and vaginal lubricative dysfunction are the principle causes of dyspareunia in the later years. For these individuals, estrogen replacement therapy provides increased quantity of vaginal secretions both in the quiescent and aroused state, while maintaining a more favorable vaginal pH to combat infection. Replacement therapy should be provided judiciously as in any other menopausal patient.

THE ADNEXAL MASS

JOSEPH C. SCOTT, Jr., M.D.

Adnexal enlargements present clinically with widely variable symptoms. Some will be asymptomatic and are first noted on abdominal or pelvic examination. Others present because of bleeding, torsion, infarction, infection, or pressure on adjacent pelvic organs. Often, the clinical history wedded to the physical findings will allow the clinician to differentiate between uterine, tubal, or ovarian lesions.

During reproductive years the most common adnexal mass will be a functional cyst. These follicle or luteal cysts ordinarily will be no larger than 5 cm in size and will undergo involution without intervention. They should be followed by monthly pelvic examinations. Complete resolution should occur in 2 or 3 months. Involution of functional cysts may be aided with the use of an oral contraceptive pill containing 50 mg of mestranol or ethinyl estradiol to suppress ovarian stimulation by pituitary hormones. Should a suspected functional cyst not resolve in 3 months, further evaluation of the patient is indicated.

Failure of a cyst to regress, or enlargement of the cyst, suggests that the mass may be neoplastic. The more common benign neoplastic cysts in the young woman are the: dermoid, cystadenoma, endometrioma, paraovarian cyst, and inflammatory cyst. The associated physical findings and the patient's history aid in the clinical evaluation. These cysts must be treated surgically.

Evaluation of the persistent adnexal mass has been aided greatly by pelvic ultrasonography. In obese patients and those patients who are clinically difficult to examine, sonography is quite helpful.

Laparoscopy for the evaluation of the persistent adnexal mass is of limited value. Should a mass persist, or be larger than 5 cm, pelvic surgery is indicated for removal. Cystectomy with conservation of the ovary if possible is the treatment of choice. At the time of operation, careful inspection of the pelvic viscera, gentle tissue handling, meticulous hemostasis, and the use of fine absorbable sutures is ideal. Should there be any suspicion of ovarian malignancy, frozen section should be done and peritoneal cytology obtained. If frozen section is not available, the more conservative operation should be done and the definitive histopathology determined later.

Cysts secondary to acute and chronic inflammation most often have adjacent tubal involvement. When inflammation is acute, aggressive antibiotic therapy is indicated. Chronic inflammation will result in hydrosalpinx or pyosalpinx often confluent with the ovary. Conservative treatment with analgesics, antibiotics, and ovulation suppression may help some patients. Those patients unresponsive to this therapy may require surgical therapy, with the operative approach tailored to the extent of the chronic disease. Solid adnexal masses always should arouse a suspicion of an ovarian neoplasm. In any age group, a solid mass deserves immediate evaluation and removal to exclude the possibility of a malignant neoplasm. Benign enlargements such as an ovarian fibroma, Brenner tumor, or leiomyoma may be treated by simple excision.

Malignant solid or cystic ovarian neoplasms deserve accurate surgical staging. The inferior diaphragm, the bowel and mesentery, peritoneal surfaces, and the omentum, should be inspected visually and any suspicious lesions biopsied. Para-aortic lymph nodes may be sampled. Cytologic sampling of the pelvis, lateral peritoneal gutters, and the upper abdomen are important. Total hysterectomy and bilateral salpingo-oophorectomy is the traditional approach for the treatment of ovarian carcinoma. This removal and accurate staging should allow for optimum treatment planning for the individual patient. Rarely in the young patient with a clinical unilateral Stage 1A category tumor, unilateral salpingo-oophorectomy may be done.

Any adnexal enlargement in the peri-menopausal and postmenopausal patient should be aggressively investigated. In these patients there is no latitude for a period of conservative observation. Following medical evaluation, surgical intervention is indicated.

CERVICITIS

DAVID PENT, M.D.

Cervicitis can be divided into two broad general categories: acute and chronic. In acute cervicitis, the clinical signs are similar to those associated with infections in other parts of the body. Chronic cervicitis, on the other hand, is a broad, descriptive term that has been applied to a wide spectrum of processes taking place in the cervix. While some authors use the term chronic cervicitis, others refer to cervical erosion, cervical ectropion, and cervical eversion. These terms have generally been used interchangeably, with no real attempt being made to establish a precise diagnosis. Fortunately, recent advances in colposcopy have contributed greatly to our understanding of the cervix and to the diagnosis and treatment of its lesions.

Acute cervicitis is usually bacterial in origin. It was classically described as arising from gonorrheal or puerperal infections, but in recent years the importance of Chlamydia infections has come to be recognized. The cervix becomes swollen and congested and the mucous membrane pouts out at the external os, with a profuse purulent discharge coming from the cervical canal. This infection in the cervix usually results in few, if any, systemic symptoms in and of itself. However, the infection can spread to the upper genital tract to involve the endometrium, endosalpinx, and pelvic peritoneum, or can spread by direct lymphatic extension to the bladder. In such a case, there are frequently generalized symptoms such as fever, pain, malaise, backache, and urinary tract symptoms, and the treatment of the more serious infection results in the treatment of the cervicitis also.

Before discussing the treatment of chronic cervicitis, it is necessary to understand something of the underlying physiologic and pathologic processes. The cervix is covered with two types of epithelium: the vaginal portion is covered with stratified squamous epithelium, and the cervical canal is lined with tall columnar mucus-secreting cells. (The latter cells apparently form glands and although there is a question as to whether or not these are true glands, they behave as glands.) Colposcopic studies have demonstrated the continuous to and fro movement of the endocervical epithelium, which advances out onto the portio of the cervix and then regresses back toward the cervical canal. This is a dynamic process that goes on throughout the life of the individual so that the endocervical epithelium can be found on the portio of the cervix in fetuses, term newborns, and prepubertal girls as well as being present in 25 per cent of nulligravida females undergoing routine examinations.

"Cervicitis" is generally used to describe the situation in which the red vascular columnar epithelium of the endocervix is clearly visible around the external os, having grown out and replaced the squamous epithelium of the vaginal portion of the cervix. "Erosion" is also commonly used to describe this condition, dating back to when the reddened area was believed to be an area where the normal, pale pink epithelium had been eroded away. (True loss of the cervical epithelium can be demonstrated colposcopically, and is a rare event, usually associated with trauma from instrumentation or from intercourse.) The columnar epithelium on the portio of the cervix frequently becomes infected with both aerobic and anaerobic bacteria, and appears reddened, edematous, hypertrophic, and vascular. It is usually covered with a mucopurulent discharge and bleeds easily on contact.

Erosion should be distinguished from ectropion, which is strictly an eversion of the lips of the cervix, which permits the endocervical epithelium to be easily seen. This eversion is seen following obstetrical delivery and in some cases a fish-mouth laceration of the cervix may allow a considerable portion of the endocervical mucosa to be visualized. Eversion is sometimes seen during pregnancy, secondary to the swelling of the cervix that can occur during gestation. True or real eversion should also be distinguished from the apparent eversion that frequently occurs when the blades of the examining vaginal speculum are separated during the pelvic examination.

On examination, the red granular columnar epithelium is, of course, seen surrounding the cervical os. As noted, the lesion bleeds easily so that some bleeding may be noted initially as a result of the trauma from the insertion of the blades of the speculum, or later when the cervix is scraped to obtain a Pap smear. This can lead to the clinical impression that the lesion is a carcinoma of the cervix, and the most central point in the management of the patient with cervicitis is indeed to rule out a carcinoma of the cervix. This must be done prior to any treatment that will alter or destroy the tissue needed for a pathological diagnosis. A Pap smear is essential, but an adequate Pap smear may be difficult to obtain because of displacement of the squamocolumnar junction and the blood and inflammatory exudate which is often present. Colposcopy should be performed if at all possible, certainly if there are any doubts as to the findings on the smear. Any areas which are suspicious, either clinically or on colposcopic examination, must be biopsied.

Cervical erosion, cervical eversion, and cervicitis are vague and ill-defined terms. They originated at a time when only a naked eye examination of the cervix was available, and that is a time that is long since past. With colposcopy the inadequacy of the naked eye examination has become obvious, and the technique now permits the rapid and specific diagnosis of the actual pathophysiologic process which is taking place. It would be much better to describe the changes that are seen in the cervix in terms of squamous metaplasia, transformation zone, columnar epithelium, and so forth, and hopefully by the time of future editions of this book, the terms erosion, eversion, and cervicitis will be eliminated from the gynecologist's vocabulary.

TREATMENT

In acute cervicitis it is necessary to rule out a gonococcal infection, using modified Thayer-Martin or one of the other special selective media. Treatment consists of aqueous procaine penicillin G, 4.8 million units intramuscularly given at two sites, along with 1.0 gram of probenecid orally. Single dose therapy with ampicillin, 3.5 grams, or amoxicillin, 3.0 grams, along with 1.0 gram of probenecid, all given orally, can also be used. For patients who are allergic to penicillin, tetracycline 500 mg orally 4 times a day for 5 days, may be used. Tetracycline is frequently used, especially if the gonorrhea culture is reported as negative, because it is effective against Chlamydia as well as against the gonococcus.

Treatment of chronic cervicitis should be reserved for those patients who are symptomatic and exhibit associated epithelial changes. Since the predominant symptom of cervicitis is due to the excess mucus production, treatment is directed towards the destruction of the abnormally located endocervical tissue. This is usually accomplished by cauterization or cryosurgery, after any acute infection has been treated and the infection has subsided.

Chemical cautery using silver nitrate is ineffective and really has no role in the definitive treatment of chronic cervicitis. Electrocautery is usually carried out using a flat blade or wire loop heated to a red hot color and with radial strokes extending out from the cervical canal to the portio of the cervix. This is usually done as an outpatient procedure without anesthesia, but it can be somewhat painful. Cauterization has largely been replaced by cryosurgery in those clinics and offices which have the appropriate equipment. The freezing results in rapid destruction of the sensory nerve endings so that the procedure is accompanied by only minimal discomfort, usually a cramping type of pain, and subsequently there is no pain from the necrotic healing area. The configuration of the cryosurgery probe allows it to be applied to a large area of the cervix, permitting rapid treatment of even quite extensive lesions. The usual technique is to freeze the cervix for 3 to 5 minutes, with the ice ball extending approximately 4 to 5 mm out from the edge of the lesion.

Since both cauterization and cryosurgery destroy the cervical tissue at risk for the future development of a malignancy, it is absolutely mandatory that the appropriate studies—Pap smear, colposcopy, biopsy—be carried out prior to treatment. Postoperatively, there is a heavy discharge following cryosurgery, starting on the first day, and this is followed by a copious watery discharge which may be foul smelling and bloody. The watery discharge peaks in approximately 2 weeks. A few patients will report some bleeding, often related to douching or intercourse, so it is probably best to restrict douching and coitus for 2 weeks, by which time the watery discharge will be subsiding.

It is rare for more elaborate procedures to be required, but occasionally a patient who has failed to respond to other measures may be benefited by a surgical approach such as a hot conization or a trachelorrhaphy. This can result in the excision of the glandular areas responsible for the discharge and restore the cervix to a more normal appearance. However, such surgery is really a bit more difficult and definitely less successful than it would appear to be.

PRURITUS VULVAE

THOMAS A. McCARTHY, M.D.

Pruritus vulvae is a term which encompasses many and various conditions of the vulva whose chief symptom is that of itching. This variety of conditions demands a precise diagnosis whenever possible to allow specific therapy. Empirical treatment on the basis of pruritus alone, without adequate diagnostic investigation, is condemned.

Specific conditions which cause intense pruritus of the vulva fall into four categories: infection, neoplasms, various vulvar dystrophies, and allergy. Differentiating these conditions can be difficult but clinical history along with the judicious use of saline and potassium hydroxide slides, culture, and biopsy is the key to diagnosis. Therapy for the common infectious diseases as well as for neoplastic changes of the vulva will not be discussed in this section. The various dystrophies, however, have been the source of much confusion in the past and deserve a more detailed discussion.

For the sake of therapeutic simplicity the International Society for the Study of Vulvar Disease suggests a standard nomenclature for various dystrophic changes. Its simplicity makes treatment of these vulvar conditions easy to understand without the need for lengthy memorization. Dystrophy, which connotes abnormal nutrition, can be either undergrowth (i.e., atrophic) or overgrowth (i.e. hyperplastic). The atrophic dystrophy is currently classified as lichen sclerosus. As an atrophic condition, lichen sclerosus is not associated with malignant potential. On the other hand, hyperplastic dystrophy may be associated with cellular atypia and as such is thought to represent a premalignant lesion. Atypia is classified as mild, moderate, or severe, much along the lines of cervical dysplasia. Occasional patients will have "mixed dystrophy," areas of lichen sclerosus mixed with areas of hyperplastic change. Since dystrophy of all types presents as a white lesion with variable amount of pruritus, biopsy is essential for accurate diagnosis.

Normal skin growth is mediated by local skin trophic hormones called chalones. The chalones work through a negative feedback mechanism upon epidermal cells. The various vulvar dystrophies occur as a result of an abnormality in this negative feedback mechanism. Hyperplastic dystrophy is due to either a decrease in production of chalones by the skin cells or a relative insensitivity of the skin to normal chalone production. Either way the negative feedback mechanism is impaired, allowing epithelial hyperplasia. Again, this may or may not be associated with cellular atypia. Atrophic changes, or lichen sclerosus, occurs when there is an excess of chalones or a relative hypersensitivity to normal chalone concentrations. Therapy for these conditions is aimed at altering this negative feedback mechanism.

In the case of lichen sclerosus, stimulation is required to reverse the atrophic changes in the skin and relieve the pruritic symptoms. The trophic hormone for skin, including skin of the vulva, is testosterone. A common misconception among gynecologists is that estrogen ought to be the stimulating hormone for the vulva. This is not the case; treatment with estrogen may result in further atrophy. The mechanism of testosterone effect is unclear. It either blocks chalone effects at the cellular level or it may have a nonspecific stimulatory effect unrelated to chalones. Topical 2 per cent testosterone ointment is the best treatment for lichen sclerosus. Unfortunately this is not commercially available and must be prepared by individual prescription. 30 cc of 10 per cent testosterone propionate is mixed with 120 grams of white petrolatum. The resultant ointment is sufficient for 8 weeks of treatment. Initially, small amounts should be rubbed in thoroughly three times a day for a period of 6 weeks. Depending on the result, a decrease in frequency of application is then appropriate, decreasing application to once or twice a week depending on the patient's symptoms. Maintenance therapy is mandatory, however, since the condition will recur if therapy is stopped.

Hyperplastic dystrophies, even those with a moderate amount of atypia, should be treated with topcial corticosteroid applications. The effect of the steroid is twofold. The first is to decrease the pruritus associated with the hyperplastic condition. Corticosteroids alone will effectively reduce pruritic symptoms but the addition of Eurax, a topical antipruritic agent, to the steroid preparation will markedly enhance its therapeutic effects. The second effect of steroids is to induce atrophic changes in the skin. The corticosteroid is thought to act as a cofactor for the epidermal chalone, thus decreasing the production rate of skin cells and reversing the hyperplasia. A 0.1 per cent corticosteroid cream such as Lidex, Halog, or Valisone is mixed 7 parts with 3 parts Eurax. The resulting cream is then applied twice daily for 4 to 8 weeks. The therapy is continued until the lesion disappears and then may be discontinued. Unlike testosterone therapy for lichen sclerosus, once the steroids are discontinued the hyperplastic changes rarely recur. If the steroid preparation is inappropriately continued the skin will continue to undergo atrophy, eventually resulting in a condition identical to lichen sclerosus.

In mixed dystrophy, which may also cause intense pruritus, a combination of the above therapies or initial steroid treatment followed by testosterone is appropriate.

Allergic reactions are responsible for vulvar itching in many women. The antigenic agents include anything from laundry detergent and bath salts to feminine deodorant sprays and scented perineal pads. Virtually anything applied to or which comes in contact with the vulva may be the culprit and must be diligently sought in patients having "nonspecific" pruritus. The agents may come from internal sources as well as external ones and include vaginitis, urinary incontinence, or enteric contamination.

Occasionally, no specific cause of the vulvar pruritus is found. In these patients, and for that matter in any patient with vulvar complaints, various nonspecific measures are helpful. A common companion of patients having vulvar symptoms is tight, clinging, synthetic underwear and pants. Obese women tend to wear pants to hide their legs; others are currently caught up in the "designer look" or use panty hose under skirts and dresses. Such garments trap moisture in the vulvar region which may induce irritation, inflammation, and pruritus. Simply advising women to avoid these whenever possible and to seek creative alternatives usually goes a long way in resolving their vulvar symptoms.

Anxiety or other psychoneurotic conditions

may induce pruritic symptoms and scratching. In addition to addressing the psychological issues, oral tranquilizers are effective for short-term relief. Hydroxyzine hydrochloride (Atarax) is quite effective as it has both tranquilizing and antipruritic effects. The usual dose of Atarax is 25 to 50 mg at bedtime or three times daily as needed. If the symptoms are chronic, an itch-scratch cycle is common. Because of itching, the patient scratches. The scratching induces chronic inflammatory and fibrotic changes in the skin which in turn produce further itching. Under these conditions the steroid/Eurax combination is helpful.

A rare patient may not respond to the above measures and have no biopsy evidence of cellular abnormality in the skin. In these patients, injection of alcohol superficially into the skin, destroying the sensory nerve endings, has proved useful. For unknown reasons alcohol injection works primarily for patients complaining of itching and has little effect on those whose primary complaint is burning or pain. The procedure must be performed under general anesthesia. The vulvar skin is marked off in a 1 cm grid pattern. 0.1 to 0.2 cc of absolute ethanol is injected into the subcutaneous tissue at the grid-crossings using a 25 gauge 1/2 inch needle. Too superficial an injection will result in skin blistering whereas too deep an injection may result in tissue necrosis and sloughing. This type of therapy is rarely indicated, however, as most patients will respond to general treatment measures with the addition of specific therapy as indicated.

UTERINE AND VAGINAL ANOMALIES

GEORGE W. MORLEY, M.D.

The sex of the embryo is genetically determined at the time of fertilization; however, the gonads do not appear until the fourth week of embryonic life when they present as undifferentiated genital or gonadal ridges. The genital ducts themselves begin to develop at 6 weeks in both male and female embryos as a pair of Wolffian ducts and Müllerian ducts respectively. At 7 to 8 weeks, gonadal differentiation occurs and at a comparable time the Müllerian ducts from either side join in the midline. This septum may persist for varying periods of time, with fusion being the ultimate goal; thus the normal development of the uterus. Lack of fusion, for whatever reason, gives rise to a variety of duplications of the uterus.

The development of the vagina begins with the caudal portion of the Müllerian duct making contact with the urogenital sinus. This stimulates the development of a sinovaginal bulb which becomes the solid vaginal plate at approximately 10 weeks. At 12 weeks, a lumen begins to develop in the vaginal plate and by the twentieth week, the vaginal plate and the uterus are entirely canalized—unless a congenital defect interferes with this process. This congenital insult usually occurs sometime after the fourth week of embryonic life and this alteration in fetal development is brought about by a variety of teratogenic conditions. Some type of uterine anomaly occurs in 1 in 350 to 500 female births, whereas congenital absence of the vagina occurs in approximately 1 in 2000 female births.

A number of diagnostic procedures should be carried out prior to any type of surgical intervention in these patients. If the patient is sex chromatin–positive as determined on buccal smear examination, then it can be assumed that this patient is a 46 XX female. Should the buccal smear examination be negative, then a more detailed karyotype study from a leukocyte culture is used to determine the exact chromosomal make-up of the patient. Certain roentgenologic studies such as intravenous pyelogram should be performed since unilateral renal agenesis is present in approximately 25 per cent of the phenotypically normal females. Of note, the renal agenesis usually occurs on the side demonstrating the more severe Müllerian defect. On occasion, a pelvic kidney is detected through this examination. Skeletal x-rays may also demonstrate abnormalities seen in association with genital anomalies in approximately 15 per cent of the patients and these abnormalities usually involve congenital changes in the vertebral spine. Diagnostic laparoscopy is seldom indicated in patients with uterine or vaginal abnormalities since an ultrasonographic evaluation can provide an accurate interpretation of the uterine anomalies if present and since the existence of any type of uterine development is extremely rare in those patients with true congenital agenesis of the vagina.

The discussion of other diagnostic studies and the management of patients with congenital anomalies of the female generative tract is divided into two sections to more clearly outline these anomalies in greater detail.

CONGENITAL UTERINE ANOMALIES

One should develop a high index of suspicion from the history given by these patients when they seek medical attention concerning their infertility or their inability to maintain a pregnancy either because of habitual abortion or repeated onset of premature labor.

The simplest morphologic classification of these uterine anomalies is as follows: (1) arcuate uterus—the uterine fundal cavity has a midline curved indentation which requires no surgical correction; (2) a septate uterus—either partial or complete, with the septum extending down to the external cervical os. In these patients, the external configuration is relatively normal; however, internally the septum is incompletely absorbed after fusion of the Müllerian ducts; (3) bicornuate uterus—the two horns are only partially fused and externally this is apparent; (4) a unicornuate uterus with a rudimentary horn—one Müllerian duct fails to descend, with the uterus and opposite tube being formed entirely from the other müllerian duct; (5) didelphic uterus—complete duplication of the uterus and cervix. On rare occasions, there is a short isthmic communication between otherwise separate uterocervical cavities.

Other investigative studies include hysterosalpingography and hysteroscopy. Hysterosalpingography aids one in determining the exact type of uterine abnormality present and hysteroscopy can oftentimes differentiate between a septate and bicornuate uterus. Furthermore, the size of the septum can be determined in this way. Excision of the septum through the hysteroscope has been reported but this approach is still in the experimental stage. If, however, one detects only the presence of a bicornuate uterus or didelphic uterus without evidence of septal prominence, then the patient can be somewhat reassured about future pregnancies since this abnormality carries with it a much better prognosis for pregnancy salvage.

The indications for surgical intervention are primarily related to the number of pregnancies the patient has experienced in the past and the time of spontaneous fetal loss of previous nonviable pregnancies. Patients who have had three successive spontaneous abortions which occurred during the first trimester of pregnancy should have a complete endocrinologic and immunologic investigation along with a thorough evaluation of the male partner before surgical intervention is considered. If, however, the abortions occurred in the second trimester of pregnancy, then one would not wish to wait beyond one or two terminations before surgically correcting the uterine abnormality. The number of fetal sacrifices a patient should undergo before surgical intervention is recommended is a most difficult decision to make and must be at the discretion of the physicians caring for these patients. It is even more difficult to decide when to surgically intervene in patients experiencing premature onset of labor during the third trimester since it is often stated that subsequent pregnancies will be maintained in utero for a longer period of time and thus approach term before the onset of the subsequent labor.

Whether or not infertility itself is an indication for surgical correction of these anomalies is still a debatable issue. Most authors feel that this is not an indication for surgical intervention; however, there are some who feel that there may be a physiologic abnormality as well as an anatomic malformation causing the infertility and thus have suggested that patients with long-term infertility in whom "all else has failed" may be candidates for a unification metroplasty. More recently, a T-shaped uterus has been demonstrated in patients exposed to diethylstilbestrol, with some having difficulty maintaining pregnancies to viability. To date, there has been very little help for these patients.

Once the indications for surgical intervention have been satisfied, then there are a number of ways to treat these patients. Before discussing the more elective treatment, it is important to discuss the emergency conditions which can arise from these developmental changes. Given a patient with a unicornuate uterus and a rudimentary horn containing a functioning endometrial lining, progressive dysmenorrhea can be related to intermittent menstruation within this rudimentary horn. On pelvic examination, this appears as an adnexal mass and is often thought to be an ovarian cyst which may be undergoing periodic torsion. Ultrasonography may aid in this differentiation. Obviously, this patient should be urgently treated with surgical excision of the rudimentary horn. Ectopic pregnancies in the rudimentary horn have also been reported with the sperm migrating through the more intact system followed by transmigration across the peritoneal cavity and into the rudimentary horn through its intact fallopian tube. Emergency surgical intervention is required.

Turning now to the more elective surgical treatment, a unification metroplasty when indicated should be performed during the proliferative phase of the patient's menstrual cycle. The original unification metroplastic procedure as described by Strassman was primarily used to correct a bicornuate or didelphic uterus. The uterine cavities are opened through a transverse incision extending from one cornua to the other and the partition between them is incised down the middle. The transverse incision in the uterus is then converted into a vertical suture line with anteroposterior closure of the incised defect.

Since this incision is in close proximity to the fallopian tubes at their junction into the cornua, one should be cautious in the closure of this defect so as not to obstruct either tubal ostium.

The Jones metroplasty effectively *excises* the uterine septum by making two vertical incisions in the shape of a "V" on either side of the septum. This, however, results in the excision of some myometrial tissue as well. Once this wedge of tissue is removed, the defect is closed in three layers in a vertical fashion using absorbable suture.

In the Tompkins metroplasty, the uterus is divided from above downward in the anteroposterior direction *through* the septum until the endometrial cavity is encountered. The septum on either side of the "bi-valved" uterus is then incised or excised without removal of myometrial tissue. The uterine walls are then approximated using appropriate sized absorbable suture. This technique is suitable for all varieties of bicornuate-unicollis uteri; the choice of metroplasty, however, may depend on the type of uterine anomaly encountered or more importantly on the preference of the physician caring for the patient.

Should there ever be an indication for metroplasty of a didelphic uterus, then one should remember only to unify the fundal portions of the myometrium without any surgical correction being directed toward either cervix since this could give rise to an incompetent internal cervical os.

One must avoid trauma to the existing myometrial tissues in attempting to enter the endometrial cavity through the uterine incision. A uterine sound inserted transvaginally can aid one in locating the uterine cavities. On occasion, these procedures can be quite vascular and the bleeding can be controlled by manual compression or by placing a soft rubber (Penrose) tourniquet around the the lower uterine segment and infundibulo-pelvic ligaments. Infiltration of a weak solution of phenelyphrine hydrochloride (Neo-Synephrine) or vasopressin (Pitressin) is appropriate. Whether or not an omental or peritoneal patch placed over the myometrial incision is necessary remains a debatable issue but is recognized by some as a prevention against the formation of adhesions.

These patients' postoperative course is usually uncomplicated and they are discharged from the hospital in 5 to 7 days. Most investigators feel that these patients should not become pregnant for at least 3 months; however, there are others who feel that a pregnancy can occur at any time in the postoperative period. Whether or not these patients should be delivered by cesarean section or be allowed a trial of labor is another debatable issue, with most physicians thinking that the risk of uterine rupture secondary to an attempt at vaginal delivery is too great for this so-called premium pregnancy; therefore, delivery at or near term by cesarean section is more frequently supported.

The existence of an incompetent internal cervical os, whether it be considered an additional anomaly or related to the uterine malformation, must be kept in mind in following these patients throughout subsequent pregnancies. Should an incompetency of the cervix be encountered, then surgical correction should be performed immediately.

The results from these various unification procedures are gratifying. From a review of the literature, it can be reported that the obstetric performance prior to unification metroplasty shows the fetal wastage to be approximately 75 per cent. The reverse is true subsequent to surgical correction, with 75 per cent fetal salvage being the usual result. Some authors have reported a 90 per cent success rate.

CONGENITAL AGENESIS OF THE VAGINA

A high index of suspicion of congenital absence of the vagina should be developed in taking a history from patients who state they are 14 to 15 years of age and have never menstruated. This speculation is further reinforced when the patient states that it is impossible for her to experience intromission during coital desires. The principal clinical characteristics of the Rokitansky-Küster-Hauser syndrome are noted on physical and pelvic examination. These patients have normal breast development, normal body contours, and normal female distribution of axillary and pubic hair. On pelvic examination, the vagina is absent and often one sees only an introital dimple or pouch which represents the urogenital sinus. Parenthetically, it should be noted that not infrequently patients participate in "urethral coitus" with progressive dilatation of the urethra from repeated intercourse. Interestingly enough, these patients do not complain of dyspareunia; they are most often continent of urine, and urinary tract infection does not occur from this type of exposure.

The uterus is absent in over 95 per cent of these patients; however, a thin fibrous band may be noted streaking across the pelvis on internal inspection. These patients experience normal ovarian function and ovulation since the ovaries are developed independently from the gonadal ridge and not from the Müllerian duct system.

The timing of the treatment of these patients is extremely important since understanding and motivation on the patient's part is necessary in anticipating a satisfactory result. These patients are usually treated after they have obtained full growth, somewhere between 17 and 20 years of age. Psychological preparation is extremely important and counseling provided either by the attending physician or by a psychologist-psychiatrist is absolutely necessary since these patients often consider themselves defective and the vaginal atresia is a threat to their body image. Unfortunately, some of these feelings are iatrogenically induced since physicians often tell these patients that they were born with no vagina and that an artificial vagina can be built for them. A more appropriate approach seems to be, "Yes, you have an incompletely developed vagina but we can create a functioning vagina for you." If handled appropriately, these patients do quite well.

These patients should be socially and sexually mature so that they are able to understand the importance and inconvenience of the operative procedure and are appropriately motivated toward carrying out the postoperative instructions. Most of these patients adjust quite satisfactorily to the fact that they will be unable to have children.

The operation itself was first described by Dupuytren in 1817; however, subsequent to this initial effort, many variations have appeared in the literature. MacIndoe in 1938 described what is currently considered the surgical treatment of choice. After the patient is placed in the lithotomy position and is appropriately prepared, a transverse incision is made in the vestibular epithelium with protection of the external urethral meatus anteriorly. In developing the neovagina, both blunt and sharp dissection are carried out through the loose fibroareolar tissue which lies between the bladder anteriorly and the rectum posteriorly and this dissection extends up to the peritoneal reflection. On occasion, one encounters a vaginal stenosis or "hour-glass vagina" postoperatively with constriction at the level of the levator muscles. This complication can be avoided by making relaxing incisions part way through the levator musculature bilaterally at 3 and 9 o'clock. Once the neovaginal vault is developed, then meticulous hemostasis must be accomplished before the donor skin graft is introduced into this area.

A split-thickness skin graft measuring 6 to 8 cm by 18 to 20 cm is taken either by a Brown or Padget dermatome set at 0.018 to 0.020 of an inch in thickness. The donor site for the skin graft is chosen after consultation with the patient and is usually taken either from the posterior thigh so that the patient does not see the scar each time she sits down or from the buttocks so that the donor site is covered by normal wearing apparel. It has always been our policy to prepare the split-thickness skin graft after preparation of the recipient site—the neovaginal vault. The skin graft is then applied to a glass, Silastic, or foam rubber obturator satisfying the individual preferences of the surgeon. The graft covers the obturator in longitudinal fashion, thus avoiding the "wrap-around" technique, and the seams are sutured along the free edges of the graft on both sides of the obturator. In this way, the apex of the obturator is covered with an uninterrupted segment of skin which improves the "take" at the vaginal apex.

Once the skin graft is applied to the obturator and again after meticulous hemostasis has been assured, the obturator is inserted into the newly developed vaginal vault without undue pressure being applied up against the urethra anteriorly. After a catheter is placed in the bladder (some prefer surprapubic drainage), the labial tissues are approximated in front of the exposed end of the obturator. This maintains the obturator in a preferred position and mobilization of the graft is minimized.

Postoperatively, it is anticipated that the obturator will remain in place for 5 to 7 days. Throughout the first 4 to 5 days, the patient is maintained on a liquid diet in an attempt to avoid colonic activity. The patient is strictly confined to bed for 3 days; however, "log-rolling" is permitted. After this 72 hour period has passed, the patient is instructed on an appropriate method of ambulation so that she can be up and about. Obviously, the patient should not sit down in a chair or sit up in bed. Prophylactic antibiotics may or may not be used, at the discretion of the attending physician.

The obturator is removed for the first time on the fifth or seventh day. The neovagina is irrigated with a standard cleansing douche solution and the patient is fitted with a more permanent obturator prepared from some type of non-breakable material. A polyfoam type of obturator is fashioned for the patient and is covered with a condom which facilitates periodic removal and insertion to allow for urination, fecal evacuation, and a cleansing douche once or twice per day. Except when the obturator must be temporarily removed, it is maintained in position 24 hours a day for a period of 3 months. The patient may become sexually active some time after the fourth postoperative week and a normal sexual response is anticipated in almost all these patients once they have become accustomed to this reconstruction.

Complications are infrequent and are usually of a minor degree. Fistulous formation is extremely uncommon and can be corrected by conventional means. On rare occasion, a distal urethral slough does occur from pressure necrosis but this can be avoided by instituting appropriate preventive measures.

An unsatisfactory result is usually reported as a "poor take." This can occur if satisfactory hemostasis is not accomplished at the time of surgery or if the recipient site becomes infected. An unsatisfactory result can also occur if the patient is not well motivated and does not cooperate with the physician in carrying out the postoperative instructions. It is estimated that the usual "take" is well over 90 per cent.

The Williams labioplasty, described in 1964, has been used as an alternative to the MacIndoe procedure primarily by our English colleagues. In this procedure, an external pouch is developed utilizing the labial tissues. A horseshoe-shaped incision is made around the posterior fourchette of the vagina with extension up either side just within the hairline of the labia majora to a point parallel to the urethral orifice. After the tissues are appropriately freed up from the underlying connective tissues, the inner skin margins are joined together using absorbable suture. The underlying tissues are united as a support to this initial closure. The lateral skin margins are then approximated in the midline in a similar fashion. Whereas this technique is quite popular in the United Kingdom, it is thought that most gynecologic surgeons in the United States do not believe it to be the treatment of choice for the correction of congenital absence of the vagina and they usually reserve this type of vulvoplasty for patients who wish to regain their sexual function after undergoing total pelvic exenteration or after experiencing foreshortening of the vagina secondary to radiation therapy of overcorrective vaginal surgery.

The Frank procedure was first described in 1938, the same year of the MacIndoe report, but as a nonsurgical treatment of congenital absence of the vagina. It has been thought that the loose fibroareolar tissue which is interposed between the bladder and the rectal tissues could be satisfactorily invaginated if patients would conscientiously carry out the physician's instructions utilizing graduated dilators. Currently this approach is becoming more and more popular in the treatment of congenital agenesis of the vagina at least initially with the hopes that the surgical correction can be avoided.

A variety of techniques have been described utilizing the nonsurgical approach with the patient sitting either on a firm chair or some other solid structure for 1 to 2 hours twice daily while studying or while watching television. These graduated dilators are made of a soft Silastic or polyethylene material, and if the patient is appropriately motivated, one can see significant progress at the time of re-examination in 4 to 8 weeks. At 16 weeks, a most satisfactory result is seen. Psychologically, these patients very much prefer the nonsurgical technique, which tends to lessen the degree of severity of the abnormality in their own minds. If, however, this technique does not bring about a satisfactory result, then time loss alone is the only delay prior to corrective surgical therapy.

As stated before, on a rare occasion, a chromosomal abnormality is detected in these patients. If the patient is a karyotypically 46 XY male pseudohermaphrodite as seen in testicular feminizing syndrome caused by androgen insensitivity, then not only does the vaginal agenesis have to be corrected but a gonadectomy must be performed in the late teens since these gonads, if retained, may undergo malignant degeneration. These gonads are usually located intra-abdominally but may be present in the inguinal or labial tissues. These patients are maintained on long-term cyclic estrogen-progesterone therapy.

Congenital absence of the vagina with some type of uterine development is rare. These patients should be considered akin to patients with transverse vaginal septa where the septum mimics congenital vaginal atresia.

A number of other vaginal anomalies must be considered in the differential diagnosis of congenital vaginal agenesis. A transverse vaginal septum is the second type of vaginal atresia. This occurs in approximately 1 in 75,000 births and most commonly appears at the junction of the upper and middle third of the vagina. On occasion, however, this septum can mimic vaginal agenesis since it can involve almost the entire vaginal tube. Most of these patients have a functioning uterus located cephalad to the vaginal septum. Symptomatically, these patients complain of increasing periodic pelvic pain which is secondary to cryptomenorrhea as well as dyspareunia which is secondary to the marked foreshortening of the vagina. As the hematometra increases, these patients may have difficulty with urination. This congenital disorder can be successfully corrected surgically through a transvaginal approach; in fact, the transabdominal approach not only is unnecessary but is undesirable. A transverse incision is made through the distal septal mucosal wall of the vagina. Once this mucosal layer is freed from the septum proper, then the body of the septum is widely excised by sharp dissection. This can be vascular on occasion. Following this, another transverse incision is made in the proximal mucosal wall of the septum. These mucosal flaps are then approximated using absorbable sutures. The healing of these repairs is uniformly satisfactory and the use of a vaginal obturator until healing is complete helps to prevent a vaginal stricture at the operative site. If properly recognized and treated, the long-term prognosis is excellent for maintaining a patent and functional vagina. On occasion, the transverse vaginal septum is perforated and pregnancies have been reported in these patients.

The longitudinal vaginal septum is much more frequently encountered and the related symptoms are less dramatic. If these patients are asymptomatic, then no treatment is required. If, however, they complain of dyspareunia, then the septum can be removed surgically utilizing standard hemostatic techniques, or if dystocia is encountered during labor, then a similar approach can be used at that time.

An imperforate hymen is the third type of vaginal atresia to be described. This abnormality can give rise to a mucocolpos shortly after birth or to a hematocolpos-hematometra-hematosalpinx complex in the menarcheal period. A high index of suspicion is the sine qua non of diagnosis, and once entertained, the treatment is straightforward. Cruciate incisions are made in the imperforate hymenal tissue with an immediate expression of a thick, chocolate-colored fluid through the incisional site. The hymenal ring is then appropriately dilated, and bleeding, if encountered, is controlled without difficulty. These patients have no problems in the future related to this defect.

A pinpoint opening in an otherwise complete hymenal membrane which allows for normal egress of menstrual fluid can give rise to unnecessary surgical intervention. A number of these patients have been operated upon hoping that an appropriate incision and dissection would bring about a direct communication with the vaginal vault. This is not only unnecessary but unwise, since scarring can develop in this area which must be excised at a later date. It is therefore suggested that these patients be examined in the office during menstruation so that the pinpoint opening can be located and recorded and the treatment can be appropriately instituted at some later date under anesthesia. These pinpoint openings are most frequently located somewhere along the periphery of the hymenal ring.

Lastly, anomalies involving malformation of both the vagina and the uterus can be diagnostically challenging, especially when a unilateral obstructive septum exists in the vagina. The diagnosis is not always easy because there may be normal menstrual bleeding from the unobstructed side. A unilateral vaginal septum that is obstructive requires surgical incision and drainage through this septal anomaly. This treatment offers the patient complete relief of symptoms while preserving reproductive capacity.

SUMMARY

Uterine and vaginal anomalies may adversely affect the sexual roles or the reproductive capabilities of patients experiencing these congenital anomalies. Therefore, these conditions merit thorough evaluation and appropriate treatment and it is incumbent upon the examining physician to be aware of these possibilities when seeing patients with chief complaints suggesting these congenital defects. Early recognition is the secret to success!

Section 4
GYNECOLOGIC ONCOLOGY

CARCINOMA OF THE VULVA

PETER E. SCHWARTZ, M.D.

The vulva is the fourth most common site for the development of a malignant lesion in the female pelvic reproductive organs. Malignant lesions occur most often in older women and usually are squamous cell cancers. Melanomas and adenocarcinomas may also arise at this site, but represent less than 5 per cent of all vulvar malignancies. Cancer developing in other pelvic organs may metastasize to the vulva, and must be distinguished from a primary vulvar lesion.

Many factors have been associated with squamous cell cancers of the vulva including infections (viral, bacterial, protozoan) and chronic vulvar dystrophies. Approximately 10 per cent of patients with cervical cancer will develop vulvar cancer. A spectrum of histopathologic changes from dysplasia to carcinoma in situ to microinvasive cancer to invasive cancer have been identified in the vulva. Although similar changes have been demonstrated to be present in the uterine cervix and progression to invasive cervical cancer established in patients with preceding cervical intraepithelial neoplasia, progression from dysplasia to invasive cancer of the vulva has infrequently been reported. Indeed, those individuals most likely to progress from carcinoma in situ to invasive cancer are either elderly or immune suppressed. The incidence of vulvar carcinoma in situ in the State of Connecticut has increased 40-fold in the past 30 years, but the incidence of invasive vulvar cancer has remained unchanged. It is possible that this is a reflection of better surveillance of women by physicians as many of the patients who are developing vulvar carcinoma in situ are under age 40.

The diagnosis of a vulvar neoplasm must be suspected in any woman with a chronic irritation which fails to respond to topical therapy, as well as in a patient in whom an ulcerative or exophytic lesion develops. The extent of a precancerous change may be determined by application of toluidine blue solution to the entire vulva and then counterstaining 1 minute later with 3 per cent acetic acid solution. Vulvar carcinoma in situ is often multifocal. The toluidine blue stain will persist in abnormal cells following the application of acetic acid. Representative biopsies should be performed in each area which retains the toluidine blue stain. Colposcopy is another technique for evaluating vulvar precancerous changes, but requires more experience than using the toluidine blue technique.

The management of vulvar squamous cell carcinoma in situ may be individualized. Patients found to have a single focus of carcinoma in situ may be treated with wide local excision of the lesion. Patients treated in this fashion must understand that the carcinoma may recur, and careful follow-up is mandatory. In addition, these patients are at higher risk for developing carcinoma in situ of the uterine cervix and should have Pap smears performed on a routine basis, at least annually, thereafter. Patients found to have multifocal vulvar carcinoma in situ require more extensive surgery in the form of a "skinning" vulvectomy. This procedure strips the vulvar skin from the underlying fatty tissue. The vulvectomy site may then be closed over primarily by mobilizing the adjacent skin, or may be covered with a split-thickness skin graft. Preservation of the underlying fatty tissue permits a cushion of tissue to cover the pubic bones, thereby avoiding or reducing dyspareunia. The need for follow-up care and evaluation of the cervix applies to patients with multifocal vulvar carcinoma in situ as well as to those with an isolated focus.

Experimental techniques to treat vulvar carcinoma in situ include laser beam treatments using colposcopic guidance to vaporize the abnormal sites, and the application of cytotoxic chemotherapeutic agents to the involved sites. Each technique appears to be less mutilating than a skinning vulvectomy, but long-term follow-up is lacking. Topical applications of 5-fluorouracil have given inconsistent results. These techniques are quite appropriate for managing recurrent carcinoma in situ for which standard treatment has failed.

Paget's disease of the vulva may be categorized as a premalignant change. It typically presents as a velvety red lesion which at times is quite extensive, extending beyond the vulva to the thighs. Often, the disease extends much further microscopically than is grossly obvious. The margins of surgical resection from tissues removed at wide local excision or vulvectomy should be evaluated microscopically before the surgical procedure is completed in order to avoid inadequate excision. Paget's disease of the vulva may be associated with an underlying apocrine gland carcinoma. The presence of the latter requires management by radical vulvectomy and bilateral superficial inguinal lymphadenectomies. The presence of metastatic adenocarcinoma to the inguinal lymph nodes is an ominous prognostic finding, as almost all patients with regional lymph node metastases succumb to the disease.

Invasive squamous cell carcinoma most often develops in the labia majora and spreads by direct extension to adjacent structures. Advanced cancers may involve the urethra, vagina, anus, rectum, or bladder. These cancers also metastasize via lymphatics and routinely involve the regional lymph nodes in the inguinal area before spreading to the deep pelvic lymph nodes. Regional lymph node involvement is an important prognostic factor. The 5-year survival for patients without lymph node metastases is approximately 80 per cent, but declines to approximately 50 to 60 per cent when 1 to 3 lymph nodes have metastatic squamous cell cancer, and to less than 25 per cent when 4 or more nodes are involved. This orderly spread to regional lymphatics allows for radical surgery to systematically remove the initial sites of local extension as well as regional lymphatics. Carcinoma of the clitoris, a disease thought in the past to spread directly to deep pelvic lymphatics without involving the superficial inguinal lymphatics, has now been shown to spread in the same orderly fashion as cancer arising in other sites in the vulva.

Recently, attention has been focused on the performance of less than radical surgery when microinvasive cancer of the vulva has been found. The definition of microinvasive cancer has yet to be established, but it is apparent that small superficially invasive cancers (<2 cm diameter, <5 mm invasion) infrequently spread to the regional lymph nodes. Patients with superficially invasive cancers may be satisfactorily treated with radical vulvectomies only; however, it would appear preferable to sample regional lymph nodes in the groins and subject them to frozen section analysis at the time of vulvectomy. If an occult metastasis is identified, the patient should undergo bilateral superficial inguinal and deep pelvic lymphadenectomy, as occasional patients have died from metastatic vulvar carcinoma following the diagnosis of microinvasive vulvar carcinoma.

Invasive squamous cell carcinoma may be associated with ulcerative or exophytic lesions. Symptoms are usually present for many months or years. Patients have frequently been treated with topical creams, including steroids, for apparent vulvar dystrophies with inconsistent results, and have then developed obvious lesions.

The management of patients with invasive squamous cancer of the vulva is based in part on clinical staging. The TNM system is most frequently employed in the United States and is shown in Table 1. The standard practice at most institutions for managing lesions confined to the vulva with clinically negative or suspicious regional lymph nodes is to perform a radical vulvectomy and bilateral superficial inguinal lymphadenectomies. Patients found to have metastases to the regional lymph nodes should undergo deep pelvic lymphadenectomies. The usual incision employed for this surgery extends from 2 cm medial to the right iliac crest, across the mons pubis to the contralateral site 2 cm medial to the left iliac crest. The lateral aspects of the skin incisions are extended caudad to each labiocrural fold and join across the perineum. The superficial inguinal lymphadenectomy is usually performed first. The margins of the lymphadenectomy are the fascia overlying the inguinal canal cranially, the sartorius muscle laterally, the adductor longus muscle medially, and the adductor canal caudally. The skin and underlying fatty tissue are excised en bloc down to and including the femoral sheath. The sartorius muscle can be readily mobilized off the inguinal ligament and transposed medially as a protective covering for the exposed femoral artery and vein. If frozen section analysis reveals cancer metastatic to the inguinal lymph nodes, a deep pelvic lymphadenectomy may be performed. The retroperitoneal space is exposed by dividing the external and internal oblique fascia overlying the inguinal canal as well as the transversalis fascia. The inferior epigastric artery and vein and the round ligament must also be divided. The limits of the deep pelvic lymphadenectomy

TABLE 1. **TNM Classification of Carcinoma of the Vulva**

T Primary tumor

T1	Tumor confined to the vulva, 2 cm or less in largest diameter
T2	Tumor confined to the vulva, more than 2 cm in diameter
T3	Tumor of any size with adjacent spread to the urethra and/or vagina and/or perineum and/or anus
T4	Tumor of any size infiltrating the bladder mucosa and/or the rectal mucosa or both, including the upper part of the urethral mucosa, and/or fixed to the bone

N Regional lymph nodes

N0	No nodes palpable
N1	Nodes palpable in either groin, not enlarged, mobile (not clinically suspicious of neoplasm)
N2	Nodes palpable in either groin or both groins, enlarged, firm and mobile (clinically suspicious of neoplasm)
N3	Fixed or ulcerated nodes.

M Distant metastases

M0	No clinical metastases
M1a	Palpable deep pelvic lymph nodes
M1b	Other distant metastases

are the common iliac artery superiorly, the psoas muscle laterally, the hypogastric artery medially, and the obturator fossa posteriorly.

The radical vulvectomy is then performed. This procedure is distinguished from a simple vulvectomy by the extent of its margins (labiocrural folds laterally, mons pubis superiorly, and perineum inferiorly) and by the depth of resection to the level of the deep fascia overlying the pubic bones.

Locally advanced vulvar cancers may require pelvic exenteration along with radical vulvectomies and superficial inguinal and deep pelvic lymphadenectomies. Vulvar lesions may extensively involve the urethra, vagina, anus, rectum or bladder. Preoperative external beam radiation therapy has been reported to dramatically reduce the size of some advanced vulvar cancers, making them susceptible to more conventional therapy and sparing the patient the need for a colostomy or urinary conduit.

Immediate complications of radical vulvectomies and superficial inguinal and deep pelvic lymphadenectomies include lymphocyst formation and wound infections. Lymphocyst formation may be reduced by using pressure dressings and suction catheters and by keeping the patient on strict bed rest for 5 to 7 days. Wound infections may be reduced with broad-spectrum prophylactic antibiotics, careful surgical technique including minimally undermining skin flaps, meticulous attention to hemostasis, and avoiding fecal contamination postoperatively by limiting oral intake for 5 to 7 days. Thrombophlebitis may be avoided by treating patients with prophylactic heparin until they are ambulatory.

Surgeons have attempted to limit wound disruption by employing ellipsoid incisions for the lymphadenectomies and leaving a bridge of skin between the lymphadenectomy sites and the vulvectomy site. Myocutaneous grafts have permitted the transposition of skin grafts with underlying fatty tissue and muscle to the groin dissection and vulvectomy sites. These grafts retain their own arterial blood supply and allow primary healing even when extensive dissections have been performed. Tensor fasciae latae and gracilis myocutaneous grafts seem well suited for this purpose.

Long-term complications of radical vulvectomies and superficial inguinal and deep pelvic lymphadenectomies include lower extremity edema and less frequently erysipelas. Edema can be managed by panty-hose type support stockings specially measured for the patient while she is still in the hospital recuperating from surgery. They should be put on in the morning when the patient is getting out of bed and worn until she retires for the evening. The foot of the bed should routinely be elevated 6 inches. Pneumomassage techniques may be useful if edema recurs. Prophylactic long-term antibiotics have been recommended to prevent erysipelas.

Malignant melanoma may infrequently present as a primary vulvar malignancy. Superficially invasive melanomas may be adequately treated with radical vulvectomies and bilateral inguinal lymphadenectomies. Most vulvar melanomas present with obvious lymph node metastases, and a chest-x-ray will usually confirm the presence of distant metastases. Once vulvar melanoma spreads to regional lymph nodes, the prognosis is invariably poor. Palliative resection of the primary lesion may play a role in providing local comfort for the patient, and chemotherapy or immunotherapy may control the disease for a period of time.

Adenocarcinomas infrequently present as primary cancers of the vulva. In addition to apocrine gland carcinoma found in association with Paget's disease of the vulva, the Bartholin's gland may be a source of a primary vulvar adenocarcinoma. Bartholin's gland adenocarcinomas have a poor prognosis, as they develop deep to the skin surface and may be quite advanced when they become clinically obvious. Carcinomas arising from Bartholin's gland ducts form squamous carcinomas. Management of these cancers is the same as for invasive squamous cell cancers arising at other sites in the vulva.

Basal cell carcinomas occasionally develop in the vulva. They are treated by wide local excision. Sarcomas rarely develop in this area and are usually treated by wide local excision. Lymphadenectomy is unnecessary as sarcomas tend to metastasize hematogenously. Cancer metastatic to the vulva may be treated with excisional biopsy and subsequent therapy directed at the primary site of the cancer. Recurrent metastases may be treated with excision or local radiation therapy, but long-term control is usually not achieved.

NEOPLASIA OF THE CERVIX

PHILIP J. DiSAIA, M.D.

The unique accessibility of the cervix to cell and tissue study and to direct physical examination has permitted intensive investigation of the nature of malignant lesions of the cervix. Its accessibility to cytologic study has contributed to the decreasing mortality of cancer of this organ.

Easy access to the cervix has also led to the skillful application of radiation techniques, which have resulted in the best overall cure rates for any malignancy found in human beings.

The cause of cervical cancer is not known, but its development seems related to the multiple insults and injuries sustained by the cervix. Cervical carcinoma is virtually nonexistent in the celibate population; only one case has been reported in the literature. It is more prevalent in women of lower socioeconomic groups, and it is correlated with first coitus at an early age and with multiple sexual partners. There is no correlation with frequency of sexual intercourse. Herpesvirus type 2 has received attention as a possible etiologic agent for cervical cancer.

The mean age of patients with carcinoma in situ of the cervix is some 10 to 15 years less than the mean age of patients with invasive disease. It should be kept in mind that the difference is, at best, a rough approximation of the duration of intraepithelial carcinoma in its assumed progression to clinical invasive cancer. However, data such as these serve to emphasize the essential nature of cytologic screening programs and possibly colposcopy performed on a periodic basis. Although these early phases may be asymptomatic, they are detectable by currently available methods. This concept of development of cervical cancer has convinced many that the control of this disease is well within our grasp in the foreseeable future. We can eradicate most deaths from cervical cancer by using the diagnostic and therapeutic techniques now available.

Evaluation of the abnormal cytologic cervical smear requires consideration of several basic premises. First, the cervical cytologic smear, or Pap test, is not a diagnostic tool but a screening device. Diagnosis rests on tissue biopsy. Secondly, while the Pap test is valid for the screening of cervical neoplasia, it is not an adequate tool for screening of other genital tract lesions. Malignant conditions of the corpus, tubes, or ovaries are infrequently associated with positive cervical cytologic findings. Third, the Pap test must be performed with care to yield optimum accuracy. The cervix must be sampled at the squamocolumnar junction where most lesions apparently originate. Fourth, and most important, several nonmalignant causes such as condyloma acuminatum, inflammation, regeneration after injury, and previous radiation therapy, may produce abnormal results on cytology.

The staging of cervical cancer is a clinical appraisal, preferably confirmed with the patient under anesthesia. Since regional involvement is typical of this disease, a careful inspection of the vagina for extension to that organ should be carried out, as well as a skillfully done rectovaginal examination to note any extension of disease to the parametrial tissues. The following diagnostic procedures are acceptable for determining a staging classification: physical examination, routine radiographs, colposcopy, cytoscopy, proctosigmoidoscopy, intravenous pyelogram, and barium studies of the lower colon and rectum. Other examinations, such as lymphangiography, arteriography, venography, laparoscopy, exploratory laparotomy, and CT scanning, are not at this time acceptable diagnostic aids for staging, although they may be utilized and treatment may be based on pertinent findings. International rules of staging require that the patient's stage not incorporate these data.

CERVICAL INTRAEPITHELIAL NEOPLASIA

The treatment of intraepithelial neoplasia of the cervix has been quite varied over the past two decades. The wide use of colposcopy for study of the transformation zone of the cervix has allowed the physician to pinpoint the abnormal cervical epithelium. Removal or destruction of this epithelium by a variety of techniques is then possible. When the physician is a skilled colposcopist and the area of involvement has been determined to be quite small, simple local excision may be an acceptable procedure performed in the office without anesthesia. Others have used hot cautery to destroy the abnormal epithelium.

During the last two decades, considerable experience with cryosurgery has been obtained in the treatment of cervical intraepithelial neoplasia (CIN). The side-effects of electrocautery, mainly pain during treatment, are not present with cryosurgery, and thus, it is an ideal outpatient modality as far as acceptance by patients is concerned. There is general agreement that cryosurgery is quite effective in treating CIN-I and CIN-II disease (mild and moderate dysplasia) as compared with other methods. The use of cryosurgery for the treatment of CIN-III lesions (severe dysplasia or carcinoma in situ) has recently been somewhat controversial. Some authors have shown a very large recurrence rate (30 to 40 per cent) when using this modality for treatment of CIN-III lesions, while other authors have reported recurrence rates (5 to 10 per cent) which are much more acceptable. Suffice it to say that the efficacy of cryosurgery for treatment of CIN-III lesions is, at this time, unsettled.

Cryosurgery is performed utilizing either nitrous oxide or carbon dioxide, and this technique appears to be effective in destroying approximately 90 per cent of the cervical epithelium of lesions treated. Although some practitioners prefer the single freeze, our experience has shown that the freeze-thaw-freeze technique has been more effective. In freezing a cervix, several conditions must be met: adequate pressure in the refrigerant tank must be present both at the beginning and at the completion of the freeze; the probe should cover the lesion identified colposcopically; a 4 to 5 mm iceball around the probe is required in order to obtain adequate freezing depth. The application of lubricating jelly to the probe facilitates the freezing process. The cervix is then allowed to thaw, which usually requires 5 to 10 minutes, and then the probe is reapplied and the process repeated. The patient is then seen in 4 months for follow-up examination and cytologic study. In some instances, 5 to 6 months is required after cryosurgery before cytologic findings will return to normal. In many instances, the initial Pap smear after cryosurgery may be abnormal, but this may only indicate the healing process and not necessarily a failure of the procedure itself.

Another promising new development in the treatment of cervical intraepithelial neoplasia has been the introduction of the surgical laser. As with any modality, time and experience are needed to see if the clinical reality will meet theoretical promise. The carbon dioxide laser, currently in clinical use, has an electrical discharge produced from a mixture of carbon dioxide, nitrogen, and helium, giving rise to an invisible continuous infrared beam. Laser therapy is followed by a much shorter healing process than cryotherapy. Perhaps even more significant, it would appear that with completion of the re-epithelialization process, the original architecture of the cervix is fully preserved after laser therapy, and the squamocolumnar junction remains visible. With cryotherapy, migration of the transformation zone up the endocervical canal is common, thus obscuring this critical diagnostic structure. It would appear that recurrence rates may be as low as or even lower than with cryosurgery. As with any new modality, long-term studies are needed before any cogent conclusion can be reached regarding laser surgery. Our experience suggests two disadvantages to the technique that we have not experienced with cryosurgery. First, the process is more painful for the office patient than cryosurgery, and secondly, the destruction of all but the smallest lesions requires much more time from both patient and physician.

Surgical conization of the cervix can be both a diagnostic and therapeutic approach to cervical intraepithelial neoplasia. This approach is always preferable where any suspicion of invasive cancer exists. Its overriding advantage lies in the fact that tissue is made available for careful histologic examination, unlike the destructive techniques described above. Most physicians currently utilize conization of the cervix for large or diffuse lesions of the cervix, especially those in the CIN-III category. In addition, conization is essential when colposcopic examination of the cervix is unsatisfactory. It remains the best method currently available for ruling out invasive disease. Cervical conization need not be a fixed technical procedure for all patients, but it should always be an adequate excision of all involved areas. Bleeding from the cone bed is usually controlled by hemostatic sutures such as anterior-posterior Sturmdorf sutures or a running-lock suture of heavy suture material encompassing the entire circumference of the cone bed. Others prefer to establish hemostasis with cautery and leave the cone bed open to healing by secondary intention. Significant cervical stenosis, cervical incompetence, and infertility due to a cervical factor are rare complications and are functions of the amount of endocervix removed. Thus, it behooves the physician to tailor the size of the cone biopsied to the extent of the disease, carefully avoiding the removal of excess tissue.

Decisions as to the choice of therapy for cervical intraepithelial neoplasia depend on many factors, including the patient's attitude and the experience of the physicians involved. Removal of the cervix or hysterectomy continues to be the definitive therapy for patients who are fully informed regarding the implications to their childbearing capacity and are in agreement in spite of the small but increased risks associated with a major operative procedure. Patients with CIN-I and II lesions who wish to maintain optimum fertility should be considered for local therapy, including cryosurgery, laser surgery, and, when possible, local excision. Conization is preferred for patients with diffuse CIN-III lesions regardless of whether the limits of the lesions can be defined colposcopically.

MICROINVASIVE CARCINOMA OF THE CERVIX

Microinvasive carcinoma of the cervix is a subject that has been associated with two decades of confusion. Diagnostic issues have been confused, and investigators have reported conflicting results on what appears to be the same subset of the patient population. Early invasion of the cervix is now recognized as a definitive entity and can be diagnosed only by microscopic examination. In almost all instances, the diagnosis should be made upon careful study of a cone biopsy specimen. In 1973, the Society of Gynecologic Oncologists accepted the following statements on microinvasive carcinoma of the cervix uteri, and these have become rather well accepted throughout the world:

1. Intraepithelial carcinoma with questionable invasion should be regarded as intraepithelial carcinoma, and

2. microinvasion should be defined as invasion in which the neoplastic epithelium invades the stroma in one or more places to a depth of 3 mm or less below the base of the membrane and in which lymphatic or vascular involvement is *not* demonstrated.

At present there is no general agreement on the type of treatment needed in this disease. Most clinicians agree that lesions that extend 1 mm or less into the stroma (early stromal invasion) may be treated with hysterectomy or possibly even cone biopsy. However, invasion to 3 mm may be associated with a 1 to 2 per cent incidence of positive pelvic nodes, and therefore a modified radical hysterectomy with pelvic lymphadenectomy should be seriously considered. The therapy of microinvasive carcinoma of the cervix should be tailored to the histological architecture of the invasive process. Experience has shown that lesions composed of isolated, scattered islands of invasive disease in the stroma are less ominous than lesions of less depth of invasion but manifest anaplasia and/or confluent tongues of invasive disease. Patients with these latter lesions should be considered for radical therapy.

INVASIVE CARCINOMA

Fortunately, more and more cases of invasive carcinoma of the cervix are discovered at an early stage (Stages I and IIA). Although 95 per cent of the lesions are of squamous cell origin and the other 5 per cent adenocarcinoma, both lesions should be treated in the same manner.

Specific therapeutic measures are often influenced by the age and general health of the patient, the extent of the malignancy, and the presence and nature of any complicating abnormalities. The controversy between surgery and radiotherapy has existed for decades and essentially surrounds the treatment of Stage I and IIA cervical cancer only. For the most part, all stages above Stage I and IIA are treated with radiotherapy. The 5-year survival data from a very large series utilizing either radiotherapy or surgery for these early lesions show rather comparable results, so that in most areas a true option for therapy exists. The advantage of radiotherapy is that it is applicable to virtually all patients, whereas radical surgery is of necessity exclusive of certain medically inoperable patients.

In most institutions, surgery for Stage I and IIA disease is reserved for younger patients in whom preservation of ovarian and vaginal function is desired. The modern operative mortality and the postoperative ureterovaginal fistula rate have both been dramatically reduced in recent years to far less than 1 per cent, making an objective decision for therapy difficult. Other reasons given for selection of radical hysterectomy over radiation include cervical cancer in pregnancy, concomitant inflammatory disease of the bowel, previous irradiation therapy for other disease, the presence of pelvic inflammatory disease or an adnexal neoplasm along with the malignancy, and patient preference. Chief among the disadvantages of radiation therapy is the permanent injury to the tissues of the normal organ bed of the neoplasm, and the possibility of second malignant lesions developing in this bed.

In the patient who has a lesion more advanced than Stage IIA, radiation therapy has been the treatment of choice since a surgical approach short of an exenteration would not provide adequate surgical margins. A host of recent data has suggested that as the stage increases, there is an increasing incidence of periaortic metastasis, which usually lies outside the field of radiation therapy. As a result, more and more patients with far advanced disease are being evaluated for surgical staging in order to identify the extent of disease, and radiation therapy fields are being drawn to encompass noted regional involvement. Unfortunately, for patients who have disease outside the true pelvis, even though the sites are identified and treated with radiation therapy, survival remains poor. The role of extended field radiation therapy remains at this point questionable and continues to be investigational. In addition, the use of adjuvant chemotherapy or immunotherapy in an effort to improve the survival of these poor-prognosis patients is also unsettled and under investigation.

RECURRENT CARCINOMA

In a very select group of patients with recurrent carcinoma of the cervix in which disease appears to be localized in the pelvis, radical surgical therapy may be applicable for salvage. In rare instances where this recurrent lesion is very small, a radical hysterectomy and pelvic lymphadenectomy may encompass the disease and give long term survival. However, in most patients, the central recurrence is such that an anterior or total exenteration must be performed in order to eradicate the disease. Modern radiotherapy has reduced the number of patients with central failure to a point where patients suitable for exenteration are becoming rare. Indeed, the only patients who are suitable for exenteration are those patients with central recurrence and no sidewall or extrapelvic disease. These procedures should be performed by skilled and experienced teams in tertiary care centers and preceded by thorough diagnostic evaluation for extrapelvic disease and extensive psychological preparation of the patient for what is a debilitating procedure. The 5-year cumulative survival after pelvic exenteration varies in the literature from 20 to 60 per cent. Both morbidity and mortality, as well as the 5-year survival rate, have steadily improved over the last two decades. Mortality in most centers is well below 5 per cent and morbidity has been similarly lowered.

Re-irradiation of pelvic recurrences of cervical cancer recurring in the previously treated field is still a subject of some controversy. However, re-irradiation for recurrent disease is usually not a worthwhile consideration in the opinion of most clinicians.

The management of disseminated cervical cancer has not significantly improved with the progress of modern chemotherapy. Recently, there have been some promising reports that cisplatinum may be a very active agent for recurrent squamous cell carcinoma of the cervix, especially for lesions occurring outside the previously irradiated field. However, to date, there have been no convincing studies suggesting that survival is prolonged by the use of any chemotherapeutic regimen in this disease. Multiple studies are under way utilizing innovating techniques such as intra-arterial infusion and drug targeting which may alter this dismal report in the future.

CARCINOMA OF THE ENDOMETRIUM

JOHN L. LEWIS, Jr., M.D.

Carcinoma of the endometrium occurs most often in women who are in the their perimenopausal years or later. It is rare before the age of 40, unless the woman has one of the following conditions: anovulation, ingestion of sequential oral contraceptives (now banned by the Food and Drug Administration), hormonal replacement with unopposed estrogens, or an estrogen-producing ovarian neoplasm. It is a very common type of malignant disease in the United States. The American Cancer Society's estimate of 38,000 new cases per year means that the incidence of endometrial cancer exceeds the combined incidence of cancers of the cervix, ovary, vulva, and vagina. The encouraging statistic is that only 3200 women in the United States die from endometrial cancer each year, whereas the number dying of ovarian cancer (11,200) and cervical cancer (7400) is far greater. This high cure rate is possible because most cases have disease limited to the fundus (stage I) and are of low histologic grade, thus making them curable with a simple hysterectomy.

DIAGNOSIS

The key to early diagnosis of this malignancy is to take a *histologic* sample of the endometrium in a woman at "high risk" as defined above and to properly evaluate any woman with abnormal uterine bleeding. Unfortunately, the regular Papanicolaou smear obtained from the cervix and vagina is positive in less than half of women with this malignant lesion. A histologic sample (by aspiration or biopsy techniques) is better than a cytologic sample (so-called "wash" techniques) because it allows the proper diagnosis not only of the cancer but also its hyperplastic precursors. Effective treatment of atypical endometrial hyperplasia can prevent this cancer from ever developing.

A fractional dilatation and curettage accompanied by examination under anesthesia is necessary for the proper staging of endometrial cancer. It is also appropriate in women with abnormal bleeding when an endometrial biopsy fails to explain the cause of the bleeding. It is important to perform the examination and fractional dilatation and curettage correctly in order to obtain the necessary information for establishing the correct stage in a given patient. Accurate staging is critical in patients with endometrial cancer, for there are few diseases in which there are such wide variations in effective treatment within a given stage. The necessary information which one should obtain is depth of endometrial cavity, presence of disease in the endocervix, grade of the tumor, and clinical evidence of disease in the parametrium, adnexal structures, bladder or rectum.

It is important to follow a standard procedure when doing a fractional dilatation and curettage in any patient with abnormal bleeding. This will ensure that all of the information needed for staging endometrial cancer will be obtained and also that there will be as little likelihood as possible that the endocervical specimen will be contaminated with tissue from the endometrial cavity. After examination under anesthesia, the patient should be prepared and draped for a sterile vaginal procedure. The cervix is first grasped with a tenaculum and the endocervical canal is briskly curetted with a narrow, sharp curette. This tissue is handled with forceps which are then placed aside and not used to handle endometrial tissue. After that the endometrium is sounded for depth. The depth of 8 cm is the dividing point for separating stages Ia and Ib when the disease is limited to the fundus. The endocervical canal is then dilated gently, after which the cavity is searched for polyps with a polyps forceps. (We use a medium sized common duct stone forceps). Sharp curettage is then carried out, but care must be taken not to use as much force as can be used safely in the endocervix.

STAGING

Assigning the proper stage to a lesion is important, for it determines what treatment will give the best chance for cure. Staging is based on the information gained by an examination under anesthesia, fractional dilatation and curettage, chest x-ray, and evaluation of any possible extension to the bladder or rectum by intravenous pyelogram, cystoscopy, and proctosigmoidoscopy. In addition, the histologic grade of the adenocarcinoma is important in determining therapy and prognosis. Unlike most "grading" classifications in other neoplasms, the one adopted by the International Federation of Obstetricians and Gynecologists (FIGO) in 1970 is based on the architecture of the tumor rather than the cytologic characteristics of the individual cells in the tumor (Table 1).

TABLE 1. **Staging of Endometrial Adenocarcinoma***

Stage I: The carcinoma is confined to the corpus.
Subdivision according to size of uterus:
Stage Ia The uterine cavity sounds to 8 cm or less.
Stage Ib The uterine cavity sounds to more than 8 cm.
Subdivision according to histology:
G1 Highly diffentiated adenomatous carcinomas
G2 Differentiated adenomatous carcinomas with partly solid areas.
G3 Predominantly solid or entirely undifferentiated carcinomas.
Stage II: The carcinoma has involved the corpus and the cervix.
Stage III: The carcinoma has extended outside the uterus but not outside the true pelvis.
Stage IV: The carcinoma has extended outside the true pelvis or has obviously involved the mucosa of the bladder or rectum. Bullous edema as such does not permit allottment of a case to Stage IV.

*Established by FIGO at Sixth World Congress, 1970

HISTOLOGY

The majority of endometrial carcinomas consist only of adenocarcinomatous elements. The presence of benign squamous elements (adenoacanthoma) does not change the prognosis or treatment. However, when there is a mixture of malignant squamous epithelium as well as malignant adenocarcinoma (adenosquamous carcinoma) the prognosis is worse. Similarly, the rare clear cell form of adenocarcinoma also has a worse prognosis.

TREATMENT

The choice of treatment in an individual patient depends on the stage and grade of her tumor as well as her individual health characteristics: age, weight, and specific health problems. When the disease is localized and the patients are considered operable, surgery is the most important form of treatment. Radiation should be added to surgery in patients with certain tumor characteristics. The vast majority of patients with endometrial cancer will have disease clinically limited to the fundus or fundus and cervix (91 per cent in our series even though we are a cancer center and tend to have advanced disease referred). Radiation therapy alone may be selected in patients with resectable disease who are considered inoperable on the basis of specific health problems, but the cure rates are cut about in half.

The type of surgery and the type (intrauterine, intravaginal, or external) and timing (preoperative, postoperative, or both) of radiation therapy are matters which are under active investigation in many centers. Those who choose preoperative radiation do so on the basis of two beliefs: (1) the staging and tumor characteristics which are known after the fractional dilatation and curettage and histologic evaluation are adequate to determine which patients need radiation in addition to surgery; and (2) the radiation therapy is more likely to be effective if the tumor is treated before it is manipulated. Those electing to use only postoperative radiation do so on the assumption that the intact surgical specimen allows them to determine important additional facts not known at the time of the staging procedure (such as depth of myometrial penetration and spread outside the uterus, particularly to lymph nodes and adnexal structures). One compromise being studied is the use of preoperative intracavitary radiation sources with an immediate hysterectomy after the sources are removed. This gives lethal radiation to the tumor in the uterus but allows preservation of the tumor architecture, so that it can be studied and the need for further radiation determined. Even those favoring preoperative radiation usually will operate first when a patient has a cystic adnexal structure which could represent an ovarian metastasis or the commonly found second primary tumor in the ovary. It is common to have the problem of trying to decide if a patient with similar tumors in the endometrium and ovary has two separate stage I cancers or stage III endometrial cancer. The patterns of growth and the presence of in situ changes are helpful but in some patients it is not possible to decide. Finally, with the possible exception of an occasional patient with stage II disease, there is no place for radical surgery in the initial treatment of endometrial cancer.

SUGGESTED TREATMENT

All *stage I, grade 1* endometrial carcinomas, regardless of size, can be adequately treated by a total abdominal hysterectomy and bilateral salpingo-oophorectomy if the patient is considered to be capable of undergoing surgery safely. The abdominal approach is preferred over the vaginal approach because of the need to remove the adnexal structures and because of the ability to evaluate spread outside the uterus. Very few patients in this category will have deep myometrial penetration or nodal spread. Low dose vaginal irradiation is advocated by some to prevent the rare vaginal recurrence.

Patients with *stage 1, grade 2* or *3* tumors require consideration of having more than surgery alone. Patients with *grade 3* lesions are at a markedly increased risk of having deep myometrial penetration, nodal spread, and failure to be cured by a simple hysterectomy alone. Although *grade 2* lesions are not as bad as *grade 3* lesions, they tend to behave more like them than the well-differentiated lesions, so we treat grade 2 and 3 lesions alike. Our own preference is to give 4000 to 4500 rads to a full pelvic port and then follow this with surgery in 4 to 6 weeks. The decision concerining postoperative vaginal radiation is based on whether the entire vagina was in the field treated preoperatively.

Stage II patients are at a higher risk of having spread outside the uterus regardless of the grade of their tumor. Those with grossly visible lesions are more likely to have nodal spread than those in whom the tumor was detected only by histologic evaluation of the endocervical curettage specimen. Because of the presence of tumor in the cervix, they are also at risk for additional spread to the parametrial tissues. For this reason some elect to treat operable patients in this stage with a radical hysterectomy, bilateral salpingo-oophorectomy, and bilateral pelvic lymphadenectomy. Our own preference is to give 4500 rads external pelvic radiation and then follow 6 weeks later with a modified radical hysterectomy and bilateral salpingo-oophorectomy. Only those nodes which are palpably enlarged are removed. If the patients are not operable because of their health problems, they receive full radiation therapy as if they had cervical cancer.

Few patients present with *stages III* and *IV* disease and because of the variations in extent of disease it is inappropriate to try to discuss them in detail in this type of presentation. An obvious exception is in those patients who are in *stage III* on the basis of spread to the ovary. That spread does not prevent them from having all of their disease removed by simple surgery which can then be followed by external pelvic radiation. If patients are in *stage IV* disease on the basis of spread outside the pelvis, they are treated in the pelvis for palliation and then given systemic therapy as if they had recurrent metastatic disease. Patients in *stages III* and *IV* whose disease is limited to the pelvis are treated with a full course of pelvic radiation and evaluated to determine if this has rendered their tumor resectable. If not, they receive intracavitary radiation or a booster dose of external radiation, depending on local factors.

RECURRENT DISEASE

With the exception of the rare patients in whom the only apparent disease is surgically removable or is localized so that it can be treated with radiation, the only hope for these patients is hormonal therapy, chemotherapy, or a combination of these. For many years progestagens have been the first choice, for they are essentially nontoxic and were the first agents to show any objective effects. However, many of us are disappointed with the low rate of sustained objective responses. Recently two observations have been made which help to explain this low rate: (1) only those tumors which contain specific progesterone-binding proteins (progesterone receptor proteins) are likely to respond to progestagen therapy; and (2) these receptor proteins are found in most grade I tumors but in few grade II and III tumors. Since most recurrences are in patients with grade II and III tumors, other therapy is needed.

In recent years there have been promising results with initial trials of cytotoxic therapy. Useful drugs include alkylating agents, 5-fluorouracil, and Adriamycin, usually given in any of several combinations. Their toxicity is a problem because of the age and general health of many of these patients. However, they have the advantage of being effective in receptor-negative tumors.

RESULTS

As noted earlier, the American Cancer Society's estimate of the number of American women dying annually of endometrial cancer (3200) is only 8.4 per cent of the number of new cases estimated to occur each year (38,000). If one assumes that the incidence remains approximately constant (ignoring a probable slight increase), this would predict a cure rate of approximately 92 per cent. This figure is in contrast with the overall cure rate of 70 to 80 per cent reported in most large series from oncology services. One explanation for this is that most women with endometrial cancers have stage I, well-differentiated lesions and have curative surgery in their local setting. Oncology services are more likely to have patients with undifferentiated tumors or those in advanced stages referred to them than those with well-differentiated tumors limited to the fundus.

Overall, endometrial cancer remains one of our most favorable gynecologic malignancies. Explanations of treatment failures and efforts to decrease the failure rate even further are now being sought by studies of occult nodal spread in the pelvic and para-aortic regions, the significance of cancer cells in peritoneal washings and the presence of specific progesterone receptor proteins. How this information will be useful in standard clinical care is yet to be determined.

OVARIAN CARCINOMA

WILLIAM T. CREASMAN, M.D.,
and DANIEL L. CLARKE-PEARSON, M.D.

Ovarian cancer kills more women in the United States than any other pelvic malignancy. Factors which account for the poor prognosis of the woman who is destined to develop this cancer include: (1) there is no screening technique to identify the patient with early cancer; (2) late stage disease is usually found at the time of diagnosis; (3) inadequate therapies are used, including inappropriate or incomplete surgery that might be of benefit to the patient; (4) to date there are no chemotherapeutic agents available which will uniformly destroy ovarian cancer, particularly if large bulky tumor remains after surgery; and (5) monitoring techniques are inadequate to predict the clinical course of the patient receiving chemotherapy.

Multiple prognostic factors must be evaluated in each patient who has ovarian carcinoma. These factors include the status of the ovarian capsule, peritoneal cytology, stage of disease, cell type and grade of tumor, the amount of residual tumor after the primary surgery, and subsequent postoperative therapy. Most of these items can only be determined with adequate surgical exploration.

Whenever cancer of the ovary is found at the time of exploratory laparotomy, the physician must be prepared to fully evaluate the extent of disease as well as be able to perform the necessary surgery. Immediately upon opening the peritoneal cavity, peritoneal cytology should be obtained. If ascites is not present, this can be accomplished by injecting 100 to 125 cc of saline into the pelvis, admixing it with a small amount of peritoneal fluid in the cul-de-sac, and then retrieving the fluid for cytologic evaluation. Peritoneal cytologic specimens from the pelvis, both lateral pericolic gutters, and the right diaphragm are recommended. Next, the surgeon must determine the full extent of the disease. It must be remembered that ovarian cancer is not a pelvic lesion but one that potentially can involve the entire peritoneal cavity. Therefore, the pelvis, peritoneal surfaces, diaphragms, omentum, and pelvic and para-aortic lymph nodes must be evaluated. Much of this can be done visually and with palpation. If suspicious areas are noted, appropriate biopsies should be made.

The surgeon must then evaluate the extent to which the malignant process may be resected, remembering that the amount of residual tumor directly correlates with the patient's prognosis. If, in the surgeon's estimation, the tumor can be completely removed, then, with rare exception, a total abdominal hysterectomy, bilateral salpingo-oophorectomy, and partial omentectomy should be performed. In addition, the pelvic and para-aortic lymph nodes should be adequately sampled to determine if metastasis to these areas has occurred. In Stage I carcinoma of the ovary, occult metastasis to the lymph nodes is present in 10 to 15 per cent of cases. Even if palpable disease is not present in the omentum, a partial omentectomy should be performed, removing the omentum at its attachment to the transverse colon. At our institution we divide the omentum into at least 10 specimens and send these separately for pathologic evaluation. By so doing, it is not unusual to find occult disease in one or two of the specimens from the omentum. In such situations, instead of Stage I disease, Stage III is now documented.

If the disease is no longer confined to the adnexal area, every attempt should be made to remove all of the gross tumor if technically feasible. This may mean removing part or all of the pelvic peritoneum as required to debulk the tumor. Survival is directly related to the amount of tumor that remains after the surgical procedure.

Even if all gross disease has been resected, adjunctive therapy is required. When the tumor is completely resected, three options are available. These include intraperitoneal isotopes, single-agent alkylating chemotherapy, or radiation therapy. Radioactive phosphorus is felt by some investigators to be the treatment of choice in this type of patient. It can be given during the immediate postoperative course and has the advantages of covering all peritoneal surfaces. Distribution of the colloid is important, and scanning techniques must be used to assure that loculation does not occur.

In the patient who is found to have many adhesions at the time of her surgical procedure, radioisotopes are contraindicated. Also, if disease has been found outside of the peritoneal cavity, including pelvic or para-aortic lymph nodes, radioisotopes will be ineffective. The toxicity from this therapy is minimal, and it has the advantage of being a one-time treatment. The use of a single agent alkylator appears to be very effective. Most investigators would use this for at least 12 to 18 months and then suggest a "second look" exploratory laparotomy. If radiation therapy is given, it must include the entire peritoneal surface from the pelvic floor to the diaphragms. Abdominal and pelvic radiation therapy requires sophisticated techniques in order to get the dosage required and minimize side-effects. This will usually require 8 to 10 weeks of therapy after surgery. It appears that the overall survival results of these three modalities are essentially the same, and should give an 85 to 90 per cent 5-year survival rate in Stage I disease.

When disease remains after surgery, but is minimal in amount (less than 2 cm in size), the therapeutic modalities of chemotherapy and radiation therapy appear to be equally effective. Experience to date has been mainly with single agent alkylating chemotherapy, although some small studies suggest that multiple agent chemotherapy may be more advantageous. For radiation therapy to be effective, the entire peritoneal surface must be covered, which requires sophisticated delivery of radiation therapy to avoid significant complications.

Unfortunately, the majority of women with ovarian cancer have bulk disease remaining after their surgical procedure. In this situation the only effective treatment is chemotherapy. Most experience has been with a single alkylating agent. Response rates of approximately 50 per cent and a median survival of about 1 year have been noted for different drugs that fall into this class. If a patient does respond to the initial chemotherapy, survival appears to be increased appreciably over those who do not respond to chemotherapy.

Because of the relatively poor survival with single-agent alkylating chemotherapy, combination chemotherapy has been evaluated. The initial studies indicated that the combinations were no better than an alkylator and did carry considerably increased toxicity. Recently, a prospective randomized study from the National Cancer Institute suggested that multiple agent chemotherapy—(hexamethymelamine, cyclophosphamide (Cytoxan), Adriamycin, and 5-fluorouracil)—was better than melphalan. This particular study has been criticized on several counts, and in evaluating the data carefully it would appear that possibly the only benefit of the combination would be in those individuals who have a Grade I or Grade II lesion. The toxicity from these multiple agents was considerable and, in fact, most patients were unable to receive the desired dose because of the side-effects.

During the last several years the use of cis-platinum in ovarian cancer has shown a rather dramatic increase in the response rate in those individuals with large residual disease. The initial data are Phase II studies, and only recently has a Phase III prospective randomized study been initiated utilizing the combination of cis-platinum, Adriamycin, and cyclophosphamide (Cytoxan) compared with Adriamycin and Cytoxan. The preliminary results from the ongoing study by the Gynecologic Oncology Group suggest that response rate is increased considerably. Although the survival rate to date is better in those individuals receiving the combination containing cis-platinum, statistical significance has not been obtained. Whether cis-platinum in combination with other drugs will be significantly more effective awaits further studies.

Immunotherapy in combination with chemotherapy has been and is currently being evaluated. *Corynebacterium parvum* and Bacillus Calmette-Guérin (BCG) have been studied. In a nonrandomized Phase-II study, *C. parvum* plus melphalan had a better response rate, progression-free interval, and survival than did melphalan by itself. This study included both optimal and suboptimal Stage III and IV disease. However, in a prospective randomized study utilizing only optimal Stage III and IV patients, the addition of *C. parvum* did not appear to improve survival. The Southwestern Oncology Group, in a prospective randomized study, evaluated Adriamycin and Cytoxan versus Adriamycin, Cytoxan, and BCG. The addition of BCG increased the progression-free interval and survival significantly. That group is currently evaluating BCG in combination with cis-platinum, Adriamycin and Cytoxan. The Gynecologic Oncology Group has begun a prospective randomized study comparing cis-platinum, Adriamycin, and Cytoxan with cis-platinum, Adriamycin, Cytoxan, and BCG. The role, if any, of nonspecific immunotherapy in ovarian cancer looks promising, but to date is unproved.

Until improvements are obtained in diagnostic and treatment modalities, ovarian cancer will remain an enigma for all gynecologists.

HYDATIDIFORM MOLE

HOWARD W. JONES, III, M.D.,
and BETH COLVIN, R.N., M.S.N.

The incidence of hydatidiform mole is approximately 1 per 1500 to 2000 pregnancies in the United States, although it is more common in other parts of the world. Recent information suggests that it is caused by deletion or inactivation of all the female chromosomes in the ovocyte with duplication of the male chromosomes from the fertilizing sperm.

Pathologically, it is important to distinguish between two different forms of hydatidiform mole which have been called the "complete" and "partial" or "incomplete" types. The "complete" hydatidiform mole is the classic form of the disease, with dilated avascular villi in the absence of membranes or fetal parts, and with at least some degree of trophoblastic proliferation. Occasionally, patients with hydropic placental villi are seen who also have an associated fetus (usually malformed) or membranes. These patients do not have trophoblastic proliferation and they are classified as having a "partial mole." This lesion is almost always benign. The classic "complete" mole has a 46XX chromosome complement, while "partial moles" usually demonstrate cytogenetic abnormalities such as triploidy.

The majority of patients with hydatidiform mole present with vaginal bleeding or passage of molar tissue. The uterus is large for dates in approximately 50 per cent of women with hydatidiform mole, but may be normal or small for dates. Fetal heart tones are not heard with the doptone.

Diagnosis is usually made today by the use of pelvic ultrasonography. With modern ultrasound techniques, hydatidiform mole can usually be diagnosed by the lack of fetal heart movement and the absence of a fetal skull or thorax. The uterus is filled instead by a rather solid mass with multiple sonolucent areas representing the hydropic villi. Although amniogram, pelvic arteriogram, and even plain x-ray have been used in the past, they are rarely used if ultrasound is available. Occasional patients will be diagnosed by the pathologist after the gynecologist has done a suction dilatation and curettage for what is presumed to be an incomplete abortion.

INITIAL EVACUATION

Once the diagnosis of probable hydatidiform mole has been established, preoperative laboratory work, including a complete blood count, blood urea nitrogen, and liver function tests, should be obtained. In addition, a serum beta-human chorionic gonadotropin (β-HCG) level should be drawn and a chest x-ray obtained to look for metastatic lesions. If there are any signs of hyperthyroidism, this should be evaluated and, of course, anemia may need to be corrected preoperatively by transfusion. A careful pelvic examination should be done to look for cervical or vaginal metastases, but these dark blue lesions are extremely vascular, and biopsy should be undertaken only with blood and an operating room immediately available.

Evacuation of the hydatidiform mole by suction evacuation is the treatment of choice. Even when the uterus is larger than 16 weeks, this can be done with minimum risk. Laminaria are not needed since the cervix is soft and dilates easily. Although regional or even local anesthesia can be used, general anesthesia is preferred. The cervix is dilated and a large (10 to 12 mm) suction cannula is inserted into the uterine cavity and suction applied. Blood and extra suction bottles should be available if the uterus is enlarged. Once evacuation has been started, a dilute solution of oxytocin should be given intravenously to maintain uterine contractions and minimize bleeding. When as much tissue as can be extracted has been removed from the uterus by suction curettage, a large curette is introduced and a gentle sharp curettage of the uterine cavity is then done. This may be helpful in removing residual molar tissue, especially in the cornual areas, and may provide the pathologist with a tissue sample more predictive of the proliferative tendencies of the mole. Care should be taken to avoid uterine perforation.

In a patient with uterine enlargement greater than 18 weeks the risk of hemorrhage and pulmonary insufficiency resulting from embolization of trophoblastic tissue must be carefully borne in mind, and these women should be very carefully monitored following evacuation.

The use of suction evacuation has greatly reduced the morbidity associated with evacuation of a hydatidiform mole, and hysterotomy or induction of labor with oxytocin or prostaglandins should be avoided if at all possible. Forceful uterine contractions or vigorous manipulation may lead to venous dissemination of the trophoblastic tissue. Hysterectomy may be an acceptable method of managing the woman with hydatidiform mole who does not desire more children. Although hysterectomy is a formidable procedure in a patient with a large vascular uterus, it may reduce the incidence of malignant sequelae, minimizing the need for chemotherapy.

At the time of evacuation of the mole, the adnexae should be carefully examined for the presence of theca lutein cysts. These ovarian cysts, which may be quite large, occur in about 30 per cent of women with hydatidiform mole and are the result of stimulation of the ovaries by high levels of gonadotropins produced by the mole. Although they require no therapy, they indicate an increased risk of malignant sequelae and occasionally rupture, causing intraperitoneal bleeding.

FOLLOW-UP CARE

Once the mole has been evacuated, careful follow-up is essential in order to diagnose and treat the 15 per cent of women who will require chemotherapy. Patients should be counseled against another pregnancy for the next year, and oral contraceptives are recommended if there are no contraindications. These are not only the most effective method of contraception, but they also suppress pituitary gonadotropins which crossreact with β-HCG at very low levels, which may produce some confusion about the origin of the elevated hormone level.

Serum β-HCG levels should be obtained every week until the levels have fallen to undetectable values. A quantitative serum assay should be used for this follow-up—there is no place for pregnancy tests which lack the sensitivity necessary to accurately follow the woman with trophoblastic disease. It usually requires about 8 to 12 weeks for the β-HCG to fall below the level of sensitivity of the assay. This is approximately 2 to 5 mIU per ml in most assays. Until the β-HCG levels have fallen to normal, pelvic examinations should be done every 2 weeks to monitor uterine involution and check on the resolution of theca lutein cysts if they are present. Routine chest x-rays or other studies are not indicated as long as the β-HCG levels are falling and the patient has not previously demonstrated a metastatic lesion, and there are no new findings on history or physical examination.

Plateaued or rising β-HCG levels or levels which have not returned to baseline values within 12 weeks require chemotherapy as outlined in the article on choriocarcinoma. Once the β-HCG level has returned to normal, the serum levels are checked at monthly intervals for 1 year. After this time, contraception may be discontinued and pregnancy permitted.

The risk of a subsequent hydatidiform mole in the same patient is not clear but is probably increased, perhaps in the neighborhood of 1 in 500 pregnancies. Therefore, early prenatal care should include ultrasonography to determine the presence of a gestational sac and fetus.

Psychological and emotional support for the woman and her family are important to help them through the crisis of this particular disease. Because this uncommon condition is often frighteningly new to the patient and her family, education is of great importance. Information at all stages in the treatment and follow-up of hydatidiform mole removes some of the mystery and allows the patient to participate in her care, assuring greater compliance with the therapeutic plan.

MANAGEMENT OF GESTATIONAL TROPHOBLASTIC DISEASE

C. PAUL MORROW, M.D.,
and JOHN B. SCHLAERTH, M.D.

A presumptive diagnosis of gestational trophoblastic disease (GTD) is made in any postmenarchal woman with an elevated serum (or urine) HCG titer in the absence of pregnancy. For practical purposes the only other consideration is the rare ovarian germ cell tumor containing trophoblastic tissue. The majority of cases of gestational trophoblastic disease result from molar pregnancy and they are detected by serial serum HCG levels utilizing a radioimmunoassay specific for the beta subunit. The normal pattern of HCG disappearance from the serum following molar pregnancy is depicted in Figure 1. The titers of patients with post molar gestational trophoblastic disease deviate from this pattern by manifesting an early plateau or rise (Figure 2). This occurs in 15 to 25 per cent of patients with true hydatid moles. Those patients having

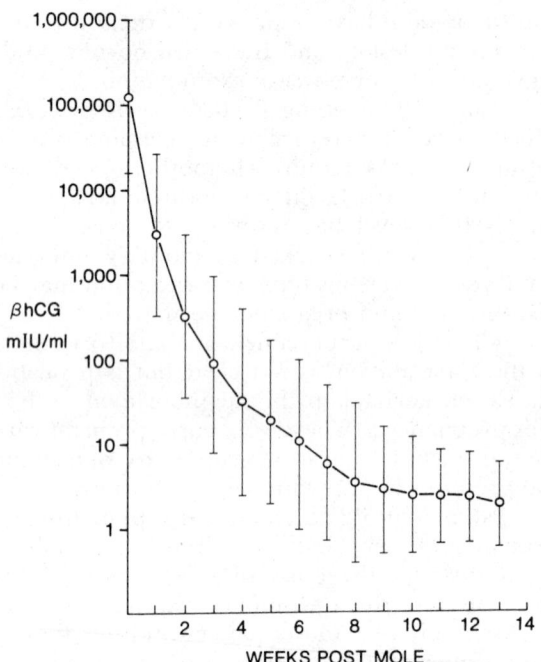

Figure 1. Normal serum β-HCG regression curve following molar pregnancy. Curve depicts mean values and 95% confidence limits. (From Schlaerth, J. B., Morrow, C. P., et al.: Prognostic characteristics of serum human chorionic gonadotropin titer regression following molar pregnancy. Obstet. Gynecol., 58:478, 1981. Reproduced with permission.)

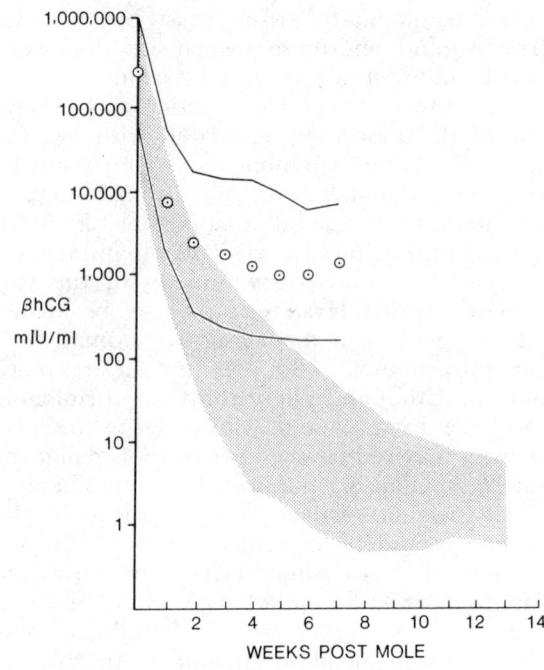

Figure 2. The stippled area represents the normal regression corridor for serum β-hCG. The mean values (circles) and 95% confidence limits for serum hCG values from patients having abnormal regression curves are superimposed. The curves separate at 5 to 6 weeks post evacuation. (From Schlaerth, J. B., Morrow, C. P., et al.: Prognostic characteristics of serum human chorionic gonadotropin titer regression following molar pregnancy. Obstet. Gynecol., 58:478, 1981. Reproduced with permission.)

an abnormal HCG regression curve following molar pregnancy have either invasive mole or choriocarcinoma, the ratio being 3 to 5 cases of invasive mole to every 1 case of choriocarcinoma. There is a tendency for invasive mole to involute spontaneously. Consequently, the ratio changes with time and by 6 to 12 months post mole the majority or even all cases of gestational trophoblastic disease will be choriocarcinoma. The presence of lung or pelvic metastases does not absolutely differentiate the two since invasive mole is capable of "deporting" to these areas.

Gestational trophoblastic disease after any pregnancy other than a molar pregnancy is always choriocarcinoma. These cases usually present with symptoms caused by bleeding from metastases to the lung, brain, liver, or genital tract. When there is choriocarcinoma in the uterus, the presentation mimics threatened abortion or ectopic pregnancy. This diagnosis must be confirmed or excluded by means of HCG testing in any woman in the reproductive age group presenting with clinical evidence of stroke, brain tumor, hemoperitoneum, gastrointestinal bleeding, pulmonary infiltrates, or threatened abortion.

The staging work-up for gestational trophoblastic disease includes a careful gynecologic and neurologic examination; chest x-ray; liver-spleen scan; CT scan of the brain; and serum β-HCG assay. Uterine curettage is reserved for patients with significant bleeding. With this data base, cases can be classified as nonmetastatic or metastatic. The latter group is further subdivided on the basis of the prognosis (good; poor) or risk for treatment failure (low; high). The traditional criteria for the high risk group are (1) time: more than 4 months since the termination of the antecedent pregnancy; (2) titer: initial 24 hour urine HCG titer greater than 100,000 IU; (3) extent: the presence of brain or liver metastases. A fourth criterion should be added to this list of high risk factors, and that is treatment by a physician inexperienced in the care of these patients.

MANAGEMENT

Nonmetastatic Gestational Trophoblastic Disease. The great majority of these cases will be the sequel to a molar gestation. The presumption is made that, in the absence of demonstrable metastases, the tumor is in the uterus. Uterine enlargement or bleeding is confirmatory evidence. In this situation the tumor is uniformly curable. The treatment of choice for those women who have completed their childbearing is a hysterectomy. This, however, is applicable to very few cases because most women with gestational trophoblastic disease are just beginning their family. For most women with this problem, then, the treatment will be chemotherapy. Traditional regimens employ methotrexate (0.4 mg per kg per day for 5 days intramuscularly or intravenously) or actinomycin D (10 µg per kg per day intravenously for 5 days). Courses are repeated about every 2 weeks as toxicity allows, until one course has been completed after the first normal HCG titer. Either regimen will induce permanent remission in 80 to 90 per cent of cases when used as the first line of treatment. The 10 to 20 per cent that prove resistant to one drug will usually respond to the other. Occasionally hysterectomy or combination drug therapy will be required. The reported end-results indicate that virtually all of these cases are curable. Follow-up HCG titers are required for 1 to 2 years before pregnancy is allowed.

Modifications of these traditional drug regimens have been employed to reduce toxicity and simplify treatment. The alternating methotrexate-citrovorum factor 8 day regimen (methotrexate, 1.0 mg per kg intramuscularly on days 1, 3, 5, and 7; citrovorum factor, 0.1 mg per kg intramuscularly on days 2, 4, 6, and 8) has the advantage of reduced toxicity. It does require 8 consecutive days of hospitalization or office visits. Patient compliance is an absolute necessity to assure that the patient is "rescued" with citrovorum factor after each dose of methotrexate. A second modified regimen is single day actinomycin D, 1.25 mg per M^2 intravenously every 2 weeks. This is extremely convenient since it requires only one office visit for each course of treatment. There is significant toxicity, however, most prominently nausea and vomiting for 1 to 2 days after treatment.

Metastatic Gestational Trophoblastic Disease. These cases should all be referred to a center with experience in the treatment of the trophoblastic tumors to assure the best possible results. Only 80 per cent will be cured in an optimal environment. Disease in patients with brain or liver metastases is much less curable.

All these patients need chemotherapy. For that relatively small group of cases diagnosed during the early follow-up period after molar pregnancy whose only metastases are pulmonary, single agent chemotherapy using actinomycin D or methotrexate is usually adequate. With an initial serum HCG titer greater than 10,000 mIU per ml, combination drug therapy with methotrexate, actinomycin D, and cyclophosphamide (MAC) is employed to shorten the treatment time and lessen the probability of treatment failure. These patients usually have considerable myometrial tumor and treatment tends to fail in the uterus, necessitating hysterectomy. The cure rate in these cases is nearly 100 per cent.

The remainder of patients with metastatic gestational trophoblastic disease almost invariably have choriocarcinoma and are at serious risk of losing their lives. For these patients MAC chemotherapy is employed roughly every 2 weeks. It is continued until 2 or 3 courses after HCG titer remission is established. Because about 10 per cent of patients will relapse after titer remission, we continue single agent therapy at 3 to 4 week intervals for an additional 6 months in some patients. Patients with brain metastases require whole brain radiation therapy. This should be initiated on an emergency basis because life-threatening hemorrhage may occur at any time. The dose recommended is 2000 to 3000 rads in 2 or 3 weeks. Brain radiation is highly effective in preventing hemorrhage and achieving a locally curative effect on the tumor.

The role of whole organ irradiation for liver metastasis is uncertain. We recommend it for patients with subcapsular metastases or extensive liver metastases, conditions in which rupture is imminent.

It is our experience that failure to cure patients with gestational trophoblastic disease is more frequently due to drug toxicity than to drug resistance, although the latter certainly occurs. Recently two regimens have proved to be useful in patients not tolerating MAC, and may even produce cures after failure with MAC. These are the multidrug Bagshawe regimen and the Einhorn triple drug therapy (vinblastine, bleomycin, and cis-platinum). Currently we reserve these regimens for second-line therapy.

EVALUATION OF THE PATIENT WITH AN ABNORMAL PAPANICOLAOU SMEAR

CHRISTOPHER P. CRUM, M.D., and RALPH M. RICHART, M.D.

The diagnostic and therapeutic approach to a patient with an abnormal Papanicolaou smear is based on the following facts: (1) invasive carcinoma of the cervix is virtually always preceded by an intraepithelial precursor lesion (cervical intraepithelial neoplasia, CIN) and the transition from cervical intraepithelial neoplasia to invasive carcinoma usually takes several years, (2) annual Papanicolaou smears will detect the vast majority of these precursor lesions prior to the development of invasive carcinoma, (3) with a colposcopically oriented out-patient examination, including cervical biopsies and endocervical curettage, invasive carcinoma can virtually always be ruled out and the size and distribution of the lesion can be determined, and (4) if the intraepithelial lesion is successfully removed, the risk of recurrence is no greater than that for a comparable high-risk population.

The proper management of the patient with cervical intraepithelial neoplasia depends primarily on careful clinical examination, cytology, colposcopy, and histology. If the results of all these examinations are consistent with a diagnosis of cervical intraepithelial neoplasia, and if invasive carcinoma is ruled out, the therapeutic approach is appropriately based primarily on the size and distribution of the neoplastic lesion. In general, low-grade lesions, including condylomata, will be small and confined to the portio, whereas high-grade lesions (CIN 3) will be larger, often circumferential, and may involve the canal. Irrespective of the specific grade of the intraepithelial lesion, if it is confined to the cervix, its limits can be visualized, the canal is confirmed to be uninvolved by a negative endocervical curettage, and thorough histologic samples contain only cervical intraepithelial neoplasia, conservative out-patient therapy is appropriate in a reliable patient. Cryotherapy is the most popular technique at present since it is inexpensive, virtually painless, does not require additional personnel, and successfully eradicates the lesion after a single application in approximately 90 per cent of cases. The carbon dioxide laser has the advantage of precise removal of tissues and careful control of tissue destruction but is expensive, associated with more side-effects, and is not necessary for the treatment of cervical intraepithelial neoplasia.

It is essential that the physician using out-patient therapy be an experienced colposcopist and that this technique not be used if the entire lesion cannot be visualized, sampled, and removed. The recommended cryotherapeutic method uses nitrous oxide as the refrigerant and a single or double freeze-thaw technique in which the ice ball at each application is allowed to advance at least 5 mm beyond the lesion. The patients are encouraged to refrain from intercourse for at least 3 weeks while the healing phase takes place. The next Papanicolaou smear is obtained 4 months following cryotherapy.

The patient is considered cured if 3 consecutive negative Papanicolaou smears are obtained in the first year following cryotherapy. Any abnormal Papanicolaou smear, colposcopic examination, or biopsy within the first year is considered a freeze-failure. A recurrence is classified as the development of a new lesion one or more years after cryotherapy following 3 negative Papanicolaou smears. In general, the cure rate is directly related to the size and distribution of the original lesion and approaches 100 per cent for low-grade cervical intraepithelial neoplasia lesions and 90 per cent for high-grade lesions after a single application.

Any patient with a large lesion which extends so deeply into the canal that the limits cannot be seen or in which a positive endocervical curettage is obtained requires conization. Conization is also mandatory if there are marked discrepancies in the cytologic, histologic, or colposcopic findings. If invasion or microinvasion is suspected cytologically, colposcopically, or histologically, or if the patient is sufficiently uncooperative that careful follow-up cannot be insured, she should be managed operatively rather than in the office.

Difficult problems in management include: (1) patients with CIN 1 Papanicolaou smears and negative colposcopy, (2) patients with squamous atypia who were exposed to diethylstilbestrol (DES) in utero, (3) cervical intraepithelial neoplasia lesions with deep gland involvement, and (4) conization specimens with positive endocervical margins. In general, if repeated colposcopy, biopsy, and endocervical curettage do not confirm the origin of a CIN 1 Papanicolaou smear, the smear should be reviewed to rule out either an inconsequential inflammatory atypia or a more severe lesion which would mandate conization. If the diagnosis is CIN 1, it is likely that the lesion is too small to be seen colposcopically, and careful follow-up with repeated Pap smears should be done until the lesion is identified. In many instances, these low-grade abnormal Pap smears are caused by human papilloma virus infection (the so-called flat condyloma), which may resolve spontaneously or may become apparent after a variable interval.

The management of patients who have been exposed to diethylstilbestrol in utero requires careful assessment of the histologic and cytologic findings inasmuch as these patients often have immature squamous metaplasia, with or without cytologic atypia, a finding which can easily be confused with cervical intraepithelial neoplasia. Unfortunately, when these patients do have cervical intraepithelial neoplasia, the lesion is often large and may extend on to the vagina. In such cases, cryotherapy may be difficult to adminis-

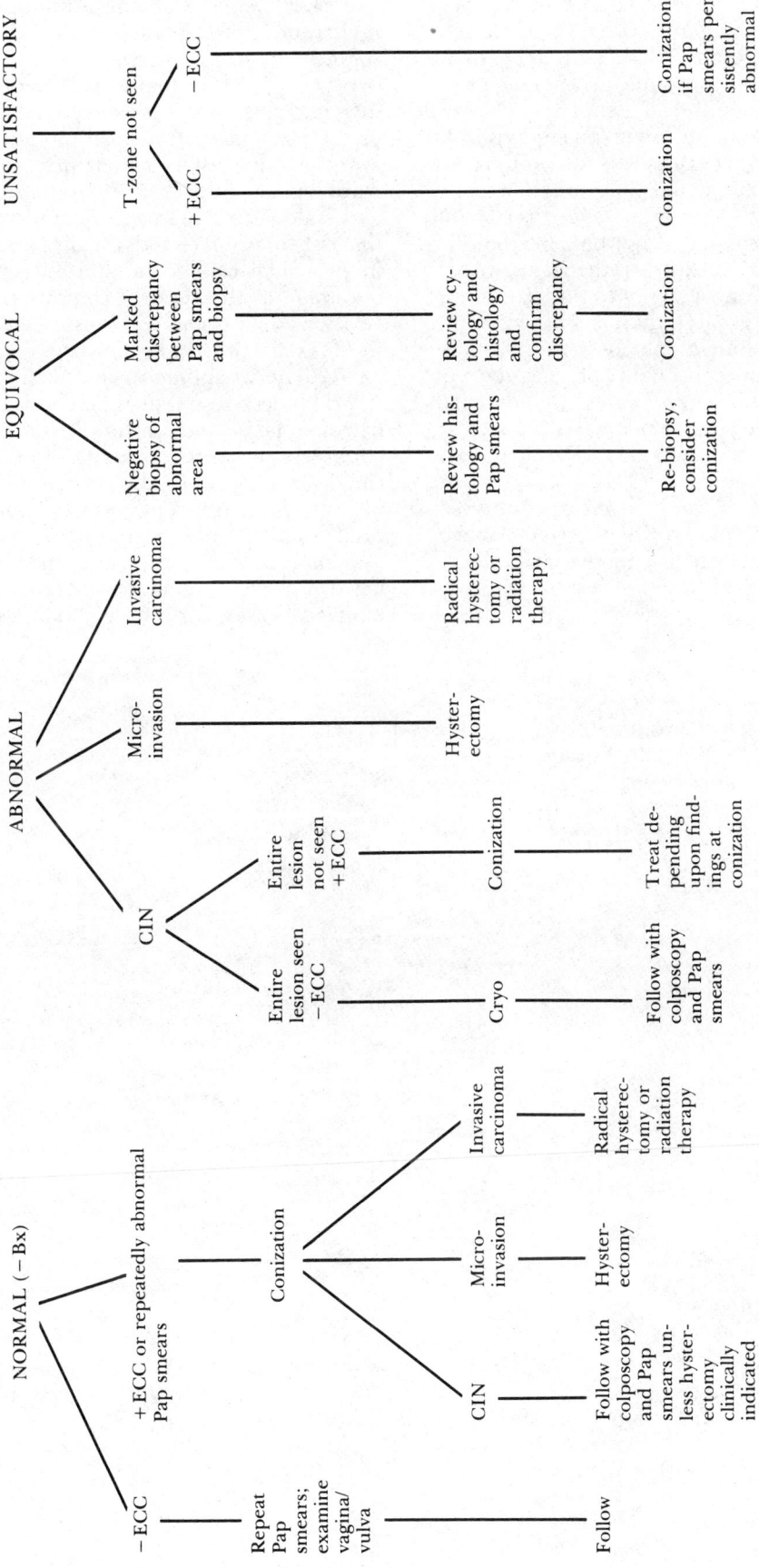

Figure 1. Evaluation of abnormal Papanicolaou (Pap) smear by colposcopy, biopsy (Bx) and endocervical curettage (ECC)

ter, and the carbon dioxide laser may appropriately be used. In patients with smaller lesions, cryotherapy is recommended, and the patients may be followed in the same manner as others with cervical intraepithelial neoplasia. Concern over deep gland involvement is expressed by some authors who feel that if the area of cryonecrosis does not extend deeply enough, residual intraglandular disease may invade directly into the underlying stroma and not be detected. Fortunately, most cervical intraepithelial neoplasms do not extend beyond 2 mm into the glands, and very few extend greater than 5 mm in depth. Lesions up to 5 mm of gland penetration are within the therapeutic field of cryotherapy. There are no documented cases of a "buried" cervical intraepithelial neoplasia following cryotherapy persisting and progressing to invasive carcinoma.

Positive endocervical margins in cone specimens is a cause of concern for the risk of recurrent cervical intraepithelial neoplasia as well as for the possibility of leaving residual invasive carcinoma higher in the canal. The former is generally not a problem. Although the risk of recurrent cervical intraepithelial neoplasia is slightly greater in patients who have positive cone margins, the majority of patients with positive margins do not have residual disease at hysterectomy and for practical purposes can be followed as any other patient post conization, i.e., with repeat endocervical curettage at 4 months and follow-up Papanicolaou smears. In general, the risk of undetected invasive carcinoma high in the canal can be minimized by endocervical curettage at the time of conization, careful correlation of cytologic, biopsy, and colposcopic findings, and careful follow-up.

Adenocarcinoma in situ of the cervix is considerably less frequent than cervical intraepithelial neoplasia and differs from its squamous counterpart by its location often high in the canal and beyond the range of colposcopy. Nevertheless, any patient with abnormal glandular cells should undergo careful colposcopy and should receive a careful endocervical curettage and colposcopically directed biopsies. In equivocal cases, conization should be done.

Section 5
GYNECOLOGIC ENDOCRINOLOGY AND INFERTILITY

PRIMARY AMENORRHEA

JAMES C. WARREN, M.D.

Primary amenorrhea is the term applied to a young woman who has not experienced menstrual periods by her sixteenth birthday. The possibility that primary amenorrhea will ensue should be suspected when there is no development of a breast bud by 12 years, or when breast development has not begun 2 to 3 years after the appearance of pubic hair (unless the latter is due to premature adrenarche). Primary amenorrhea is a symptom; therefore, before therapy is considered, a specific diagnosis must be made. Establishing menstrual periods depends upon a hypothalamus that episodically secretes the decapeptide luteinizing hormone–releasing hormone (LH-RH); a pituitary that secretes gonadotropins; ovaries that make steroid hormones; a uterus with an endometrial cavity that responds to hormonal withdrawal by bleeding; and a patent conduit of egress. The absence of any of these components may be responsible for a given case of primary amenorrhea.

The history, physical, and laboratory examination should focus on answering the five relevant questions: Does the patient have a uterus and a patent conduit of egress? Has she developed female secondary sexual characteristics? Is she now making estrogen? Has she ever had any hormonal therapy? Does she have peculiarities of body habitus or signs of massive androgen production? Clinical examination must establish the presence or absence of the uterus and vagina, quantitate breast development by the Tanner score, and evaluate quantity of pubic hair and body habitus. Pertinent laboratory testing includes determination of serum FSH (and on occasion, serum LH), serum testosterone, serum prolactin, and a maturation index. An extremely useful clinical test for the production of estrogen (if the uterus is present) is to administer 100 mg of progesterone intramuscularly and see the patient 3 weeks later to ascertain the presence or absence of significant withdrawal bleeding. The bleeding should always be quantitated (i.e., if a normal menstrual period is a dollar's worth, how much did the patient have? A penny's worth or 5¢ worth indicates low estrogen production. If in doubt, the progesterone challenge should be repeated with 10 mg of medroxyprogesterone acetate (Provera) daily for 5 days.

The patient's mother usually brings her to the physician. By the age this occurs, it is almost always possible to decide as to the presence or absence of the uterus and vagina. While occasionally vaginal examination cannot be conducted (for indeed, some of these patients have only a rudimentary vagina), a careful rectal examination will allow a definite decision. Only rarely is one forced to conduct an examination under anesthesia.

If the uterus is absent and the patient has secondary sexual characteristics (areolar pigmentation and good ductal tissue in the breast), two possible diagnoses must be considered: congenital absence of the uterus and testicular feminization syndrome. Clinically, the diagnosis of testicular feminization can usually be made by the striking paucity of pubic hair in an otherwise well-developed young woman. The diagnosis is confirmed by evaluation of serum testosterone which approximates a normal female level in patients with congenital absence of the uterus and more nearly approximates a normal male range in the patient with testicular feminization. In the patient with congenital absence of the uterus, it is important to decide whether any endometrial cavity is present. The critical question is whether the patient has periodic pelvic cramping. Given a patient without a visible cervix who indicates that she has menstrual-type cramps, there must be a strong suspicion that an endometrial cavity exists.

Absence of both uterus and secondary sexual characteristics is extremely rare. These patients often have enzyme abnormalities which preclude steroid production or gonads which once made müllerian inhibiting substance but underwent some type of "self-destruction," leaving the patient agonadal. These patients are best referred to centers where specialized studies can be done.

The patient who presents with a uterus but absence of secondary sexual characteristics and no sign of estrogen production requires a quantitation of serum FSH. The critical number here is 40 mIU per ml if the patient has reached her twelfth year of age. Lower values indicate hypogonadotropism which may be due to any one of several causes (see below). Higher values indicate ovarian failure (typical of the dysgenetic gonad) or, more rarely, a resistant ovary syndrome.

The patient who presents with a uterus and secondary sexual characteristics may simply have failed to ovulate (as a result of polycystic ovary syndrome or "so-called" hypothalamic anovulation); she may also have a failing ovary or may be hypogonadotropic. Here, ascertaining whether the patient is producing estrogen is extremely important. While breast development generally suggests production of estrogen, this may have occurred by endogenous secretion which has since fallen, or may have occurred as the result of administered hormones, sometimes unknown even to the patient. For that reason it is important to confirm presence or absence of estrogen production by the maturation index and the administration of progesterone. A menstrual period within 14 days after the administration of progesterone in oil and a maturation index with greater than 20 per cent superficial cells indicates that she is making estrogen. Some breast development in the absence of the other estrogen parameters may indicate that she is now producing only subnormal amounts of estrogen.

It is important to evaluate serum prolactin in any woman with abnormal menstrual periods. The only exceptions are patients who have an elevated serum FSH (above 40 mIU per ml), or who have the polycystic ovary syndrome, well established by bilaterally enlarged ovaries or a serum LH:FSH ratio (expressed in mIU per ml) of 3 or more. Hyperprolactinemia may be a cause of primary amenorrhea. Indeed, in some patients presenting with this disorder, pituitary adenomas have already developed. Remember that primary hypothyroidism may cause serum prolactin elevation because TRH also induces release of prolactin. In every patient with an elevated prolactin level, quantitation of serum TSH should be carried out. The best favor a gynecologist can do for his patient with hyperprolactinemia is to prove primary hypothyroidism as the etiology. While it is responsible only 2 to 3 per cent of the time, making this diagnosis, treating with thyroid, and lowering prolactin removes the patient from that group of girls with hyperprolactinemias who require long-term follow-up, waiting for the possible appearance of a prolactinoma.

Based upon the studies above, several definitive diagnoses can be made. They are listed in Table 1 (with the exception of those that fall into the uterus absent, breasts absent category).

TABLE 1. **Diagnosis of Primary Amenorrhea**

Uterus and Breasts Present
Imperforate hymen
Vaginal septum
Ovulation failure ("hypothalamic")
Polycystic ovary syndrome

Uterus Absent, Breasts Present
Congenital absence of the uterus (partial or complete)
Testicular feminization syndrome

Uterus Present, Breasts Absent (or Subnormal with Low Estrogen Production)
Hypogonadotropinism—idiopathic
Hypogonadotropinism with elevated prolactin
Hypogonadotropinism secondary to weight loss and exercise
Ovarian failure
Resistant ovary syndrome

Uterus Present, Breasts Absent (or very subnormal), with Signs of Massive Androgen Overproduction
Congential adrenal hyperplasia
Virilizing adrenal tumor

Below we discuss parameters upon which each of these diagnoses is made and the appropriate therapy.

Imperforate Hymen. The patient has normal secondary sexual characteristics and a bulging, often darkened hymen. Usually a uterus can be felt high up on rectal examination. The diagnosis can usually be made easily on the first visit. Therapy is to incise the hymen (conducted in the office or under general anesthesia) and maintain patency.

Vaginal Transverse Septum. The patient presents with normal secondary sexual characteristics. There is a blind vagina without a visible cervix. There are often two dimples in the septum, which may be bulging. It should not be needled in the office, as blood is a wonderful culture medium. On rectal examination, the upper vagina is felt to be full. Sometimes the uterus can be defined separately, sometimes it cannot. Therapy is to incise and partially remove the septum, and anastomose the upper and lower vagina. General anesthesia and careful attention to maintaining patency are required. When the septum is close to the cervix, one may have trouble even with carefully placed stents, and sometimes the physician, the patient, or her husband has to use his or her fingers to maintain dilation of this septal area and prevent "scarring down." If it scars down to the point where it does not allow menstrual egress or intercourse at some future date, a second surgical reconstruction will be considerably more difficult.

Hypothalamic Anovulation. These patients present with good breast development, have a uterus (cervix visible), and are making estrogen. They bleed following administration of progesterone. They are not hirsute and have a normal serum free testosterone concentration. Once the diagnosis of ovulation failure is established, the strategy is to look for a specific cause and, if found, treat it. Specific causes include polycystic ovary syndrome (discussed in detail in another article), hypothyroidism and hyperprolactinemia. Most often a specific cause will not be found. In this case, the strategy is to give the patient synthetic progestins for the first 10 days of each calendar month to induce withdrawal bleeding and avoid the endometrial hyperplasia which may bring later problems of menometrorrhagia. Continued unopposed estrogen carries a risk of endometrial carcinoma, so synthetic progestins should be used the full 10 days. Using the same days in all patients based upon calendar months is invaluable in a large practice. When a patient phones, one needs only a calendar to know what is going on. Should a patient in this category desire pregnancy, she, by virtue of her estrogen production, is the one in which pregnancy yields are most favorable. Finally, in some patients who originally appear to have hypothalamic anovulation, over a period of time, a characteristic polycystic ovary syndrome will develop.

Polycystic Ovary Syndrome. These patients usually have erratic bleeding secondary to anovulation, but occasionally present with primary amenorrhea. When that is the case, they have normal secondary sexual characteristics, the uterus is present (cervix visible), and they bleed on progesterone withdrawal and show evidence of androgen overproduction: mid-line body hair, acne, and oily skin. Cover hair on arms and legs does not indicate androgen overproduction. These patients have elevated serum free testosterone levels. Sooner or later they will have serum LH:FSH ratios of 3 or greater. Treatment depends on the extent of hirsutism. If it is not a problem, monthly administration of synthetic progestins on the first 10 days of each calendar month is satisfactory therapy. If it is a problem, serum free testosterone levels may be suppressed with low-dose contraceptives about 95 per cent of the time, or glucocorticoids (such as Decadron, 0.5 mg at bedtime) about 40 per cent of the time. In those instances in which the above medications are contraindicated, spironolactone will be successful in doses of 50 to 100 mg bid. Glucocorticoids and spironolactone may or may not establish ovulatory menstrual periods. If they fail to do so, progestin should be given for the first 10 days of each calendar month. Moderate hirsutism, present for short periods (2 to 3 years) will usually regress markedly with suppression therapy. In passing, it is pertinent to consider the possibility of early Cushing's syndrome. If Cushing's disease is suggested (by hypertension, glucose in the urine, striae, or centripetal obesity) screening tests should be done: 24-hour urinary free cortisol collected on a quiet day (should not exceed 80 mcg per 24 hours); a study of diurnal variation where serum cortisol levels are quantitated at 8:00 AM and 4:00 PM (afternoon values should be half the morning value); and the Nugent test, wherein one gives 1 mg of Decadron at bedtime and quantitates serum cortisol the next morning (should be below 5 mcg per dl). When the patient with polycystic ovary syndrome desires pregnancy, clomiphene citrate is administered as for the patient with hypothalamic anovulation.

Congenital Absence of the Uterus. This patient presents with normal secondary sexual characteristics (particularly normal pubic hair) but the vagina is absent or there is a shallow vaginal opening. On rectal examination, one of two findings is noted. In those who deny monthly pelvic pain, have nothing in the upper vagina, and have no uterus or perhaps a small marble-sized nodule, laparoscopy is not indicated. In those who complain of real and persistent monthly pain, laparoscopy is indicated. It is best scheduled at a time when the patient has or expects to have her monthly pain. The presence of a uterine remnant with blood issuing from the fallopian tubes indicates that the uterine remnant does bear an endometrial cavity and will have to be extirpated.

The literature contains descriptions of procedures used to attempt reconstruction and promote fertility. They often fail and should be tried only after considerable discussion, as loss of surgically induced patency requires a second operation. On occasion the uterine cavity will not communicate with the fallopian tubes and an enlarging abdominal mass and persistent worsening pain will signal extirpation. A vagina must be created. In our experience, the best method for doing this is the Frank procedure (nonsurgical). Young's rectal dilators are inserted into the small dimple or shallow vagina and it is progressively enlarged by having the patient push them into this dimple for 20 to 30 minutes twice daily, utilizing pressure to the point of minimal discomfort. Patients can usually make a functional vagina in 3 to 4 months. One will not do this until the patient approaches a possible marriage, or an age of maturity where she will maintain the patent vagina once it is constructed. We prefer the Frank procedure because it works so nicely. Should the patient allow the vaginal size to dissipate, resumption of dilator therapy or surgical reconstruction is done more easily than in those instances where a surgically constructed vagina has scarred down by neglect. In only a small number of patients is the Frank procedure not possible. These are patients with a "dash board perineum" where there is no dimple or shallow vagina to serve as a point to fix the rectal dilator for insertion. In this small number of patients, surgical construction of a vagina is indicated.

Testicular Feminization Syndrome. The patient presents with uterus absent and normal (sometimes even supernormal) breast development. The vagina is small and shallow. On rectal examination, nothing is felt in the upper vagina, and no uterus is present. An impressive feature is the reduced quantity of pubic and axillary hair. Serum testosterone determination will usually approximate the male level and a chromosomal analysis of peripheral blood will reveal the Y chromosome. This disorder results from absence of a biologically effective androgen receptor protein. Two therapeutic steps are indicated. The first is the creation of a functional vagina. Here the Frank procedure can always be used. The second is removal of the gonads because of the high incidence of tumors arising in intra-abdominal testes. Gonadal removal should be accomplished after puberty, but by the eighteenth year of life. There is debate as to whether to tell these patients that their gonad is a testis and that they bear a Y chromosome. Our general attitude has been to describe an abnormal gonad that is not making the right kind of hormones and only go into full details when requested by the patient or her family.

Idiopathic Hypogonadotropinism. The patient has a uterus but it is small. Breast development is usually absent, sometimes subnormal. Maturation index and failure to bleed after progesterone shows lack of estrogen production. Serum FSH determinations are below 40 mIU per ml. The problem is failure of the pituitary to release enough gonadotropin. This may be because the hypothalamus is not carrying out episodic release of LHRH or because gonadotropes in the pituitary do not synthesize biologically active gonadotropins. Therapy consists of cycling the patient with estrogen and progestin. We use conjugated estrogens (Premarin, 1.25 mg tablet) on the first 25 days of each calendar month, with medroxyprogesterone acetate (Provera, 10 mg tablet) from day 16 to 25 of each calendar month. Usually by the second or third cycle the patient will begin to have menstrual periods and over several months will notice the development of breasts and adult body contours. Unopposed estrogen should not be given to these individuals. The progestin should be given monthly in the above doses and for a 10 day period. If response is not adequate, Premarin may be increased to 2.5 mg daily for the first 25 days of each month. Every 2 years, therapy is stopped for 4 to 6 months to see if the patient establishes her own cycles. Occasionally one does, and we conclude that she was really just a "late bloomer." When such patients do not "turn on" but desire pregnancy one may use episodic LHRH or gonadotropins.

Hypogonadotropinism Secondary to Prolactin Elevation. A patient in this category may resemble the patient in the above paragraph but will have elevated serum prolactin levels. (It cannot be stressed too much that every patient with primary amenorrhea should have a serum prolactin determination unless her gonadotropin levels are elevated above 40 mIU per ml or polycystic ovary syndrome can be established.) If the thyroid cannot be implicated, coned-down Sellar views, polytomograms, and CT scans (in sequence) should be carried out and will often disclose a prolactinoma or craniopharyngioma. If they do not, we administer bromocriptine (Parlodel), 1.25 mg twice daily and reevaluate serum prolactin in 2 weeks. This dose (or multiples thereof) will usually return prolactin to normal levels, defining the etiology and demonstrating to the patient that she can, indeed, "turn on." After 6 months of therapy we stop and talk. The choices are: no therapy, estrogen and progestin, or more bromocriptine. No one really knows the best choice. We favor Premarin and Provera to maintain development and serial serum prolactin every 6 months with repeat radiologic studies on significant rise of prolactin or at intervals of 1 to 2 years.

Hypogonadotropinism Secondary to Weight Loss and Exercise. Although weight loss amenorrhea and exercise amenorrhea (associated with running, swimming, gymnastics, and ballet) most commonly present as secondary amenorrhea, one occasionally encounters it among young women with primary amenorrhea. Several of the patients we have seen had commenced sexual development and appeared to be on the verge of instituting menses when exercise or weight loss induced a regressive hypogonadotropic, hypoestrogenic state. These women are hypoestrogenic as shown by breast development and response to progesterone. Their gonadotropin levels are below 40 mIU per ml and their prolactin levels are normal. The best way to handle this problem (after laboratory testing, including serum prolactin determination) is to encourage the patient to gain back her weight or to stop her exercise. Weight loss amenorrhea (which is probably a variant of anorexia nervosa) and exercise amenorrhea are the most commonly unrecognized kinds of hypogonadotropic amenorrhea that we see. Thus, a careful review of the patient's weight and exercise activity is of extreme importance. We suggest that the patient stop her exercise and/or gain her weight back over 6 months. We advise her that once she has done this, return or establishment of normal menstrual periods establishes the etiology, and she can then recommence exercise or diet. This has worked in all but a few patients, who were "world-class runners" who would not stop their workouts.

Ovarian Failure. These patients have a uterus, are hypoestrogenic, lack development of secondary sexual characteristics (or at least have them at subnormal levels), fail to bleed in response to progesterone, and have serum FSH values above 40 mIU per ml. They do not need prolactin determinations or skull x-rays. They do need chromosomal studies to look for the presence of the Y chromosome, under which circumstances the gonads should be removed.

The problem results from absence of primary follicles in the ovary. Some patients are normal or eunuchoid in appearance. Most present as "Turner's syndrome" with short stature, shield chest, multiple nevi, and low hairline. Chromosome studies are variable, but only the presence of a Y chromosome calls for removal of the small or "streak" gonads. Therapy consists of cyclic estrogen and progestin as described above for idiopathic hypogonadotropic amenorrhea. Development of secondary sexual characteristics and menses will follow. While a few of these patients have had a few follicles lurking in the ovary and a lesser few have even attained a pregnancy, one should tell the patient to meet the desire for motherhood by adoption.

Resistant Ovary Syndrome. This patient presents with a uterus, is hypoestrogenic, and lacks significant breast development. Her serum FSH is above 40 mIU per ml (which usually is associated with the absence of primary follicles from the ovary). Actually she has follicles, but they are not responsive even to the high endogenous gonadotropin levels. The etiology remains undetermined. One of the earliest descriptions of this syndrome was as the "Savage syndrome." Distinguishing between the more common situation of ovarian failure and the resistant ovary is possible by biopsy of the ovary. (If the gonad is bereft of primary follicles, one has ovarian failure; if ovarian follicles are present in reasonable numbers, one has ovarian resistance.) Recently a treatment has evolved from anecdotal experiences. Patients are cycled for a period of 3 to 6 months, after which the cyclic Premarin and Provera are discontinued. Several patients who began spontaneously producing estrogen, ovulated, and attained pregnancy following this therapy have been reported. Therefore, ovarian biopsy is generally not done to differentiate between ovarian failure and ovarian resistance; rather, all patients are cycled and, should they want pregnancy, the medication is stopped to see if they will ovulate spontaneously.

Congenital Adrenal Hyperplasia and Virilizing Adrenal Tumor. The former disorder is usually recognized and treated in childhood; the latter is extremely rare. Nevertheless, when one sees primary amenorrhea in a patient presenting with signs of severe hirsutism and virilization (clitoral enlargement, deepening voice, temporal balding), these disorders should be considered. Urinary 17-ketosteroids and plasma dehydroepiandrosterone sulfate will be strikingly elevated in both disorders. The former, in which heterosexual development is of long duration, also displays clear-cut elevation of urinary pregnanetriol and serum 17α-hydroxyprogesterone, while in the latter these values are normal. Further, in the former disorder glucocorticoids suppress 17-ketosteroids and serum dehydroepiandrosterone to normal, while in the patient with tumor they are not suppressed. Therapy of congenital adrenal hyperplasia is medical (glucocorticoids and often mineralocorticoids), which, when all steroid values are returned to and kept at normal concentrations, institutes ovulatory menses. Therapy of adrenal tumor is, of course, surgical.

SUMMARY

Primary amenorrhea is a symptom. Definite diagnosis depends upon identification of obstruction of reproductive tract outflow, ascertaining the presence or absence of a uterus, and deciding whether estrogen is being produced or not. In the patient who has a uterus and is clearly not producing estrogen, it is the serum FSH value (after age 12 years) which most clearly differentiates between ovarian and pituitary failure. When the uterus is absent, a serum testosterone determination is indicated. Serum prolactin levels should be determined in all these patients, except those with clearly established polycystic ovary syndrome and those who are hypergonadotropic. Ductal tissue in the breast, more than 20 per cent superficial cells on maturation index, and a bleeding episode equal to half the normal menstrual flow or more means estrogen is being produced.

By careful application of the above principles, the gynecologist should be able to diagnose and adequately treat at least 90 per cent of the cases of primary amenorrhea encountered. The patient with primary amenorrhea must have a definitive diagnosis established before therapy is started. Any patient with primary amenorrhea who has a uterus can be treated with birth control pills and will respond by bleeding, removing the major symptom which brought her to the physician's office; but this is clearly not in her best interest. We have seen patients in whom this "shot-gun" therapy, continued over several years, has allowed prolactin-secreting microadenomas to progress to macroadenomas: a genuine and serious error in judgment.

SECONDARY AMENORRHEA

JOSE P. BALMACEDA, M.D.

The diagnostic evaluation and management of the patient with secondary amenorrhea must follow an orderly, step-by-step approach based upon a clear understanding of the physiopathology of the various clinical conditions that may underlie this symptom.

The presence of normal menstrual function implies:

1. that the endometrium is capable of responding to steroid stimulation (estrogen and progesterone);

2. that the ovaries are producing estrogen

and progesterone in a cyclic manner that results from ovulation;

3. that FSH and LH are being secreted by the anterior pituitary in a sequence that determines ovulation to occur;

4. that the hypothalamus is producing sufficient gonadotropin-releasing hormone and its vascular communications with the pituitary are intact.

The procedure presented in this chapter excludes patients with secondary amenorrhea and signs of excessive androgen production (hirsutism, virilization) or hyperprolactinemia.

A complete history and physical examination should be performed, the most important objectives being to establish the presence of normal secondary sexual characteristics and rule out pregnancy. We do not consider it necessary to routinely screen patients for thyroid dysfunction with TSH, T_3, and T_4 tests, and do so only in the presence of a suggestive history or physical findings. Because prolactin-secreting adenomas do not invariably present with galactorrhea, serum prolactin levels should be measured. Patients with elevated prolactin are discussed in detail in another article.

After the first visit the patient should be given a progestational agent to induce withdrawal bleeding. We use medroxyprogesterone (Provera, 10 mg daily for 5 days). Progesterone in oil, 100 or 200 mg, administered by intramuscular injection can also be used. The patient is instructed to expect vaginal bleeding 2 to 7 days after the last tablet is ingested. The amount of vaginal bleeding can vary from very heavy passage of large blood clots to light spotting, the interpretation being the same: "The patient who has withdrawal bleeding in response to the administration of a progestational agent has normal levels of endogenous estrogen and an endometrium capable of responding to them."

POSITIVE PROGESTATIONAL CHALLENGE TEST

If the patient responds to the administration of Provera with vaginal bleeding and has a normal serum prolactin level, no further workup is needed and the diagnosis of amenorrhea secondary to anovulation can be made. This group includes patients with anovulation secondary to hypothalamic dysfunction and polycystic ovary syndrome.

Hypothalamic Dysfunction

Hypothalamic dysfunction may be the most frequent cause of secondary amenorrhea. The pathophysiology of this syndrome is not completely understood. Pituitary secretion of follicle-stimulating hormone (FSH) and luteinizing hormone (LH) is controlled by gonadotropin-releasing hormone (GnRH) liberated by the hypothalamus following a determinate pattern combining a tonic and pulsating secretion. A qualitative more than a quantitative change in the secretion of GnRH must occur because circulating FSH and LH levels are normal in these patients. Although in the majority of the cases no specific etiology can be found, a well taken history may reveal the precipitating factor.

Stress and Drugs. Amenorrhea may be related to stressful situations sometimes poorly recognized by the patients (examinations, moving to college, breaking of a relationship, economic problems, and so forth). Prolonged drug use can also cause amenorrhea. Among those most commonly cited are phenothiazines and tricyclic antidepressants, which are commonly associated with elevated prolactin levels. The mechanism of action probably affects the dopaminergic systems in the central nervous system.

Post-Pill Amenorrhea. Amenorrhea starting after the use of oral contraceptives, or post-pill amenorrhea, is also due to hypothalamic dysfunction. The diagnosis should not be made until 6 months elapse after the oral contraceptives are discontinued. During this interval more than 90 per cent of patients recover menstrual function. Patients presenting galactorrhea are an exception to this rule and should be investigated without delay. Post-pill amenorrhea should not be confused with "amenorrhea" starting while the patient is still taking oral contraceptives. In this situation, the failure to demonstrate withdrawal bleeding signifies lack of sufficient proliferation of the endometrium. After ruling out pregnancy, the treatment of this condition may consist of either changing the oral contraceptive to one with a higher estrogen content, or supplementing the one she is using with estrogen tablets (e.g., adding ethinyl estradiol, 0.05 mg daily for 21 days, for one or two cycles).

Weight Change and Amenorrhea. Loss of more than 15 per cent of ideal body weight may be associated with abnormal menstrual function. These patients present all the characteristics of hypothalamic dysfunction with normal FSH and LH, and positive response to progesterone challenge. As the weight loss gets to be severe (e.g., anorexia nervosa with more than 25 per cent of ideal body weight lost) low levels of gonadotropins and estrogens are more common, accompanied by alterations of thyroid function. The practicing physician should be able to recognize that, although most of the patients with amenorrhea due to weight loss will respond to counseling and regain weight, there is a group with serious psychological alterations that need psychiatric treatment.

On the other hand, excessive weight gain can also be associated with amenorrhea. Whether obesity itself causes the menstrual alteration or whether stress underlies both the amenorrhea and the compulsive eating is not clear. The majority of these patients recover menstrual function after losing weight.

Polycystic Ovary Syndrome

A second group of patients with secondary amenorrhea who respond to progesterone withdrawal are those with polycystic ovarian disease. Although classically described as presenting with hirsutism and obesity, these two stigmata may be absent. The exact cause of polycystic ovary syndrome is still unknown. The syndrome is associated with abnormal gonadotropin secretion with increased LH:FSH ratio, which differentiates these patients from patients with hypothalamic dysfunction.

Ovarian steroidogenesis is abnormal, with increased production of androstenedione and testosterone. The ovaries have a thickened capsule, a large number of follicular cysts, and hyperplasia of the stroma. Excessive circulating androgens and hypothalamic insensitivity to estrogens are possible causes.

Treatment

Treatment of the patient with secondary amenorrhea and normal levels of endogenous estrogen (hypothalamic dysfunction or polycystic ovary syndrome) can be initiated after the progesterone challenge test. Specific therapy will depend mainly on the desire for fertility at the time of consultation.

If the patient desires fertility, then the treatment of choice is induction of ovulation with clomiphene citrate (Clomid). It is in these patients that Clomid gives the best results. If clomiphene therapy is not successful, the use of postmenopausal gonadotropins is indicated. Induction of ovulation is discussed in detail in another article.

On the other hand, if the patient does not desire fertility one should induce periodic withdrawal bleeding with a progestational agent. Medroxyprogesterone acetate (Provera), 10 mg daily, should be given for 7 to 10 days every 2 months. This treatment alleviates the effects of prolonged unopposed estrogenic action on the endometrium, that is, endometrial hyperplasia and increased risk of endometrial adenocarcinoma.

Some form of contraception (diaphragm, condoms, and so forth) is recommended for patients who wish to avoid pregnancy in case spontaneous recovery of menstrual function or occasional ovulation occurs. Low-dose oral contraceptives are not contraindicated as long as the patient understands that amenorrhea will recur after discontinuation of the birth control pills.

Long term follow-up should include a serum prolactin level every 5 to 6 months and instructions to report to the physician if periodic withdrawal to medroxyprogesterone fails to occur.

NEGATIVE PROGESTATIONAL CHALLENGE TEST

Failure to demonstrate withdrawal bleeding after administration of a progestational agent is due to a lack of proliferation of the endometrium secondary to uterine synechiae formed as a complication of infection or curettages (Asherman's syndrome) or to insufficient or low circulating estrogens.

Asherman's Syndrome

The majority of patients with Asherman's syndrome have uterine synechiae formed after curettages following delivery or abortion especially in the presence of infection (endometritis). If the amenorrhea started after a curettage, hysterosalpingogram and/or hysteroscopy should be performed without further work-up. The hysteroscope permits direct visualization and sometimes resection of the scar tissue. Tuberculous endometritis can also cause sufficient endometrial destruction to cause lack of proliferation. This entity is very rare in the United States but should be considered in the differential diagnosis of patients from the Middle East, Africa, and Latin America. The majority of the cases are secondary to a pulmonary focus. Chest x-ray often reveals the characteristic lesions.

The lack of response to high doses of estrogen (e.g., conjugated estrogens, 2.5 mg daily for 21 days) followed by medroxyprogesterone (10 mg daily for 5 days) can also be used as a diagnostic test for Asherman's syndrome. In our experience, though, the history of these patients is always clear enough to justify a hysterosalpingogram or hysteroscopy.

Secondary Amenorrhea with Low Circulating Estrogens

This group includes patients with ovarian failure and patients with hypothalamic-pituitary failure. Serum FSH concentrations will differentiate between these two groups. If low circulating estrogen levels are due to ovarian failure,

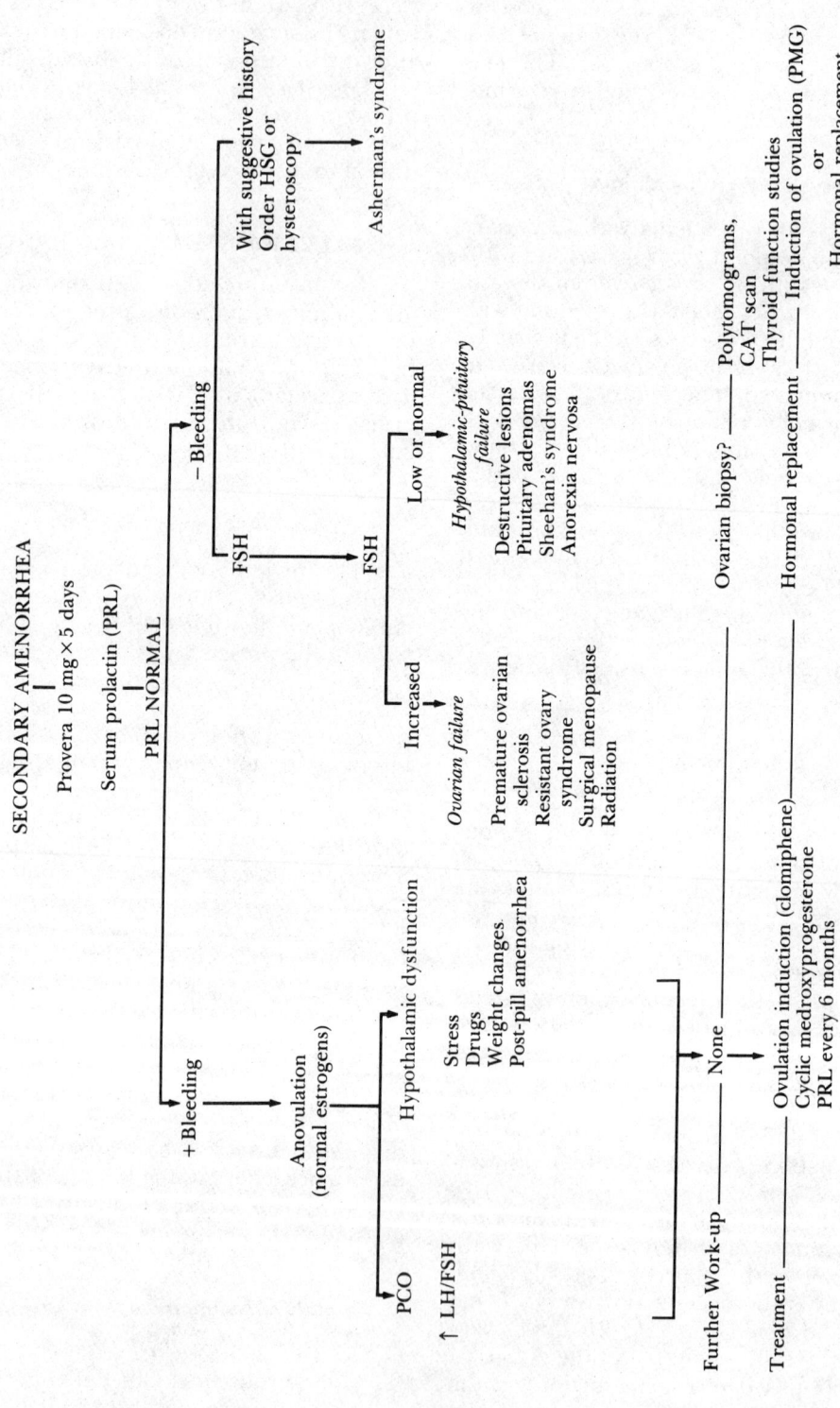

Figure 1. Evaluation and treatment of secondary amenorrhea.

FSH is elevated (over 40 mIU per ml); if due to hypothalamic-pituitary failure, FSH will be low or normal.

Amenorrhea Secondary to Ovarian Failure (↑ FSH). Ovarian failure is more commonly found in patients presenting with primary amenorrhea, but in a small number of patients ovarian insufficiency causes secondary cessation of menstrual function.

PREMATURE OVARIAN FAILURE. By definition, ovarian failure which occurs before age 35 after a period of apparent normal activity is termed "premature ovarian failure." This entity is also known as premature menopause and premature ovarian sclerosis. Most commonly, the onset of premature ovarian failure is in the early 20s, although it can occur earlier (e.g., before menarche, presenting as primary amenorrhea). The karyotype of these patients is 46XX. No hereditary tendency has been noted. The diagnosis is established by laparoscopy. The ovaries appear small. Follicles are scanty or absent on ovarian biopsy.

Premature ovarian failure is irreversible and there is no possibility of pregnancy in the future. Therapy consists of hormonal replacement.

RESISTANT OVARY SYNDROME. This syndrome was first described by Jones and Moraes Reuhsen in 1969 in patients with primary amenorrhea. Since then, a few cases of secondary amenorrhea have been found with the same ovarian characteristics. These patients also have 46XX karyotypes, and normal secondary sexual characteristics, but demonstrate low estrogen levels and elevated gonadotropins. They differ from patients with premature sclerosis in that the ovaries are usually larger and smooth. Biopsy reveals normal histology with numerous primordial follicles.

The only justification for ovarian biopsy to differentiate these patients from patients with ovarian sclerosis is that some of these women ovulate after wedge-resection of the ovaries, high-dose estrogen therapy, or human menopausal gonadotropin therapy.

MISCELLANEOUS. Patients who have been surgically castrated (e.g., surgery for extensive endometriosis pelvic inflammatory disease not responsive to antibiotic therapy) or who have received pelvic irradiation to treat malignant tumors (causing ovarian fibrosis) are included in the group with amenorrhea due to ovarian failure.

In a small number of women, ovarian infection (e.g., tubo-ovarian abscess) and endometriosis may cause enough destruction to produce ovarian failure. More frequently, though, these entities result in anovulation with dysfunctional bleeding or amenorrhea.

TREATMENT OF OVARIAN FAILURE BY HORMONAL REPLACEMENT. After the diagnosis of ovarian failure as the cause of secondary amenorrhea, no further work-up is needed. With the exception of the few cases reported in the literature where high estrogen or gonadotropin therapy has resulted in ovulation, treatment consists of hormonal replacement.

The most common replacement regimen is a combination of conjugated estrogens (0.3 to 1.25 mg daily for 21 days) with medroxyprogesterone (10 mg daily added from days 15 to 25). The patient should experience withdrawal bleeding after the last tablet of Provera. The dose of estrogen is adjusted, guided by the amount of vaginal bleeding, by symptoms of estrogen deficiency (e.g., hot flushes), and by symptoms of estrogen intolerance (e.g., nausea, fluid retention). These patients should be seen by the physician every 6 months.

Amenorrhea Secondary to Hypothalamic-Hypophyseal Failure (FSH Low or "Normal"). Patients included in this group are those with low circulatory estrogens resulting from a lack of ovarian stimulation secondary to insufficient gonadotropin secretion. Although a single measurement of FSH or LH in serum may appear to be normal, serial blood samples demonstrate lower levels of gonadotropin than in patients with normal circulatory estrogens. In many of the cases amenorrhea forms part of more complex syndromes where signs of deficiency of other tropic hormones produced by the anterior pituitary are present.

HYPOTHALAMIC HYPOFUNCTION (HYPOTHALAMIC HYPOPITUITARISM). Hypothalamic function may be affected by a variety of diseases that cause a decrease in GnRH production or that deform the anatomy to interfere with GnRH transport to the pituitary gland. Destruction of the hypothalamus may occur secondary to tumors. Craniopharyngiomas and germinomas are among the most common tumors causing hypothalamic hypofunction. Lesions originating in other organs can also metastasize to the hypothalamus. Encephalitis and chronic granulomatous diseases such as tuberculosis and sarcoidosis also affect hypothalamic function. Other causes include degenerative diseases, irradiation, and head injuries.

HYPOPHYSEAL HYPOFUNCTION (PRIMARY HYPOPITUITARISM). Irradiation, surgical ablation, and tumors, among other things, may cause pituitary destruction and gonadotropin deficiency. All tumors that can cause hypothalamic compression can, by extension to the sella turcica, affect the hypophysis, but the most common causes are pituitary adenomas, probably the most common intracranial tumors. Many of them are so small that they do not affect the endocrine function of the gland. The most frequent cell type is the cromophobe. Many adenomas are endocrinologically active, producing one or more hormones (e.g., basophilic adenomas can produce ACTH and cause Cushing's disease) including the complex glycoprotein hormones (FSH, LH, TSH). Patients with prolactin-secreting adenomas may present with amenorrhea without galactorrhea. For this reason a serum prolactin level should be ordered on the first visit.

Another well known cause of primary hypopituitarism is Sheehan's syndrome. The enlarged pituitary gland of term pregnancy is very susceptible to ischemia and necrosis secondary to postpartum hemorrhage. The degree of hypofunction seen in these patients varies. The most severe cases may present rapid mammary involution, loss of axillary and pubic hair, fatigue, hypotension, and even diabetes insipidus. Milder cases may present only with amenorrhea and low gonadotropins. Thorough evaluation of all pituitary functions should be done in every case.

TREATMENT AND FURTHER WORK-UP. Patients with hypothalamic-pituitary failure should have further evaluation before therapy for amenorrhea is initiated. Because tumors are frequent in this group, most of the work-up is designed to rule out neoplasia. A second objective is to determine whether or not there is a deficiency of other tropic hormones.

These patients should undergo: (1) radiologic evaluation of the sella turcica (polytomograms, CT scan); (2) evaluation of thyroid function (TSH, T_3, T_4) and growth hormones; and (3) insulin tolerance test. By inducing hypoglycemia with insulin one can gain an idea of the pituitary reserve of ACTH and growth hormone.

Therapy for the patient with hypothalamic pituitary failure depends upon whether or not pregnancy is desired. In those who desire pregnancy, induction of ovulation is indicated. These patients are good candidates for postmenopausal gonadotropin (e.g., Pergonal) therapy. If pregnancy is not a goal, hormonal replacement with estrogen and medroxyprogesterone is recommended.

INDUCTION OF OVULATION

DANIEL R. MISHELL, JR., M.D.

Ovulation-inducing drugs should only be given to those women who are infertile and either do not ovulate at all or ovulate infrequently. Their use should be restricted to patients who are infertile and also have oligomenorrhea or amenorrhea. Currently there are three drugs available for inducing ovulation: clomiphene citrate (Clomid), bromoergocriptine (Parlodel), and human menopausal gonadotropin (Pergonal). Of these the one that has been in use the longest and is the safest and easiest to administer is clomiphene citrate. The drug is usually administered for 5 days beginning on the first to fifth day of spontaneous or induced menses.

Clomiphene Citrate. Clomiphene citrate is a weak estrogen with a chemical structure similar to that of diethylstilbestrol. As such, this agent binds to the estrogen receptor sites in the hypothalamus and pituitary, preventing endogenous estrogens from reaching these sites. Because clomiphene has a weaker estrogenic action than estradiol, it does not exert a negative feedback on the release of GnRH. Thus when it is ingested, gonadotropin levels rise and stimulate the ovary to make increasing levels of endogenous estradiol. Following discontinuation of the drug, the endogenous estrogens continue to rise and exert a negative feedback on the hypothalamic-pituitary axis, resulting in a decrease in circulating gonadotropin levels. At the same time estradiol levels from the dominant ovarian follicle rise and eventually by positive feedback stimulate the gonadotropin surge that induces ovulation. Ovulation occurs at a varying time interval after the drug is stopped, usually between 5 and 9 days with an average of about 7 days.

In order to determine not only that ovulation has occurred but when it has occurred, it is important that patients take their basal body temperature for 2 weeks after stopping Clomid. If it is impossible for them to take basal body temperature, then serum progesterone should be determined 2 weeks after stopping the agent to determine that ovulation has occurred. The presence of bleeding 3 weeks after stopping the drug does not indicate that ovulation has occurred, since this may just be estrogen withdrawal bleeding. Because of the mechanism of action of clomiphene citrate it is necessary that patients treated with this drug have circulating endogenous estradiol levels of about 40 pg per ml or greater. In practicality, this means that if they are amenorrheic or oligomenorrheic, they should have withdrawal bleeding following either intramuscular progesterone in oil or orally administered progestins or else clomiphene will not induce ovulation.

Clomiphene citrate was extensively studied clinically prior to its being approved for use by the United States Food and Drug Administration in 1965. In the pre-marketing studies, varying dosages and duration of administration were used. Of all patients treated, the average incidence of ovulation was about 70 per cent and incidence of pregnancy was about 30 per cent. It was found that the dosages of 50 mg for 5 days and 100 mg for 5 days were the most effective dosages with the least number of side effects, and these doses are those that are now recommended for use in the product brochure. Analysis of 2369 pregnancies that occurred prior to marketing showed that the rates of spontaneous abortion, stillbirths, and ectopic pregnancy were similar to rates of other groups of infertility patients who subsequently conceived.

There were 9 per cent multiple live births, of which more than 90 per cent were twins. There were a few triplets, quadruplets, and quintuplets. With the use of the fixed dosage regimen for five days, the incidence of multiple gestation has been diminished and consists nearly entirely of twins. A recently published review of 10 years' experience with this individualized graduated treatment regimen in one large clinic revealed that the incidence of multiple births, nearly all twins, was less than 5 per cent and the first trimester abortion rate was about 15 per cent.

The congenital anomaly rate was about 2.5 per cent. In the pre-marketing studies the overall incidence of birth defects was also 2.4 per cent which is similar to that in the general population. These consisted of various types of defects such as congenital heart defects, Down's syndrome, clubbed feet, and gut defects. However, when clomiphene was administered in the first 6 weeks of gestation the incidence of birth defects was 5.1 per cent. Although not significantly higher than the 2.4 per cent observed in patients in whom the drug was administered prior to conception, the increase is of concern. Therefore, it is important that clomiphene citrate not be administered when a patient is pregnant and that the drug be administered only after the patient has an episode of withdrawal bleeding.

Side effects noted with clomiphene citrate in the pre-marketing studies showed a 14 per cent incidence of ovarian enlargement, 11 per cent incidence of vasomotor symptoms, and a 7 per cent incidence of abdominal discomfort. In addition, a few patients had problems with blurring of vision, urticaria, or hair loss. The incidence of ovarian enlargement and other symptoms is much less with the fixed dosage and fixed days of treatment. The ovarian cysts are generally less than 10 cm in size and will resolve spontaneously provided there is no further stimulation of the gonads by another treatment course. Cyst formation can occur after any cycle of treatment, even if the same dosage is being administered. Therefore, it is advisable that prior to each treatment course the patient have a bimanual examination to be certain that ovarian enlargement is not present. If ovarian enlargement is present, the next treatment course should be withheld until the ovarian cyst resolves spontaneously.

Patients should be initially treated with 50 mg a day for 5 days. If ovulation does not occur, then the dose should be increased to 100 mg a day for 5 days in the next treatment course. If patients do not ovulate with this dosage, then the dose should be sequentially increased to 150, 200, and then 250 mg a day for 5 days in subsequent treatment cycles. With the last dosage regimen, an additional 10,000 units of HCG is given 7 days following the last pill to stimulate the LH surge. If the patient ovulates at any one of the lower dosages, that dosage is maintained until pregnancy occurs.

Utilizing this graduated sequential dosage regimen, one can expect about a 90 per cent ovulation rate in patients with oligomenorrhea, and about a 70 per cent ovulation rate in patients with amenorrhea who have withdrawal bleeding following progesterone, whether or not they have hyperprolactinemia. Overall about half the oligomenorrheic patients treated who ovulate will conceive, and about 40 per cent of the amenorrheic women who ovulate will conceive. About half of all those patients treated with the 50 mg dose will ovulate and about half of these ovulating patients will conceive. About a third of those treated with the 100 mg dose will ovulate and half of those who ovulate will conceive. Of the patients treated with all dosage regimens, about 70 per cent of those who ovulate and/or conceive will be treated with the 50 or 100 mg dosage. Therefore, about 30 per cent of all those patients treated with clomiphene who ovulate will do so only if they are treated with dosages greater than 100 mg for 5 days. In addition, about 30 per cent of patients conceiving after clomiphene treatment will only have done so when treated with greater than the 100 mg dosage.

About half the pregnancies occur following the first ovulatory cycle of treatment and about 25 per cent of the pregnancies occur following the second ovulatory cycle of treatment. Thereafter, the incidence of conception declines, with only about 5 per cent of those patients who eventually conceive doing so after treatment for more than five ovulatory cycles. Since patients who conceive with this treatment usually do so after the first few ovulatory treatment cycles, it is recommended to postpone the remainder of the infertility work-up, other than a semen analysis, until after 3 ovulatory treatment cycles have taken place. Clomiphene citrate does not cause poor cervical mucus and does not produce an inadequate luteal phase. This agent thus does not cause infertility. Patients whose only infertility factor is anovulation should have a conception rate of 90 per cent following clomiphene treatment. However, if other infertility factors are present, the conception rates are less than 10 per cent.

Patients with adequate endogenous estrogen who do not ovulate after treatment with 250 mg of clomiphene for 5 days followed by HCG can be treated in one of two ways. If their dehydroepiandrosterone sulfate (DHEAS) level is elevated, they should be treated with dexamethasone, 0.5 mg at bed time for 2 weeks prior to, concomitantly with, and following the administration of clomiphene at the 250 a day for 5 day dosage. The dexamethasone should be continued until the patient receives the HCG, 1 week later. For those patients who do not have an elevated DHEAS, clomiphene citrate, 250 mg, should be administered for 8 days with 10,000 units of HCG given 1 week after the last clomiphene tablet. Use of these two regimens will increase the incidence of ovulation in amenorrheic patients with progestin withdrawal bleeding treated with clomiphene citrate.

Human Menopausal Gonadotropin. For patients who do not ovulate after these regimens, or for initial therapy of patients who have amenorrhea with absence of withdrawal bleeding following progesterone who also do not have hyperprolactinemia, the therapy of choice is human menopausal gonadotropin (HMG). It is difficult to administer HMG because each patient responds individually in each treatment cycle and the amount of medication and duration of therapy may differ from course to course. Therefore, estrogen monitoring is mandatory.

Prior to treatment with HMG, it is essential that a full infertility work-up be performed including a laparoscopy, and the patient should only be treated if the entire infertility work-up reveals no other causes of infertility. While receiving HMG, patients should be seen initially once a day and examined to determine the amount of cervical mucus. In addition, a serum sample or 24-hour urine should be obtained for measurement of immunoreactive estrogens. Ultrasonic monitoring of the size of the ovarian follicle is very helpful.

Initially, 2 ampules of HMG a day should be administered, and the dose increased sequentially until the estrogen levels reach between 500 and 1000 picograms per ml and/or the dominant follicle is greater than 18 mm in diameter as measured by ultrasonography. At this time the HMG is stopped and 10,000 units of HCG is given 24 to 36 hours after the last injection to induce ovulation.

With HMG therapy, ovulation should be induced in nearly 100 per cent of the cycles but the pregnancy rate without other infertility factors is only about 60 per cent. The multiple gestation rate ranges between 10 and 15 per cent and the spontaneous abortion rate is between 25 and 30 per cent. With estrogen monitoring, post-treatment ovarian enlargement should occur in less than 5 per cent of patients, and the hyperstimulation syndrome should be less than 1 per cent. Patients should be counseled that it takes an average of about 3 ovulatory cycles to conceive with HMG, and that the spontaneous abortion rate is high. However, the incidence of congenital anomalies in infants born following HMG is no higher than in spontaneous ovulatory cycles.

Bromoergocriptine. The last drug currently approved for induction of ovulation is bromoergocriptine, a dopamine agonist. The use of this agent should be limited to those patients who have amenorrhea with low endogenous estrogen levels and elevated prolactin levels. Bromoergocriptine is given in a dosage of 2.5 mg twice a day and the ovulation rate should be about 90 per cent, with the pregnancy rate varying between 50 and 80 per cent. The incidence of multiple gestation, abortion, and congenital abnormalities is no greater than in a normal ovulating population. However, about 25 per cent of the patients will have side effects consisting mainly of nausea, headache, and dizziness, although some patients also develop abdominal pain and nasal congestion. Because clomiphene has fewer side effects than bromoergocriptine and is as effective, clomiphene should be used to treat anovulatory patients with hyperprolactinemia who do not have very low endogenous estrogen levels.

POLYCYSTIC OVARY SYNDROME

JOSEPH P. HOLT, JR., MD., Ph.D., and BRIAN LITTLE, M.D.

Polycystic ovarian disease encompasses a spectrum of signs and symptoms, the two principal characteristics of which are (1) anovulation and (2) androgen overproduction. Peripheral conversion of the elevated androgen leads to elevated levels of estrogens, primarily estrone, and thus this condition has also been termed "continuous estrous syndrome." The overproduction of androgens is seen in a wide spectrum of clinical conditions including hirsutism, polycystic ovaries, ovarian hyperthecosis, rare ovarian tumors, hypothyroidism, congenital adrenal hyperplasia, and Cushing's syndrome. The clinical features of patients with polycystic ovary syndrome were described by Stein and Leventhal in 1935 and include oligoamenorrhea, hirsutism, infertility, and obesity. The ovaries are generally, but not always, enlarged and oblong, with a thickened smooth capsule beneath which are numerous primary and atretic follicles.

The etiology of the polycystic ovary syndrome is unresolved. The syndrome can probably result from a number of derangements in the hypothalamic-pituitary-ovarian axis. Furthermore, it has been shown by vein catheterization studies that the source of the increased circulating androgens may result from either adrenal or ovarian overproduction of androgen, or a combination thereof. The increased production of androgen in turn increases the estrone level by peripheral conversion. This may cause the increased tonic luteinizing hormone (LH) level which completes the cycle by stimulating further production of androgen.

Laboratory confirmation of the polycystic ovary syndrome can be done by documenting an elevation of the serum level of LH and a normal or low follicle stimulating hormone (FSH) level, resulting in a 3:1 or greater gonadotropin ratio. One or more serum androgens, dehydroepiandrosterone sulfate, androstenedione, or total testosterone, are frequently elevated in this condition. The free serum testosterone level is elevated in patients with hirsutism, and the serum sex steroid binding globulin level, also known as testosterone-estradiol binding globulin (TeBG), is low. Urinary 17-ketosteroids have been found to be at the upper limit of normal or elevated in over 20 per cent of patients with polycystic ovaries. Urinary 17-ketosteroids are useful only in excluding androgen-producing tumors since they do not correlate well with the elevated serum androgen levels found in hirsute patients. Serum prolactin is determined because hyperprolactinemia may be associated with polycystic ovary disease.

TREATMENT OF THE INFERTILE PATIENT

The treatment of the infertile or hirsute patient with polycystic ovary syndrome is diagrammed in Figure 1. Patients desiring pregnancy undergo an infertility evaluation including (1) basal body temperature graphs, (2) tubal patency test, (3) post-coital test, (4) endometrial biopsy, and (5) a midluteal serum progesterone determination. The diagnosis of polycystic ovary syndrome is confirmed in the anovulatory hirsute woman with enlarged ovaries by the finding of an elevated luteinizing hormone level with a 3:1 or greater LH:FSH ratio. The initial measurement of the abnormal elevation of serum androgens (e.g., serum free testosterone) confirms and documents the baseline pretreatment level of the hyperandrogen state.

The hyperandrogen state in many patients may be ameliorated by glucocorticoid administration and adrenal suppression. As shown in Figure 1, an initial trial of dexamethasone (0.5 mg daily at bedtime) will usually suffice. Determination of the serum free testosterone and dehydroepiandrosterone sulfate levels after one month of therapy will determine those patients that respond with a lowering of their androgen levels; subsequent spontaneous ovulation will frequently occur. Dexamethasone is discontinued in patients who fail to normalize their hyperandrogen state. Patients who do not ovulate should be treated with clomiphene citrate. Care must be exercised to be sure the patient is not pregnant before initiating therapy. Progesterone (100 mg in oil intramuscularly) is given to initiate a menstrual period, prior to therapy. Both dexamethasone and clomiphene citrate may be required at the same time to stimulate ovulation.

Clomiphene citrate causes a temporary elevation of FSH and LH, stimulating follicular development. The rising 17-β-estradiol subsequently initiates, by positive feedback at the pituitary, the mid-cycle LH and FSH surge with subsequent ovulation. The patient is given clomiphene citrate beginning with 50 mg per day on days 5 through 9 of the menstrual cycle. This dosage should be tried for at least two cycles, and if ovulation is not achieved, then increasing increments of 50 mg should be given per cycle to a maximum dosage of 200 mg. If ovulation still does not occur, human chorionic gonadotropin, 5000 to 10,000 units intramuscularly, is added to the regimen and administered once between days 16 and 18 of the menstrual cycle.

One should remember that patients with polycystic ovary disease are particularly sensitive to clomiphene citrate and require pelvic examinations at the end of each cycle to determine if cystic enlargement of the ovaries has developed. Further stimulation of such cysts could result in the ovarian hyperstimulation syndrome. Clomiphene citrate treatment must be discontinued if visual or central nervous system symptoms develop. Most studies demonstrate that the majority of patients with polycystic ovary syndrome will ovulate on clomiphene citrate therapy and about 50 per cent will conceive.

The unusual patient who fails to ovulate on clomiphene citrate therapy may occasionally be considered for human menopausal gonadotropin (HMG, Pergonal) therapy. Historically, wedge resection of the ovaries was found to be associated with clinical improvement of hirsutism, spontaneous ovulation, and in some patients

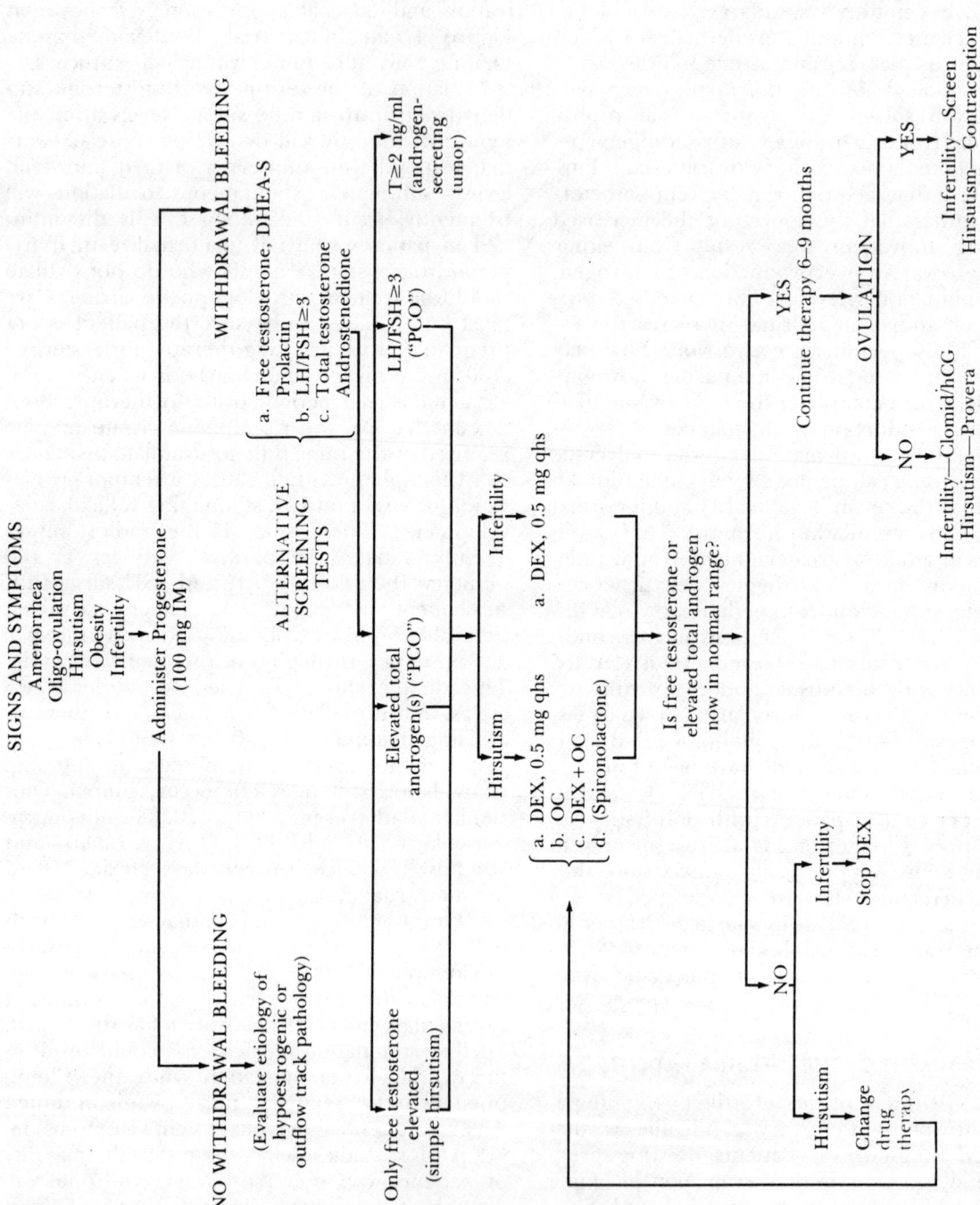

Figure 1. Treatment of polycystic ovary syndrome. DEX, dexamethasone; OC, oral contraceptives.

subsequent pregnancy. Although the testosterone level is initially lowered by removing significant amounts of ovarian tissue, clinical response to this treatment is variable. This surgical approach also involves the risk of forming pelvic adhesions which could additionally contribute to infertility.

TREATMENT OF HIRSUTISM

Glucocorticoids, oral contraceptive pills, and possibly spironolactone are available for the treatment of the hirsute patient. The treatment of the hirsute patient as shown in Figure 1 is individualized and determined by the response of the patient's serum androgen level to single or combination drug therapy. The source of the androgen overproduction in an individual patient may be either adrenal or ovarian, or both. Currently an accurate method of predicting which patient will respond to glucocorticoid or oral contraceptive therapy is not available, and therefore either treatment may be utilized initially.

Glucocorticoids and Oral Contraceptives. The treatment of hirsutism diagrammed in Figure 1 initially utilizes dexamethasone, 0.5 mg taken daily at bedtime for 1 month. At the end of that month of therapy, the previously abnormal serum androgens are again measured. If the dexamethasone therapy is successful in suppressing the androgen level to the normal range, then therapy is continued for 6 to 9 months and modest improvement in the hirsutism is expected to be seen within 5 to 6 months. If androgen suppression with dexamethasone is not achieved, then an "estrogenic" oral contraceptive may be substituted for or may be added in combination with the dexamethasone. In either case, after another month of therapy, serum androgen levels are measured and the therapy continued only if adequate suppression of serum androgens has been obtained.

Patients on dexamethasone therapy may have significant adrenal suppression and should be appropriately managed by tapering therapy at withdrawal and increasing dosage in the face of stress such as infection or disease. The dose of dexamethasone may be reduced in some patients if the androgen levels remain in the normal range. After terminating drug treatment, the patient is monitored clinically for the continued regression or resumption of hirsutism and is also monitored by following the serum free testosterone levels so that therapy may be reinstituted when the patient is no longer in remission. Patients responding to dexamethasone single drug therapy frequently resume ovulatory cycles and therefore will need appropriate contraception. The patient who remains anovulatory on dexamethasone and has unopposed estrogen secretion to the endometrium should be treated with cyclic medroxyprogesterone acetate (Provera), 10 mg per day for 10 days each month, to decrease the risk of endometrial cancer.

Spironolactone. The diuretic spironolactone has been used for many years in the treatment of mild hypertension. Recently there have been reports in the literature (Cumming, D.C., et al.: JAMA., 247:1295, 1982) that spironolactone has anti-androgenic activity, causing marked improvement in the hirsutism of patients with polycystic ovary disease. A decrease in the quantity of hirsutism as well as a reduction in the diameter of the individual hair shaft has been noted.

The mechanism of action of spironolactone appears to involve both a lowering of the serum total and free testosterone and androstenedione levels in patients with polycystic ovary disease and possibly competitive inhibition of testosterone at the androgen receptor level in the hair follicle. Spironolactone does not appear to affect dehydroepiandrosterone sulfate levels. This relatively new therapeutic approach to the treatment of hirsutism may lead to the resumption of ovulatory menstrual cycles. Since the anti-androgenic effect of this drug on a fetus is unclear, the medication should be used only in the hirsute patient with appropriate contraception.

Three pharmacologic therapies—glucocorticoid, oral contraceptive pills, and possibly spironolactone—are available to treat and diminish the hirsutism associated with the polycystic ovary syndrome. The treatment should be tailored to the individual patient, determining that patient's serum androgen response to the medication. Anovulatory patients not on oral contraceptives must be cycled with progestins since they are at increased risk for endometrial cancer. Since our knowledge of the complex biochemistry involved in hair growth is incomplete and pharmacologic treatment yields variable results, electrolysis is still useful therapy for the hirsute patient.

GALACTORRHEA AND HYPERPROLACTINEMIA

VAL DAVAJAN, M.D.,
and OSCAR A. KLETZKY, M.D.

Galactorrhea is the nonpuerperal secretion of breast fluid noted either spontaneously or following manual expression. It can be either unilateral or bilateral. In looking for galactorrhea, the breast should be compressed in a concentric manner from its periphery toward the nipple. The fluid is usually milky or watery in appearance and contains fat globules when examined under a microscope. Microscopic examination is a simple and accurate diagnostic test for galactorrhea and should be utilized if there is any question when breast fluid is expressed. The exact incidence of galactorrhea in women of the reproductive age group is unknown.

Prolactin is the key hormone involved in the pathophysiology of galactorrhea. Prolactin secretion is controlled mainly by the hypothalamus, which has an inhibitory effect on release of prolactin from the pituitary through the action of dopamine. In animals, but not in humans, a prolactin-releasing factor related probably to serotonin has also been reported.

In human beings, prolactin secretion is enhanced by sleep, stress, exercise, nipple stimulation, thyrotropin-releasing hormone, insulin-induced hypoglycemia, and tranquilizers. Prolactin secretion is inhibited by levodopa, dopamine, and certain ergot alkaloids such as bromocryptine.

DIFFERENTIAL DIAGNOSIS

Galactorrhea and hyperprolactinemia have been associated with drugs, prolactin-secreting pituitary adenomas, hypothyroidism, acromegaly, Cushing's disease, and chest trauma, lesions such as herpes zoster or extensive breast manipulation.

Drugs. Drugs are the most common cause of galactorrhea. Drugs causing galactorrhea include: most tranquilizers, antihypertensive drugs, and narcotics. Oral contraceptive steroids and estrogens alone have been shown to stimulate prolactin secretion, but estrogens are also known to interfere with the action of prolactin on breast glands and thus inhibit galactorrhea. Thus, it is unlikely that ingestion of estrogen is a cause of galactorrhea.

Pituitary Tumors. The work-up of patients with galactorrhea is always focused on whether or not a pituitary tumor is present because of the serious nature of this disease. Approximately two thirds of the patients with galactorrhea have hyperprolactinemia (>20 ng per ml). A small percentage of women with amenorrhea but no galactorrhea (< 10 per cent) will also have hyperprolactinemia. Approximately 50 per cent of patients with oligomenorrhea or amenorrhea have hyperprolactinemia. Of these, approximately half will have radiographic changes in the sella turcica compatible with a pituitary adenoma. Pituitary tumors smaller than 10 mm in diameter have been referred to as microadenomas, and those larger than 10 mm are called macradenomas. In approximately 10 per cent of galactorrheic patients who have abnormal x-rays, serum prolactin levels have been reported to be normal. At this medical center, to date all of these patients have been found to have an empty sella turcica.

Gonadotropin levels are low in some patients with pituitary tumors but in many of these patients the baseline levels of luteinizing hormone and follicle-stimulating hormone have been found to be in the normal range and therefore not helpful in making the correct diagnosis.

In patients who have radiographic evidence of a pituitary adenoma, the lack of response of prolactin to induced hypoglycemia, chlorpromazine, or administration of thyrotropin releasing hormone suggests independent secretion of prolactin from an adenoma when compared to normal prolactin-secreting pituitary cells. In contrast, bromocriptine in most patients with adenomas (and levodopa in some patients) does lower the circulating levels of prolactin.

Hypothyroidism. Primary hypothyroidism is the cause of galactorrhea in 2 to 5 per cent of patients presenting with this finding. These patients have diminished thyroid hormone and lack the negative feedback on the hypothalamic-pituitary axis. This failure results in an increased secretion of endogenous thyrotropin releasing hormone which not only overstimulates the thyrotrophs to produce more thyroid stimulating hormone but also stimulates the lactotrophs, thus causing an increase in release of prolactin. The best way to make the diagnosis of primary hypothyroidism is to measure serum thyroid stimulating hormone by radioimmunoassay. The diagnosis is made when the value of thyroid stimulating hormone is elevated above the normal range (the upper normal level ranges between 5 and 10 mU per ml in most laboratories). In addition to thyroid stimulating hormones, a serum T_4 and free thyroxine index (FTI) should be obtained in order to rule out the rare case of TSH-producing pituitary adenoma. Patients with this latter diagnosis have elevated T_4 and free thyroxine levels.

Acromegaly and Cushing's Disease. Galactorrhea in these diseases is of secondary importance and, therefore, the diagnosis and treatment is directed toward the primary disease and will not be discussed here.

Chest Trauma, Herpes Zoster, or Extensive Breast Manipulation. The exact mechanism by which these conditions cause galactorrhea has not been clearly defined. It has been shown that in normal women breast manipulation does increase the serum levels of prolactin. If the manipulation or irritation of the breast is constant, the resultant hyperprolactinemia most likely will lead to galactorrhea.

THE RELATIONSHIP BETWEEN MENSTRUAL CYCLES AND PROLACTIN LEVELS

Galactorrhea can be present in women with both normal and abnormal menses. Galactorrhea associated with a pituitary tumor has even been reported in postmenopausal women. Therefore, in normal menstruating women with galactorrhea a complete work-up cannot be ignored. The menstrual history in conjunction with a single serum prolactin value has been used to identify patients as being in a low or a high risk category for pituitary adenoma.

The low risk group of galactorrheic patients are those with normal menses and normal serum prolactin levels (less than 20 ng per ml). In this clinic none of the patients with the above findings has been found to have abnormal hypocycloidal tomograms of the sella turcica. However, in galactorrheic patients with normal menses and hyperprolactinemia, abnormal tomograms compatible with the presence of microadenomas have been found. Because of these findings, it is recommended that all galactorrheic patients with hyperprolactinemia have a work-up while galactorrheic patients with normal menses and normal prolactin need no further diagnostic evaluation. The high risk group of patients were found to be: (1) those with prolactin levels greater than 200 ng per ml and (2) those with amenorrhea-galactorrhea and low circulating levels of estrogen as determined by failure to have uterine bleeding following administration of progesterone. Approximately two thirds of these patients were found to have abnormal x-rays compatible with pituitary adenomas.

Patients with galactorrhea who give a history of using tranquilizers, or amphetamines, or are taking oral steroid contraceptives, should stop the medication if at all possible for at least 3 months. After being off the medication for 1 to 2 months, if the galactorrhea persists the patient should undergo a work-up. If the patient is taking tranquilizers or antihypertensive drugs and cannot stop the medication, the work-up only should be initiated if the prolactin level is elevated and the TRH stimulation is abnormal.

Patients with galactorrhea should first have a serum thyroid stimulating hormone determination to see if they have hypothyroidism. If the TSH is elevated the diagnosis can be confirmed by measurement of T_4 and free thyroxine index (FTI). Patients with primary hypothyroidism will have elevated TSH and low FTI values. These patients are then treated with thyroxine starting at a dose of 0.05 mg for 2 weeks and then increased to 0.1 mg daily. The TSH should then be repeated in one month and if it is still elevated the thyroxine should be increased to 0.15 mg daily and the TSH rechecked in 1 month. Seldom will a patient require more than 0.2 mg of synthroid daily.

All patients with galactorrhea who have a normal serum TSH value should then have the serum prolactin measured. If the prolactin is normal and the patient has a normal menstrual cycle she needs no further evaluation except that her prolactin should be checked every six months.

Recently we demonstrated that with the use of a single serum prolactin determination and anteroposterior and lateral plain x-ray of the sella turcica, it is possible to identify patients with galactorrhea who do not need sellar tomography or computed tomography (CT) scan to establish the diagnosis of pituitary microadenoma. The patients who do not need tomograms or CT scans are those who have a normal anteroposterior and lateral plain film of the sella turcica and who have normal serum prolactin levels. This is true even if they have oligomenorrhea or amenorrhea. In addition, patients with abnormal plain films of the sella do not need tomograms but only a CT scan with 2 mm cuts. Patients with galactorrhea who have elevated serum prolactin level greater than 60 ng per ml or who have an abnormal prolactin response to TRH stimulation test should have a CT scan of the sella turcica. In our clinic, to date, no patient with prolactin of >60 ng per ml has had a normal TRH stimulation test. To do a TRH stimulation test, 500 µg of TRH is given intravenously after a baseline blood sample is obtained. A second blood sample is drawn 20 minutes later and serum prolactin concentrations measured in both samples. An increase of 200 per cent or more over the baseline in the prolactin concentration is considered a normal response. All patients with abnormal x-rays should have CT scans. If a patient has an abnormal CT scan and a normal prolactin value, then metrizamide should be used to determine if the patient has an empty sella syndrome. The adrenocorticotropic hormone and growth hormone reserves should also be tested by using insulin to induce hypoglycemia in all patients who are found to have a large pituitary tumor.

At our Medical Center, surgical therapy is recommended only for patients with macroadenomas or those with evidence of extrasellar extension of the tumor who failed to respond to bromocriptine therapy. Following surgery, if the pituitary tumor is thought to be incompletely resected, these patients should be placed on bromocriptine therapy.

The recommended dose of bromocriptine (Parlodel) is 2.5 mg daily at bedtime for 7 days, then 2.5 mg bid. Some patients may need higher doses of the drug to make them euprolactinemic. The effects of this drug appear to be only temporary since the majority of patients following the discontinuation of the medication revert back to having amenorrhea, hyperprolactinemia, and galactorrhea. No definitive information is yet available as to the long-term effect of this mode of therapy in patients with known prolactin-secreting pituitary adenomas although some reports of tumor regression have been published.

For all patients with microadenomas, conservative management is now being recommended. These patients are being followed every 6 months with prolactin measurements and every 24 months with a CT scan. If an enlargement of the adenoma is noted during the follow-up, then surgery should be performed.

Patients with microadenomas who desire to conceive and who are willing to take a very small risk of having a sudden growth of the tumor during pregnancy are being managed conservatively in most medical centers. If the tumor expands during the pregnancy, the patient should be treated immediately with high doses of bromocriptine and followed closely with a CT scan. During pregnancy, patients should have visual field examinations performed at 20, 28, and 34 weeks of gestation. Utilizing this approach, over 20 patients at this Medical Center with abnormal x-rays have been delivered at term without complications.

CONTRACEPTION

PAUL F. BRENNER, M.D.

Contraception is a reversible method for the prevention of pregnancy used by either or both partners. A 100 per cent effective, risk-free method of contraception does not exist even for one person. Each subject requesting a contraceptive method must be prepared to make a compromise. This compromise can only be reached when the person requesting the method clearly understands the risks and benefits associated with each of the available forms of contraception.

ORAL CONTRACEPTIVES

The combination oral contraceptives contain both a synthetic estrogen and a synthetic gestagen in each active tablet. Some formulations are marketed so that the user ingests a single tablet every day, going from one packet directly to another without tablet free days. These packets contain 21 tablets with the estrogen-gestagen combination followed by 7 tablets void of any hormone. Oral contraceptives are a highly effective method of contraception with a pregnancy rate of 0.2 per 100 women-years of use. As long as tablets are not omitted, the effectiveness of the combination birth control pills is the same irrespective of the specific hormones or the dose of the hormones in the formulation. The risks in selecting birth control pills as a method of contraception may be grouped as the common minor untoward effects and the very rare but serious clinical sequelae.

The common side effects associated with the synthetic estrogen component of the pill include nausea, breast tenderness, fluid retention, reversible hypertension, mood changes, and depression. In some individuals angiotensinogen increases in response to the administration of exogenous estrogen. Approximately 5 per cent of women who use birth control pills for 5 years are observed to have a significant rise in their blood pressure to hypertensive levels. When the pills are discontinued the levels of angiotensinogen fall and the blood pressure returns to normal. A very important aspect of monitoring women who take birth control pills is to take their blood pressure at each visit. Weight gain, acne, amenorrhea, and nervousness are side effects attributed to the synthetic gestagen. The failure to have withdrawal bleeding in the hormone-free period of each cycle can be very alarming to the user because the reassuring monthly signal that she is not pregnant has disappeared. The individual who fails to have withdrawal bleeding while using birth control pills, can be managed by increasing the amount of estrogen or decreasing the amount of gestagen administered each cycle. Irregular bleeding and melasma are adverse effects related to both components of the combination pills.

There are several rare but very serious side effects associated with the use of oral contraceptives. The risk of cholelithiasis is doubled in pill users, and the annual incidence is one in every 1250 women taking birth control pills. A significant increased risk of myocardial infarction, three-fold, is found in pill users over the age of 35 who are smokers. Women under the age of 35 years, regardless of whether they smoke or not, do not have a significant risk of heart attacks if they elect to use birth control pills, and nonsmokers over the age of 35 may use the pill without significantly increasing their chances of a heart attack. While smoking appears to be the most important risk factor for heart attacks, other compounding factors include diabetes, hyperlipidemia, and hypertension. All of these factors seem to act synergistically with birth control pill use to increase the risk of ischemic heart disease.

The latest report of the Royal College of General Practitioners Contraception Study indicates that at the end of 10 years of observation there is no increased risk of heart disease related to the duration of use of the pill. These data are based on a much greater experience and contradict their earlier report. Deep vein thrombophlebitis is increased 3 times in birth control pill users and occurs in 1 out of every 10,000 users annually. The risk of pulmonary embolism is increased four-fold in pill users with a yearly incidence of 1 in every 30,000 pill takers. Cerebral vascular accidents occur 3 times more frequently in pill users. One in every 30,000 women using the pill is hospitalized each year with a stroke, and 1 in every 200,000 women using the pill dies, each year from a cerebrovascular accident. Liver adenomas are found in 1 out of every 50,000 oral contraceptive users each year. It should be stressed that while these side effects are very serious, they are also very infrequent. Pill users who complain of headaches, visual disturbances, chest pain, and unilateral lower extremity pain should discontinue their pills immediately, until the etiology of the complaint is ascertained and the possibility of stroke, pulmonary embolus, heart attack, and deep vein thrombosis has been excluded.

False statements not supported by scientific evidence have appeared in the lay literature and sometimes even in the medical journals concerning the side effects of oral contraceptive use. One set of erroneous statements has linked pill use to cancer. Women have been informed that pill increases the risk of cancer of the breast, endometrium, cervix, and liver as well as causing prolactin-secreting pituitary adenomas. There is no evidence that combination oral contraceptives increase the risk of breast cancer. There is a trend which has not reached statistical significance in some of the prospective pill studies that pill users have less breast cancer. In December 1975, articles first appeared which concluded that postmenopausal women taking estrogen without any gestagen had an increased incidence of endometrial carcinoma. Women selecting combination oral contraceptives are reported to have significantly less endometrial cancer in two recent prospective studies. Some investigations indicate that pill users have an increase in cervical dysplasia. When these studies are corrected for the confounding factors of early age at first intercourse and number of sexual partners this risk disappears. While the increase in hepatic adenomas has been associated with birth control pill use, there is no association between their use and liver carcinoma. In the last 5 years many medical centers throughout the world have collected a large number of women with prolactin-secreting pituitary adenomas. A suggestion has been put forth that these tumors are related to birth control pill use. There is no evidence to support this conjecture, and most probably the large increase in the women with these microadenomas reflects new diagnostic methodology including the radioimmunoassay for prolactin, tomograms, and CT scans.

Additional false statements have been written about the pill. Ingestion of birth control pills has been said to cause diabetes mellitus, secondary amenorrhea, and sterility. Pill users have been advised to use a vitamin supplement, to take pill-free "rest periods" every few years, and to avoid pregnancy immediately after discontinuing oral contraceptives in order to reduce the chance of the pregnancy ending in a spontaneous abortion or producing a child with a congenital anomaly.

Ingestion of oral contraceptives does not cause diabetes mellitus. Women taking birth control pills have impaired carbohydrate metabolism, and diabetic women using the pill may notice an increase in their insulin requirements, but these changes are reversible and disappear when the oral contraceptives are discontinued.

Recent studies question whether there is a distinct entity of post-pill amenorrhea. It may well be that women destined to have secondary amenorrhea who use birth control pills mask the development of amenorrhea during the period the pills are taken. Former users of oral contraceptives have no greater incidence of amenorrhea than non-pill users.

Birth control pill users have lower concentrations of the B complex vitamins and vitamin C, but these levels remain in the normal range. Pill users do not routinely need a vitamin supplement.

One of the biggest errors a contraceptive counselor can make is to advocate rest periods of 2 to 3 months duration every few years of pill use in order to reduce the risk of complications. The only real benefactor of rest periods for pill users are the abortionists who terminate the unwanted pregnancies which result. Women who wish to conceive after using oral contraceptives on the average have a 2 to 3 month delay in becoming pregnant compared with women discontinuing barrier methods. Two to three years following the cessation of oral contraceptives or the cessation of barrier methods, the same number of women become pregnant. There is no evidence that birth control pills cause sterility.

There has been great concern for the outcome of pregnancy for those women who become pregnant after stopping the use of oral contraceptives. These women do not have an increase in spontaneous abortions or an increased risk of babies with congenital malformations. Women are best advised not to conceive immediately after stopping oral contraceptives because the length of the follicular phase in the first cycle is so unpredictable and this makes dating of the pregnancy more difficult, not because of concerns over spontaneous abortions and congenital anomalies.

The rare but very serious clinical sequelae have received widespread coverage in both the medical and the lay press. The benefits to using oral contraceptives other than protection against unwanted pregnancy have been almost totally ignored. These benefits are equally as important as the risks. Women using birth control pills have fewer functional ovarian cysts and less benign breast disease. These two benefits account for 270 less surgical procedures per 100,000 pill users annually compared with an equal number of non-pill users. Other benefits associated with birth control pill use include regular menstrual cycles, less premenstrual tension, less dysmenorrhea, less anemia, and less salpingitis. This last benefit as it relates to infertility and ectopic pregnancy cannot be emphasized enough. Pelvic inflammatory disease approaches epidemic proportions in some parts of our population and the protection against this disease afforded by the pill has great clinical significance. Life-saving benefits of pill use include less endometrial cancer, less ovarian cancer, and less rheumatoid arthritis.

For some women the risks of taking oral contraceptives are clearly greater than the benefits. Absolute contraindications to the use of oral contraceptives include women with a history of vascular disease, hypertension, diabetes, hyperlipidemia, breast cancer, endometrial cancer, pregnancy, heart disease, and liver disease. Women with a history of deep vein thrombosis or thrombophlebitis, pulmonary embolus, stroke, sickle cell disease, and systemic lupus erythematosus should not take birth control pills. Women with sickle cell trait or varicose veins are suitable candidates for the pill. Hypertension increases the risk for both heart attacks and strokes and seems to act synergistically with birth control pill use in enhancing the risk of these deadly diseases. The diabetic is one of the most difficult patients to counsel regarding family planning. Diabetes is a vascular disease and therefore pill use in diabetic women is associated with a significantly increased risk of ischemic heart disease. Diabetics are known to have decreased defense mechanisms against infection and thus they are not good candidates for an IUD. On the other hand pregnancy can be devastating to diabetic women, and they need adequate protection from unplanned pregnancy. As a compromise, they can use either an IUD or a sub 50 mcg synthetic estrogen pill, some of which do not adversely alter carbohydrate metabolism. Women with active liver disease should not ingest the pill but women with a past history of liver disease who now have normal liver function may use birth control pills. Relative contraindications to oral contraceptives include migraine headaches, heavy smoking, oligomenorrhea, and severe depression.

Teenage pregnancy is an important medical and social problem facing our society. The magnitude of this problem seems to be growing each year. More than one million pregnancies in women under the age of 20 years occur in this country annually. Most of these are premarital pregnancies, the majority of which are unintended and the result of the absence of or inadequate information about reproduction and contraception. Family planning counselors have had major concerns about prescribing birth control pills to teenagers. One effect of estrogen is to fuse the distal epiphyses of the long bones. One concern pertaining to the administration of the potent synthetic estrogen to women in their early teens is that it will cause premature fusion of the distal epiphyses and reduce that individual's potential height. Once menarche has occurred, the final height can not be altered by the administration of exogenous estrogen. Therefore, the ingestion of birth control pills by menstruating teenagers will not affect their ultimate height. Another concern is that the ingestion of the pill by a young woman before her reproductive axis has fully matured will permanently damage that axis. Once a woman has 3 consecutive, spontaneous, ovulatory menstrual cycles, oral contraceptives will not alter hypothalamic-pituitary-ovarian function.

Teenage compliance in the use of birth control pills has always been a problem for contraceptive counselors. Some of the common side effects associated with pill use, which include nausea, weight gain, breast tenderness, breakthrough bleeding, amenorrhea and acne, are apt to discourage the very young contraceptive acceptor and lead to discontinuation of the method. In an effort to achieve the greatest compliance of pill use among teenagers, a formulation should be selected which is dispensed in a 28-day pill packet, contains less than 50 mcg of synthetic estrogen, and contains a synthetic gestagen other than norgestrel, which is the most androgenic of the five available synthetic gestagens. The more androgenic the formulation is, the more likely the pill user will develop acne, which is a serious deterrent to the cosmetically conscious teenager.

When a woman first uses birth control pills, a formulation with less than 50 mcg of synthetic estrogen is preferred. This oral contraceptives containing less than 50 mcg of estrogen are equally as effective as the birth control pills which contain 50 mcg of estrogen or more, as long as tablets are not omitted. Clinical evidence now supports the theoretical supposition that the lower-dose formulations are associated with fewer serious clinical sequelae than the pills containing more estrogen. If a pill user is already taking a formulation with 50 mcg of estrogen, particularly if that estrogen is mestranol, and is not experiencing any side effects, no attempt is made to change her to a product containing less estrogen. If a pill user is presently ingesting a formulation containing more than 50 mcg of estrogen, she should be switched to a lower dose pill even if she is experiencing no untoward effects.

When first starting to use oral contraceptives, acceptors commonly ingest the first tablet on the fifth day of their cycle or on the first Sunday after menses begins. Women can also start taking birth control pills the first day of their menstrual cycle, and this offers greater protection in the first cycle of pill use to women with short menstrual cycles and negates any need to consider the use of a concomitant method in the first cycle. Women electing to use oral contraceptives following a first trimester abortion should begin pill use within 48 hours of the termination of the pregnancy. The very first cycle is most likely to be an ovulatory one with a normal cycle length. Following a second trimester abortion, birth control pills should be started 1 week after the termination of the pregnancy. This first cycle is also most likely to be an ovulatory one, but ovulation is usually delayed 1 week. A week's delay in beginning pill ingestion may reduce the chance of thromboembolic disease.

Birth control pills should not be given to lactating women. The use of pills reduces the quantity of the milk and alters the quality of the milk. Non-nursing mothers following a term delivery can start to use birth control pills 2 weeks after the birth of the child. This delay also is to reduce the occurrence of thromboemboli.

Once birth control pills have been prescribed, patients are asked to return at 3 months and annually thereafter. At all return visits a non-directed history and blood pressure are obtained. In addition, at the annual visits breast, abdominal, and pelvic examinations are performed, and a Papanicolaou smear is obtained. Women less than 35 years of age who have a significant past history of immediate family members sustaining a myocardial infarction at an early age or young women who have physical findings suggestive of hyperlipidemia should have a lipid panel determined before starting oral contraceptives. Women who by past history are at increased risk for diabetes mellitus should have their ability to metabolize carbohydrates measured before receiving pills. All women over 35 years of age who are presently using or about to initiate the use of birth control pills should have their circulatory lipids and carbohydrate tolerance tested. Women with a past history of liver disease require liver function studies before they elect to use birth control pills as their method of family planning. Serum chemistries are not measured in all women desiring to use oral contraceptives or at specific intervals for those patients currently using birth control pills.

INTRAUTERINE DEVICES

The intrauterine device (IUD) is slightly less effective than oral contraceptives, with a pregnancy rate of 2 to 3 per 100 women-years of use. While the intrauterine device is free of the alterations in protein, carbohydrate, and lipid metabolism found in pill users, the IUD can produce uterine side effects. The uterine device is a particularly convenient method of family planning, as it does not interrupt coitus and foreplay, and requires very little patient motivation for monitoring. Currently, 5 IUDs are available for use in the United States. The Lippes Loop and the Saf-T-Coil are first generation, nonmedicated devices whose effectiveness is related to the size of the IUD. These devices do not require removal at a designated time interval. More than half the removals of nonmedicated devices are related to uterine bleeding and/or pain. A second generation of smaller IUDs were developed in an attempt to lessen the bleeding and pain associated with IUD use. In order to obtain an acceptable level of effectiveness these medicated devices were designed to release either copper or progesterone. The Copper T-200 and Copper-7 devices contain 200 square millimeters of copper surface area, and the manufacturer recommends removal at the end of 3 years of use. The Progestasert system releases 65 μg of progesterone daily and annual removal is recommended.

Clinical problems associated with the use of

intrauterine devices include perforation, expulsion, uterine bleeding and pain, accidental pregnancy, infection, and missing strings.

Perforation. Both fundal and cervical perforations occur in IUD acceptors. Fundal perforations almost always happen at the time of insertion and occur in approximately 1 in every 1000 to 2000 insertions. Fundal perforations may be reduced by careful determination of the size and position of the uterus by palpation, and confirmation of the size and position of the uterus by use of a sound prior to any attempt at insertion. Flexion of the uterus may be decreased by steady traction on the cervical tenaculum. All extrauterine IUDs should be removed as soon after the diagnosis is established as possible. Adhesions, bowel obstruction, and bowel perforation have resulted from the presence of IUDs in the peritoneal cavity, even with the nonmedicated devices made of nonreactive Silastic. Cervical embedments and perforations have followed the insertion of "T" and "7" shaped devices in nulliparous women. The vertical stems of these devices are forced by uterine contractions into the posterior lip of the cervix. The tip of an embedded device is palpable during the bimanual examination. These devices are removed by cervical dilatation, repositioning of the device in the fundus, and then withdrawal of the IUD through the cervical canal. An iatrogenic fistula serves as a conduit between the nonsterile vagina and sterile endometrial cavity and should be avoided.

Expulsions. The expulsion rate of IUDs decreases as the interval since insertion increases. Following first and second expulsions, if the patient is agreeable, another attempt at insertion of an IUD can be made. After second insertions, two thirds of the devices are retained, and following the third insertion one out of three IUD users retains their devices. The possibility of success is too low to justify more than three attempts at insertion of an IUD for any one individual. The overall expulsion rate for IUDs after the third attempt at insertion is 6 to 7 per cent. One fifth of all IUD expulsions are unnoticed by the user. This has great clinical significance, as one third of all accidental pregnancies are the result of unnoticed expulsions. An IUD must be placed in close proximity to the top of the fundus for maximal effectiveness. Partial expulsions of the IUD occur and are an indication for the removal of the device, as a partially expelled IUD will be less than optimally effective in the prevention of pregnancy. Any history of uterine bleeding and/or pain, or of the strings suddenly becoming longer is an indication to examine the patient for the possibility of an expulsion and to sound the cervical canal to the internal os looking for a partial expulsion.

Uterine Bleeding and/or Pain. IUD users have menses which are heavier and last a greater number of days compared with their menses prior to selecting an IUD. An average of 35 ml of menstrual blood is lost during a cycle in which no contraceptive modality is used. The ingestion of oral contraceptives decreases the amount of blood lost each menstrual cycle, and nonmedicated and copper IUDs increase the amount of blood lost each cycle. Women receiving nonmedicated devices lose 70 to 80 ml of blood each cycle and women using the Copper 7 or Copper T lose 50 to 60 ml of blood each cycle. The use of the Progestasert system decreases the amount of menstrual blood loss.

Uterine bleeding and/or pain is more common in the initial months following an IUD insertion. If evaluation fails to indicate an organic cause of the bleeding and pain, the patient is encouraged to continue using the device. Every IUD user with uterine bleeding or pain must be carefully assessed for the presence of accidental pregnancy, pelvic infection, and complete or partial expulsion of the IUD.

Accidental Pregnancy. Current IUD users who become pregnant with an IUD in utero require special counseling. An accidental pregnancy with the IUD present in the endometrial cavity is more likely to terminate in a spontaneous abortion than a pregnancy not associated with IUD use, or a pregnancy that resulted from an unnoticed expulsion of an IUD. Forty-five to 60 per cent of pregnancies which occur with the IUD within the uterus end in spontaneous abortion. If an accidental pregnancy occurs with the IUD in utero in a patient who desires to continue the pregnancy, and the appendage is easily accessible in the vaginal vault, the IUD should be removed. Removal of the IUD does not increase the possibility that the pregnancy will terminate in abortion, but actually decreases the risk. If the strings of the IUD are not readily accessible in the vagina and the patient wishes to continue the pregnancy probing for the IUD is contraindicated.

Women selecting an IUD have 90 per cent fewer tubal pregnancies than if they used no method of family planning. The IUD is even more effective in preventing an intrauterine pregnancy than an ectopic pregnancy. For patients pregnant with IUDs retained within the uterus, the ratio of ectopic pregnancy to intrauterine pregnancy is increased and the patients are instructed there is a greater chance that an accidental pregnancy associated with IUD use is a tubal pregnancy.

A woman who becomes pregnant while using a Dalkon Shield IUD has an increased risk of serious sepsis. All pregnancies resulting from the use of the Dalkon Shield should be terminated as early as feasible. Any patient, pregnant or non-pregnant, found to be using the Dalkon Shield, even if completely asymptomatic, should have the device removed. The risk of sepsis during pregnancies with other IUDs is much less clear. Patients are not advised to terminate their pregnancies in order to avoid the dangers of septic abortion, but they do require careful observation during their pregnancy.

Women who become pregnant while using an IUD envision the device in close proximity to the fetus and the cause of fetal malformations. The IUD is found between the placental membranes when pregnancies occur with the device in utero, and there is no increased risk of congenital anomalies with either the medicated or nonmedicated IUDs.

Infection. Even since IUDs manufactured from non–tissue reactive Silastic were introduced clinically there was concern that their use would be associated with an increased risk of symptomatic pelvic infection. Serious infections and death occurred with earlier devices made of tissue-reactive substances. Insertion of IUDs necessitates carrying bacteria from the vagina into the endometrial cavity. The appendage of the device is a theoretical conduit for bacteria from the vagina to the uterine cavity. Transfundal cultures at various intervals following IUD insertions, at the time of abdominal hysterectomy, indicated the endometrial cavity was sterile 30 days or longer after the placement of the IUD, and that host resistance prevented clinical infection in the first month after insertion. Many multiparous women who received nonmedicated devices were followed 6 years or longer and no increase in pelvic infection was detected. Starting in the mid 1970s several studies demonstrated an increased risk of pelvic inflammatory disease in IUD users. These studies have been criticized for the lack of a uniform criterion for the diagnosis of this disease, and the selection of patients using barrier methods of contraception or oral contraceptives as controls, both of which are known to decrease the risk of pelvic infection, and in some studies a large number of the subjects were using the Dalkon Shield.

There is a specific group of women which appears to be at a high risk for pelvic infection if an IUD is used. Women with a past history of a symptomatic pelvic infection and the young, nulliparous woman with multiple sexual partners have a 3-fold increased risk for symptomatic pelvic infection if they receive the IUD. These women are best advised not to use an IUD.

Current IUD users who have endometritis and/or salpingitis are treated aggressively with antibiotic therapy which covers both aerobic and anaerobic organisms. Removal of the IUD does not appear to alter the clinical response to antibiotics. If the IUD is removed, adequate circulating levels of antibiotics should be obtained before the device is extracted from the uterus.

Actinomycosis has been reported in IUD users, particularly in women who have used an IUD for 5 years or longer. This organism is most commonly found where there is tissue damage or a foreign body present. Although the presence of actinomycosis associated with an IUD is frequently asymptomatic, it may be associated with symptoms of leukorrhea, uterine bleeding, and pain. The same symptoms usually present with women with pelvic infections. When obtaining a Papanicolaou smear for women using an IUD, the pathologist should be instructed to look for actinomycosis. Asymptomatic IUD users who are found to have actinomycosis should have their IUD removed but do not require antibiotics. IUD users with symptomatic actinomycosis require antibiotics and removal of the device. Penicillin is the drug of choice.

Missing Strings. Some IUD acceptors report that they no longer can feel the threads of the IUD and this is confirmed by inspection of the cervix. The diagnostic possibilities include unnoticed expulsions, a device in utero, and an extrauterine location of the device. Pregnancy should be excluded before invading the uterine cavity. The cervical canal is probed and frequently the strings are found curled up in the canal. If the threads are not in the cervical canal, a flat plate film of the abdomen and pelvis is obtained. When the device is not seen on the x-ray, an unnoticed expulsion occurred. If the device is present on the flat plate film the IUD is either intrauterine or extrauterine in location. Probing of the uterine cavity with a sound detects some of the intrauterine devices. If the IUD is not palpated by a sound, the position of the device is determined by ultrasonography or a hysterogram. Whether extrauterine or intrauterine, all devices with missing strings should be removed. Intrauterine devices with missing strings are frequently malpositioned and do not afford maximal effectiveness.

Some women have absolute or relative contraindications to IUD use. Absolute contraindications to an IUD include a past history of symptomatic endometritis and salpingitis; women with markedly impaired defense mechanisms to infection; and women with a past history of ectopic pregnancy, current pregnancy, a uterine cavity less than 5.5 cm in length, a uterine cavity deformed by submucus fibroids, or a congenital anomaly. The rare women allergic to copper should not use a copper IUD. Relative contraindications to an IUD include anemia, a heavy menstrual flow, and dysmenorrhea. A woman with heavy menses or dysmenorrhea who insists on using an IUD may be a candidate for the Progestasert system.

DIAPHRAGM

In actual use the diaphragm is less effective than either birth control pills or intrauterine devices. The pregnancy rate is related to the motivation of the user as well as the motivation of the contraceptive counselor. Even teenagers can use a diaphragm and achieve a pregnancy rate comparable to IUD acceptors. Subjects are fitted with actual diaphragms rather than the fitting rings. Diaphragms of increasing diameter are placed in the vagina until one which is too large for the patient is determined. The next smallest diaphragm is selected, and its presence in the vagina should not produce discomfort. The patient should practice several times inserting and removing the diaphragm. After each insertion the position of the diaphragm is checked to ascertain that the cervix is entirely covered. The arcing diaphragm is used for women with a markedly flexed uterus. The patient is instructed to inspect the diaphragm before each insertion, looking for perforations, and if there is any question the diaphragm is filled with water to detect any leaks. Each time the subject uses her diaphragm, spermicidal jelly or cream is placed in the center of the dome and spread around the outer edge. The diaphragm is left in the vagina a minimum of 8 hours after the last coital exposure. If the subject has more than one act of coitus in a short period of time additional jelly is placed in the vagina before each coitus, but the diaphragm is not removed to place spermicidal agent in the center of the dome. The patient selecting a diaphragm is examined during her first cycle of use to ascertain that she is using the method properly. At each annual visit, following a spontaneous or therapeutic abortion, after a term delivery, subsequent to significant weight change, and when symptoms are present of vaginal discomfort, bladder or urethral pain, difficulty voiding, and urinary tract infection, the patient is examined to determine if she requires a change in the size of her diaphragm.

CONDOM

The condom is a method of contraception which has the additional advantage of preventing the transmission of venereal disease. Other advantages of the condom include the fact that it is a method of family planning which is free of systemic effects and except for local irritation and the rare individual who is allergic to a component of the condom, it does not produce local side effects. There are disadvantages of this method. It requires motivation and responsibility on the part of the male partner to use the method each time intercourse occurs. It may interrupt sexual foreplay, and the male partner has decreased sensation during coitus. The condom is an inconvenient method of contraception which, when used alone, has a rather high failure rate, but when condoms and foam are used together the effectiveness of the method approaches that of the oral contraceptives. To properly use this method before an attempt at vaginal penetration is made, a condom is applied over the entire length of the erect penis, leaving a reservoir at the end for the collection of sperm. The penis and condom are withdrawn from the vagina simultaneously before the penis becomes flaccid. Lubricant prevents tearing the condom and reduces vaginal irritation, but Vaseline is not used, as it causes rubber to deteriorate.

VAGINAL FOAM, SUPPOSITORIES, AND CREAMS

Vaginal foam, suppositories, and creams have two components, a spermicidal agent and the carrier substance such as the foam, suppository, or cream. The spermicidal agent most commonly used is nonoxynol-9 (nonylphenoxy polyoxyethylene ethanol). The advantages of using vaginal foam, suppositories, or creams are that they do not cause systemic alterations and, except for the rare individual who has an allergic reaction, there are no local untoward reactions. The disadvantages associated with this method include that it is considered messy and it may interrupt sexual foreplay. This method of family planning also requires strong patient motivation, as the vaginal spermicide must be placed in the vagina prior to each act of coitus. These agents are inserted as close to the cervix as possible and not more than 1 hour before sexual contact. The subject is instructed not to douche for at least 8 hours after intercourse. The vaginal foam container must be shaken well before use, and a second full container of foam should be available as a back-up. The use of vaginal suppositories requires an interval of 10 minutes from the placement of the suppository in the vagina and coitus to allow the suppository to melt. The failure rate of vaginal spermicides is too high to recommend their use as a single agent general method of contraception. There are specific indications for the use of vaginal spermicides. These include women having very infrequent coitus, an unplanned act of coitus when an alternative method is not available, women immediately postpartum or perimenopausal when their fertility is reduced, and as a concomitant method with other contraceptive modalities.

RHYTHM METHOD

A woman using the rhythm method abstains from intercourse during the time when fertilization is most likely to occur. The ovum can be fertilized for 48 hours or less following ovulation, and the sperm can fertilize an ovum for 48 hours or less after ejaculation. The fertile period is extended 3 additional days beyond which the ovum can be fertilized and 3 days beyond which ejaculated sperm can fertilize the ovum. In the idealized 28-day menstrual cycle ovulation and fertilization would most likely occur between day 9 and day 19. For women with variable menstrual cycle length the fertile period is defined as starting the nineteenth day before the earliest likely menses and extending through the ninth day before the latest likely menses. The rhythm method of family planning is contraindicated for women whose menstrual cycle length varies 8 or more days from cycle to cycle or whose menstrual cycles are equal to or less than 25 days. The use of the basal body temperature (BBT) graph is a practical means of estimating the time of ovulation in each cycle. Abstinence from intercourse until there are 3 consecutive days of a sustained temperature elevation in the BBT will greatly increase the effectiveness of the rhythm method.

TREATMENT OF DYSFUNCTIONAL UTERINE BLEEDING

ANTONIO SCOMMEGNA, M.D.

Dysfunctional uterine bleeding is abnormal bleeding caused by *endocrine dysfunction* and not organic causes. The diagnosis of dysfunctional uterine bleeding is usually made through exclusion of all local or systemic organic causes of uterine bleeding, which include most gynecologic disorders, complications of early pregnancy, and some systemic diseases. The term "dysfunctional" refers to alterations in the physiologic mechanism controlling normal menstrual function.

Anovulatory dysfunctional uterine bleeding is characterized by disruption of the cyclicity of the patient's usual menstrual pattern. *Ovulatory* dysfunctional uterine bleeding is characterized by menstrual bleeding which, although cyclic, is excessive in amount (more than 80 ml) or in duration (longer than 7 days).

In over 80 per cent of all cases of dysfunctional uterine bleeding, anovulation, prolonged stimulation of the endometrium, and estrogen breakthrough are the etiologic factors. The remaining patients have ovulatory cycles and ovulatory-type dysfunctional uterine bleeding. Dysfunctional uterine bleeding in the latter group is related to an abnormal estrogen or progesterone secretion such as persistence of the corpus luteum or other defects in corpus luteum or to altered endometrial function. Anovulatory dysfunctional uterine bleeding is most common at both extremes of the reproductive life: immediately following menarche and just preceding menopause. About 50 per cent of patients with dysfunctional uterine bleeding are over 45 years of age, about 20 per cent are adolescents, and the remaining 30 per cent are in their reproductive years. Ovulatory dysfunctional uterine bleeding on the other hand is most common during reproductive years and, when not associated with altered corpus luteum function, is related to local endometrial causes such as overactive endometrial fibrinolysis and/or alteration in the production of prostanoids by the endometrium or myometrium.

Diagnosis. A careful history will differentiate cyclic from acyclic bleeding. In addition, a complete blood count, a sensitive pregnancy test, and, except in the very young, a fundal endometrial biopsy should be performed. These tests in conjunction with a complete physical and pelvic examination will help identify women with organic gynecologic disorders, complications of early pregnancy, and other systemic organic diseases. Appropriate hormonal evaluations should be performed in women who show signs of thyroid, adrenal, or pituitary diseases. In women who complain mainly of menorrhagia, profuse or prolonged menstrual cycles, or in whom the endometrial biopsy reveals secretory endometrium, a hysterosalpingogram and/or hysteroscopy should be performed to exclude a submucous myoma or polyp.

TREATMENT

Expectant Management

If the patient presents herself with the first episode of dysfunctional uterine bleeding, the bleeding is minimal or moderate, and the hemoglobin is normal, expectant management is indicated. Isolated episodes of dysfunctional uterine bleeding are frequent in the menstrual history of many women. The patient should be instructed to record her basal body temperature and keep an accurate menstrual calendar to help determine whether subsequent cycles are ovulatory.

Ambulatory Treatment

Most episodes of dysfunctional uterine bleeding can be managed on an ambulatory basis. Therapeutic objectives consist of arrest of the bleeding episode, prevention of its recurrence, and correction of the anemia if present. For the treatment of the acute episode of bleeding, three hormonal regimens are indicated: oral contraceptives, progestins alone, and sequential estrogen-progestin therapy.

For the arrest of the bleeding episode, *oral contraceptives* (estrogen with a 19-nor progestational steroid) should be given in doses higher than those used for birth control. A preferred regimen consists of Enovid, 5 mg, or Ortho Novum, 2 mg, administered 4 times daily for the first 4 days, 3 times daily for the next 4 days, twice daily for the following 4 days, and once daily for the last 4 days, a total of 16 days of therapy. The episode of bleeding is arrested with this regimen within the first 72 hours in more than 90 per cent of patients. About 1 to 4 days after discontinuation of treatment, withdrawal bleeding takes place and is usually short, lasting no longer than 6 days, and resembles normal menstrual bleeding.

An alternative method for control of anovulatory bleeding consists of the administration of a *progestin alone* (e.g., medroxyprogesterone acetate or norethindrone acetate, 10 mg a day for 3 weeks). This treatment is employed in women who have relative contraindications to estrogen therapy and it is useful when the bleeding is from a proliferative or hyperplastic endometrium. This treatment is effective in about 50 per cent of the patients, a success rate which is lower than that observed with oral contraceptives, but which has fewer side-effects.

Sequential estrogen-progestin therapy is particularly useful in the treatment of adolescent girls with prolonged episodes of dysfunctional uterine bleeding in whom endogenous estrogen production may be low. Conjugated estrogens (2.5 mg 4 times daily) are given for a period of 3 weeks. During the last week of treatment, medroxyprogesterone acetate, 10 mg a day, is added to the regimen. This treatment is as effective in arresting the bleeding as oral contraceptives and it may be more effective in preventing the recurrence of dysfunctional uterine bleeding. Irrespective of the treatment used, about half of the patients will complain of side-effects, nausea being the most prominent symptom.

Hospitalization

Because of the possibility of serious intrauterine pathology, women over 35 years old as well as those in whom hormonal therapy has failed, should undergo endometrial curettage. This procedure is usually performed as a dilatation and curetagge under general anesthesia in the hospital. However, office endometrial curettage (vacutage or similar procedures) may be adequate.

Hospitalization is indicated in women who show signs of hypovolemia or have very profuse vaginal bleeding which, unless promptly arrested, will lead to hypovolemia. In such patients, rapid arrest of the bleeding episode is very important. Intravenous estrogens are effective in inducing rapid hemostasis because of their immediate stabilizing effect upon the endometrium. Conjugated estrogens (Premarin) are administered intravenously in 25 mg doses. The initial dose is repeated at 2 hours and then every 4 hours. The bleeding is controlled within 6 hours in about 75 per cent of patients; otherwise a dilatation and curettage is performed.

After the bleeding has stopped, intravenous estrogens are replaced with oral estrogen-progestogens given either as sequential or combination therapy as previously described.

PREVENTION OF RECURRENT DYSFUNCTIONAL UTERINE BLEEDING

If the endometrial biopsy reveals proliferative or simple hyperplastic endometrium indicative of anovulatory bleeding, the patient should receive 5 to 10 mg of medroxyprogesterone acetate daily for the first 10 days of every month to prevent unopposed estrogen stimulation of the endometrium and thus avoid recurrences. The patient should be advised that this regimen does not interfere with spontaneous ovulation, should it occur, and a mechanical method of contraception is advised in sexually active patients.

Synthetic progestogens should be avoided if there is a possibility of pregnancy since a relationship has been suggested between certain congenital malformations of the VACTERL type and synthetic progestin administration early in pregnancy. If the biopsy reveals secretory or mixed endometrium indicative of ovulatory dysfunctional uterine bleeding, oral contraceptives should be administered in the usual doses, particularly in women who desire contraception. The use of oral contraceptives, however, may mask the development of more profound alteration of hypothalamic-pituitary-ovarian function and should be avoided in anovulatory patients. Should such women desire to become pregnant, induction of ovulation with clomiphene citrate is the treatment of choice.

Women with recurrent ovulatory dysfunctional uterine bleeding may also benefit from administration of a prostaglandin inhibitor at the time of the period. Mefanamic acid in doses of 500 mg 3 times daily from the onset until the end of menstruation, but not to exceed 1 week, will decrease blood loss by one third in about 75 per cent of women with menorrhagia.

Danazol in a dose of 200 mg daily given continuously will also reduce markedly menstrual blood loss in women with ovulatory dysfunctional uterine bleeding. The mechanism of action is related to a direct effect of the drug on the endometrium and at this dose it does not interfere with ovulation. Both of these treatment modalities may be useful in women in whom oral contraceptives are contraindicated. When so treated, sexually active women should use a barrier method of contraception.

When thorough diagnostic evaluation has failed to reveal specific or correctable pathology, and dysfunctional uterine bleeding recurs or cannot be controlled by hormonal and iron therapy, hysterectomy is the therapy of choice in those women in whom childbearing is no longer important.

MENOPAUSE

DAVID R. MELDRUM, M.D.

Following the menopause, the ovary ceases its production of estrogen, resulting in estrogen deficiency. Ovarian androgen production continues, leading to relative androgen excess and often to mild hirsutism and defeminization. Luteal activity no longer occurs, allowing continuous estrogen stimulation of responsive tissues. The extent of estrogen deficiency varies greatly, since the source of estrogen, the conversion of androstenedione in adipose and muscle tissue, varies directly with body weight. The concentration of sex hormone–binding globulin varies inversely with body weight, thus further exaggerating the effects of body size on availability of estrogen to tissues. Clinical problems associated with estrogen deficiency, such as hot flashes and osteoporosis, are more likely to occur in women who are thin or normal in weight. On the other hand, endometrial and breast cancer are more common in obese postmenopausal women.

Hot flashes are due to hypothalamic dysfunction caused by loss of ovarian feedback signals, with cyclic activation of thermoregulatory pathways resulting in flushing and perspiration. In many patients homeostatic adjustment occurs with time, with spontaneous disappearance of symptoms, although in about 25 per cent of cases the hot flashes persist for more than 5 years. Feedback inhibition of the hypothalamic centers controlling gonadotropin secretion can be partially restored with estrogen or progestin replacement. Theoretically, the use of both estrogen and progestin during part of the replacement cycle may have an additive or even synergistic effect, resulting in better control of hot flashes than with estrogen alone. In some patients higher doses of estrogen are needed to control hot flashes than appear to be necessary for treatment of the remaining effects of estrogen deficiency. Empirically, the estrogen dose can be gradually decreased or even discontinued after control of symptoms has been achieved. Other medications such as Bellergal and clonidine have been shown to reduce symptoms, although clinically these agents are less effective than adequate sex steroid replacement.

Osteoporosis is the most significant health problem caused by gonadal insufficiency. Loss of bone density can be prevented with adequate estrogen replacement. The incidence of fractures of the wrist and hip is reduced in association with estrogen treatment. Loss of bone density is greatest in the first 4 years following menopause, and a similar acceleration of calcium loss has been noted following discontinuation of estrogen. The maximum effect in preserving bone will be achieved if estrogen is begun soon after menopause and continued on an extended or even permanent basis. Obese women and black women have a much lower incidence of osteoporosis and therefore minimal potential benefit from estrogen prophylaxis. All other women must be considered to be at significant risk. Calcium supplementation (2.5 gm of calcium carbonate at bedtime) has been shown to retard bone loss and should be considered when estrogen is contraindicated.

Recent randomized double-blind studies of the effect of estrogen on psychological symptoms have shown significant beneficial effects on memory, anxiety, and irritability. Estrogen also relieves insomia and has been shown to decrease sleep latency and to increase the depth and duration of sleep and the amount of rapid-eye-movement (REM) sleep. Hot flashes during sleep have a close temporal relationship to waking episodes and may be a principal cause of the sleep disturbance associated with estrogen deficiency. The chronic sleep disturbance may in turn underlie other disturbances of affective and cognitive function.

Risks of estrogen replacement relate to unopposed estrogen stimulation of estrogen-responsive glandular tissues and to an exaggerated effect of oral estrogen on hepatic lipid and protein metabolism. The risk of endometrial cancer is 3 to 8 times more common with estrogen replacement and is related to dose and duration of treatment. Cyclic use of progestin reduces this risk, in one study to a level below that of untreated women. Endometrial biopsies during treatment have shown a reduction of hyperplasia with cyclic progestins, the most prominent effect being seen with use of a progestin for 10 or more days. Bleeding during drug treatment is more likely to be associated with endometrial abnormalities than with bleeding confined to the medication-free interval. The risk of breast cancer may be increased 2 to 3-fold, again relating to dose and duration of treatment. Patients with a history of cystic mastitis have been found to be at even greater risk when replacement estrogen is given. Women with prior oophorectomy appear to not be at increased risk.

Hepatic effects of estrogen result in an increased rate of gallbladder disease (2.5-fold), and increases in mean blood pressure and serum triglycerides, presumably owing to the stimulation of renin substrate and alteration of lipoprotein metabolism by estrogen. Thrombophlebitis, myocardial infarction, and stroke have not been found to be increased at currently recommended doses. A recent case-control study associated a reduction of cardiovascular disease by about one-half with prior estrogen use.

The choice of whether to replace estrogen must be individualized according to the benefits and risks of treatment following a thorough discussion with the patient. Since estrogen preparations vary markedly in potency, the best choice is one on which there are the most data about dose levels associated with benefits and risks. Administration of conjugated equine estrogens at a dose of 0.625 mg appears to confer the benefits for most women, while at the same time limiting risk. As information becomes available on systemic replacement, routes avoiding absorption through the portal circulation will likely prevail. A progestin given for at least 10 days will confer maximum benefit in opposing estrogen stimulation. A C-21 derivative, such as medroxyprogesterone acetate, 10 mg, should be chosen, since 19-nortestosterone derivatives decrease high density lipoprotein (HDL) cholesterol. A convenient regimen is to give estrogen on days 1 to 25 of each calendar month, with the progestin given on days 16 to 25. In patients at increased risk for endometrial cancer, a pretreatment biopsy should be considered. Endometrial sampling should also be considered when bleeding starts during the medication portion of the cycle, and should always be carried out when bleeding occurs with the use of estrogen unopposed by cyclic progestin.

ANDROGEN EXCESS OF ADRENAL ORIGIN

SERGIO C. STONE, M.D.

In a patient with symptoms or signs of increased androgen production, which include oily skin, acne, hirsutism, or virilism (muscle development, weight gain, deep voice, temporal baldness, enlarged clitoris, decreased breast size), the adrenal gland may be the source of the extra androgen.

ANDROGEN OF ADRENAL ORIGIN

The adrenal gland produces weak androgen, categorized by the presence of a keto group in position 17 in a 19C steroid, 17 ketosteroids. They are readily measured in 24 hour urine collections. Recently, measurement of dehidroepiandrosterone sulfate (DHEA-S) has been replacing 17 ketosteroids as a marker of adrenal androgen production. Since the ovary produces very little DHEA-S, this is a good marker of the adrenal contribution to androgen production. The adrenal also contributes to testosterone production, mainly through synthesis of androstenedione and its peripheral conversion mechanism, but most testosterone results from ovarian function (direct secretion and peripheral conversion of ovarian androstenedione).

The adrenal gland can produce excess androgen by three basic mechanisms: (1) adrenal hyperfunction, or excess adrenal production, possibly due to mild forms of steroid metabolism dysfunctions, not due to any of the characteristic congenital adrenal hyperplasia syndromes; (2) congenital adrenal hyperplasia or typical steroid metabolism deficiencies that result in typical recognizable syndromes; and (3) adrenal tumor, adenoma or carcinoma.

Adrenal Hyperfunction

The most common clinical form is adrenal hyperfunction, followed by congenital adrenal hyperplasia and very rarely by an adrenal tumor. Mild progression of symptoms over a period of years is typical. The initial diagnostic step after a complete history and physical-pelvic examination is to determine plasma levels of testosterone and DHEA-S. In most cases of adrenal hyperfunction, the DHEA-S will be elevated (normals for most laboratories, 95 to 230 μg per dl) and testosterone will be normal or slightly elevated (normal 0.1 to 0.9 ng per ml). Recommended methods of diagnosis are testosterone and DHEA-S in plasma, though 17-α-hydroxyprogesterone (or pregnanetriol in urine) can be used to rule out congenital adrenal hyperplasia.

CONGENITAL ADRENAL HYPERPLASIA

In adult women, the possibility of undiagnosed congenital adrenal hyperplasia is remote. There are five recognized metabolic errors in the adrenal steroid metabolic pathway. Only two of these produce excess androgen in adult women: 21-hydroxylase and 11-hydroxylase deficiency. Of these rare conditions, 21 hydroxylase deficiency is the most common. A simple blood level of 17-α-hydroxy-progesterone or urinary pregnanetriol should be enough to rule out this deficiency.

The individual with 11-hydroxylase deficiency cannot produce cortisol, corticosterone, or aldosterone; has excess Desoxycorticosterone (DOC) with sodium retention and hypertension; and has excess androgen, 21-OH hydroxylase deficiency, low cortisol, and hypertension. Fifty per cent have various degrees of the salt-losing syndrome. They produce excess androgen and excess 17-α hydroxyprogesterone (pregnanetriol). These patients, encountered only rarely by the practicing physician, are best treated by proper referral to an experienced endocrinologist.

OVARIAN CONTRIBUTION

If testosterone is moderately to highly elevated and especially if DHEA-S is normal, the ovary is the most likely source of the extra androgen and the adrenal involvement may be nil or minimal. For diagnosis, ovarian suppression for 3 weeks with birth control pills is recommended. Testosterone and DHEA-S should be measured again to document adequate suppression and rule out an ovarian tumor.

Adrenal Tumor

If DHEA-S is markedly elevated, the possibility of an adrenal tumor should be ruled out with a suppression test. There are multiple suppression regimens. We recommend the following plan: DHEA-S plasma level (base line), dexamethazone, 0.5 mg orally every 6 hours for 3 days; DHEA-S plasma determination on day 4. If DHEA-S is suppressed to normal levels an adrenal tumor is very unlikely. With partial or lack of suppression, the patient work-up should include a stimulation test, adrenal scan, intravenous pyelogram, and so forth. Referral is strongly recommended.

TREATMENT

Once the diagnosis of adrenal hyperfunction is made, the therapeutic decision must consider the need for long-term therapy and possible side effects or complications. These factors must be carefully explained to the patient. The logical step is to suppress the hyperfunctioning adrenal with glucocorticoids. We have found dexamethasone most useful, easy to administer, and fairly free of side effects and complications.

Usually, 0.25 to 0.75 mg per day is enough to reduce both testosterone and DHEA-S to normal. It is possible to further decrease these doses by using an alternative-day method of administration, which should reduce the problems of side effects and complications. We measure DHEA-S and testosterone 3 weeks after the initiation of the therapy to evaluate the results of our treatment and to adjust it accordingly. We start with 0.5 mg orally at bedtime and we increase it to 0.75 if the suppression is inadequate or decrease it 0.25 mg if we oversuppressed. The aim is to keep DHEA-S and hopefully testosterone at their low normal level and to avoid oversuppression and the possible side effects and complications of long-term therapy, by using the lowest possible dose.

If testosterone is not suppressed, the ovarian source should be suspected, and 3 weeks suppression with oral contraceptives should lower testosterone to normal. Dual suppression may be needed in some patients.

An important consideration is the need for long-term treatment in order to obtain clinical results. Most patients will find it difficult to accept months or years of therapy before any demonstrable effect on symptoms. It is not unusual to encounter anxiety and impatience. On occasions, the best of treatments will only arrest further progression of the condition and will not produce any major remission.

The treatment of congenital adrenal hyperplasia and adrenal tumors is best accomplished in centers used to see a fair number of these patients, and referral is again strongly recommended.

NEW DEVELOPMENTS

Recently, new drugs have been used with variable success, especially in hirsutism. Tagamet (cimetidine), Aldactone (spironolactone), and ciproterone acetate reportedly block testosterone receptors, increase estradiol levels, decrease plasma testosterone, and have dramatic effects in hirsutism. They are not FDA-approved and the clinical experience is still rather narrow. My own experience in a limited number of patients has been disappointing, but the reports in the literature are encouraging. Aldactone, the most widely used, can be given in doses of 100 mg (25 mg tablets) for several months, as a therapeutic trial. Dramatic results are reported, with rapid loss of hair, but the treatment must be kept for many years to avoid rebound when stopped. More information is certainly needed.

ASHERMAN'S SYNDROME

RICHARD C. BUMP, M.D.,
and MOON H. KIM, M.D.

Asherman's syndrome (post-traumatic intrauterine synechiae) represents the permanent adherence of the anterior and posterior uterine walls with resulting partial or complete obliteration of the uterine cavity. The placement of the adhesions is variable, with the clinical presentation being dependent on both the location and extent of the adhesions. Cervical-isthmic adhesions can result in secondary amenorrhea and cyclic pain with hematometria and hematosalpinx. Corporeal adhesions may be manifested by hypomenorrhea (partial obstruction) or amenorrhea (total atresia), as well as by infertility (total atresia or cornual adhesions) or pregnancy wastage (partial obliteration).

Traumatic insult to the basal endometrium of the infected pregnant or recently pregnant uterus has been the clinical circumstance observed to precede the formation of intrauterine adhesions most consistently. Puerperal dilatation and curettage more than 48 hours post partum and particularly in the second through the fourth postpartum week results in Asherman's syndrome in up to 25 per cent of cases.

Intrauterine adhesions have also been described more commonly following hydatidiform mole evacuation, uterine packing for postpartum hemorrhage, and manual removal of the placenta. Rarely, adhesions result from operative procedures such as myomectomy, metroplasty, or cesarean section. Of significant concern is the fact that a large proportion of cases in recent series of Asherman's syndrome reported in the United States and Japan have followed the termination of uncomplicated first trimester pregnancy by both sharp and suction curettage.

Adhesions rarely result from inflammation in the absence of trauma, a rare but notable exception being tuberculous endometritis. Similarly simple diagnostic curettage of the nonpregnant uterus seldom results in adhesion formation.

HYSTEROSCOPY FOR DIAGNOSIS AND THERAPY

Direct observation of intrauterine adhesions with determination of their severity and extent can be achieved with either the contact or the panoramic hysteroscope. The former is simple and less expensive but offers a more limited view and may not be suitable for treating extensive adhesions. Pressure sufficient to rupture bridging synechiae may be applied with the contact scope, or the completeness of blind curettage or probing may be assessed. The panoramic scope is more complicated and requires the use of a distending medium (CO_2 or one of various dextran solutions) but does allow better visualization for operative manipulations and sharp adhesion lysis. For this reason it is preferred for operative lysis of adhesions, particularly for patients with extensive adhesions. With extreme obliteration of the uterine cavity, simultaneous laparoscopy is indicated to guide hysteroscopic manipulation and to monitor for uterine perforation during the hysteroscopic dissection. Rarely, it is necessary to resort to hysterotomy in an attempt to restore the cavity in patients with total atresia.

Following restoration of cavity patency, the cavity is distended with either an inflated 3 cc Foley catheter balloon for 5 to 7 days or an IUD for 2 months. We prefer a No. 14 Foley catheter with a 3 cc balloon inflated. Antibiotic coverage is advocated for the duration of the catheter placement. Exogenous estrogen-progestin administration (Premarin, 2.5 to 5.0 mg per day, with Provera, 10 mg for 10 days every 30 to 60 days) is maintained for one or two cycles in an effort to promote endometrial regeneration. Adjunctive use of corticosteroids and other anti-inflammatory agents has been advocated by some but is not of proven benefit. The use of Hyskon (Pharmacia Co.) solution as a distending media may be of benefit in preventing recurrence of adhesions.

PROGNOSIS

Success of therapy is usually measured by restoration of menses and obstetric performance, and depends upon the severity of the adhesions. Historically, with blind curettage to break down adhesions, menstrual function was restored in only about 65 to 75 per cent of cases. Much higher rates of menstrual restoration have been reported by hysteroscopic lysis, with some series reporting 100 per cent success.

Pregnancy rates historically have been reported at 30 to 60 per cent, with increased risks of spontaneous abortion, ectopic pregnancy, and premature labor and delivery. Overall, about 50 per cent of reported pregnancies have resulted in term delivery, with only 40 per cent of treated women realizing a living child. The rate of placenta accreta is increased and should be anticipated at delivery. Early reports of obstetric performance following hysteroscopic therapy have shown no significant improvement in obstetric outcome to date.

FEMALE STERILIZATION

KEITH P. RUSSELL, M.D.

During the past decade, female sterilization has become one of the most frequently performed gynecologic operations, exceeded only by dilatation and curettage and biopsy procedures. It is estimated that over 700,000 female sterilizations are now performed annually in the United States. This increased utilization of a method of contraception and family planning has been the result of a number of factors: clarification of the legal status of the procedure, with elimination of previously vague legal impositions; the development of technically simpler operative procedures; and changes in the social mores and reproductive patterns of large segments of the population. Although in the past there were no clear-cut legal restrictions against female sterilization, the considered opinion of many legal advisers was that the physician could be charged with "mayhem" if the procedure was not carried out for strictly medical indications. This concept was anachronistic, since these caveats were applied only to female sterilization, male sterilization in the form of vasectomy being carried out on request of the patient in most communities. It has now been clearly established that female sterilization is legally permissible and justifiable with consent of only the patient herself, just as is true of other surgical procedures. The courts have established that, except for mentally handicapped individuals, it is not necessary to secure the consent of other parties such as the husband or consort, in order to carry out the procedure, other requirements such as informed consent by the patient being satisfied.

Sterilization procedures offer the female patient a certain means of permanently limiting her family and provide a form of contraception that is effective when other methods are unsatisfactory or contraindicated. For example, serious side-effects from oral contraceptives in women over 35 years of age who are smokers or who have complicating factors such as hypertension, obesity, or certain vascular problems can be contravened by the performance of sterilization. Patients who have intolerance to hormone contraception or who have had difficulties with intrauterine devices, the other two most reliable methods of contraception presently available, may turn to sterilization as a safe and effective alternative. Failed contraception with other methods may also lead to decision for sterilization.

The Federal government has instituted certain restrictions on female sterilization for those patients for whom the government subsidizes medical care. These restrictions include a waiting period of 30 days (which may be reduced to 72 hours with acquiescence of the patient) and a lower age limit of 18 years. It should be noted that there are no requirements pertaining to parity or age-plus-parity, which were previous general guidelines.

TYPES OF STERILIZATION

Partial Tubal Resection. This method is usually combined with tubal ligation. The cut ends of the tubes are usually buried in adjacent tissues such as the mesosalpinx (broad ligament) or uterine musculature. Fimbriectomy is a form of partial tubal resection in which the outer third of the tube, including the fimbria, is totally excised. This latter method has been reported to have some serious disadvantages, including subsequent development of hydrosalpinx in the remaining segment of tube, and failed sterilization.

Tubal Occlusion. This may be accomplished by simple ligation (Madlener), tubal cauterization, mechanical obstructive devices applied to the tubes, or the use of tubal occlusive substances instilled through the endometrial cavity. The latter methods are still investigational at the present time; the objective is that they will permit reversal of the sterilization status, when desired.

The most common forms of tubal coagulation or other occlusive methods are those utilizing the laparoscope, under general or (less desirably) local anesthesia, with unipolar or bipolar electrocoagulation of the tubes. It has been shown that the coagulation is best carried out a distance of 1 cm or so from the cornual insertion of the tube. Subsequent ectopic pregnancies have occurred with greater frequency when the tubes are coagulated flush at the cornual junction, permitting the development of endosalpingiosis extending from the uterine segment of the tube and growing outward, providing a nidus for implantation of a fertilized egg.

By means of laparoscopy the tubes may also be transected or, more commonly, occluded by the application of plastic rings (Falope) or clips (metal or plastic).

It should be noted that laparoscopic techniques have a higher failure rate if they are performed immediately after abortion. In general, this caution applies to all sterilization procedures, with regard to the pregnant state. For instance, it has been shown that there is a higher failure rate when the Pomeroy method of tubal ligation and resection is carried out at the time of cesarean section than when it is carried out as an interval or delayed procedure.

Hysterectomy. Although sterilization is usually a byproduct of hysterectomy, there are certain indications in which hysterectomy may be the preferred method of sterilization. These latter conditions are usually associated with uterine disease, pelvic discomfort, menstrual abnormalities, or other situations in which a hysterectomy might not otherwise be recommended but when combined with the need for sterilization may be a justifiable procedure. Each case must be evaluated on its merits. When there are questionable or borderline indications, the prudent physician will usually seek consultation for the purpose of justifiable support of his decision to perform hysterectomy. It should be noted that most third party payers do not consider that hysterectomy, when performed purely for sterilization purposes, is a compensable procedure.

MOST COMMONLY USED PROCEDURES

Laparoscopic Fulguration. By either closed or open laparoscopy the tube is grasped and coagulated. If desired, in addition, the tube may be cut. The method usually requires a portal of entry in addition to the laparoscopic incision, for the use of grasping or operating instruments. If plastic rings or metal clips are to be applied, this is usually carried out via the two-portal technique.

Mini-laparotomy. In this technique, a small transverse incision is made, usually at the pubic hairline. A small self-retaining retractor can be placed after the peritoneum is opened, for visualization. Visualization is further enhanced by the use of an indwelling intrauterine probe placed transvaginally, thus allowing for uterine manipulation during the procedure. This self-retaining probe is placed at the beginning of the procedure, prior to laparotomy.

Mini-laparotomy allows for direct visualization and greater availability of the tubes for resection, in addition to visualization of each ovary for gross abnormalities. In general, an attempt is made to resect approximately 1.5 cm of each tube in its midportion. In addition, the tube is usually ligated with either chromic catgut or a nonabsorbable suture. If desired, cauterization of the ligated and cut ends of the tubes can also be carried out, in a further effort to achieve permanent tubal occlusion. In the Irving technique, the cut ends of the proximal segments of the remaining tubes are buried in the wall of the uterus posteriorly. Other methods simply bury the cut ends in the mesosalpinx. The Uchida procedure calls for delineation of the mesosalpinx by injection of fluid (saline), thereby allowing the oviduct itself to be more clearly visualized and resected.

Vaginal Approach. In this method, the tubes are approached through a posterior culdotomy incision. Although the method may usually be easily performed on a multiparous patient, particularly if retroversion exists, there are frequent difficulties in visualizing the entire length of the tubes in many cases. This latter aspect is exceedingly important, in order to delineate the tube from the round ligament, a structure that not only closely resembles the tube in its midportion but also lies closely adjacent to the tube. It is imperative that each tube be clearly identified to its fimbriated end when performing any sterilization procedure, including all of the above. Failures have occurred when this consideration has been overlooked.

HAZARDS

The hazards of female sterilization embrace all those that are associated with any surgical procedure, including excessive postoperative bleeding, infection, and prolonged pelvic pain. In addition, it has been reported that there is an increased rate of subsequent ovarian malfunction, often leading to uterine bleeding problems, as a consequence of female sterilization. Every effort should be made to avoid compromising ovarian circulation and to prevent ovarian fixation or constriction in the pelvis, when carrying out sterilization procedures. Although a "postligation syndrome" has been postulated, which includes menorrhagia and associated problems such as dysmenorrhea and pelvic pain, the exact etiology or even existence of such a clinical condition has not been established.

The essentially permanent nature of the sterilization procedure may lead to a subsequent "regret" reaction in some patients. The most common cause for such result is a changed marital or parental status. Other reasons are largely psychological, and may be associated with inadequate discussion and counseling prior to the procedure, marital stresses, sexual problems, or the timing of the procedure (interval procedures are associated with fewer regret reactions than those performed with delivery or abortion). Prior psychological problems and improper motivation for the procedure (external pressures) also account for increased regret reactions.

FAILURE OF STERILIZATION

Failure rates vary slightly for different procedures. The overall failure rate including all commonly acceptable methods is probably in the range of 1 per cent. The patient should always be cautioned that there is no method which has proved to be 100 per cent effective, including hysterectomy (there have been rare instances of abdominal pregnancy occurring following hysterectomy). On the other hand, the patient should not be led to believe that the method she may elect, in consultation with the physician, can likely be reversed at some future time. The procedure should be approached with the consideration that the decision has been made for permanent sterilization. Although tubal patency may be attained through surgical repair of previously ligated or partially resected tubes, the success rate for term pregnancies under such circumstances approaches only 10 to 20 per cent.

The major reasons for failure of sterilization are: (1) a pre-existing undetected pregnancy; (2) errors in surgical technique; and (3) actual method failures. Failures associated with pre-existing pregnancy can usually be avoided by performing the procedure shortly following normal menstruation or by the performance of sensitive pregnancy tests preoperatively. Technical errors are avoided by careful attention to tubal identification and utilization of standard surgical procedures. True method failures probably occur in 2 to 3 instances per 1000 sterilizations. There is a higher failure rate when the procedure is carried out in association with delivery or abortion.

When sterilization failure occurs, as evidenced by a subsequent pregnancy, the patient may be offered abortion as a back-up procedure. Should the patient elect to carry the subsequent pregnancy to term, consideration should be given to a repeat sterilization procedure at that time.

All patients should be warned that there is an increased risk of ectopic pregnancy in patients who have been sterilized, relative to those who have not. Ectopic pregnancy is far more frequent after cautery laparoscopic techniques than following other methods. Tubal recanalization, with resultant impaired oviductal function, undoubtedly plays a major role in such occurrences. Fulguration of a tube too close to its cornual entrance into the uterus may permit the development of endosalpingiosis and subsequent ectopic pregnancy.

It has been shown that the incidence of this complication can be reduced by fulgurating the tubes at least 3 to 4 cm from the cornua, or excising and ligating the tubes as described under mini-laparotomy.

ANOREXIA NERVOSA
(Starvation-Amenorrhea Syndrome)

STEVE N. LONDON, M.D.,
and CHARLES B. HAMMOND, M.D.

Although anorexia nervosa is a psychiatric disorder, patients with this disease often present initially to gynecologists. Since the choice of therapy and probably the final outcome for patients with anorexia nervosa depends upon early recognition, early diagnosis must be the first line of therapy.

Generally speaking, the woman at greatest risk for developing anorexia nervosa is in adolescence or her early 20s, is usually from a higher socioeconomic class, and has a personality background of that of an "overachiever." Anorexia nervosa is a rare disorder but in certain populations the incidence may approach 1 in 200 to 300 women. More important is the fact that mortality for patients with anorexia nervosa still ranges between 5 and 20 per cent despite all modes of therapy.

Amenorrhea is a common presenting symptom of anorexia nervosa. Of interest is that up to 75 per cent of all patients with anorexia nervosa will develop amenorrhea before demonstrable weight loss. This suggests that the weight loss in and of itself is not responsible for the cessation of menses. Unfortunately no laboratory test is diagnostic for anorexia nervosa. However, almost all anorectics exhibit the following endocrine profile: normal follicle-stimulating hormone, low luteinizing hormone, 17-hydroxy and 17-ketosteroids normal to minimally elevated, serum cortisol elevated up to two times normal, low T_3, normal T_4, and normal prolactin. Given the general range for most laboratories, these amenorrheic young women may be categorized as having "eugonadotropic" amenorrhea, often with rather striking hypoestrogenism. All these items are variable. The diagnosis of anorexia nervosa must be considered in any patient seen for primary or secondary amenorrhea.

Casper and Davis divided anorexia nervosa into three phases which allows an understanding of the psychopathology and facilitates early diagnosis. In Phase I some external event impacts upon the patient's self-esteem so she becomes preoccupied with her appearance. In Phase II the patient begins to reduce her weight successfully and systematically. During Phase II most patients develop a "restless hypermotility." Also, in Phase II, the patient becomes preoccupied with food and develops the fear that one day she will be fat. Phase III is the physically moribund end of the spectrum. When patients reach this phase, the diagnostic criteria of Feighner are usually fulfilled.

A modified version of Feighner's criteria for establishing the diagnosis of anorexia nervosa is (1) a weight loss greater than 25 per cent of original body weight; (2) no medical or psychiatric illness that can account for the weight loss; (3) "a distorted, implacable attitude toward eating food or weight that overrides hunger, admonition, reassurance and threats;" and (4) at least two of the following signs or symptoms: amenorrhea, an increase in lanugo hair, bradycardia, periodic overactivity, vomiting, or episodic bulimia.

Patients in Phase I and II of anorexia nervosa can usually be treated successfully as outpatients, but if the disorder progresses to Phase III hospitalization is generally required. Once the patient is hospitalized, therapy is directed toward restoring adequate nutrition and treating the underlying psychological disorder. Unfortunately, the restrictive and sometimes punitive nature of hospital therapy discourages voluntary admission. It thus may become necessary on occasion to admit the patient against her will. The method of psychotherapy employed upon admission varies from institution to institution. Unfortunately, there are no controlled studies which indicate whether psychoanalysis, family therapy, or behavioral therapy is the optimal treatment form. Behavior therapy in conjunction with medical therapy probably is the most popular form of therapy for patients in Phase III of anorexia nervosa.

Behavioral therapy is based on the premise stated concisely by Blinder that "the impairment of food intake in patients with anorexia nervosa can be viewed as a specific learned behavior perpetuated by environmental reinforcements." In essence, all social and emotional reinforcement for fasting must be withdrawn. To accomplish this the patient should be isolated in a stripped room and not permitted to receive visitors or to have recreational activities. A personal hierarchy of rewards is established and usually a weight gain of half a pound per day is rewarded by the return of privileges. The exact number of calories necessary to gain 1 kg varies but depends upon the weight of the patient at the start of treatment and a history of prior obesity. Approximately 7500 excess calories are necessary to increase an anorectic's weight by 1 kilogram. It is important to realize in severely affected patients that nutritional resuscitation is necessary before psychotherapy can be useful. If conventional methods fail and the patient manifests life-threatening weight loss, then total parenteral nutrition (TPN) must be considered. The two main contraindications for TPN are the likelihood of a patient-induced air embolus and the inability of the family and patient to participate in psychotherapy.

In conjunction with behavioral therapy, chlorpromazine or cyproheptadine is often used to facilitate weight gain. The relationship between weight gain and these drugs is not fully understood. Numerous other medical approaches have been tried during the past 50 years, but none has approached the success of combined behavioral and medical therapy.

Although the short-term success rate with behavioral therapy in some series is up to 85 per cent, the long-term results are most pessimistic. Bruch has estimated that fewer than half of anorectic patients achieve a satisfactory adjustment. The remainder suffer recurrent episodes, other psychopathology, or even death. It is obvious that all patients require continued intensive psychotherapy following discharge. It must be noted that follow-up studies have not demonstrated any particular treatment regimens to be superior. More importantly, there is no correlation between short-term success and ultimate outcomes.

Even if body weight returns to normal and is maintained after treatment in patients with anorexia nervosa, menstrual function may not return. This again emphasizes that the weight loss in and of itself is not necessarily responsible for the amenorrhea. Substitutional therapy with estrogen and added progestin will result in cyclic bleeding and amelioration of hypoestrogenic symptoms, but is usually not indicated in patients with anorexia nervosa. Most therapists prefer to await spontaneous cycles that result from the combined weight gain and psychotherapy, and thus which serve as an indicator of improvement.

However, if fertility is desired in the improved patient in whom amenorrhea persists, then ovulation induction with clomiphene citrate, human menopausal gonadotropin (HMG), or gonadotropin-releasing hormone (GnRH) can be utilized. In general, clomiphene has proven unsatisfactory in inducing ovulation in these patients. However, one or two 7-day courses of 100 mg per day should be tried, in view of the expense and problems of the other methods. HMG therapy has resulted in the restoration of menses and fertility in most anorectics. This agent acts directly upon the ovary, by-passing the defective hypothalamus. HMG is currently the most successful and popular method of inducing ovulation in anorectics. GnRH therapy may result in the future in reliable ovulation in hypogonadotropic hypoestrogenic patients, by-passing the hazards of HMG, mainly the hyperstimulation syndrome and multiple births. However, not enough data are present at this time to assess its final place.

XY GONADAL DYSGENESIS

JOE LEIGH SIMPSON, M.D.

Although most often associated with monosomy X (45,X) or X-structural abnormalities, gonadal dysgenesis may occur in individuals with an apparently normal male (46,XY) chromosomal complement—XY gonadal dysgenesis. Gonadoblastomas or dysgerminomas occur frequently (20 to 30 per cent). At least one form is inherited in X-linked recessive fashion.

Patients will frequently present with primary amenorrhea. Because short stature is not characteristic, ascertainment before puberty will ordinarily be possible only if screening studies have been performed. Affected individuals are of normal female appearance, but show no development of secondary sexual characteristics. No breast development is evident; pubic hair is scant or absent; external genitalia are normal but unstimulated. Vagina, cervix, and uterus are small but likewise well-differentiated. Thus, findings on pelvic examination will not differ from those of individuals who have gonadal dysgenesis with other chromosomal complements [e.g., 45,X,46,XX, or 46,X,i(Xq)]. Somatic anomalies are usually not present.

Chromosomal studies are necessary to exclude other types of gonadal dysgenesis. One should count 50 cells to exclude 45,X/46,XY mosaicism, a sporadic condition that no other family members would be expected to have. X-chromatin studies (buccal smear) will not suffice because they do not permit XY gonadal dysgenesis to be distinguished from 45,X. Distinction is important because gonadal extirpation is necessary only in the former.

Endocrine studies confirm gonadal failure. FSH and LH are increased. Other studies, such as serum estrogen, are not obligatory. H-Y antigen may or may not be present. There is some suggestion that XY gonadal dysgenesis with H-Y antigen is more likely to be associated with neoplasia than XY gonadal dysgenesis without H-Y; however, more data are necessary.

More than one family member with gonadal dysgenesis suggests either XY or XX gonadal dysgenesis. XX gonadal dysgenesis is inherited in an autosomal recessive fashion, whereas XY gonadal dysgenesis is inherited in X-linked recessive fashion. Thus, affected male siblings, maternal uncles, or maternal male first cousins (actually all phenotypically female) suggest XY gonadal dysgenesis.

MANAGEMENT

The first step in managment is diagnostic confirmation.

Detailed Pedigree. X-linked recessive inheritance places certain relatives at risk for the same disorder as the index case, as noted already. These relatives should be identified, for they would benefit from therapy and counseling concerning risk of neoplasia. The presence of amenorrhea in individuals at risk warrants chromosomal studies. Such studies also would be appropriate for relatives who have not yet undergone puberty.

Once the diagnosis is confirmed, patients need to be reassured that sexual adequacy can be anticipated in all areas except childbearing. (Embryo transfer techniques are a formal possibility even here.) It is not obligatory to divulge the genetic sex. One can merely say that the gonads (or the ovaries) failed to develop, or developed abnormally. This approach will also provide a useful introduction for discussing gonadal extirpation. However, individualization with respect to communicating the true karyotype is necessary, especially if medical personnel or other widely read individuals are involved.

Gonadal Extirpation. Laparoscopy or laparotomy is not necessary for diagnostic confirmation, but the latter is necessary for gonadal extirpation. Little is gained by delaying extirpation indefinitely because (1) germ cell neoplasias arise as early as the first decade and (2) gonads are only streaks, which cannot feminize patients. If breast development or pubic hair is present, gonadal extirpation is a matter of some haste. Secondary sexual development in XY gonadal dysgenesis is almost always the result of estrogen production by a gonadoblastoma or dysgerminoma. These tumors may be verified on the basis of roentgenography (calcification) or ultrasonography (masses).

Streak gonads, typically present on the posterior aspect of the broad ligament, are 3 to 4 cm long and 0.5 cm wide. Sequential clamping and suture ligation can remove the organs; however, the procedure may not be so simple as it would appear, particularly if the broad ligament contains prominent vessels. In fact, total abdominal hysterectomy with bilateral removal of the streaks is technically easier. For psychological reasons, however, it is preferable not to remove the uterus.

Hormonal Replacement Therapy. This author begins treatment with conjugated estrogen, 0.625 mg daily on days 1 through 20 each calendar month. This is increased to 1.25 mg per day, possibly to a maximum of 2.50 mg per day, again in cyclic fashion. After an initial period of treatment with estrogens alone, medroxyprogesterone is added (10 to 20 mg) on days 16 to 20. Other regimens are equally appropriate, including use of combined oral contraceptives; however, progestins should always be administered as well as estrogens. Response can be monitored on the basis of side-effects, withdrawal bleeding, or endometrial biopsies. Breast development, pubic hair, and enlargement of pelvic structures should occur.

General Physical Examination. Somatic anomalies are sometimes associated with XY gonadal dysgenesis. Some are doubtless coincidental, whereas others indicate a distinct malformation syndrome in which streak gonads are merely one component. Anomalies reminiscent of 45,X Turner syndrome suggest 45,X/46,XY mosaicism. Of importance is that individuals with otherwise typical XY gonadal dysgenesis may show renal parenchymal abnormalities (nephritis, nephrosis). Thus, renal status should be assessed periodically.

TESTICULAR FEMINIZATION

JOE LEIGH SIMPSON, M.D.

Complete testicular feminization (complete androgen insensitivity) is an X-linked recessive disorder in which 46,XY individuals have bilateral testes but female external genitalia, a blindly ending vagina, and no müllerian derivatives. Affected individuals undergo breast development and puberal feminization, and hence present as well-developed females. Most cases result from a deficiency of the cytosol receptor for androgen (receptor-negative), but other mechanisms can be responsible because some patients have cytosol receptors (receptor-positive). In addition, some individuals with androgen insensitivity show clitoral hypertrophy and labial-scrotal fusions; the term "incomplete androgen insensitivity" is applied to these individuals. This will not be considered further.

Gynecologists will usually detect patients with complete testicular feminization because of primary amenorrhea. Physical examination reveals females of normal appearance. Some are quite attractive and have pronounced breast development, but others are similar in appearance to unaffected females. Statural growth and body proportions are usually normal. Pubic and axillary hair are sparse, but scalp hair is normal. External genitalia are normal for females. The vagina terminates blindly and is shorter than usual, presumably because the müllerian ducts fail to contribute to formation of the vagina. Occasionally the vagina is very short or represented merely by a dimple. Neither a uterus nor fallopian tubes are usually present, although occasionally fibromuscular remnants or rudimentary fallopian tubes persist. Testes are usually normal in size and located in the abdomen, inguinal canal, or labia.

The most important physical finding is absence of a uterus and cervix. Such a finding in a female with normal external genitalia almost always indicates either testicular feminization or müllerian aplasia. Individuals with both conditions show breast development. In both, the vagina ends blindly, although it is more often foreshortened in müllerian aplasia. The sole differentiating feature upon physical examination is lack of pubic hair in complete testicular feminization.

X-linked recessive inheritance for complete androgen insensitivity implies risk for brothers, uncles, and maternal first cousins of the index case. (Of course, all affected individuals would be phenotypic females.) Not every affected individual will have other affected relatives, for some will represent new mutations. In addition, familial aggregates of müllerian aplasia have been reported; thus, identification of other affected family members without a uterus should not obviate appropriate diagnostic procedures.

Cytogenetic studies are obligatory in differentiating between müllerian aplasia and complete androgen insensitivity. Chromosomal analysis of lymphocytes should be performed, rather than relying upon a buccal smear. Mosaicism is not to be expected; thus, a routine study of 20 cells should suffice.

Endocrine studies are ordinarily not obligatory, for the diagnosis should be apparent on the basis of physical findings and cytogenetic studies. Plasma testosterone is normal or slightly increased. LH is slightly increased, presumably because Leydig cells are somewhat unresponsive. Analysis of cultured fibroplasts is necessary to determine whether cytosol receptors are present or not, but such tests can be confined to research protocols.

MANAGEMENT

Diagnostic confirmation is necessary, taking advantage of the methods listed above. Laparotomy or even laparoscopy is not necessary to make the diagnosis.

Pedigree. A complete pedigree should be taken, with particular emphasis on individuals expected to be affected on the basis of an X-linked recessive condition: brothers, maternal uncles, and maternal male first cousins (all phenotypic females). Affected individuals past the age of puberty would show primary amenorrhea; prepubertal phenotypic females could benefit from routine cytogenetic studies that could reveal them to be genetically male and, hence, affected.

Psychological Considerations. A reasonable policy is not to divulge the genetic sex. Candor does not always seem to be the best policy. One may relate that the gonads are abnormal, or that "ovaries" failed to develop, facts that will prepare the patient for further discussion concerning gonadal extirpation. Reassure the patient, or the patient and parents if the patient is a minor, that feminine development and sexual adequacy (save childbearing) can be anticipated in all. A foreshortened vagina may require attention, but optimistic long-term outcome can be anticipated.

If the patient is a child, it may sometimes be appropriate to communicate the true genetic sex to the parents, again with the caveat that it would perhaps not be wise for them to relay such information further. Likewise, medical personnel will probably be sufficiently versed to know the differential diagnosis. In these circumstances, I find it helpful to inquire of such individuals the extent of their reading. If the differential diagnosis—complete androgen insensitivity (testicular feminization) or müllerian aplasia—is provided, candor is obviously essential.

Gonadal Extirpation. Testes must be removed because they can undergo neoplastic transformation. The prevalence of neoplasia, initially believed as high as 20 per cent, actually seems much lower, perhaps only that expected with intra-abdominal testes. Neoplasia rarely occurs before the late second or early third decade. For this reason this author prefers postpubertal orchiectomy in order to permit spontaneous feminization during adolescence. Alternatively, some authorities prefer gonadal extirpation at a younger age because "fewer questions" are asked.

Testes are softer than ovaries and may be surrounded by vessels that impart a reddish appearance. Their removal requires laparotomy, except in the rare circumstances in which testes are labial. Testes are usually identified in the posterior pelvis or in the inguinal canal. Failure to locate testes readily probably indicates an inguinal location. An exploration of the internal inguinal rings may demonstrate a vas deferens which, upon gentle tugging, may bring a testes into view and permit removal. Dissection of the inguinal region is probably not advisable for the average gynecologist. Extirpation requires clamping and suture-ligating vascular pedicles.

Vagina. Vaginal depth is usually satisfactory, only occasionally requiring surgical attention. Should the vagina be foreshortened, dilators will generally suffice to produce normal depth. Rarely is it necessary to construct a vagina by the McIndoe procedure or a modification thereof.

Hormonal Treatment after Gonadal Extirpation. This author prefers 1.25 mg conjugated estrogens on days 1 to 20 each calendar month, supplemented by 10 to 20 mg of medroxyprogesterone on days 16 to 20. Other hormones and other regimens can be used; however, in all, cyclic estrogens supplemented by progestins should be employed. Oral contraceptives can be used, provided sufficient estrogen levels can be maintained. If gonads have been extirpated prior to puberty, treatment should be begun at approximately 12 years of age.

HYPOPITUITARISM

PAUL F. BRENNER, M.D.

Hypofunction of the pituitary gland may be either secondary or primary. Secondary pituitary failure is the result of hypothalamic disease which alters the interactions of the hypothalamic pituitary hormones. Medications, stress, weight loss, anorexia nervosa, and aberrations in neurotransmitter signals have the potential to adversely affect hypothalamic function and in turn the release of pituitary hormones. The synthesis of hypothalamic releasing hormones may be impaired without any of these other extrinsic factors being present. Medications may be discontinued, the effects of stress on the central nervous system usually abate with time and the effects of weight loss are reversed when the individual returns to her ideal body weight. Patients with anorexia nervosa have a greater problem than just the severe loss of weight. They have an inappropriate concept of their body image and require psychiatric therapy.

Primary pituitary failure is caused either by a destructive lesion or a tumor of the pituitary gland. Pituitary tumors which are macroadenomas (>10 mm), which cause visual disturbances, or which extend beyond the confines of the sella turcica require surgical extirpation. The management of prolactin-secreting microadenomas will be considered in the section on galactorrhea.

The most common non-tumorous cause of spontaneous hypopituitarism in adult women is Sheehan's syndrome. This syndrome is the hypofunction of the hypophysis which occurs as the result of infarction following severe postpartum hemorrhage, circulatory collapse, and shock. Usually only the anterior pituitary gland is affected and the neurohypophysis is not involved. In extreme cases the neurohypophysis may be affected, and in response to a vasopressin deficiency, diabetes insipidus occurs. The extent of the ischemic necrosis of the anterior pituitary gland is related to the length of time the postpartum woman is hypotensive. The longer the individual is hypotensive, the greater the amount of the hypophysis which is infarcted.

Clinical findings of hypopituitarism are not present unless 75 per cent or more of the anterior pituitary gland is destroyed. The earliest signs of Sheehan's syndrome are the inability of the postpartum mother to breast feed, and if she had a perineal shave during labor the hair fails to reappear. The affect on the target organs of the decreased secretion of the tropic hormones ACTH, TSH, prolactin, FSH and LH by the anterior pituitary gland leads to lower circulating levels of cortisol, thyroxines and estrogen. Nausea, vomiting, weakness, lethargy, apathy, hypothermia, hypotension, and even vascular collapse are clinical manifestations of lowered cortisol. Cold skin, dry skin, constipation, depilation of the eyebrows, and myxedema are findings which result from hypothyroidism. Amenorrhea, decrease in breast tissue, and atrophy of the vagina result from hypoestrogenism. The fall in the circulating levels of androgens of both adrenal and ovarian origin causes a decrease in axillary, pubic, and body hair and a decline in libido. Melanin is also produced by the anterior pituitary gland, and when melanin production falls, the skin pigmentation and the color of the breast areolas fades and the patient fails to tan when exposed to sunlight.

Hypopituitarism has a deleterious effect on erythropoiesis which results in a moderate normocytic, normochromic anemia.

Not all of the tropic hormones are necessarily deficient in hypopituitarism. In some cases there is a decrease of only one anterior pituitary gland hormone. With a lesser degree of anterior pituitary destruction clinical symptoms may appear very gradually, and several months or even years may pass before they are apparent. In some forms of hypopituitarism, there are no overt manifestations of the disease, but there is a decrease in tropic hormone reserve. At times of great stress, a decrease in ACTH reserve may be life-threatening.

The treatment of Sheehan's syndrome consists of multiglandular hormone replacement therapy for the remainder of the patient's life. Before embarking on this involved and expensive long-term therapy, the diagnosis of Sheehan's syndrome must be confirmed beyond any reasonable doubt. The evaluation of adrenal function and particularly ACTH reserve is essential for the individual suspected of having Sheehan's syndrome. Baseline serum cortisol determinations will not confirm or exclude the presence of this disease. An 8-hour ACTH infusion test is performed for patients throught to have long-standing Sheehan's syndrome. Either the insulin-induced hypoglycemia test or the metyrapone test may be used to evaluate ACTH reserve. The cortisol response to the hypoglycemia induced by insulin administration is the preferred test of ACTH reserve. Hypoglycemia followed by an abnormal blunted cortisol response is indicative of insufficient ACTH reserve. Serum thyroxin (T_4) and free thyroxine index are tests used to diagnose secondary hypothyroidism. TSH levels are a sensitive indicator of primary hypothyroidism but cannot be used to diagnose secondary hypothyroidism. Symptoms of hypothyroidism can appear years after the episode of postpartum hemorrhage and vascular instability. Subjects suspected of having Sheehan's syndrome should have their thyroid function tested at least annually. Secondary hypogonadism may be tested by the gonadotropin-releasing hormone test, serum estradiol or the progesterone challenge test.

Treatment of Sheehan's syndrome involves the administration of hormones in order to replace those of the target organs which are deficient. Hydrocortisone is used to treat the cortisol insufficiency. One regimen of corticosteroid therapy is to prescribe 10 mg of hydrocortisone in the morning and the same dose in the evening. Other regimens attempt to simulate the diurnal variation in cortisol concentrations by giving a higher dose in the morning than in the evening. Either regimen is acceptable. Patients ingesting corticosteroid should always carry some form of identification with them indicating the nature of their disease, the specific medication, and dose they are receiving. They also should have available at all times an extra dose of medication to be used in an emergency. Only during times of severe stress or surgery will an increase in their corticosteroid therapy be necessary.

Hypothyroidism, if present, is treated with thyroid hormone replacement. Fifty μg of L-thyroxine is given daily and the dose is increased 50 μg every 2 to 3 weeks until the patient is euthyroid. Usually a normal serum thyroxine and the free thyroxine index can be achieved with a daily dose of 150 μg of L-thyroxine.

Patients with Sheehan's syndrome with secondary hypogonadism should receive cyclic estrogen therapy with the addition of a gestagen in the latter part of the cycle in order to prevent osteoporotic fractures and vaginal mucosa atrophy. One regimen is to administer conjugated equine estrogen, 0.625 mg daily for the first 25 days each calendar month. Oral medroxyprogesterone, 10 mg a day, is added to the regimen from day 16 through day 25 each calendar month. Women of child-bearing age with Sheehan's syndrome who desire to conceive are candidates for human menopausal gonadotropin therapy for induction of ovulation. In very rare cases of partial disease, spontaneous recovery of pituitary function has occurred and even pregnancy has been reported.

LUTEAL PHASE DEFECTS

GEORGEANNA SEEGAR JONES, M.D.

Since the corpus luteum is a continuum of the follicle, any etiology which leads to follicular dysfunction may also, in more muted forms, result in luteal dysfunction. Progesterone dysfunction at the end-organ endometrial level may also occur in relation to specific endometrial defects, scarring, and progesterone receptor deficiency. The clinical manifestations are infertility, or early pregnancy wastage. The diagnosis is best made by properly timed, properly taken, endometrial biopsy, and must be documented by repeat biopsy. Although correction of the cause is always desirable therapy, an etiologic diagnosis is not always possible.

The diagnosis of a luteal phase defect, defined as a disturbance of *progesterone production* or *response*, can theoretically be made on the basis of any quantitative measure of progesterone. Traditionally, the clinical method of choice has been the endometrial biopsy. The properly taken and properly diagnosed biopsy serves as a bioassay of the patient's response to her own luteal function and therefore measures both the production of the hormone and the end-organ effect of progesterone. Three serum progesterone assays taken during peak luteal function are also adequate, provided the assay laboratory has a properly standardized hormonal assay curve for the entire normal menstrual cycle.

Corpus luteum insufficiency may be categorized by a description of the defect: (1) a short luteal span with normal steroid secretion, (2) a normal luteal span with low steroid secretion, or (3) a short luteal span with abnormal steroid secretion. The luteal span which is short with normal steroidogenesis characteristically occurs in the early menarcheal years, and in my experience may be of no clinical significance. Classification by etiologic factors is more meaningful, and should always be attempted. Since the corpus luteum is a continuum of the follicle, any factor that will cause anovulation will, when it occurs in a more muted form, cause a corpus luteum defect. The following outline by anatomic areas is a convenient classification:

1. Central nervous system factors causing an initial low FSH early in the cycle, a low LH surge, or a deficient tonic LH residual
   a. Psychogenic causes, usually stress-induced
   b. Anatomic lesions
      (1) Drug-induced
      (2) Weight/height disparities (anorexia nervosa, constitutional)
      (3) Athletic training programs
      (4) Hyperprolactinemia
2. Diseases of intermediate metabolism
   a. Chronic illness
   b. Diabetes
   c. Hypothyroidism or hyperthyroidism
   d. Adrenal disease
   e. Self-induced or inadvertent weight gain or loss, unrelated to anorexia nervosa
3. Gonadal factors
   a. The perimenopausal phase of premature menopause
   b. Excessive prostaglandin $f_2\alpha$
   c. Iatrogenic drug administration, Clomid, Pergonal, or related gonadotropin stimulators, causing excessive estradiol in relation to progesterone
4. End-organ—uterine
   a. Progesterone receptor defect
   b. Endometrial sclerosis

It has been shown that disturbances of hypothalamic pituitary function which cause (1) too little FSH early on in the cycle, (2) inadequate LH surge, or (3) an inadequate tonic LH following the surge may all be associated with luteal phase defects. Such defects are extremely difficult to document in a clinical practice situation. The history and physical examination should always include questions which will indicate the possibility of chronic illness or metabolic disease; weight gain or loss; psychogenic stress; and drug ingestion, including excessive smoking, caffeine, and alcohol consumption. A prolactin assay should always be ordered, and if one plans to attempt gonadotropin augmentation with Clomid or replacement with hCG or hMG, an FSH or LH assay should be obtained prior to therapy.

Specific Tests for Diagnosis of the Luteal Phase Defect. An endometrial biopsy for the diagnosis of a luteal phase defect should always be taken in conjunction with a properly kept basal body temperature chart. Although the basal body temperature chart can alert one's suspicion of the diagnosis, it is unreliable as a diagnostic method, but necessary in order to properly interpret the biopsy. The endometrial biopsy must be taken close to the end of the menstrual cycle; the 26th day of a 28 day cycle is ideal. In this way, the biopsy is used as a bioassay which the patient performs on herself. It is obvious from the shape of the progesterone curve that the serum progesterone assay should not be obtained on this date, as the progesterone values by this time have reached a low level.

A full-thickness piece of endometrium must be obtained from the top of the fundus. The curette should be inserted gently to the fundus. With a firm, single stroke a biopsy should be taken from the posterior surface or the lateral uterine wall. In this way, the possibility of interrupting an early implantation is remote. If either the operator or the patient is concerned about this possibility, the patient should be asked to refrain from intercourse or use a barrier method of contraception in the cycle in which the biopsy will be taken. If the surface epithelium is not included in the histologic sample, or the endometrial sample is from the lower uterine segment, it cannot be dated.

It is wise for every gynecologist who is interested in making this diagnosis to learn to date the endometrium by the method of Hertig, Noyes, and Rock (Fertil. Steril., 1:1, 1950). The patient should return to the office the week after the biopsy is taken, with her basal body temperature chart. The biopsy is then read according to the histologic dating, the day of onset of menses being assigned as day 28, and the day of estimated ovulation being assigned as day 14. If the biopsy is normal, the histologic dating should be within 2 days of the date according to the presumed ovulation and according to the count back from the onset of menses. If there is more than a 2 day discrepancy between the histologic dating and the menstrual calendar dating, a luteal defect is diagnosed. Any patient may have a sporadic luteal defect related to stress or incidental factors. Therefore, an endometrial biopsy must be obtained in a second menstrual cycle for this finding to be of clinical significance. Since each monthly corpus luteum is a unique endocrine organ, the luteal phase defect cannot be of clinical importance unless it is repetitive.

Serial serum radioimmunoassays for progesterone can be used as a diagnostic method or to confirm the diagnosis of a luteal phase defect. A single progesterone assay, however, can be misleading. It is obvious from the shape of the progesterone curve that the serum progesterone assays should not be obtained on the day the endometrial biopsy is taken. Abraham has indicated that if three serum progesterone assays are obtained at the peak of the progesterone secretory phase, this is a satisfactory method for diagnosing a luteal defect. However, this takes for granted that one can identify the ovulation date without knowing the exact date of the LH surge, and this is sometimes difficult. It also makes the assumption that one is dealing with a laboratory which has a well established progesterone curve for the normal menstrual cycle.

Although, in our experience, hyperprolactinemia is an unusual cause of the luteal phase defect, it is one which responds readily to specific therapy and which is easily diagnosed. It should therefore not be overlooked.

TREATMENT

Correction of the etiologic defect is, of course, always the preferred therapy. However, as the luteal phase defect is multifactorial, it is sometimes difficult to make this etiologic diagnosis.

Experience has shown that substitution progesterone therapy is the simplest and most universally successful treatment. Clomid therapy will sometimes prove successful, and human chorionic gonadotropin, hCG, may also be effective. A repeat endometrial biopsy on therapy must be obtained to determine the efficacy of any therapy.

General Supportive Measures. If specific factors can be defined, these should be corrected. Drug excess including caffeine and nicotine, compulsive jogging, nutritional abnormalities causing height/weight discrepancies, underweight or obesity, and diseases of intermediate metabolism must not be overlooked, as all of these should be specifically corrected.

Bromocriptine. Luteal defects associated with hyperprolactinemia, usually respond very rapidly to bromocriptine (Parlodel), 2.5 mg given at night. This dose is usually quite sufficient. The prolactin assay should be repeated after 3 weeks of therapy, and if it is not within normal range the dosage can be gradually increased to 7.5 mg.

Gonadotropin Stimulation. If an FSH or tonic LH defect is suspected, clomiphene citrate (Clomid) will sometimes be corrective by causing an increased pituitary hormone secretion. Again, clomiphene is usually effective in the lowest possible dose, 50 mg a day for 5 days. In our experience, if this is not effective as judged by a repeat endometrial biopsy during the first treatment cycle, it is useless to increase the dosage.

Human chorionic gonadotropin, (hCG) stimulation will correct either an insufficient LH surge or a deficient tonic LH stimulation; 5,000 IU at the time of the LH surge is a satisfactory supplement for the mid-cycle defect and 2,500 IU every second day will serve to supplement a tonic LH deficiency.

Correction of End-Organ Deficiency. The only end-organ deficiency which will respond to corrective measures is endometrial sclerosis, and under these circumstances surgical treatment, preferably removal of synechiae under hysteroscopic direct vision with insertion of a prosthesis to prevent recurrence of synechiae, is most effective. However, when the synechiae are marked, the treatment is notoriously unsuccessful, and end-organ deficiency, associated with progesterone receptor defect, is not amenable to therapy.

Substitution Therapy. Replacement therapy with progesterone in oil, 12.5 mg daily, beginning as soon as it can be determined that ovulation has occurred, will usually correct the deficiency regardless of the etiology. This is a sufficient dosage to adequately supplement most luteal phase defects and restore the normal hormonal pattern. It is not sufficiently large to unduly prolong the menstrual cycle and delay a menstrual period. If significantly more than 12.5 mg of progesterone per day are administered a pseudopregnancy can be produced. Progesterone vaginal or rectal suppositories, 25 mg twice a day or 50 mg once a day, can also be used. These, however, are not commercially available and must be compounded by the individual pharmacist.

*progesterone powder	11 grams
polyethylene glycol 400	524 grams
polyethylene glycol 6000	348 grams

It should be noted that oral progestational drugs cannot be substituted for physiologic progesterone and many of these because of their long circulation are luteolytic rather than additive. Progesterone supplementation is preferred to corpus luteum stimulation with human chorionic gonadotropin because it does not produce a pseudopregnancy and it does not interfere with a quantitative beta hCG serum pregnancy test. This is especially important in the treatment of patients with a history of repeated miscarriages, when the early documentation of normal trophoblastic growth and development is desirable.

The question of teratogenicity of progesterone has been confused by the tendency to use the term interchangeably for progestational drugs. A symposium in 1978 reported in *Fertility and Sterility* (*30*:16) found no evidence for teratogenicity, and in November, 1981 the Food and Drug Administration Drug Advisory Committee on Fertility and Maternal Health unanimously voted to exclude progesterone and 17-hydroxyprogesterone from the list of teratogenic progestational drugs.

PRECOCIOUS PUBERTY

PAUL D. MANGANIELLO, M.D.

Precocious puberty is that condition which results in inappropriate, accelerated development of an individual's secondary sexual characteristics. Precocious development may be isolated, involving the breasts (thelarche), menses (menarche), sexual hair (pubarche), and growth, or these changes can occur simultaneously. If one takes 2.5 standard deviations from the mean for these developmental milestones as normal for the female in North America, breast development would be considered precocious if it occurred before the age of 8; pubic hair and accelerated growth velocity if it occurred before age 9; and menarche if it occurred before age 10.

Precocious puberty when true, or constitutional, is due to early activation of the hypothalamic-pituitary-gonadal axis. Pseudoprecocious puberty occurs secondary to either ingestion of exogenous sex steroids or increased endogenous sex steroid production. Precocious development may be consistent with gonadal and chromosomal sexual development, isosexual, or, as seen in females with congenital adrenal hyperplasia, heterosexual.

Precocious development, when due to increased gonadotropins, may be a result of a tumor involving the hypothalamic or pituitary region. This would be the inciting cause in 5 per cent of females and is seen in approximately 25 per cent of males. Other causes for early activation of the hypothalamus are the McCune-Albright syndrome, or polyostotic fibrous dysplasia; ectopic gonadotropin production; and primary hypothyroidism. Constitutional or idiopathic activation is seen in approximately 55 per cent of females and 40 per cent of males.

Precocious development may be secondary to a primary ovarian or adrenal lesion, i.e., a tumor, or an enzyme defect with resultant increased steroid production. Exogenous sources of estrogens and androgens should always be considered.

Once a careful history and physical examination have been performed, appropriate laboratory tests should be obtained to separate the individual with constitutional precocious puberty from the individual with an organic lesion. The diagnosis of constitutional precocious puberty is generally one of exclusion.

Limiting our discussion to the female, if a child presents with precocious puberty, short stature, and a delayed bone age, hypothyroidism should be considered. This would be confirmed by a low serum T_4 and an elevated TSH. Gonadotropins may be consistent with the bone age or in the pubertal range.

Isosexual precocious development with an accelerated bone age, depressed gonadotropins, and normal to elevated estrogen levels may indicate the presence of an ovarian or an extremely rare feminizing adrenal tumor. Ultrasonography should prove helpful in the evaluation of the ovary. An intravenous pyelogram with computed tomographic scanning of the adrenal should be revealing.

Heterosexual precocious development with accelerated bone age and depressed gonadotropins may be secondary either to a masculinizing ovarian tumor which would be reflected in elevated levels of testosterone; elevated 24-hour urinary 17-ketosteroids, pregnanetriol, serum dehydroepiandrosterone sulfate (DHEA sulfate), and 17-hydroxy-progesterone (17-OH-P_4) would implicate either an enzyme defect or the presence of neoplasia in the adrenal.

Isosexual development with accelerated bone age, pubertal levels for gonadotropins, estrogens, DHEA sulfate, and 24-hour urinary 17-ketosteroids point to a central source as a basis for precocious development. Neurologic examination, skull radiographs, and a cerebral CT scan should disclose a central nervous system lesion. Finally, a beta-HCG determination should be obtained in order to detect a tumor elaborating human chorionic gonadotropins.

TREATMENT

The effectiveness of therapy depends upon the abnormality uncovered. Hypothyroidism is readily treated with thyroid replacement; congenital adrenal hyperplasia with adrenal suppression; and ovarian, adrenal, or central nervous system neoplasia with surgical extirpation when indicated.

To date, treatment of constitutional precocious puberty has been far from satisfactory in attempting to allow the individual to attain an ultimate adult height of more than 5 feet. At the present, three preparations have been used extensively; medroxyprogesterone acetate (Depo-Provera); danazol (an isoxazole derivative of 17α-ethinyltestosterone); and cyproterone acetate.

Depo-Provera has probably been the most commonly used preparation in the United States. It is generally administered intramuscularly in doses ranging from 100 to 200 mg per M^2 per week, and, although some investigators would disagree, it is usually considered a potent gonadotropin suppressant. Its suppressive effect on breast and pubic development is variable. Although it does inhibit menstruation, it has not been shown to prevent the progression of skeletal maturation. Undesirable secondary effects from chronic usage have included adrenal insufficiency secondary to the drug's adrenal suppressive ability, and the development of cushingoid changes at higher dosages. Its use should be limited to suppressing menses, if deemed necessary psychologically, and as a means of contraception.

Danazol, along with other biologic properties, exhibits an anti-gonadotropic effect and, as such, was initially felt to hold some promise for the treatment of precocious puberty. This early optimism has waned; although the majority of investigators have noted a reduction of breast size and the cessation of menses, therapy does not appear to decrease bone maturation.

Cyproterone acetate (CPA), although not available in the United States, has been used clinically in Europe. It has been noted to have both anti-androgenic properties, competing with testosterone receptors, and progestational properties, suppressing gonadotropin release. With oral doses of from 65 to 150 mg per M^2 per day, some investigators claim a beneficial effect of cyproterone acetate on prognosis for adult height. As with the two preceding agents, CPA does inhibit menses as well as breast and pubic development. Although it induces dose-related evidence of biochemical adrenal insufficiency, no patients have reportedly manifested clinical evidence of adrenal insufficiency. Various adrenal function studies indicate reversal of adrenal suppression within 3 months of discontinuation of the drug.

Recently, it has been noted that either chronic, continuous infusion of GnRH, or the administration of a long-acting analogue of GnRH, will have a paradoxical effect, suppressing the pulsatile release of gonadotropins. Crowley's group has shown that subcutaneous administration of 4 mcg per kg per day of the GnRH agonist analogue (D-Trp^6-Pro^9-NEt-GnRH) significantly decreases both the basal gonadotropin levels and the response to exogenous GnRH. No vaginal bleeding was noted during therapy in any of the subjects studied and, within 4 months of treatment, regression was noted in breast size and pubic hair growth for several patients. It will require, however, several years before enough information is obtained concerning the effects of GnRH analogues on bone maturation and any undesirable side-effects resulting from their administration.

Section 6
BREAST DISEASES

FIBROCYSTIC DISEASE

GORDON K. JIMERSON, M.D.

The term fibrocystic disease is used by most physicians to describe a clinical entity consisting of nodular breast tissue and/or breast pain and/or breast cysts. Many prefer the term mammary dysplasia though this term does not seem to add specificity. Histologic findings included under this heading are adenosis, fibrosis, and cysts. Ductal ectasia and papillomas are not usually included under this heading and are not included in this discussion.

The etiology of fibrocystic changes is not clear, though the importance of estrogen seems apparent. The nodularity and discomfort characteristically increase in the premenstrual phase and subside in the postmenstrual phase of the cycle. Estrogen therapy will often exaggerate the symptoms. Some degree of adenosis, fibrosis, and cystic changes occur normally as females progress through the reproductive years. It is only when these changes become clinically apparent that the diagnosis of fibrocystic disease is appropriate. The findings and symptoms usually become progressively more severe through the fifth decade and then typically disappear after the menopause.

TREATMENT

A logical approach to therapy presumes an understanding of the desired results. There is no convincing evidence that the histologic tissue changes can be reversed by any means short of castration or mastectomy. The therapeutic goal is therefore symptomatic relief. The most common symptom is anxiety. Unfortunately the anxiety is often induced by a casual comment by a physician telling the patient she has "fibrocystic disease." Many times the patient has nothing more than small breasts with minimal fatty tissue, thus allowing the normal nodular breast tissue to be palpated. Women with small breasts are therefore more often told of the "fibrocystic disease." Physicians should avoid making the diagnosis of fibrocystic disease casually. Patients who do not have dominant masses, severe pain, or cysts should be managed by a combination of careful examination, instruction in self-examination, and reassurance.

Severe pain is far more difficult to manage successfully. Therapy still begins with careful examination, instruction in self-examination, and reassurance but may require more active management. Sometimes adequate relief may be obtained from mild analgesics and a firm bra providing good support. When these measures do not suffice, additional therapy may be attempted. Several reports have suggested significant relief may be obtained by avoiding methylxanthines (caffeine, theophylline, and theobromine) and nicotine. Methylxanthines are present in significant amounts in tea, coffee, cola, chocolate, analgesics containing caffeine and certain respiratory drugs. Pharmacologic agents used for relief of painful fibrocystic disease include progestins, vitamin E, bromocriptine, and androgens. Of these the most promising treatment is danazol in doses of 100 to 400 mg daily for 3 to 6 months. This treatment is very effective in most patients in reducing both nodularity and pain but has as disadvantages high cost and significant recurrence of symptoms after the medication is discontinued.

Cysts should be treated by aspiration. Aspiration can be accomplished very easily with a small bore needle and syringe. When clear fluid is obtained the patient should be re-examined in one month. If the cyst recurs, repeat aspiration is acceptable. If brown, green, or grossly bloody fluid is obtained, biopsy is indicated.

Some studies indicate that patients with fibrocystic disease have an increased risk of malignancy. Studies have not uniformly shown this increased risk and there remains some controversy. Nevertheless it seems prudent to emphasize frequent breast examinations and self-examination in these patients. The role of mammography as a routine screening procedure in patients under 50 years of age with or without fibrocystic disease remains unclear.

BREAST MASS AND NIPPLE DISCHARGE

GORDON K. JIMERSON, M.D.

BREAST MASS

The first and most crucial step in proper management of the patient with a breast mass is accurate diagnosis. Although biopsy is commonly the most important diagnostic tool, other diagnostic or therapeutic steps are sometimes indicated. For the purpose of this discussion, breast masses are classified as vague masses, cystic masses, subclinical masses, and solid masses.

Vague Mass. A "questionable" mass, fullness, or prominent area of breast tissue is frequently found during palpation of the breast. This vague type of mass is most often encountered in women with small breasts. Two common areas of such findings are the inframammary ridge at the lower edge of the breast and the upper outer quadrant of the breast. Examination of the breast in the immediate postmenstrual phase of the cycle will decrease the frequency of such findings. Most often, when the area seems vague or questionable after meticulous examination, it is nothing more than prominent breast tissue. Repeat examination by the physician at monthly intervals over several months or regular self-examination by the patient is often sufficient investigation. In high-risk patients, in patients more than 40 years of age, and in patients in whom the mass is "probable" as opposed to "doubtful," radiologic evaluation (mammography or xeromammography) is indicated. Biopsy is indicated if the radiologic findings confirm the presence of a mass.

An alternative approach to the management of vague masses not considered worrisome enough for open biopsy is needle aspiration biopsy. The technique is simple and only mildly painful. A 10.0 or 20.0 ml syringe is used and a 20 gauge needle inserted into the area to be investigated. Vacuum is applied and the needle is moved back and forth in the tissue several times prior to withdrawal. This technique requires the availability of a pathologist with interest and expertise in cytologic techniques.

Cystic Mass. The presumptive diagnosis of breast cyst is made when examination reveals a well-defined, smooth, symmetric, tense breast mass. Although breast cysts are sometimes tender, they are frequently asymptomatic. Simple aspiration of the cyst with a relatively small-gauge needle (e.g., 21 gauge) under sterile conditions usually suffices for both diagnosis and therapy. If clear or straw-colored fluid is obtained and no palpable mass remains, no further therapy is indicated. The patient should be instructed in self-examination so that she may observe for recurrences. When aspiration yields bloody or dark fluid, biopsy is indicated, as these findings are occasionally associated with malignancy. The role of cytologic study in breast cysts is controversial, but there is no convincing evidence that it is helpful when the guidelines just discussed are followed. Recurrence of a cyst may be treated by reaspiration or excision. If there are multiple recurrences in the same area, surgical excision is indicated.

Subclinical Mass. The subclinical mass is defined as a mass discovered by radiologic examination in the absence of a palpable mass. The accuracy of mammography and xeromammography is such that biopsies are indicated when suspicious or "positive" findings are present. In the absence of a palpable mass, the area should be localized by the radiologist and a wedge of breast tissue should be removed. If any doubt remains, the removed tissue may be examined by x-ray prior to histologic examination in an effort to guarantee that the abnormal area has been removed.

Solid Mass. Management of the well-defined, noncystic breast mass requires histologic examination. In young women with firm, regular tumors suggesting fibroadenoma, excisional biopsy should be the first, and usually the only, diagnostic and therapeutic step. When the mass is irregular or accompanied by signs suggestive of malignancy (skin retraction, local edema, enlarged nodes, skin ulceration, or nipple retraction) it is helpful if the diagnosis can be made by needle biopsy. This allows the diagnosis to be established prior to administration of general anesthetic and with minimal trauma. Having the definitive diagnosis prior to surgery allows proper preoperative evaluation, including radiographic studies of the opposite breast, skeletal surveys, blood chemistry determinations, and chest x-ray.

NIPPLE DISCHARGE

The evaluation and management of the patient with nipple discharge begins with proper classification into milky discharge (galactorrhea or abnormal lactation) or nonmilky discharge. This classification is usually not difficult, as abnormal lactation is usually bilateral and milky in appearance. If doubt remains after gross examination, a simple fat stain will differentiate the lipid-laden milky discharge from the lipid-free nonmilky discharge.

Milky Discharge. The frequency of abnormal lactation varies considerably, according to the vigor used in looking for it. Secretions discovered with vigorous manipulation of the breast are commonly seen and of little significance. Abnormal lactation that is discovered by the patient or by the physician during a routine breast examination requires investigation.

The first diagnostic and therapeutic effort should consist of identifying and discontinuing drugs that may be the cause of lactation. These include tranquilizers, antihypertensive medications, and sex hormone steroids. If there is no history of recent drug ingestion or if abnormal lactation continues after discontinuance of drug therapy, the next step should be to rule out a mechanical or neural reflex stimulation. This includes such entities as thoracic herpes zoster infection, recent thoracotomy, chest wall trauma or burns, suckling, manual stimulation, and spinal cord lesions.

When mechanical and drug-related causes for milk secretion have been excluded, a serum prolactin level should be obtained. If the prolactin level is normal, reassurance and simple observation suffice. If serum prolactin levels are elevated, the evaluation should include thyroid profile studies, serum cortisol levels, and polytomographic studies of the sella turcica.

Pituitary microadenomas are diagnosed in many such patients. The therapy for microadenoma of the pituitary is controversial at present. Some favor trans-sphenoidal surgical excision of the microadenoma. This is especially useful when the primary goal is fertility. Irradiation has been used with some success, but many months are required before the return of ovulatory cycles. The long-term follow-up of these patients is not yet sufficient to permit comparison of the two methods of therapy for microadenomas. Some authors presently recommend bromocriptine therapy even with radiographic evidence of microadenoma if visual field examinations and other pituitary functions are normal.

Abnormal lactation associated with elevated prolactin levels in the absence of a microadenoma should be treated with bromocriptine. Bromocriptine is very successful in suppressing lactation and allowing normal ovulation and fertility in such patients. Bromocriptine mesylate should be given in doses of 2.5 mg 3 times daily with meals for 6 months. Long-term results from bromocriptine treatment are not yet available and it is mandatory that yearly polytomograms be obtained since there are numerous reports of pituitary adenomas diagnosed years after the initial appearance of abnormal lactation.

Nonmilky Discharge. Nonmilky discharge of the nipple that escapes spontaneously may be serous, grossly bloody, brown, or green. The colors green and brown represent blood pigment. Both serous and bloody discharge may be associated with ductal papillomas, carcinoma, ductal ectasia, or cystic disease. Careful palpation will sometimes reveal an associated mass requiring excisional biopsy. Sometimes a "pressure point" producing discharge with palpation and pressure will be identified in patients in whom there is no palpable mass. Wedge biopsy is indicated in such instances. In the absence of a palpable mass or pressure point, mammography, cytologic studies, and repeat examinations are indicated. If multiple duct orifices are involved, some authors have recommended complete excision of the major duct system. This may be accomplished through a circumareolar incision with isolation of the major duct system using blunt and sharp dissection, separation from the nipple, and removal of an inverted cone of tissue following the ducts for approximately 3 to 5 cm. Others would recommend careful follow-up with repeated manual and radiologic examinations in patients without palpable or radiologic abnormalities. This conservative approach seems especially wise in young patients.

MASTALGIA

EDWARD A. GRABER, M.D.

Mastalgia (breast pain) is a common symptom complex that is controversial as to etiology as well as therapy. It affects about 10 per cent of the adult female population. In most cases it is hormonally mediated, but in others its cause may be either local or systemic pathology.

Many physicians believe that almost all mastalgia is of psychological origin and is found especially in introspective, high-strung women with an underlying cancerphobia. This explanation, while it may apply to a minority, is far too simplistic. Many underlying pathologic conditions produce breast pain. Credence for the psychosomatic explanation, however, can be augmented by the fact that in many studies the response to specific therapy is no better than to a placebo. Furthermore 50 per cent of women with mild to moderate mastalgia, with or without mastopathy, will become asymptomatic within 2 years from the onset of symptoms without therapy. This, of course may be explained on the basis of an endogenous hormonal upsets being corrected spontaneously.

Many existing textbooks confine their discussion concerning breast pain to one paragraph consisting of few statements about the psychic background of these women. In all fairness, however, it must be stated that on somatic psychometric analysis, 25 per cent of the cases have scores outside the normal range. Whether this is the cause or effect is open to debate.

In order to make a more rational approach to diagnosis and successful therapy, one must first classify the cause of mastalgia. This is not simple. It covers an extensive array of local and general disorders.

The most common syndrome is that of cyclic breast pain. This is probably hormonally induced, but disparate results are found in different studies reporting hormone analysis. The most consistent findings indicate that most patients with mastalgia have normal estradiol levels, plus significantly lower progesterone levels in days 3 to 7 of the luteal phase (inadequate corpus luteum?). There is an increase in breast pain with anovulatory cycles as well (decreased or absent progesterone?). The relationship between abnormal levels of progesterone to benign mastopathy and mastalgia, if any, has not been proved. Progesterone has no effect on the breast unless combined with estrogen. Any condition that produces an upset of the estrogen-progesterone ratio will probably produce mastalgia. This includes chronic disease, adrenal tumors, estrogen-secreting ovarian tumors, and the use of exogenous estrogen in post menopausal women.

There is elevation of gonadotropins, especially FSH, in the luteal phase in some women with mastalgia. Patients recovering from severe debilitating illness or starvation have an elevated FSH (refeeding gynecomastia). In these patients, mastalgia indicates recovery. In conditions associated with elevated human pituitary gonadotropins such as hypergonadotrophic hypogonadism or pituitary tumors, breast tenderness is also a prominent symptom. It should alert the physician to pursue a further work-up. Adolescent mastalgia is an indication of increased sensitivity to the physiologic changes in pituitary secretion.

Recent work has indicated that the serum level of prolactin is chronically elevated in the luteal phase of women with mastalgia. Prolactin controls the movement of water and electrolytes into breast tissue and controls physiologic interstitial edema. This usually occurs in the 7 to 10 premenstrual days, but can exist for a longer period. This finding is the basis for bromocriptine therapy which will be part of the subsequent discussion on therapy. Prolactin suppression normalizes the hypothalamic-pituitary-ovarian axis. Elevated prolactin alone, as is seen in the galactorrhea-amenorrhea syndrome, does not produce mastalgia. The patient must have an intact cyclical hormonal pattern. With hyperprolactinemia, there is usually anovulation or induced luteal insufficiency with premenstrual breast pain.

Breast pain may arise from mechanical stretching accompanying breasts which are large, heavy, and pendulous. At the other extreme, it may result from breast cancer. In patients with previous trauma or previous removal of a benign tumor, abnormal tenderness may be produced by excess fibrosis or underlying fat necroses.

Tietze's syndrome producing pain over the costrochondral junction may be confused with breast pain. The etiology is unknown and there is no specific therapy.

Monders' syndrome (thrombophlebitis of the superficial mammary veins) will cause breast tenderness which will resolve with resolution of the pathologic process.

Moderate to serious chronic cystic disease of the breast as well as adenosis and duct ectasia cause breast discomfort which diminishes with treatment and improvement of the underlying disease.

Certain drugs definitely increase mastalgia either because their chemical configuration is very close to that of estrogen or because they increase serum levels of prolactin. These include marihuana, aldactone, reserpine, phenothiazines, digitalis, and some psychotropic compounds.

Spinal cervical root compromise with pain referred into the breast area because of nerve compression is seen in some cases. Cervical spondylosis responds to cervical traction.

With Graves' disease, mastalgia is thought to be due to the secretion of LATS. Control of the disease causes regression of the pain.

Patients with chronic neurologic stimulation of the breast (chest wall disease, nipple stimulation, and so forth) will frequently complain of breast discomfort. Removal of the underlying cause causes improvement of the local symptoms.

Finally, breast infection must be considered. Acute mastitis may result from sucking of the nipple during sexual encounters as well as with normal puerperal breast feeding. In the presence of a breast abscess, in addition to the usual *Staphylococcus albus*, one must consider tuberculosis and actinomycosis as the infectious processes.

THERAPY

Before discussing any medical therapy, one important fact must be emphasized. If a discrete breast mass is palpated as the cause of mastalgia, the treatment should consist of a mammogram plus biopsy.

A mammogram may also be of value if granular and shotty modularity is palpated in relation to breast pain. Radiologic evaluation may suggest a definitive direction for therapy, but should not be accepted as gospel. Clinical judgment is still the most important factor in making one's ultimate decision.

Most patients will respond to observation, reassurance, adequate breast support, and, if necessary, mild analgesia. A cantilever brassiere which distributes most of the weight to the back rather than the shoulders has considerable therapeutic value. If the symptoms do not improve, further therapy is indicated.

Until recently the use of progesterone during the secretory phase of the cycle was standard therapy. In fact, in Europe, breast massage using progesterone cream is advocated. The use of progesterone (100 mg weekly intramuscularly for the last 2 weeks of the cycle or 10 mg of Provera OD orally for the 15th to 25th day of the cycle) in the United States has become less popular because of the spotty response. As a matter of fact, some patients have maintained that their symptoms were accentuated.

Another popular therapeutic modality has been the use of premenstrual diuretics and salt restriction. This form of therapy has also fallen into discard because most women showed no decrease in breast or total body water and had no relief of their symptoms. In some that did, the placebo effect may have been active.

Two basic medical approaches have proven to be statistically more effective than placebo. Unfortunately, neither has been cleared by the United States Food and Drug Administration at the time of this writing. If used, at least an informed consent by the patient should be a requirement. In the hands of almost all physicians who have used them, no permanent damage has resulted. Hopefully, the Food and Drug Administration will issue permission for their use for mastalgia in the near future.

It has been known for many years that antiestrogens caused marked improvement of cystic disease and mastodynia. The use of testosterone resulted in marked improvement of pain. The main problem was that it had an undesirable masculinizing effect. Danazol (Danocrine), a testosterone derivative, has proved to be therapeutically effective. It decreases estrogen by its hypothalamic-pituitary action as well as by the blocking estrogen receptor sites locally. It produces a low, non-fluctuating estrogen level, lower prolactin levels, and produces rather spectacular regression of symptoms and mammographic and physical findings. The suggested dose is 400 mg daily, but some patients react favorably to 100 mg daily, for 6 months. The main disadvantage is the rather significant menstrual disturbance and other side reactions if higher doses are required. The high cost is also a major factor in some situations.

Usually, therapy can be terminated after 6 months. If the condition returns and causes further significant symptoms, therapy can be repeated, but this is unusual. Most cases remain in remission at least one year, and if symptoms return, they are usually mild and can be treated less drastically.

The other drug that produces statistically valid improvement is bromocriptine (Parlodel). In many cases, 1.25 mg twice daily for 3 to 6 months will produce marked alleviation of symptoms. Some patients require 2.5 mg twice daily. Bromocriptine normalizes the hypothalamic-pituitary-ovarian axis, and drops the level of prolactin to the normal range. Unfortunately when bromocriptine is discontinued there is generally a relapse within few months. Since the FDA has not approved this drug for this use in the United States, pyridoxine (vitamin B_6), which is supposed to be a prolactin inhibitor, has been prescribed in doses of 600 to 800 mg daily. The therapeutic results have been inconsistent.

Finally, vitamin E in doses of 400 IU three times daily is advocated. The rationale is not explained but it has been reported to produce improvement in a small series. How much of this is psychosomatic or due to pure chance is unknown.

BREAST CANCER

DOUGLAS J. MARCHANT, M.D.

Breast cancer is the most common cancer in women, representing 28 per cent of all malignant diseases. More than 100,000 women in the United States develop breast cancer and approximately 35,000 die of the metastatic disease each year. One in 11 newborn females is destined to develop breast cancer. Every 17 minutes, three new cases are diagnosed and one woman dies of breast cancer in the United States.

Eighty per cent of the lesions are detected in patients over 40 years of age, and less than 1.5 per cent are found in those under 30. The recent breast cancer detection program sponsored by the National Cancer Institute and the American Cancer Society have dramatically demonstrated that a significant number of early breast lesions are found in patients 40 to 50 years of age.

EPIDEMIOLOGY

The descriptive epidemiology of breast cancer divides patients into high-risk and low-risk groups. The most important risk factors are related to race, age at first birth, previous breast disease, family history, and endocrine status. Numerous studies have shown that the risk of developing breast cancer is extremely low for Orientals living in the Orient. A woman who has her first full-term pregnancy at age 16 has one-half the risk of developing breast cancer as the woman who is pregnant for the first time at 30 years of age or older. Early menarche and late menopause place the patient in the high-risk group. The degree to which previous breast disease increases the risk of breast cancer has not been clearly determined. It is suggested however that the *degree* of dysplasia can be correlated with the subsequent risk of breast cancer. Family history is significant, particularly for those women in whom breast cancer develops during their reproductive years. In women whose mother or sister develops breast cancer premenopausally, the risk is increased 8-fold.

Analytic epidemiology explores several causal hypotheses. The most prominent are related to genetic, viral, and endocrine factors. Among endocrine factors, the relationship of estrogen to the development of breast cancer is the most important. The importance of early age at menarche and delayed menopause clearly indicate that ovarian activity is an important determinant of risk. Much additional research is required and will focus on other endogenous and exogenous factors such as diet and drugs that can alter the effect of estrogens and the subsequent risk of breast cancer. Clearly, the goal of epidemiologic research is to provide the basis for preventive intervention. Our present state of knowledge of the analytic epidemiology of breast cancer suggests a very limited approach to such prevention. For example, it would be difficult to alter the age of menarche and to promote early pregnancy to protect against breast cancer. These approaches are not consistent with the present goals of our society. One risk factor that may be alterable is obesity. This is particularly true in postmenopausal women for whom the risk is much greater.

EVALUATION OF THE PATIENT

From a practical standpoint, the proper evaluation of the patient with breast disease begins with an accurate and thorough history which must include the patient's age, menstrual history, family history of breast disease, use of medication, pregnancy history, including the date of the birth of the first child, and treatment of previous breast disease.

Examination of the breasts consists of a careful and methodical evaluation which, when combined with instruction in breast self-examination, takes 4 or 5 minutes. Palpation is performed with the flat of the hand. Even minor abnormalities in the substance of the breast tissue can be appreciated by wetting the breasts using pHisohex or similar soapy material. The breasts should be examined at every gynecologic visit and particularly at the time of the first prenatal visit and monthly thereafter if symptoms or initial physical findings warrant. Adjuncts to the physical examination include thermography and mammography, or xeroradiography. While the thermogram is not a specific test for cancer, it is a useful marker and may direct the examiner's attention to a particular area of the breast. Thermography should always be used as an extension of the physical examination, and suspicion confirmed by mammography or xeroradiography.

It is important to distinguish between a screening examination and a diagnostic evaluation of the symptomatic patient. Women with clinical signs of cancer should always have a mammogram regardless of age. Every woman with *obvious* cancer should have a mammogram, since the rate of synchronous bilateral cancer is approximately 4 per cent. In screening the asymptomatic patient, mammography has a sensitivity rate of about 90 per cent. Forty-five per cent of all cancers are detected by mammography alone, that is, they are clinically occult. Physical examination discovers 55 per cent of the cancers, but physical examination alone is positive in 10 per cent of the cases. It is therefore important to use both physical examination and mammography in screening for breast cancer. A negative mammogram in the presence of a real three-dimensional mass that does not yield fluid on aspiration should not deter the surgeon from biopsy. Approximately 10 to 15 per cent of palpable carcinomas may be missed by mammography. Conversely, a suspicious mammogram in the absence of clinical findings deserves a biopsy.

It is clear that if we are to improve the survival of patients with breast cancer, we must find the lesion before it has metastasized. Occult lesions discovered by mammography are best localized by the radiologist and removed using either local or general anesthesia. The usual technique is for the radiologist to insert a needle or wire using x-ray control. The surgeon then follows the wire to the suspected lesion. Obviously, the lesion, when removed, must be x-rayed to verify removal of the suspicious area.

SELECTIVE TREATMENT

With the appreciation that cancer of the breast is often a systemic disease with approximately 50 per cent or more of patients presenting with metastatic disease, previously held concepts and therapeutic approaches must be reassessed and placed in proper perspective. Three forms of treatment are available for curable breast cancer:

1. the radical mastectomy of Halsted;
2. the modified radical mastectomy, either preserving or removing the pectoralis minor muscle;
3. removal of the lesion followed by radiotherapy.

Today few patients will undergo the classic

radical mastectomy of Halsted. Present evidence clearly indicates that the modified radical mastectomy properly performed is equivalent to the radical mastectomy. Exceptions include lesions deep in the breast involving the pectoralis fascia or muscle. The modified mastectomy is more difficult to perform because of the limited exposure due to the preservation of the pectoral muscles. It is however more cosmetic and results in less edema of the arm and earlier return to normal function. Breast reconstruction is also facilitated by the use of the transverse incision and preservation of the pectoralis major muscle. Removal of the breast and axillary dissection are common to both the radical and modified radical procedures. In the Madden modification, the pectoralis major and minor muscles are both preserved. This makes a complete dissection of Level 1 and 2 nodes difficult. The Patey modification, favored by most surgeons, removes the pectoralis minor muscle to facilitate exposure of the axilla.

Radiation therapy as an alternative to surgery has the chief advantage of better functional cosmetic results with equal or less morbidity. Complete tumor excision, although not necessarily wide surgical resection, is important for good local control. With gross removal of the tumor which in some clinics amounts to a quadrantectomy, modest doses of radiation (5000 rads) can control microscopic disease with adequate preservation of function and cosmesis. Boost therapy to the area of excision can be performed with the electron beam or with interstitial implantation of radionucleotides. Most radiotherapists believe that primary radiotherapy should be restricted to patients whose lesions are relatively small in comparison to the size of the breast. In premenopausal patients who are clinically Stage I, it is important to have axillary sampling to identify those women with positive nodes who might benefit from adjuvant chemotherapy.

Postoperative adjuvant radiotherapy is infrequently used in most clinics, although there is no question that it decreases local and regional recurrence and may have a small effect on survival in certain subsets of patients. On the other hand *routine* adjuvant radiotherapy does not appear to improve survival.

Several studies have indicated that more than 70 per cent of all breast cancer patients will die of or with their disease in a 30 year period following the initial diagnosis. Using NSAPB data, it has been estimated that less than one fourth of all patients had disease confined to the breast at the time of diagnosis. Another 15 per cent had disease limited to the breast in the node-bearing areas. Almost two thirds of these patients had distant metastases prior to mastectomy. It is clear that a significant increase in survival of patients with breast cancer will depend upon diagnosis prior to the occurrence of metastases or treatment of such metastases immediately following local therapy, i.e., adjuvant chemotherapy.

The following statements can be made from recent reports:

1. No single form of adjuvant therapy may be considered as an established form of therapy.

2. The long-term costs of adjuvant chemotherapy have only begun to be evaluated. Among patients receiving adjuvant thiotepa, there does not seem to be an increased incidence of second malignant lesions. However the long-term toxicity of the more intensive therapy with alkylating agents could conceivably be greater.

3. Patients with clinical Stage I and II lesions with no histologic evidence of nodal involvement should not be treated with antineoplastic agents at the present time.

4. Adjuvant regimens designed for individual patients and significantly different from published regimens are to be discouraged.

It is now well-established that estrogen-positive tumors are associated with a clinical response to therapeutic hormonal manipulation, and with a prolonged interval between diagnosis of breast cancer and recurrence. If the estrogen receptor is greater than 10 femtomoles per mg of protein, the likelihood of response is greater than 50 per cent. If the receptor result is negative or less than 10 femtomoles per mg of protein, the response is less than 8 per cent. A high content, greater than 100 femtomoles per mg of protein, is associated with an increased response rate—greater than 80 per cent. The estrogen receptor assay should be utilized along with other clinical factors that predict response in selected patients for hormone treatment. These include a tumor-free interval of greater than 2 years, postmenopausal status, prior response to hormone treatment, and metastatic or recurrent disease predominantly in skin or lymph nodes. The relationship of the estrogen receptor assay to clinical response to cytotoxic chemotherapy remains controversial. Tumor specimens collected for the assay should include at least 500 mg of tissue. The specimen should be placed on dry ice or liquid nitrogen within 20 minutes of surgical removal since the estrogen receptor protein is very heat labile. A representative specimen must always be submitted for histologic verification.

In practical terms, this means that when an outpatient biopsy is performed, either under local anesthesia or on a day surgery basis under general anesthesia, a frozen section must be obtained to verify the presence of cancer and the need for estrogen receptor protein analysis.

The treatment of recurrent or metastatic breast cancer consists of hormone manipulation based upon the endocrine receptor values, the menopausal status of the patient, and the location of the metastatic disease. For example, oophorectomy is indicated in the premenopausal patient who is estrogen-positive. Additional response may follow adrenalectomy or hypophysectomy. If the estrogen receptor assay is negative, or if there is rapidly advancing visceral disease, chemotherapy should be started immediately. For postmenopausal patients who are estrogen-positive, estrogens or tamoxifen may be employed. Combination chemotherapy given either weekly or cyclically seems to achieve the highest response rate, the greatest complete response, and the longest remission duration, and the greatest increase in survival. Single drugs, either as part of a sequence or randomly used, appear to be less effective than combination chemotherapy. A recent article suggests that tamoxifen offers the best choice of therapy for patients with metastatic breast cancer after conventional endocrine therapy and combination chemotherapy have failed.

It is unfortunately true that even with Stage I and II so-called curable breast cancer, after a 20 year period only 20 per cent of patients with Stage I disease survive. Thus as stated previously, more than half presenting with "early" breast cancer actually have systemic disease. The cure must depend upon the earlier diagnosis of subclinical disease and appropriate systemic therapy.

Section 7
GENERAL MEDICAL AND SURGICAL PROBLEMS

HYPERALIMENTATION FOR THE CANCER PATIENT

JOHN B. SCHLAERTH, M.D.

There is an obvious place for hyperalimentation in a malnourished patient who presents with complications from a potentially curable cancer. When cancer is recurrent or metastatic, hyperalimentation becomes controversial. Its use has been tempered by the fears that growth of the tumor will be enhanced and that pain and suffering may be needlessly prolonged by such support. Added to this are the considerations of morbidity from the procedure and the considerable expense involved. However, in debilitated cancer patients it can increase strength, decrease pain and analgesic requirements, increase tolerance of chemotherapy, improve appetite and wound healing, facilitate fistula closure, and produce a feeling of well-being.

It is likely that, in the future, the use of antineoplastic combination chemotherapy, with or without radiation therapy, in advanced ovarian and endometrial carcinoma will demonstrate long-term remissions with significant prolongation of useful life. It is also possible that reductive surgery and extended field radiation therapy, with or without chemotherapy or immunotherapy, hold the same promise in advanced cancers of the lower genital tract. For such radical therapies, patients will need to be in the best possible nutritional status.

GENERAL INDICATIONS

Practical guidelines for implementing nutritional therapy have been suggested and include the following: a loss of 10 lb over a period of 3 months, a 5 per cent decrease in ideal weight, a serum albumin level of less than 3.5 mg per dl, a low total lymphocyte count, anergy to skin test antigens (streptokinase-streptodornase, mumps virus, Candida); a low serum transferrin level, a low lean body mass-creatinine height index, and a low triceps skinfold measurement. In addition, it is well to consider some form of nutritional support for any patient who will be without oral intake for 5 days or longer.

The remainder of this article discusses the various methods of therapeutic nutrition available and their suggested uses in gynecologic oncology.

ENTERAL NUTRITION

Whenever possible, the gastrointestinal tract should be utilized for nutrition. In gynecologic oncology, situations for management by enteral nutrition include malnutrition, anorexia, or both; the short bowel syndrome; and support during radiation therapy or chemotherapy.

At times, high-protein, high-calorie diet supplements will suffice. Anorexia and early satiety are common in cancer, however, and adequate oral nutrition is often not possible.

Nasogastric feeding using narrow polyvinyl tubes (2.0 mm in diameter) minimizes the problems of rhinitis, pharyngitis, parotitis, otitis media, and patient acceptance that occur with ordinary nasogastric tubes. (Keofeed Tube, Flow Med. Co., Sunnyvale, CA; Dobhoff Feeding Tube, Bioresearch Medical Productions, Inc., Raritan, NJ) The small diameter tube may require the use of a low-viscosity fluid (Isocal, Precision Isotonic) and/or a constant flow pump. The rate of administration and the concentration used are gradually increased over 3 to 4 days.

Complications of the elemental diet include: (1) nausea, vomiting, cramps, and diarrhea, which are usually related to the rate of administration and concentration of the diet; (2) gastric retention and aspiration, which are avoided by elevation of the head and periodic aspiration to confirm gastric emptying; and (3) hypertonic dehydration, which is best avoided by monitoring urine output and specific gravity, and allowing access to additional water.

Occasionally, a nasogastric feeding tube cannot be continued because of patient intolerance or bleeding. In this case gastrostomy or jejunostomy tube feeding may be applicable.

INTRAVENOUS HYPERALIMENTATION

This term refers to the administration of a hyperosmolar solution of nutrients into the superior vena cava. Its primary indication is the malnourished patient whose gastrointestinal tract is not suitable for oral or tube feeding. Common clinical settings for its use in gynecologic oncology are (1) in patients who have undergone radiotherapy, chemotherapy, or both and who have severe gastrointestinal symptoms; (2) in patients with complications following radical or ultra-radical surgery (evisceration, sepsis, fistula, bowel obstruction); and (3) in patients with anorexia and tube feeding intolerance who require nutritional improvement prior to, or as part of, medical therapy.

Intravenous hyperalimentation is considered a temporary measure to maintain or regain adequate nutrition. There are patients with irreparable bowel damage, however, who would die without parenteral feeding. The development of permanent indwelling subclavian catheters (Broviac, Hickman) has made it possible to establish a program for home administration of hyperalimentation solutions. Some patients have been maintained in good health with only parenteral hyperalimentation for several years.

To avoid the many and potentially serious complications that can arise with hyperalimentation, specially trained personnel are required. Included in the treatment team are physicians skilled in the technique of inserting and maintaining the central venous (usually subclavian) catheter and aware of the metabolic requirements and complications of hyperalimentation; pharmacists well acquainted with the preparation and handling of the hyperalimentation solutions; and nurses versed in the administration of the solutions and the care of hyperalimentation patients. Experience has shown that complications rise in relation to the inexperience of the team members. The central venous catheter requires specialized care and is never used for drawing blood or for administration of solutions, blood, or medications, other than the intravenous nutrients.

The hyperalimentation solutions are administered by a constant infusion pump with a built-in safeguard against air embolism. Generally, 1 gm of protein per kg of body weight per day and 30 calories per kg of body weight per day are given. Age, state of malnutrition, and the magnitude of the pathologic process will require changes in these guidelines.

Usually, a standard solution containing 25.0 per cent glucose and 4.25 per cent aminoacids is used. Suggested electrolyte additions are as follows: sodium chloride, 50 mEq per liter; potassium acid phosphate, 20 mEq per liter; potassium acetate, 40 mEq per liter; magnesium sulfate, 8 mEq per liter; and calcium gluconate, 10 mEq per liter. These however may need to be changed on a daily basis.

A multivitamin infusion containing water-soluble vitamins A, D, and E is added to 1 liter of intravenous solution per day. If hyperalimentation continues longer than 1 week, vitamin K, 10 mg per week intramuscularly, folic acid, 10 mg per week, and vitamin B_{12}, 1 mg intramuscularly per month are given. The trace elements zinc, copper, and iodine are best given by weekly infusions of plasma. Likewise, to prevent essential fatty acid deficiency, 1000 ml of 10 per cent intravenous fat emulsion (Intralipid, Liposyn) are given weekly through a peripheral vein.

The hyperalimentation infusion is begun slowly with 1 liter given over the first 12 hours. Thereafter, 2500 to 3000 ml can be administered every 24 hours. This suggested formula provides 106 to 127 gm of amino acids and 2500 to 3000 nonprotein calories. The infusion rate and glucose and the aminoacid concentrations can be changed as needed. Insulin may have to be added to the regimen if hyperglycemia or glycosuria develops.

Whenever the hyperalimentation solution is stopped, a 10 per cent dextrose infusion should be given through the central catheter or through a separate peripheral vein. There is a lag in the fall of high endogenous insulin levels, and withdrawing the concentrated dextrose infusion can lead to insulin shock. Discontinuation of the hyperalimentation should be done by gradual lessening of the glucose concentration over 48 hours. The catheter should be assessed daily, and the patient examined daily for signs of complications (pneumothorax, hydrothorax, or hemothorax; thoracic duct or brachial plexus injury; catheter misplacement).

The basic routine to be followed during hyperalimentation includes accurate assessment of intake, output, and daily weight; recording of temperature 4 times daily; and determination of urinary levels of sugar and acetone four times daily. Concentrations of blood glucose, blood urea nitrogen, sodium, potassium, bicarbonate, and chloride should be determined daily until stable, then every other day. Serum albumin, calcium, phosphorus, and magnesium levels should be determined twice a week. Constituents of the hyperalimentation solution are altered in amount daily as indicated. An optional assessment is the determination of nitrogen balance, although a false-positive nitrogen balance is possible in cancer patients.

The most common complication of intravenous hyperalimentation is catheter sepsis. If no other source for fever is determined, the solutions and the catheter should be cultured and the catheter removed. In patients with fever secondary to a known preexisting infection, it is wise to preemptively remove and replace the catheter, perhaps every 5 days. *Candida albicans* has been reported to cause fungemia in patients receiving hyperalimentation. Pneumothorax, brachial plexus injury, and an embolism can complicate catheter insertion. Prolonged catheter placement may cause thrombosis or emboli.

Metabolic imbalances are a constant threat and must be guarded against by frequent blood tests. A particularly dangerous disorder is hyperosmolar hyperglycemia, which presents as mental confusion or coma. Emergency treatment consists of rapid infusion of 5 per cent dextrose with one-quarter or one-half normal saline. Insulin is given concomitantly to treat the hyperglycemia.

PERIPHERAL PARENTERAL NUTRITION

In well-nourished patients exposed to a short-term health hazard (elective surgery, infection), peripheral intravenous administration of dextrose (D_5W), amino acids, or both, can prevent or reduce protein catabolism. For another group of patients, those characterized by a good nutritional status but who are undergoing extensive surgery with the prospect of a long postoperative recovery period during which the gastrointestinal tract cannot be used (e.g., because of pelvic exenteration or resection of irradiated bowel), more intensive nutritional support is necessary. Parenteral nutrition through peripheral veins fills this gap between central venous hyperalimentation and routine administration of intravenous fluids.

This program utilizes amino acids, carbohydrates, and fat (Intralipid, Liposyn). Two liters of intravenous solution containing 4.25 per cent amino acids combined with 5 per cent dextrose are given over a 24 hour period. Simultaneously, 1 liter of 10 per cent intravenous fat emulsion is given through a Y connector over 24 hours. Electrolytes need to be added to the amino acid–glucose solution. Suggested initial amounts are 20 mEq of sodium chloride per liter and 20 mEq of potassium acid phosphate per liter. A multivitamin infusion preparation is added to 1 intravenous liter daily. Five hundred units of sodium heparin are also added to each liter of amino acid–glucose. With an increase in volume, amino acid, or glucose concentration, or amount of lipid infusion, the amount of protein and calories can be changed. With this regimen, 0.85 gram of amino acids and 1500 nonprotein calories are provided daily.

Several precautions must be observed when using intravenous lipid. The serum should be examined daily to guarantee that the lipidemia clears between infusions. In-line filters cannot be used with the lipid, and nothing can be added to the lipid solution. Contraindications to the use of intravenous fat emulsion include hyperlipidemia and lipoid nephrosis, severe liver damage, coagulation disorder, and severe pulmonary disease.

HYPERTENSION IN THE NON-PREGNANT PATIENT

WILLIAM M. BARRON, M.D., and MARSHALL D. LINDHEIMER, M.D.

While physicians of the last century recognized the importance of elevated blood pressure in the pathogenesis of arteriosclerotic cardiovascular disease, intensive systematic investigation into the problem of hypertension has occurred only in the past 20 to 30 years. Most recently there has been a serious attempt to standardize the approach to both diagnosis and therapy. In concert with such attempts, many of the recommendations to follow are consonant with those of the 1980 report of the Joint National Committee on the detection, evaluation and treatment of high blood pressure sponsored by the National Institutes of Health.*

The initial step in the management of any patient with elevated blood pressure is establishing a sound diagnosis, a task which necessitates considerable attention to the technical details of measurement. Determinations are best made with the subject seated after a period of rest of at least 10 minutes. Allowance should be made for the size of the patient's arm, as syphygmomanometer cuffs which are either too small or too large may produce significant measurement errors. The American Heart Association recommends that the width of the inflatable bladder be 40 per cent and the bladder length 80 per cent of the circumference of the arm. The diastolic blood pressure is noted as that level where the Korotkoff sounds disappear (phase V) since such values, in adults, correspond most closely to intra-arterial diastolic pressure measurements.

The Joint National Committee has stated that the diagnosis of hypertension is confirmed when the average of multiple blood pressure measurements made on at least three visits is 90 mm Hg or higher. However, these lower limits are currently being re-evaluated at the National Institutes of Health and a preliminary report has suggested that patients with diastolic levels between 80 and 89 be regarded as a group with minimally increased risk. Certainly, any given level of blood pressure elevation is of greater concern in younger women, and the extent of both diagnostic evaluation and therapeutic intervention will depend greatly upon the age of the patient.

Following the confirmation of a diagnosis of hypertension, a history, physical examination, and a limited number of laboratory tests should be performed in order to evaluate the following:

1. Are there additional, perhaps remediable factors present which place the patient at further increased risk for cardiovascular disease? Of importance are the coexistence of diabetes, hyperlipidemia, cigarette smoking, and a family history of cardiovascular disorders.

2. Has the elevated blood pressure resulted in end-organ damage? Specifically, is there evidence of retinal, cardiac, renal, or cerebrovas-

---

*The full report may be obtained from the High Blood Pressure Center, 12080 National Institutes of Health, Bethesda, Maryland.

cular disease? Such findings suggest significant hypertension of prolonged duration and indicate the need for treatment.

3. Does the patient have a secondary, perhaps correctable cause of hypertension? Since less than 5 per cent of all patients with elevated blood pressure have a curable cause of their disease, exhaustive and expensive investigations should be undertaken only when suspicion of a specific disorder is suggested by the history, physical examination and/or screening laboratory tests.

The history and physical examination provide major clues to the diagnosis of many types of secondary hypertension. Use of oral contraceptives is probably the most common endocrine cause of hypertension, and the history of past or present use should always be sought. Most patients with pheochromocytoma will complain of sudden attacks of headaches, nervousness, palpitations, or excessive sweating. It is usually not productive to pursue laboratory investigation in the absence of such symptoms or other evidence to suggest the diagnosis. Cushing's syndrome, thyroid disease, and coarctation of the aorta can all be excluded at the bedside in the usual patient. Renal artery stenosis secondary to fibromuscular dysplasia is suggested by a history of onset of hypertension below the age of 30, presence of a bruit in the flank or upper abdomen, or a poor response to medical therapy. A strong family history suggests essential (idiopathic) hypertension.

Routine laboratory investigation should include a urinalysis and serum creatinine, since renal disease may be both the cause as well as the result of chronically elevated blood pressure. A serum potassium determination is also indicated in all patients both to help exclude hyperaldosteronism and to serve as a baseline in the event that diuretics are used as therapy. Additional tests which are recommended as part of the routine evaluation include serum cholesterol, glucose, uric acid, and an electrocardiogram.

TREATMENT

Indications and Goals for Therapy. It is widely agreed that individuals with diastolic pressures greater than 104 mm Hg should receive antihypertensive therapy including drug treatment, if necessary, to maintain acceptable levels of blood pressure. However, precisely which patients with mildly elevated pressures (diastolic 90 to 104 mm Hg) should be treated remains a matter of debate. The question is whether there is a reasonable chance that a given therapy will reduce the cardiovascular risk associated with hypertension sufficiently to outweigh any potential adverse effects (costs, inconvenience, psychological and physical side-effects) of the treatment itself. In the case of the young woman with a diastolic blood pressure of 90 to 100 mm Hg for whom 40 years of diuretic or anti-adrenergic therapy is being considered, the question of benefits and risks has not been unequivocally answered.

It is reasonable to offer non-drug therapy to patients with even the mildest elevation of blood pressure. Beyond this one must evaluate each woman's overall cardiovascular risk, considering such factors as hypercholesterolemia, cigarette smoking, diabetes, race (blacks tend to suffer more from the consequences of hypertension), and family history of premature cardiovascular disease. In general, the greater the risk, the more aggressive one should be in attempting to lower the patient's blood pressure since hypertension is often the most readily correctable risk factor. Regardless of additional risk factors we feel that pharmacologic treatment is indicated if diastolic blood pressure persists at levels of 95 mm Hg or greater despite the use of non-drug therapy.

Once the necessity for pharmacologic therapy has been determined, goals of treatment should be decided upon. A reasonable initial goal is to achieve and maintain diastolic pressures at less than 90 mm Hg. The ultimate aim should be the lowest diastolic pressure consistent with safety and tolerance. In this regard, in women with moderate or severe hypertension it may be extremely difficult to achieve levels of 85 to 90 mm Hg without undue side-effects. In such situations diastolic values of 90 to 100 mm Hg may be acceptable end-points, since even partial reduction of the blood pressure will be in the patient's best interest.

Patient Education. Assuring optimal control of hypertension demands more than just prescribing specific therapy. The physician must educate the patient as to the nature of her disease, treatment regimens available, goals of therapy, the potential adverse effects of the treatments selected, and, importantly, the serious consequences of untreated chronic hypertension. It should be kept in mind that poor compliance is probably the most common cause for failure of antihypertensive therapy, a situation which may be avoided if the patient is appropriately informed and involved in the treatment regimen from the beginning.

Non-Pharmacologic Intervention. Non-drug treatment is indicated in all subjects with hypertension. The general measures employed are (1) dietary management, (2) aerobic exercise (e.g., swimming, bicycling, jogging), (3) relief of stress, and importantly (4) control of other factors which place the patient at increased risk for cardiovascular disease.

Dietary therapy should include modest reduction of salt intake to approximately 5 gm per day (2 gm or 85 mEq of sodium). Although such mild restriction usually does not, in and of itself, lower blood pressure, it significantly potentiates the effects of nearly all antihypertensive medications and will also lessen the urinary potassium losses consequent to diuretic therapy.

Weight reduction in obese subjects may yield a substantial improvement in blood pressure levels. This is best accomplished gradually by means of a conservative dietary program and regular exercise. If hyperlipidemia is present, appropriate restriction of cholesterol and saturated fats is also indicated. Too much alcohol may be harmful, and reduction to a maximum of about two ounces per day should be advised. Since moderate alcohol intake of 1 to 2 ounces a day may actually improve the cardiovascular prognosis by elevating high density lipoprotein cholesterol levels, hypertensive patients need not be forced to eliminate alcohol completely from their diets.

While neither reduction of stress nor exercise should be regarded as primary therapy for hypertension, both modalities may contribute to blood pressure control and help reduce the risk of cardiovascular disease. The problem of stress, however, should not be approached by prescribing tranquilizers or sedatives. These drugs have little effect on blood pressure but are associated with significant risks, and are thus rarely useful in the long term treatment of hypertension.

Additional non-pharmacologic therapy includes the elimination of cigarette smoking, a step which is often the most significant one in terms of reducing the patient's risk of future cardiovascular disease. Finally, oral contraceptives should never be prescribed to women with elevated blood pressure.

Drug Therapy. The stepped-care approach to the pharmacologic management of hypertension is widely practiced and strongly recommended both because of its logical simplicity and demonstrated efficacy (Tables 1 and 2). It entails initiating therapy with a small dose of an antihypertensive drug, gradually increasing the dosage of that drug, and then sequentially adding further agents as they are needed to achieve the desired goal. A new agent is added when the maximum dosage of medication being utilized is reached and/or unacceptable side-effects occur. Because of the difficulty in manipulating dosage, combination agents should be considered only after an unacceptable level of blood pressure has been maintained for several months using single component antihypertensives.

Before additional medication is added the physician should assess why previous therapy has been unsuccessful. Explanations for this problem include poor patient compliance, excessive sodium intake, weight gain, insufficient dosage of antihypertensives, use of "competing" drugs (e.g., nasal decongestants, appetite suppressants), and secondary causes of hypertension such as renal artery stenosis and pheochromocytoma.

TABLE 1. **Stepped-Care Approach to Antihypertensive Drug Therapy**

STEP	DRUGS
1	Diuretic
2	Adrenergic inhibiting agents*
	Beta blockers
	Methyldopa
	Prazosin
	Reserpine
3	Vasodilator
	Hydralazine
4	Additional adrenergic inhibiting agents
	Clonidine†
	Guanethidine
Resistant patients	Minoxidil, Captopril (see text)

*These drugs are listed in alphabetical order. This does not indicate preferential order of usage.

†Some include clonidine as a Step 2 agent, however we rarely use it prior to vasodilator (hydralazine) therapy and prefer to consider it a Step 4 drug.

Step 1. A thiazide-type diuretic is the initial drug of choice as it will lower diastolic pressure to less than 90 mm Hg in approximately half of all hypertensives while causing relatively few adverse effects. It should be noted that the dose-response curves of these agents plateau near the usually recommended starting dosages. Therefore, increasing amounts of, for example, hydrochlorthiazide beyond 50 mg daily results in little additional decrement in blood pressure while causing considerably more unwanted effects such as hypokalemia, hyperuricemia, and hyperglycemia.

Decrements in serum potassium secondary to diuretic therapy may be minimized if the physician prescribes a diet low in sodium and high in potassium. Administration of potassium chloride supplements or potassium-retaining agents such as triamterene or spironolactone is unwarranted as long as blood levels remain above 3.0 mEq per liter. However, even mild degrees of hypokalemia should be avoided in women with heart disease of the type that predisposes to arrhythmias or requires digitalis therapy.

Hyperuricemia frequently accompanies thiazide therapy. However, increments are usually small and do not require alterations in medication as long as the patient is asymptomatic and serum levels remain below 10 mg per dl. Similarly, the effects of thiazides on glucose tolerance are small and these drugs may be used in insulin-dependent diabetics.

Furosemide is a potent diuretic, the use of

Table 2. Drugs Used in the Treatment of Hypertension

DRUG	USUAL DAILY DOSAGE	ADVERSE EFFECTS*
Step 1		
Hydrochlorthiazide†	25–50 mg in 1 or 2 doses	Hypokalemia, hyperuricemia, hyperglycemia
Step 2		
Nadolol	40–320 mg in 1 dose	Effects shared by beta blockers: bradycardia, heart failure, bronchospasm, fatigue, depression, gastrointestinal disturbance
Propranolol	40–240 mg in 2 doses	
Metoprolol	50–225 mg in 2 doses	
Atenolol	50–100 mg in 1 dose	
Timolol	10–20 mg in 2 doses	
Methyldopa	500 mg–2 gm in 2–4 doses	Sedation, postural hypotension, liver toxicity, lactation, Coombs' positive hemolytic anemia
Prazosin	2–20 mg in 2 doses	Syncope with initial doses, postural hypotension, sedation, headache
Reserpine	0.1–0.25 mg in 1 dose	Psychic depression, aggravation of peptic ulcer disease, nasal congestion, postural hypotension
Step 3		
Hydralazine	20–200 mg in 2–4 doses	Headache, tachycardia, may aggravate angina, lupus-like syndrome
Step 4		
Clonidine	0.2–2.4 mg in 2–4 doses	Severe rebound hypertension after abrupt withdrawal, sedation, dry mouth, postural hypotension
Guanethidine	10–300 mg in 1 dose	Postural hypotension, weakness, bradycardia, diarrhea
For resistant patients		
Minoxidil	5–40 mg in 1 dose	Tachycardia, marked fluid retention, hypertrichosis
Captopril	75–450 mg in 3 doses	Pancytopenia, nephrotic syndrome, renal failure, loss of taste, tachycardia

*These are selected effects and the physician should consult a pharmacology text and/or the Physicians Desk Reference for more complete information.

†One example of many available thiazide-type diuretics.

which may lead rapidly to volume depletion, hyponatremia, and other serious electrolyte disturbances. This drug should be reserved for individuals with renal insufficiency.

A beta blocking agent (usually a Step 2 agent) may be used as alternative initial therapy in selected younger women, particularly those with a rapid heart rate and increased pulse pressure. If adequate control of blood pressure is not achieved, a thiazide-type diuretic is then added.

Step 2. This group comprises a large number of anti-adrenergic agents, all of which have roughly equal potency in lowering blood pressure. With the exception of beta blockers, sustained efficacy of these drugs necessitates the concomitant use of diuretics. Failure to prescribe a saluretic agent leads to sodium retention which in itself may increase blood pressure or make the vasculature refractory to the vasodilating action of the adrenergic inhibiting drugs.

We prefer to use a long-acting beta blocker such as nadolol. Prescription of such a medication, which is taken but once daily, will significantly increase patient compliance. Beta-adrenergic blocking agents are contraindicated in women with heart failure, heart block, or significant peripheral vascular disease. We also avoid the use of these drugs in insulin-dependent diabetics, but some authorities feel that $beta_1$ selective agents (e.g. metoprolol, atenolol) can be utilized in this population with acceptable risks.

Prazosin, a post-synaptic alpha-adrenergic blocker, is an attractive alternative Step 2 agent. Cardiac output and renal blood flow are maintained when this drug is prescribed, a distinct advantage over the beta blockers. The major problem associated with prazosin is that severe postural hypotension and syncope may occur after the initial dose or following a rapid increase in dosage. Such problems may be minimized by prescribing the very first dose (1 mg) at bedtime and increasing subsequent medication slowly. Postural hypotension is also an occasional adverse effect of methyldopa and reserpine. For this reason blood pressure should be measured in both the supine and standing positions in women taking any of these antihypertensives. Reserpine is currently unpopular, particularly as it is more prone to produce life-threatening psychic depression than other Step 2 drugs and because it may also cause serious exacerbation of peptic ulcer disease. Still, it can be administered in a single daily dose and is occasionally useful in selected patients.

Finally, although all the adrenergic blocking medications are associated with sexual dysfunction in male subjects, relatively little is known about such effects in women. Therefore, it is important to include a sexual history in the initial evaluation and to maintain awareness for such problems after drug therapy is begun.

Step 3. Hydralazine, which acts directly on vascular smooth muscle, is a potent vasodilator. It is especially useful when combined with beta blocking agents. The latter drugs decrease cardiac output, reduce heart rate, and may lead to an increase in peripheral resistance. All of these effects are reversed with the use of hydralazine. Furthermore, this medication is usually well tolerated, the hydralazine-induced lupus-like reaction being rare in dosage schedules below 200 mg per day.

Step 4. If Step 3 therapy is unsuccessful and remediable causes of blood pressure unresponsiveness have been considered, clonidine or guanethidine may be added to or substituted for the Step 2 agent being used. Clonidine, a central acting alpha$_2$ (presynaptic) receptor agonist, appears to lower blood pressure by reducing sympathetic outflow from the brain. Severe rebound hypertension may occur if this drug is withdrawn abruptly, and thus if therapy is discontinued the dose should be gradually tapered over 4 to 7 days. Guanethidine, a potent postganglionic blocking agent, is rarely used in our practice as adverse effects are substantial. These include marked postural hypotension, weakness, diarrhea, and bradycardia.

Most patients requiring Step 4 care are best handled by physicians specializing in hypertension. This is especially true for the newer medications that are utilized more rarely such as captopril, an angiotensin-converting enzyme inhibitor, and minoxidil, a potent direct-acting peripheral vasodilator.

HYPERTENSION IN THE POST-MENOPAUSAL PATIENT

Recent data indicate that hypertension in elderly women should not be ignored and that such patients benefit substantially from therapy. However, it should be noted that older individuals, particularly those over the age of 60, are generally more sensitive to the adverse effects of antihypertensive drugs, particularly volume depletion, postural hypotension, and alterations in mental function. For this reason treatment is best initiated with drug dosages that are half those recommended for younger women, and subsequent increases should be made more slowly.

Isolated systolic hypertension, frequently encountered in the elderly, is most commonly a consequence of sclerosis of the aorta and large arteries, although other causes such as hyperthyroidism, severe anemia, Paget's disease, and arteriovenous fistula should also be ruled out. While elevated systolic blood pressure correlates closely with cardiovascular morbidity and mortality, there are no clear data to confirm that treating this disorder actually benefits the patient. Nonetheless, because of the association with stroke and heart failure we believe that a cautious attempt to lower levels below 160 mm Hg is reasonable. With the exception of the reduction in drug dosages mentioned above the approach to treatment is generally the same as outlined previously.

ACHIEVING LONG-TERM CONTROL OF HYPERTENSION

The prognosis for patients with hypertension has improved dramatically in the past decade and should continue to do so if we are able to succeed in maintaining long-term control of blood pressure at levels as close to "normal" as possible. Such therapy, which is often life-long, is difficult and demands substantial commitment on the part of both physician and patient. In this regard treatment and follow-up should be made as convenient as possible. In addition, ongoing frank discussions regarding adherence to diet and drug regimens, side-effects of medication, and the need for continued therapy are extremely important. It cannot be overly emphasized that careful attention to these issues plays an essential role in the management of these patients.

ACNE VULGARIS

MARINA BALL, M.D.,
and JOHN VALENTIC, M.D.

Acne is a disease resulting from hair follicle impactions. The impaction is due both to retention and to increased production of squamous epithelial cells. Impactions form in the superficial portion of the hair follicle (open and closed comedones) and may eventually rupture into the dermis resulting in inflammatory lesions (papules, pustules, nodules). Even though these morphogenetic events are widely accepted, the precise primary pathogenetic event(s) eludes us. Heredity, androgens, 5-alpha-reductase, sebum, free fatty acids, microorganisms and their enzymes, intercellular cement, and so forth, all have ill-defined and controversial roles. While questions remain and research continues, we already have extremely effective therapy for this condition.

Treatment of acne is not difficult in most patients, especially if a regimen can be appropriately individualized. Implicit in this statement is the concept that both the disease and the patient vary considerably. As a result, acne is usually treated with more than one active agent and a number of adjunctive measures.

A vital aspect of the successful management of acne is the first office visit. It is during this critical, formative interchange that the bonds of mutual trust and understanding are formed. Adequate time should be allotted during this first visit to sit quietly and discuss, in simple terms and with the help of a drawing, the basic anatomy of the obstructive and inflammatory lesions of acne. Explanations of the chronicity of acne, its waxing and waning course, and, most importantly, the fact that amelioration and control rather than cure are the only realistic goals with presently available therapy will prevent later disappointment over expectations of cure. This interview then serves as a basis for the greater acceptance of required therapies which all require cooperation of the patient over many months or years.

Patients with numerous open and closed comedones (blackheads and whiteheads) without inflammatory papules require "unplugging" of the occluded follicles. Such unplugging agents include topical retinoic acid and topical benzoyl peroxide.

Retinoic acid is available in several strengths—cream base, 0.05 and 0.1 per cent, and gel base, 0.025 and 0.01 per cent. Retinoic acid can cause mild irritation and dryness of the face initially. This is usually due to one or more of the following: (1) application of too much medicine; it should be applied in a very thin film gently smoothed in, and should be applied in strengths and frequencies no greater than those which just begin to produce erythema and peeling; (2) failure to avoid pooling in natural crevices; care should be taken to avoid the crevices of the mouth, eyes, nasal-facial junction, and the nasolabial fold; (3) application too soon after washing the face; since retinoic acid will penetrate hydrated skin more readily, the patient should wait at least 20 minutes after washing before applying the medication; (4) additive effects of other irritants; the patient may still be using various over-the-counter peeling agents containing sulfur and/or salicylic acid and/or resorcinol, abrasive cleansers, excessively frequent washing with soap and water, and frequent use of astringents; (5) injudicious sun exposure; retinoic acid increases the sensitivity of the skin to sunburn; retinoic acid should be applied only at night and use of a sunscreen with an SPF (sun protection factor) of 8 or greater is recommended.

Benzoyl peroxide has keratolytic properties as well as being antibacterial and reducing the surface free fatty acid level. It also can hasten the involution of some pre-existing lesions. This product is available by both prescription and over-the-counter sale. Benzoyl peroxide is marketed in several strengths—2.5, 5, and 10 per cent. It is best to start with the lowest concentration to avoid excessive irritation until the skin begins to "harden" (not to be confused with resistance which does not occur). The incidence of allergic contact dermatitis due to benzoyl peroxide is quite low, about 1 to 2 per cent. With the exception of enhanced sensitivity to sun exposure, the same usage patterns which tend to produce problems with retinoic acid–induced irritation should be looked for with benzoyl peroxide. Additional benefit can usually be achieved by using benzoyl peroxide in combination with retinoic acid; e.g., benzoyl peroxide in the morning and retinoic acid at night. One may find that pretreating for one week with benzoyl peroxide alone may decrease the irritancy of the retinoic acid used subsequently. It is not known whether benzoyl peroxide or retinoic acid can cause fetal harm when administered to a pregnant woman; nor is it known whether either of these drugs is excreted in human milk.

A mild soap is recommended initially so that the patient will not experience further dryness of the face from normal cleansing. Expression of comedones with a comedone extractor (acne surgery) can be beneficial in comedonal acne. Often it is best to use the comedone extractor after therapy with an unplugging agent has already been initiated for two to four weeks. By this time, an early "softening" of the lesions occurs and their mechanical removal is facilitated. If too heavy a hand is used, the possibility exists of creating deeper, more inflammatory lesions by rupturing the comedones.

When the acne patient presents with comedones as well as inflammatory papules or pinhead-sized pustules, therapy is initiated with an antibiotic along with either retinoic acid or benzoyl peroxide. Antibiotics can now, of course, be given by either the oral or topical route for acne. Oral antibiotics most often used are tetracycline, erythromycin, or minocycline. Topical antibiotics for acne that are now FDA-approved include clindamycin phosphate (Cleocin-T), erythromycin (Staticin and A.T.S.), meclocycline (Meclan), and tetracycline (Topicycline), the first two being the most widely used.

The most common cause of apparent failure with topical antibiotics is the expectation that these medications will clear up existing lesions. Their role is prophylactic, preventing or decreasing the formation of new inflammatory lesions. Therefore, little or no effect can be seen before about 4 to 8 weeks, a similar time period as for retinoic acid and benzoyl peroxide. Use of topical antibiotics for mild to moderate inflammatory acne ordinarily will be more effective if combined in a regimen including retinoic acid and/or benzoyl peroxide, e.g., topical antibiotics applied in the morning and afternoon, with retinoic acid or benzoyl peroxide applied at night.

There are no adequate and well-controlled studies of any of the topical antibiotics in pregnant women and it is not known whether any of them is excreted in human milk. Nevertheless, a recent preliminary controlled human study on the in vivo percutaneous absorption of several anti-acne drugs has shown that each of the three topical antibiotics, clindamycin phosphate, erythromycin, and tetracycline, was absorbed less than 1 per cent through the skin and less than 0.1 mg of each was detected in the urine. There are no known cases of pseudomembranous colitis directly attributable to any of the above mentioned three topical antibiotics. Still, patients should be instructed to stop the antibiotic if diarrhea occurs and to call the physician if it persists. The treatment of pseudomembranous colitis is vancomycin.

If, in the opinion of the physician, pitted scarring may develop from the active acne lesions, oral antibiotics are preferred initially, along with an unplugging agent. When prescribing the use of oral antibiotics, it is important to check for drug allergies and to make sure the female patient is not pregnant and is not considering pregnancy in the near future. Tetracycline is usually prescribed in a divided dosage of 1 gm per day to be taken on an empty stomach (one hour before a meal or two hours after a meal). Side-effects include nausea, diarrhea, phototoxicity, and onycholysis. The drug is contraindicated in pregnancy and in children less than 12 years of age because of permanent staining of teeth. It is also contraindicated in patients with liver or kidney disease. Erythromycin is usually prescribed in a divided dosage of 1 gm per day, not necessarily on an empty stomach. Epigastric distress is a not uncommon side-effect. Minocycline is a potent tetracycline which does not need to be taken on an empty stomach and is prescribed in a divided dosage of 100 to 200 mg per day. It carries the same contraindication in pregnancy and in children that tetracycline does because of the permanent staining of teeth. In addition, dizziness and cutaneous pigmentation are dose-related side-effects.

Breakthrough bleeding and, rarely, pregnancy have been reported in women who were taking oral contraceptives and antibiotics concurrently. Such interactions have been reported for rifampin, ampicillin, and tetracycline. The antibiotics induce microsomal enzymes in the liver that presumably accelerate the metabolism of estrogen. In some cases, this apparently has resulted in subtherapeutic blood levels of the estrogen component of the oral contraceptive. Oral contraceptive therapy is not considered a contraindication to antibiotic therapy, but the physician and patient should be aware of the potential interaction. The problem would be expected to occur more frequently with the low-estrogen preparations. While receiving concurrent, long-term antibiotic therapy and oral contraceptives, mechanical contraception could be used near mid-cycle as a precaution, if desired. Breakthrough bleeding first occurring with oral contraceptives after initiating antibiotic therapy suggests that re-evaluation of the contraceptive preparation used by the patient would be appropriate.

With all of the above mentioned oral antibiotics used to treat acne over a long period of time, candidal vaginitis is a frequent side-effect. More rarely, a gram-negative folliculitis superinfection may result.

Cystic acne can be most difficult to treat. Initially, therapy with oral antibiotics is begun (tetracycline, 1 gm per day up to 3 gm per day, in divided doses on an empty stomach, or minocycline, 100 mg twice a day). The topical treatment depends on various factors including the severity of the cystic acne, the degree of skin oiliness, the presence of comedones, inflammatory papules, or nodules. Therefore, either retinoic acid, benzoyl peroxide, or soaks may be suggested. Triamcinolone suspension in a concentration of 2.5 to 5 mg/ml is often beneficial when injected directly into the cyst with a 30 gauge needle. Because of potential skin atrophy, injections of this nature should not be performed into the same cyst more often than once every 3 weeks. Incision and drainage of the cyst is not recommended because of its scarring potential.

Despite strict adherence to the therapeutic principles outlined here, a small group of patients truly seem refractory to treatment. In these patients, careful evaluation is required to rule out additional aggravating factors. These include hormonal imbalance, overgrowth of resistant organisms (gram-negative folliculitis), emotional stress, and a variety of external factors such as abusive cleansing, friction, and cosmetics.

Hormonal imbalance may be suggested by hirsutism, as well as by aggravation of acne, and requires evaluation for adrenal 11- and/or 21-hydroxylase deficiency as well as other causes of increased androgen secretion.

One should also verify whether the patient is taking an "androgen-dominant" oral contraceptive such as those containing the progestational agent norgestrel or very low estrogen-containing drugs with the progestational agent norethindrone.

Crops of recurrent pustules on the chin and perinasal area as well as indolent nodulocystic lesions in the same location should lead one to suspect overgrowth of gram-negative organisms resistant to the antibiotic being administered. These can readily be identified by culture and appropriate therapy instituted according to the sensitivity of the organism cultured. One should also look for the source of the organism, not infrequently the nares or the external auditory canal (otitis externa).

Emotional stress can frequently aggravate existing acne and can, at times, be explosive in its onset. While one can attempt to assist the patient with this emotional stress, brief courses of treatment with prednisone (20 to 40 mg/day) may be required. The drug should be tapered rapidly over a period usually of not more than three weeks.

A variety of external factors have been implicated either in the initiation or aggravation of acne. Occupational exposure to halogenated hydrocarbons has long been known to be acnegenic. More recently, it has been demonstrated that hair pomades and occlusive, oily cosmetics also may induce or aggravate acne. In addition, inflammatory acne is partially aggravated by the use of abrasive cleansers or devices, and all forms of acne can be aggravated by heat, humidity, and friction such as may occur under athletic equipment or when the patient constantly rests his or her chin in the palm of the hand. These are easily treated by advising the patient of their nature and avoidance.

Finally, in particularly severe cases, the judicious use of anti-inflammatory agents may be indicated. We already have referred to brief courses of prednisone. Those physicians familiar with its use might also try treatment with sulfones.

Pending FDA approval,* 13-*cis* retinoic acid will prove to be a valuable tool in the treatment of severe cystic acne. This drug, given orally in dosages of 0.5 to 2 mg per kg per day, decreases sebaceous gland activity up to 90 per cent. Remissions of up to 30 months following 12 weeks of therapy occur in cases of severe cystic acne. Clinical toxicity, which is dose-dependent and reversible, is limited principally to the skin and mucous membranes (cheilitis, xerosis, dry nasal mucosa, conjunctivitis). A transient, dose-dependent elevation of serum triglycerides occurs in 70 per cent of patients, the greatest risk being in those with elevated levels prior to therapy or with predisposing medical conditions (diabetes, obesity, etc.). Even though the half-life of 13-*cis* retinoic acid is relatively short (about one day) the drug has been shown to be teratogenic in laboratory animals. Therefore, females should be on oral contraceptives during therapy and for 1 month following discontinuance of therapy.

ILEUS

A. GERSON GREENBURG, M.D., Ph.D.

Ileus is a failure of peristalsis. It is a *functional* impairment of downward propulsion of intestinal contents not associated with mechanical obstruction. Ileus results from a variety of causes. Ileus is *a sign* of other disease processes: it is not by itself a disease. Beyond general management, specific therapy is directed at elimination of causitive problems. The differentiation of ileus from mechanical small bowel obstruction is crucial: different diagnostic and therapeutic paradigms are required and specific therapy is unique.

The gut is presumed to have a pacemaker responsible for its normal peristalsis. Whether it is a true anatomic structure or a manifestation of the balance between sympathetic (paralytic) and parasympathetic (stimulating) innervation is not known. Following most intra-abdominal and pelvic surgery, small bowel motility is rapidly restored, usually within hours. The stomach regains its tone and function within 24 hours, the right colon with 48 hours and the left colon within 72 hours of surgical intervention. Some impairment of function, delayed gastric emptying, and late appearance of flatus is expected following abdominal surgery. The more extensive the surgery (e.g., radical hysterectomy, pelvic exenteration, retroperitoneal node dissection) the longer the delay in return of function to be expected. Ileus is that situation which ex-

---

*The FDA has approved 13-*cis* retinoic acid (Accutane, Roche Laboratories) for the treatment of severe, recalcitrant cystic acne. The drug is available in 10 mg and 40 mg capsules.

tends beyond the expected time of return of function for a given operation or which appears after function has seemingly returned.

Ileus is primarily a clinical diagnosis; it is a sign and not a disease entity. It is usually seen in the postoperative period. It is most often a sign associated with a significant complication. Presentation is usually with abdominal distention, most often painless. The abdomen is non-tender unless there is peritoneal irritation in which case peritoneal signs will be present. Bowel sounds are decreased or absent and the patient experiences nausea and frequently vomits.

GENERAL MANAGEMENT

Two classes of ileus are considered. First, the expected prolongation of return of bowel function associated with extensive operations and second, ileus associated with a major complication. Prevention and knowledge of postoperative course manage the former while intervention is often required for the latter.

If a long and extensive operation is planned, maintenance of nasogastric suction in the postoperative period until the output is less than 500 ml per day or the patient has active bowel sounds and passes flatus is necessary. Monitoring of electrolytes and adequate replacement of all ionic and volume losses along with maintenance of adequate red cell volume is essential. If the patient is expected to be "starved" for more than 4 days, nutritional supplement is most helpful. Indeed, if preoperative nutritional replacement is used, as in the situation of extensive malignancy with malnutrition, this must be continued through the operation and well into the postoperative period. Serum electrolytes (sodium, potassium, chloride, calcium, magnesium), arterial blood gases, and routine chemistries (glucose, BUN, creatinine and amylase) help in identification of problems needing correction. Gastric alkalinization not only prevents stress bleeding it decreases secretions and fluid load to the small bowel. Cimetidine, 300 mg intravenously every 8 hours, is a good starting dose.

ILEUS ASSOCIATED WITH COMPLICATIONS

The common causes of ileus are grouped into categories: reflex, peritonitis, neurogenic, vascular, and metabolic. Since ileus arises from different causes, the therapy is more specific and directed, sharing all of the aspects of general management and more.

When ileus is diagnosed on clinical grounds and radiologically, intestinal decompression with long and short tubes is necessary. This not only decreases the load of fluid and gas to the nonfunctional small bowel, it prevents distention and decreases the risk for some vascular injuries. A long mercury-weighted tube is passed into the duodenum under fluoroscopic control to aid its downward passage. A short tube is also passed. Electrolytes and blood chemistries are assessed, if only for baseline reference. Treatment is directed at the basic underlying illness and not specifically directed at attaining return of bowel function.

Reflex ileus usually results from an infectious process remote from the operative site. Pneumonia and urinary tract infections are the most commonly encountered. Aggressive tracheobronchial toilet and attention to asepsis in placing catheters help to prevent the situation. Treatment of the remote infection is indicated. Ileus resulting from retroperitoneal or pelvic hematoma, themselves the result of extensive surgical procedures, usually clears later in the postoperative course, in 5 to 7 days. This would be a normal, expected, yet delayed recovery of function.

Peritonitis as a cause of ileus must be recognized and treated early. This could result from anastomotic or suture line leak, intraoperative soilage, or recognized or unrecognized injury to the bowel during surgery. Peritoneal signs (pain, tenderness, guarding, and rigidity) usually accompany peritonitis associated with ileus. Drainage of serosanguinous fluid from the wound or frank dehiscence may be associated. Therapy is based on identification of the causative event and its prompt and direct correction. Re-operation for drainage of abscesses (sump drains) and definition of suture line dehiscence is often required. Abdominal ultrasonography or CT scanning is helpful in defining abscesses which require drainage. Percutaneous drainage under radiologic control, interventional radiology, is on the horizon for the treatment of single and localized lesions.

Postoperative pancreatitis as a cause of ileus is rare following pelvic surgery but can be seen with retroperitoneal dissections. Its management requires prompt and aggressive fluid replacement and full multisystem support, primarily pulmonary, metabolic, and nutritional. As with other forms of peritonitis, the ileus is associated with bowel wall edema and localized accumulation of extracellular fluid.

Neurogenic causes of ileus are rarely encountered in the obstetric and gynecologic patient population. Except for ileus related to operative intervention, most other causes are not encountered (e.g., head or spinal cord injury, major trauma, pelvic or lumbar spine fracture). Bleeding into the abdominal wall can delay return of bowel function similar to pelvic or retroperitoneal hematomas.

Vascular accidents, mesenteric thrombosis, and embolus to the mesenteric vessels are unusual yet real causes of ileus. The debilitated, often cancer-ridden patient with malnutrition is most frequently at risk. Whether these patients are truely hypercoagulable or simply have altered microhemodynamics due to tumor burden is not known. Ileus associated with vascular compromise has a poor prognosis. In the suspected high-risk patient, low-dose heparin is indicated (5000 units subcutaneously pre-operatively and every 6 hours postoperatively for 7 to 10 days). Infarcted bowel presents similarly to ileus except that there is a significant elevation in white blood cell count out of proportion to the clinical findings. When ischemia progresses to infarction, peritonitis from perforation is apparent. Fortunately, these are rare events. If there is suspicion of vascular compromise as the cause of ileus, then mesenteric angiography is indicated.

Postoperative ileus is most commonly the result of altered metabolic factors. Deficiencies in specific electrolytes responsible for smooth muscle function significantly delay the reappearance of bowel activity. Proper attention to maintenance and replacement fluid and electrolyte therapy all but eliminates this group as a significant factor. Deficits in ionized potassium, calcium, or magnesium are the most commonly seen abnormalities. The latter are frequently associated with hepatic disease or malnutrition. Hypokalemia most frequently results from inadequate replacement of potassium losses through gastric drainage, fistulas, or the urinary tract. Monitoring and replacement of electrolyte losses and deficits decreases the incidence of this cause of ileus. Unsuspected renal failure or diabetic ketoacidosis can also produce an ileus. Both conditions require specific therapeutic intervention.

PHARMACOLOGIC CAUSES OF ILEUS

Any event which impairs the myoneural junction or the acetylcholine mechanism resulting in altered neurogenic stimulation of the bowel with loss of muscle tone produces ileus. In addition to the categories noted above, pharmacologic toxicity of individual drugs or drug-drug interactions must be considered. Certain drugs in large doses (e.g., dopamine, diphenoxylate hydrochloride) decrease bowel motility. Psychotropics and anticholinergics also slow gut activity. Postoperative ileus may result from these agents singly or in combination.

It is attractive to consider the use of pharmacologic sympathetic blockade and parasympathetic stimulation to effect return of bowel function in patients with ileus. Obviously, this regimen would apply to only a small population of patients who have failed to regain bowel function after 2 or 3 weeks, all other causes of ileus having been dismissed. For early ileus, pharmacologic therapy with adrenergic blockage and neostigmine stimulation or metaclopramide fails logically. Early ileus often reflects a problem elsewhere. Treatment of the "sign" does not get at the underlying problem and adds an additional risk factor for the patient. These pharmacologic regimens have not been fully documented in a scientific manner in specific populations. They are to be reserved for "intractable" cases where all else seems to fail.

HEADACHE

MARY C. TAYLOR, M.D.

Headache is one of the most frequently encountered complaints in almost any type of primary care medical practice. Most often it is of a benign nature, but it may also signal the presence of significant underlying general medical or central nervous system pathology. The pericranial structures such as the eyes, ears, sinuses, dentition, joints, cervical spine, cranium, and vascular structures of the head may also be sources of pain. In other instances, headache may indicate psychogenic rather than physical factors.

Clues to the more malignant nature of the headache include recent onset, sameness of location, increasing duration or severity, early morning predominance, nocturnal awakenings from headache, exacerbation by coughing or Valsalva maneuvers, failure of conventional treatments, and a history of associated neurologic signs and symptoms. Although none of these factors alone is necessarily predictive of structural intracranial pathology, they can be reliable guides to further neurodiagnostic evaluation when used in combination with the neurologic examination. The forms of headache most frequently encountered are vascular and migraine headache, cluster headache, muscle contraction (tension) headaches, and inflammatory or traction headaches.

VASCULAR AND MIGRAINE HEADACHES

It should be kept in mind that not all that throbs is migraine. Etiologic factors in the production of throbbing headaches include toxins (e.g., lead, carbon monoxide, insecticides), drugs (e.g., theophylline, monosodium glutamate, nitrates, alcohol), drug withdrawal (e.g., caffeine, ergots, amphetamines), hypertension, muscle contraction headache, and structural (e.g. arteriovenous malformations) defects, among others.

There are two basic types of migraine—a prodromal or classic form and nonprodromal or common migraine. The former are thought to constitute about 10 to 20 per cent of migrainous patients and are characterized by episodes of visual disturbances or focal neurologic symptoms preceding the headache by 15 to 30 minutes. The headache may be followed by drowsiness. Common migraine has few premonitory symptoms or signs and is frequently associated with nonspecific complaints of nausea, vomiting, and photophobia. In both instances, there is frequently a family history, onset prior to age 20, a history of food allergies (e.g., red wine, tyramine-containing foodstuffs, nitrites, monosodium glutamate), and a throbbing unilateral though alternating hemicranial headache. In both instances, females outnumber males and the frequency and intensity of headache may be exacerbated by premenstrual tension and exogenous estrogens. Symptoms are frequently ameliorated during late pregnancy.

Vascular changes are felt to play a significant role in producing the migraine syndrome. The initial prodromal phase is thought to be due to intense vasocontriction with resulting focal ischemia; vasodilation and vessel distention may account for the throbbing or pounding component.

Therapy may be abortive if the headache occurs only once a month. Very often, mild analgesia such as aspirin or acetaminophen is sufficient, but in patients with more severe acute attacks, the ergot alkaloids remain the mainstays of therapy. In the patient with prodromal or classic migraine, ergotamine alone or in combination (Cafergot) orally, sublingually, by inhaler, or by rectum may be effective in aborting the headache altogether if taken early during the prodrome. In cases of established headache, the same preparation, or in severe cases, parenteral ergot preparations such as ergotamine tartrate (Gynergen), 0.25 to 0.5 mg intramuscularly initially, with the possibility of a repeat dose in 1 hour, or dehydroergotamine, 1 mg intramuscularly or intravenously, repeated in 1 hour, may be given. No more than 0.5 mg of ergotamine should be given intravenously in 24 hours, or 1 to 2 mg by any parenteral route in one week. Up to a total dose of 3 mg of dehydroergotamine may be given in divided doses at 1 hour intervals. In those patients intolerant of ergots, Midrin, 2 capsules in 12 hours, may be prescribed.

Though ergotamine tartrate and dehydroergotamine have fewer oxytocic effects than ergonovine or methylergonovine, the ergots have been implicated as teratogenic agents and it is best to avoid all ergot preparations during pregnancy. Other contraindications include complicated migraine (e.g., hemiplegic, hemianesthetic migraine, etc.), peripheral vascular disease, thrombophlebitis, hypertension, heart disease, recent infection or sepsis, and the presence of significant gastrointestinal or hepatorenal disease.

Other acute measures include bed rest in a quiet darkened room and abstinence from food or drink. If these combinations of measures fail, resorting to conventional narcotic analgesics is appropriate in treating the acute attack.

In patients with more frequent or severe headaches, prophylactic measures must be taken. In addition to avoidance of those circumstances or foods that precipitate the headache, a number of pharmacologic agents are available. Ergotamine tartrate, 1 mg twice a day for 6 days of each week, or ergotamine in combination with phenobarbital and belladona (Bellergal), 1 tablet 4 times daily, is sometimes helpful. Of the nonergot compounds, propranolol in divided doses up to 160 mg per day appears to be most effective for patients with migraine alone. Amitriptyline (Elavil) is also effective, especially in patients with mixed migrainous-contraction headache syndromes. Clonidine, 0.1 mg 3 times daily, or cyproheptadine (Periactin), up to 16 mg per day, may also be used. Caution must be exercised in the use of any of these drugs. Even discontinuation can be associated with complications such as ergot withdrawal headache, sudden death with propranolol, and hypertensive crisis with clonidine.

In those patients unresponsive to any of the more conventional drug therapies, methysergide (Sansert) is administered orally in 2 mg doses up to 6 mg per day. This drug has a high incidence of such side effects as retroperitoneal and cardiac fibrosis and is usually discontinued for 6 to 8 weeks after 3 to 4 months of continuous usage, with monitoring of cardiac and renal function.

CLUSTER HEADACHE

Cluster headache, or histamine cephalgia, is predominantly a disease of adult males without hereditary implications. Typically, after the ingestion of vasodilatory substances, especially alcohol, the patient is awakened from a sound sleep by a severe, always unilateral, rapidly peaking pain behind or around the eye associated with ipsilateral facial flushing, conjunctival injection, nasal congestion or rhinorrhea, or Horner's syndrome. The pain is of short duration, lasting from minutes to several hours, and the attacks have a tendency to cluster over a period of several weeks.

The pain of cluster headache is generally severe, but because of the sometimes infrequent and unpredictable nature of the attacks prophylactic treatment may be difficult or unwarranted. The same ergotamine preparations used to treat acute migraine may be used to treat cluster headaches. Methysergide, 2 mg 3 times per day, alone or in combination with cyproheptadine, 4 mg four times daily, is frequently effective. Nitrates, alcohol, and foods containing vasodilator substances are avoided. Corticosteroids such as triamcinolone, 4 mg 4 times daily, or prednisone, 30 mg every other day for up to 10 to 14 days, may be useful adjuncts should other therapeutic measures fail.

Methysergide can not be used for prolonged prophylaxis because of its side effects. However, cyproheptadine is an effective preventive agent with fewer side effects. Lithium, 900 mg per day, or serum drug levels less than 2.0 mEq per liter, is also an effective means of prophylaxis. Rarely all of these measures meet with failure and cryotherapy of the sphenopalatine ganglion may be considered.

MUSCLE CONTRACTION HEADACHE

The patient with muscle contraction headache is distinguished by the presence of a constant, day in–day out, bilateral, frequently nuchal-occipital, tight, bandlike pressure pain associated with contraction of the head and neck muscles and the presence of ongoing emotional conflicts. Frequently, migraine and muscle contraction headache syndromes occur together.

Patients with mild muscle contraction headaches may be treated with analgesics such as aspirin, acetaminophen, or Fiorinal. Caution must be exercised in the use of the latter as well as any other sedative-tranquilizer or narcotic analgesics with addictive potential. Because of underlying emotional factors, these patients and others with chronic headache syndromes may be more susceptible to drug dependency. The pharmacologic agent of choice in more refractory cases is amitriptyline, 50 to 150 mg per day. This agent appears to have analgesic actions independent of its antidepressant effect. In instances where amitriptyline is ineffective, imipramine may be tried. Zomepirac sodium, 50 to 150 mg per day, is one of the newer agents found effective in muscle contraction headache. Any of these agents should be combined with more simple procedures such as neck and shoulder massage, local heat, and relaxation techniques such as yoga, meditation, and hypnosis. Biofeedback, utilizing feedback of electromyographic (EMG) activity from the frontalis or temporalis muscles, appears to be a very useful adjunctive form of therapy.

INFLAMMATORY OR TRACTION HEADACHES

Of the headaches of inflammatory or traction etiology, two deserve special mention. These are giant cell or temporal arteritis, and post–lumbar puncture headache. The former is an inflammatory, obliterative disorder of medium and large-sized vessels which may result in a sharp, boring headache with or without pain and stiffness in the limb girdles. Associated complaints may include fever, malaise, jaw claudication, weight loss, and blindness. The majority of patients are women over the age of 50. Laboratory studies may show an elevated erythrocyte sedimentation rate (ESR) and a positive temporal artery biopsy. It should be pointed out that neither a normal sedimentation rate nor a normal biopsy excludes the diagnosis of giant cell arteritis. In order to prevent the visual and neurologic complications of giant cell arteritis, therapy should be instituted as soon as possible with prednisone, 60 to 80 mg per day for 4 to 6 weeks, followed by gradually tapering dosages to the lowest maintenance dose.

The post–lumbar puncture headache is a dull or throbbing headache of variable intensity appearing a few hours to days after a lumbar puncture and of variable duration. It is usually present in the upright position and relieved by recumbency and is associated with low cerebrospinal fluid pressure. Treatment is usually preventive, and its incidence can be reduced by utilizing smaller bore needles and rehydration techniques. Also, there is evidence that employing autologous blood patches may reduce its incidence in patients at greater risk, such as those undergoing radiologic or anesthetic procedures.

PNEUMONIA

THOMAS C. CESARIO, M.D.

Pneumonia may occur in a variety of syndromes related to the nature of the specific causative agent. Indeed, a wide ranging number of organisms, varying from viruses and bacteria to fungi and parasitic agents, may cause pneumonia. Strictly speaking, pneumonia should be defined on the basis of the x-ray film. Thus, infections producing a roentgenographically demonstrable infiltrate may be said to produce pneumonia. Utilization of these more rigid criteria permits a more accurate and more specific discussion.

From a therapeutic standpoint, an understanding of pneumonia would involve an appreciation of the causative organisms. Of all pneumonias occurring in the population as a whole, the majority are caused by organisms other than true bacteria. Thus *Mycoplasma pneumoniae* accounts for a substantial percentage of the pneumonias diagnosed.

Mycoplasma pneumoniae is an agent capable of growth on artificial media. It is also an agent which, while similar to bacteria in many ways, still has some distinctive properties. Belonging to the family Mycoplasmataceae, it requires sterols for growth, is capable of metabolizing glucose, and lacks a rigid cell wall. It has a rather distinctive appearance when grown on artificial media. This appearance has been referred to as resembling a fried egg. While a number of different mycoplasma species have been isolated from humans, *M. pneumoniae* is the only one known to regularly produce pulmonary infections.

From an epidemiologic viewpoint, infections caused by *M. pneumoniae* are often endemic, although well-defined epidemics may occur. Infections can occur in all age groups although the greatest incidence of pneumonia seems to occur in the 5 to 19 year age group. Spread occurs within closed populations, especially families. The risk of pneumonia following infection with this agent is approximately 5 to 10 per cent. Overall, *M. pneumoniae* accounts for 20 per cent of all pneumonias observed in the community based upon an extensive survey conducted in Seattle.

Probably of importance in the epidemiology of *M. pneumoniae* infections is the fact that prolonged excretion occurs following acquisition of the organism.

The incubation period following exposure to this agent is about 3 weeks and the spectrum of disease produced includes both upper and lower respiratory tract manifestations.

Pneumonia produced by *M. pneumoniae* tends to be milder than that produced by the bacterial organisms discussed below. Usually there is an insidious onset over several days followed by cough. The cough is usually dry and may be associated with substernal soreness, coryza, sore throat, and otalgia. Fever generally ranges from 102 to 104° F.

Patients with infections due to this organism are often not severely ill. Physical findings often include rhonchi and rales, but findings are occasionally observed on the tympanic membranes (bullous myringitis), and occasional patients have skin rashes.

Death from *M. pneumoniae* infections is very rare, and fever generally lasts up to two weeks. Cough and infiltrates on x-ray films last up to 6 weeks.

Total leukocyte counts are generally below 10,000 cells per cu mm, but higher counts are occasionally observed. Sputum Gram stains show either no organisms or only normal throat flora. Either lymphocytes or polymorphonuclear leukocytes can be observed in the sputum smears.

A number of nonspecific reactions have been associated with mycoplasma infections, of which the best known is the appearance of a positive cold agglutinin test. While low titered reactions (i.e., less than 1:40) are occasionally found in normals, higher titers are often associated with infections due to *M. pneumoniae*. Approximately half of United States Marines with infections caused by this organism had positive tests, and usually patients with more severe disease are more often positive. Cold agglutinins usually develop at the end of the first week or at the beginning of the second week of illness.

Radiographically, the most typical appearance of pneumonia caused by this organism is a unilateral lower lobe segmental bronchopneumonia, although more severe involvement may occur.

Complications from *M. pneumoniae* include relapsing pneumonia, erythema multiforme, meningoencephalitis, and rarely hemolysis. Other complications are unusual but include myopericardial involvement, arthralgias, and mild hepatitis.

Both erythromycin (500 mg every 6 hours) and tetracycline (250 mg every 6 hours) are effective therapy for *M. pneumoniae*, but the latter is contraindicated in pregnancy. Reinfections with *M. penumoniae* are known to occur.

Other nonbacterial agents capable of causing pneumonia include influenza virus, adenoviruses, and rarely rickettsia or chlamydia. Respiratory syncytial virus, while responsible for a significant number of pneumonia cases in young children, does not often produce this disease in older children or adults.

Influenza A virus typically occurs during the winter months and often occurs in periodic cycles. Pandemic influenza, which is due to a major antigenic variation in this virus, comes in cycles of approximately 10 years. Lesser epidemics occur in intervals of about 2 years.

The typical syndrome of influenza includes severe myalgias as the most distinctive feature, but arthralgias, fever, dry cough, and ocular symptoms are common.

One significant complication of influenza is primary influenzal pneumonia. Indeed many of the deaths in the 1918–1919 pandemic were associated with this complication. Primary influenzal pneumonia is pneumonia caused by the virus itself. While secondary bacterial pneumonias as described below are generally more common, influenzal pneumonia is often catastrophic. Typically, primary influenzal pneumonia occurs in individuals with cardiac disease, especially mitral stenosis, or individuals with other chronic underlying processes. Pregnancy has been considered a predisposing factor in some cases.

Primary influenzal pneumonia follows the onset of the influenza syndrome by 2 or 3 days and rapidly progresses to dyspnea, cyanosis, and often death from respiratory failure.

Unfortunately no effective treatment exists for influenzal pneumonia at this time, and only supportive treatment may be offered. The role of amantadine in influenzal pneumonia is not yet known.

The other major known viral etiologic agent causing pneumonia in the adult is the adenovirus group. While certain adenovirus strains are endemic in the population, others are known to produce distinctive epidemics. This has been especially true in military populations. The most distinctive adenovirus syndromes include pharyngoconjunctival fever, keratoconjunctivitis, acute respiratory distress syndrome (ARDS), and pneumonia. The latter produces a syndrome resembling that produced by mycoplasma but is often less severe. Adenovirus pneumonia is not typically associated with the development of cold agglutinating antibodies. Treatment is again supportive.

Coxiella burnetii is responsible for Q fever and is acquired through contact with hooved animals. The organism contaminates the excreta and placenta of these animals and is highly resistant to drying. Man acquires the organism through inhalation.

The clinical manifestations of Q fever include myalgias, fever, chills, and sweats. A nonproductive cough is common. Approximately half of the cases of infection attributed to this organism are associated with pneumonia. Hepatitis is also encountered. Diagnosis of Q fever is typically made using serologic methods. Tetracycline has been considered the standard of treatment for Q fever, but chloramphenicol has also been suggested. The latter in pregnancy may be the only alternative to tetracyclines.

Psittacosis is an infectious disease of birds which may be communicated to man.

The organism, which infects a wide variety of avian species, is present in the excreta, on the feathers, and in the tissues of infected birds. Man inhales the organism and acquires a systemic disease with pulmonary involvement.

After an incubation period of 1 to 2 weeks, the clinical manifestations begin. Headache, malaise, myalgias, arthralgias, and rash may all be observed. Cough, altered mental status, and gastrointestinal findings all occur. Rales, splenomegaly, and hepatomegaly are relatively common physical findings, but jaundice is only occasionally encountered.

While the organism may be isolated from clinical specimens, serologic studies remain the standard means of diagnosis.

Tetracycline is considered the most effective therapy in doses of 2 grams per day. The role of other antibiotics, including erythromycin and chloramphenicol, is less clear.

Mortality in untreated psittacosis has been reported to range from 20 to 40 per cent, thus underscoring the importance of treatment which appears to reduce the death rate to approximately 1 per cent.

While nonbacterial causes of pneumonia are the most common causes of pneumonia overall, bacteria are the most common causes observed in hospital practice. Among the bacterial causes of pneumonia, *Streptococcus pneumoniae* accounts for the majority of cases (about 70 per cent of cases of pneumonia admitted to the hospital).

Streptococcus pneumoniae is a gram-positive organism which grows in short chains and produces alpha hemolysis when cultured on blood agar. This organism is generally identified by sensitivity to Optochin.

Pneumococcal pneumonia can be seen in all age groups and has a higher incidence in patients over the age of 40. While *Streptococcus pneumoniae* may be commonly isolated from normal carriers, strains normally colonizing the upper airways are often higher serotypes and are less often associated with disease production. The majority of pneumococcal disease is sporadic in nature and often results after prior injury has compromised pulmonary defenses. Thus viral infection may be an important factor predisposing to *Streptococcus pneumoniae* infection by altering subsequent bacterial clearance.

The incubation period of pneumococcal pneumonia is 1 to 3 days. Subsequently the clinical syndrome is ushered in by a shaking chill followed by fever. Patients commonly begin to produce rust colored sputum and complain of a unilateral pleuritic type of chest pain. Dyspnea, malaise, and even prostration are common. On physical examination the patients often have rales and signs of consolidation. Gastric distention is common.

Patients with pneumococcal pneumonia characteristically exhibit leukocytosis and may also have hyperbilirubinemia and hypoxemia Appropriately collected sputum will often demonstrate the characteristic lancet-shaped diplococci.

Penicillin G is considered the most appropriate antibiotic for patients with pneumococcal pneumonia. Intramuscular administration of 1.6 to 2.4 million units per day in divided doses will generally suffice, although intravenous treatment may be indicated for toxic patients with extensive disease. Even oral administration of penicillin V, 500 mg every 6 hours, will usually suffice if the patient is not toxic, has limited disease, and is capable of taking oral medication. Erythromycin is a suitable alternative to penicillin, as are most of the cephalosporins.

The complications of pneumococcal pneumonia include empyema, lung abscess (especially with disease due to Type II pneumococcus), bacteremia, meningitis, endocarditis, septic arthritis, and rarely peritonitis. Mortality from pneumococcal pneumonia ranges from 5 to 10 per cent. *Hemophilus influenzae* is another of the bacterial agents associated with pneumonia. *Hemophilus influenzae* is a gram-negative bacillus. Both encapsulated and nonencapsulated strains exist, but systemic disease is usually associated with the former. Several serotypes exist, of which type B tends to be most often associated with invasive disease. Infections with *Hemophilus influenzae* usually are rather strikingly related to age, with disease states seen predominantly under age 3. Other diseases which impair some element of normal host defenses may also predispose to hemophilus infections. Pneumonia caused by this agent may be either bronchopneumonias or lobar pneumonias. Viral upper respiratory infections are common antecedent factors predisposing to this type of bacterial infection. Fever, chills, purulent sputum, and dyspnea are all part of the clinical syndrome.

The diagnosis of *Hemophilus influenzae* infections is facilitated by Gram-stained smears of sputum. Cultures of sputum, blood, or pleural exudate are all useful from a diagnostic standpoint.

Therapeutically, ampicillin (6 to 12 grams per day) remains a useful agent, but since about 5 per cent of strains isolated from patients with disease due to hemophilus are resistant to this antibiotic, individuals with life-threatening disease should be treated with ampicillin and chloramphenicol until sensitivities are known. Cefamandol and other newer cephalosporins may also be useful to treat infections caused by *H. influenzae*.

Staphylococcus aureus is another bacterium that occasionally causes pneumonia, but in the present era it accounts for less than 1 per cent of all pneumonias. Most typically staphylococcal pneumonias are seen following influenza virus infections. This fact is attributable to the major alterations induced by this virus in the respiratory tract epithelium. Characteristically, secondary bacterial pneumonias will have their onset 5 to 7 days following the initial influenzal symptoms. Staphylococcal pneumonias may also occur in patients debilitated by other diseases. Pneumonias caused by this bacterial agent often involve multiple lobes and may progress rapidly to produce lung abscess and empyema. Pneumatoceles so characteristic of staphylococcal disease in children are not often seen in adults.

Sputum examination by Gram stain and culture is critical to the diagnosis, and cultures of blood should always be undertaken prior to treatment.

The drug of choice for staphylococcal pneumonia is a semisynthetic penicillin (nafcillin perhaps being the best) given intravenously in a dose of 6 to 18 grams per day. Cephalothin would be a suitable choice in the patient with a past history of penicillin rash, and vancomycin might be considered in the patient with a previous history of anaphylactic reaction to penicillin.

Gram-negative bacilli such as *Escherichia coli, Klebsiella pneumoniae,* and *Pseudomonas aeruginosa* may also cause pulmonary infection. These organisms are generally seen in hospital-acquired infections in individuals with other disease processes. Patients with malignant diseases, especially leukemia, and patients with respiratory failure requiring ventilatory assistance may be especially predisposed to *Pseudomonas aeruginosa* infections. Infections of the lung with gram-negative bacilli often leads to necrosis with subsequent abscess production. Gram stain of an appropriately obtained sputum should facilitate the diagnosis once again.

Initial therapy should include an aminoglycoside antibiotic (gentamicin or tobramycin in a dose of 5 mg per kg per day either intravenously or intramuscularly). Often a second antibiotic will be required to eradicate pulmonary infections due to these agents. Carbenicillin or ticarcillin might be appropriately added for *Pseudomonas aeruginosa* and a cephalosporin for Klebsiella or *Escherichia coli* infections).

In recent years, *Legionella pneumophila* has been added to the list of agents capable of producing pneumonia. A gram-negative bacillus, this organism can affect persons of almost any age group but most cases occur after middle age. The organism is acquired from environmental sources, with person-to-person spread occuring infrequently if at all. Persons at highest risk would appear to be those who are immunosuppressed.

The onset of Legionnaires' disease is associated with malaise, myalgias, headache, fever, and chills. A dry initial cough is observed, often associated with pleuritic chest pain. Symptoms referable to other organs are a distinctive feature. Thus diarrhea, abdominal pain, and delirium are frequent. Physical findings usually include rales and ronchi. Laboratory examinations reveal slightly elevated total white blood cell count, abnormal liver function tests, hematuria and hypoxemia.

The radiologic appearance of Legionnaires' disease is often a patchy alveolar infiltrate which progresses to consolidation. The diagnosis of this disease can be made by culture, demonstration of the organism in the sputum or biopsy material or by serological change.

In addition to supportive therapy, erythromycin appears to be the drug of choice. Erythromycin should be used in a dose of 500 mg to 1 gram every 6 hours. Rifampin may also be clinically useful but experience with this drug in Legionnaires' disease is lacking.

Mixed anaerobic organisms may also produce pneumonia after aspiration of oral contents into the lung. The latter situation occurs during episodes of unconsciousness, protracted vomiting, seizures, or through accidental aspiration of foreign bodies. Necrosis of lung is common in this circumstance with resultant lung abscesses.

In addition to fever and cough, halitosis is frequent in these patients.

Gram stain of the sputum in patients with aspiration will reveal mixed organisms.

Treatment will generally involves penicillin in divided doses of 2.4 to 6 million units per day. Clindamycin may be the most effective alternative to penicillin, but erythromycin is also a reasonable choice in the patient allergic to penicillin.

Lastly in the investigation of patients with pneumonia consideration should always be given to the possibility of underlying fungal infections or even tuberculosis if the epidemiologic circumstances are appropriate and no other organism can be incriminated.

ATELECTASIS

G. ROBERT MASON, M.D., Ph.D.

Atelectasis is derived from two Greek stems; the first of these, "ateles", describes that which is imperfect or incomplete, and the second, "ectasis", refers to a stretching out and may also refer to the dilatation of a hollow organ or of a canal. Combined, these stems are used to describe the incomplete aeration of a portion of lung tissue. Two clinical conditions in which this finding is most common are in the incomplete expansion of the lung of the newborn and, similarly, in patients immediately following an operative procedure. We shall concern ourselves here specifically with the latter.

If the airway leading to a major pulmonary segment is obstructed completely, the gases contained in that segment will, over a time, be absorbed gradually down their concentration gradient into the circulation, leading to complete collapse or atelectasis of that segment. Thus, it has been assumed that the major cause of atelectasis is obstruction of the airway, presumably by retained secretions. The most common observation, however, is that atelectasis is subsegmental, or "platter-like," rather than lobar. In the experimental laboratory, obstruction must be complete to cause atelectasis. Collateral aeration through the pores of Kohn is adequate to prevent collapse in subsegmental occlusion. Thus the "bronchial plug" theory of causation must be regarded as an unusual cause of atelectasis.

It has been shown that constant tidal volume ventilation results in decreased lung volume, decreased compliance, and increased arteriovenous shunting. This apparent decrease in functioning pulmonary volume appears to occur on the basis of collapse of small functional units from hypoventilation, and may be reversed by hyperventilation, even after considerable delay.

A major factor in maintaining expansion of alveolar units is the presence of a surface active agent or "surfactant" which reduces surface tension of the alveolus. Agents or diseases which reduce the concentration of this substance will tend to promote pulmonary collapse. Chronic lung disease such as bronchitis, emphysema, asthma, and chronic smoking are associated with an increased incidence of atelectasis, presumably related to altered quantities of surfactant.

Atelectasis is said to be the most common postoperative complication. It occurs more commonly with upper abdominal operative procedures than with lower abdominal or extremity procedures. Clinical manifestations customarily noted are increased pulse rate and elevated temperature, usually occurring within the first 12 to 24 hours following completion of an operative procedure. Chest examination will sometimes reveal localized areas of decreased breath sounds or rales to auscultation, and in some cases some bronchial mucous wheezing sounds heard more centrally. Frequently, however, there will be little or no auscultatory or other physical findings. The diagnosis may then be made on many occasions with a chest x-ray which will show a small segmental or subsegmental "platter" atelectasis, or in some cases collapse of a larger portion of lung as in a segment or lobe. Any patient with an otherwise clean operative procedure who shows increased pulse and temperature to over 38°C or 101°F in the immediate postoperative period should be suspected of having atelectasis.

THERAPY

Considering that prevention is often the best cure, attention should be given to cessation of smoking at least 2 weeks preoperatively and to varying the depths of respiration during the course of the operative procedure. Prior to the termination of the operative procedure, several efforts should be made to hyperinflate the lung and to completely suction the tracheobronchial tree of whatever mucous secretions might be residual. Similarly, in the postoperative period, efforts to have the patient breathe deeply either by self-induced negative pressure or by externally induced positive pressure will be helpful in expanding the atelectatic areas. In those cases in which there is residual mucus in smaller bronchioles, efforts should be turned to encouraging the patient to cough vigorously. The coughing effort is perhaps one of the most effective in increasing intra-pulmonary pressure. Patients who are unwilling to cough and rid themselves of secretions must frequently be assisted by nasotracheal suction and may require a more vigorous effort such as fiberoptic or rigid bronchoscopy to eliminate residual secretions. A technique which is often helpful is to place a small polethylene catheter into the trachea through the cricothyroid membrane and inject 15 to 20 cc of normal saline. This often will assist in lubricating the secretions and will encourage the patient to cough. Many times, however, the normal saline solution is reasonably well tolerated by the patient without coughing. In these cases approximately 0.5 cc of distilled water is often very effective in eliciting a vigorous cough.

Various devices are in use in this country for the purpose of pulmonary expansion and in decreasing atelectasis. Devices such as intermittent positive pressure breathing (IPPB) have not been shown scientifically to have consistent value. However, breathing against various forms of resistance, both positively and negatively, such as incentive spirometry and "blow-bottles" may be of benefit. Various medications such as expectorants and mucolytic solutions are available to liquefy bronchial secretions. Bronchodilators may also be of use in some patients. These various techniques may be tailored to the patients particular problem. If one of them is to be chosen in a consistent way clinically, it would be prudent to choose the cheapest of them. A relatively new development, high frequency ventilation may be of benefit, although sufficient clinical experience is not yet available.

Index

Note: Page numbers in *italics* refer to illustrations; page numbers followed by (t) refer to tables.

Abdomen, examination of, in newborn, 135
Abortion, and septic shock, 174
    recurrent, 27–29, 27(t)
    spontaneous, 27
    therapeutic, 29–30
Abruptio placentae, 10–11
Abscess(es), of Bartholin's gland, 167, 168
Abstinence syndromes, after withdrawal from alcohol, 81–82, 81(t)
    after withdrawal from drugs, 76
    in offspring of drug abuser, 75, 75(t), 132
Acne, 271–274
Actinomycin D, for gestational trophoblastic disease, 203
Actinomycosis, IUD use and, 231
Acyclovir (Zovirax), in treatment of herpes genitalis, 33, 163
Adenocarcinoma, of cervix, 206
    of vulva, 191
Adenoma(s), of pituitary gland, 217–218, 224, 246
    and galactorrhea, 257
    treatment of, 225, 226
Adenosis, vaginal, 144–146
Adnexa uteri, masses of, 177
Adrenal gland(s), congenital hyperplasia of, 213, 237
    hyperfunctioning of, 236–237
    tumor of, 237
    and virilization, 213
Afrit (oxymetazoline), for rhinitis, 107
Agar, for neonatal hyperbilirubinemia, 129–130
Airway, patency of, in newborn, 117
Alcohol, for premature labor, 23
    for pruritus vulvae, 144, 181
Alcohol abuse, diagnosis of, 78–79, 79(t)
    in pregnancy, 77–82
    as risk to fetus, 78, 78(t)
Alcoholic hallucinosis, 81, 81(t)
Alcohol intoxication, 80–81, 80(t)
Aldactone (spironolactone), for hirsutism, in adrenal disorders, 238
    in polycystic ovary syndrome, 211, 223
Aldomet (methyldopa), for hypertension, 270(t)
    in pregnancy, 5
Amenorrhea, primary, 209–213, 210(t)
    secondary, 213–218, *216*
Amino acids, in intravenous hyperalimentation, 266
    in peripheral parenteral nutrition, 267

Aminophylline, for asthma, in pregnancy, 108(t)
    for pulmonary embolism, 51
Amitriptyline (Elavil), for headache, 277, 278
Amniocentesis, in diagnosis of genetic defects, 111–113
Amnionitis, premature rupture of extraembryonic membranes and, 19–20, 35, 82–83
Amniorrhexis, 19–20, *20*, 35
    and amnionitis, 19–20, 35, 82–83
    oxytocin induction of uterine contractions after, 20, 35, 83
Amniotic fluid, cytologic studies of, in diagnosis of genetic defects, 111–113
    extrusion of, into maternal vasculature, 49–50
    meconium in, 41
Amniotic fluid embolism, 49–50
Amniotomy, uterine contractions after, 37
Amobarbital, for convulsions, 3
Amoxicillin, for bacterial bronchitis, in pregnant asthmatic patient, 108
    for bacterial rhinosinusitis, 107
    for cervicitis, 179
    for gonorrhea, 158(t)–160(t)
    for salpingitis (PID), 156, 159(t)
    for urinary tract infection, 31
Amphetamine(s), teratogenic potential of, 74(t)
    withdrawal from, 76
Ampicillin, for amnionitis, 83
    for bacterial bronchitis, in pregnant asthmatic patient, 108
    for bacterial rhinosinusitis, 107
    for cervicitis, 179
    for gonorrhea, 158(t)–160(t)
    for pneumonia, 281
    for salpingitis (PID), 156, 159(t)
    for urinary tract infection, 31
Amytal, for convulsions, in status epilepticus, 63
Analgesia, in labor, 84–86
Anaprox (naproxen), for dysmenorrhea, 151(t)
Androgen, overproduction of, 236–238
Anemia(s), in pregnancy, 70–74, *72*
    iron-deficiency, 71, 73
    laboratory findings in, 73(t)
    megaloblastic, 71
Anesthesia, in cesarean section, 86–87
    in labor/delivery, 83–87
    in rheumatic heart disease patient, 60
Anorexia nervosa, 241–243
Anovulation, hypothalamic, 210–211

INDEX

Antacid(s), administration of, before induction of general anesthesia, 87
Antepartum fetal heart rate testing, 16–18, *18, 19*
Antibiotic(s). See also specific agents, e.g., *Erythromycin.*
  for acne, 272–273
  for urinary tract infection, 31
  in prophylaxis against bacteremia, in pregnant patient with rheumatic heart disease, 59
Anticoagulant(s). See also specific agents, e.g., *Heparin.*
  for venous thrombosis, 51–54
  in prophylaxis against venous thrombosis, 55
    in pregnant patient with rheumatic heart disease, 59–60
Anticonvulsant(s), 3, 5, 61, 62(t), 63
  dosage of, for newborn, 133(t)
Antiplatelet agents, for venous thrombosis, 54
Anus, examination of, in newborn, 135
Apresoline (hydralazine), for hypertension, 270(t), 271
  in pregnancy, 3, 5
Arcuate uterus, 182
Arthritis, rheumatoid, in pregnancy, 69
Ascorbic acid, in treatment of drug overdose, 77
Asherman's syndrome, 215, 238–239
Asphyxia, perinatal, and seizures in newborn, 131
Aspirin, for dysmenorrhea, 151(t)
  for premature labor, 23
  for rheumatoid arthritis, 69
Asthma, in pregnancy, 106–109, 108(t)
Atarax (hydroxyzine), for pruritus vulvae, 181
  in improvement of analgesia, in first stage of labor, 84
Atelectasis, 282–283
Atenolol, for hypertension, 270(t)
Atropine, in resuscitation of newborn, 119

Back, examination of, in newborn, 135
Bacteremia, antibiotic prophylaxis against, in pregnant patient with rheumatic heart disease, 59
Barbiturate(s), teratogenic potential of, 74(t)
  withdrawal from, 76
Barbiturate clearance, 77
Bartholin's gland, cysts of, 167–168
Basal cell carcinoma, of vulva, 191
Beclomethasone, for asthma, in pregnancy, 108
  for rhinitis, 107
Behavioral therapy, for anorexia nervosa, 242
Bellergal, for headache, 277
Bentyl (dicyclomine), for urinary incontinence, 149
Benzathine penicillin G, for syphilis, 161(t)
Benzodiazepine(s), teratogenic potential of, 74(t)
  withdrawal from, 76
Benzoyl peroxide, for acne, 272
Beta-adrenergic agonists, in prevention of premature labor, 22
  in treatment of premature labor, 23–24
Bichloracetic acid, for condyloma acuminatum, 90
Bicornuate uterus, 182
Biliary colic, in pregnancy, 99, 100
Biliary tract, inflammation of, in pregnancy, 99, 100
Birth canal, obstruction of, 37
Birth control, 226–233
  counseling of collagen disease patients on, 70
Bladder, unstable, 149

Bleeding, intracranial, and seizures in newborn, 131
  postpartum, 87–89
  uterine, dysfunctional, 233–235
    IUD use and, 230
  vaginal, in third trimester of pregnancy, 9–11
Bowel. See *Intestine.*
Bradycardia, fetal, eclampsia and, 3
Breast(s), cancer of, 259–262
  disease(s) of, 255–262
  fibrocystic disease of, 255
  fluid secretion by, nonpuerperal, 223–226, 256–257
  mass(es) of, 255–256
  pain in, 257–259
  resection of, for cancer, 261
Breast-feeding, and hyperbilirubinemia, 130
Breech presentation, 11–13
Bromocriptine (Parlodel), for galactorrhea, 257
  for hyperprolactinemia, 226
  for hypogonadotropinism, secondary to hyperprolactinemia, 212
  for luteal phase defects, 249
  for mastalgia, 259
  in induction of ovulation, 220
Bronchitis, treatment of, in pregnant patient with asthma, 108–109

Cafergot, for headache, 277
Calcium, diminished serum levels of, in newborn, 125
  and seizures, 132
Calcium carbonate, in prophylaxis against osteoporosis, 235
Calcium chloride, in resuscitation of newborn, 119
Calcium gluconate, for magnesium sulfate toxicity, 4
  for neonatal hypocalcemia, 125, 132
Calorie supply, in intravenous hyperalimentation, 266
  in peripheral parenteral nutrition, 267
Cancer. See also *Carcinoma.*
  hyperalimentation for patient with, 265–267
  of breast, 259–262
Candidal infection, of vagina, 141, 141(t), 165–166
Captopril, for hypertension, 270(t)
Carbamazepine (Tegretol), for convulsions, 62(t)
Carcinoma. See also *Cancer.*
  cervical, 191–195
  endometrial, 195–198, 196(t)
  ovarian, 198–200
  vulvar, 189–191, 190(t)
Cardiac massage, in resuscitation of newborn, 119
Cardiogenic shock, 172(t)
Cardiovascular monitoring, of pregnant patient with rheumatic heart disease, 60
Cefaclor, for bacterial rhinosinusitis, 107
  for urinary tract infection, 31
Cefoxitin (Mefoxin), for gonorrhea, 158(t)–160(t)
  for salpingitis (PID), 156, 159(t)
Cephalosporin(s), for bacterial bronchitis, in pregnant asthmatic patient, 108
  for urinary tract infection, 31–32
Cerclage, in prevention of premature labor, 22
Cervicitis, 177–179
Cervix, adenocarcinoma of, 206
  carcinoma of, 191–195
  chlamydial infection of, in pregnancy, 164

INDEX

Cervix *(Continued)*
   conization of, for intraepithelial neoplasia, 193, 204
   inflammation of, 177–179
   intraepithelial neoplasia of, 192–193, 204, 206
   perforation of, IUD use and, 230
Cesarean delivery, anesthesia in, 86–87
Chemotherapy, for breast cancer, 261, 262
   for endometrial carcinoma, 197–198
   for gestational trophoblastic disease, 203
   for ovarian carcinoma, 199–200
Chest, examination of, in newborn, 134–135
Chest physiotherapy, and respiratory support, in respiratory distress syndrome, 122
Chin, examination of, in newborn, 134
Chlamydial infection, of female genital tract, 141(t), 142–143, 164–165
2-Chloroprocaine, epidural block with, in labor, 85, 86
Cholangitis, in pregnancy, 99, 100
Cholecystitis, acute, in pregnancy, 99, 100
Cholelithiasis, in pregnancy, 99, 100, 102
Choriocarcinoma, 202
Chromosomal abnormalities, 135–136
   antenatal diagnosis of, 111–112
Citrovorum factor, for gestational trophoblastic disease, 203
Class A diabetes, 6, 8
Cleft lip/palate, 138
Clindamycin, for amnionitis, 83
   for salpingitis (PID), 156, 159(t)
Clinoril (sulindac), for dysmenorrhea, 151(t)
Clomid. See *Clomiphene citrate (Clomid)*.
Clomiphene citrate (Clomid), for corpus luteum deficiency, 28, 249
   in induction of ovulation, 218–220
   in polycystic ovary syndrome, 221
   in treated anorexia patient, 243
Clonidine, for headache, 277
   for hypertension, 270(t), 271
Clotrimazole, for infectious vaginitis, 141(t), 142, 166
Cluster headache, 277–278
Cocaine, withdrawal from, 76
Coitus, painful, 174–176
Colic, biliary, in pregnancy, 99, 100
Colitis, ulcerative, in pregnancy, 100
Collagen diseases, in pregnancy, 68–70
Colpoperineorrhaphy, for uterine prolapse, 146, 147
   for vaginal prolapse, 148
Colporrhaphy, for cystocele, 147
Coma, alcohol-induced, treatment of, 80(t)
   myxedema, 44
   treatment of, 45
Condom, 232
Condyloma acuminatum, 90
Conization, of cervix, for intraepitheal neoplasia, 193, 204
Constipation, in pregnancy, 101–102
Contraception, 226–233
   counseling of collagen disease patients on, 70
Contraceptive(s), oral, 226–229
   and amenorrhea, 214
Contraction stress test, 16–18, *18*
   in postterm pregnancy, 40
Convulsion(s), 60–64
   alcohol withdrawal and, 81–82, 81(t)
   drug overdose and, diazepam for, 77
   drugs for control of, 3, 5, 61, 62(t), 63
      in newborn, 133(t)
   in newborn, 130–133

Corpus luteum deficiency, 28, 247–249
Corticosteroid(s). See also specific agents, e.g., *Prednisone*.
   for inflammatory bowel disease, 101
   for systemic lupus erythematosus, 69
   for vulvar hyperplastic dystrophy, 180
Coumarin, for venous thrombosis, 53–54
Cream, spermicidal, 232
Cri-du-chat syndrome, 136
Crohn's disease, in pregnancy, 100
Cromolyn, for asthma, in pregnancy, 108
Cryosurgery, for cervical intraepithelial neoplasia, 192–193, 204, 206
   for chronic cervicitis, 179
   for condyloma acuminatum, 90
Curettage, in removal of products of conception, in treatment of postpartum hemorrhage, 89
   suction, after fetal death, 25, 26
     and abortion, 30
     in removal of hydatidiform mole, 200
Cyclicillin, for urinary tract infection, 31
Cyclophosphamide, for gestational trophoblastic disease, 203
Cyproheptadine (Periactin), for headache, 277, 278
Cyproterone acetate, for precocious puberty, 250
Cyst(s), of Bartholin's gland, 167–168
   of uterine adnexa, 177
Cystic fibrosis, 137
Cystocele, 147

Danazol (Danocrine), for dysfunctional uterine bleeding, 235
   for endometriosis, 171
   for fibrocystic breast disease, 255
   for mastalgia, 259
   for precocious puberty, 250
Danocrine. See *Danazol (Danocrine)*.
Decadron (dexamethasone), for adrenal hyperfunction, 237
   for polycystic ovary syndrome, 211, 221, 223
   for shock, 173
   in lowering of androgen levels, 220
Dehydroergotamine, for headache, 277
Delirium tremens, 81(t), 82
Delivery, abnormal presentations and, 36
   abruptio placentae and, 11
   anesthesia in, 83–87
     in rheumatic heart disease patient, 60
   breech presentation and, 11–13
   cesarean, anesthesia in, 86–87
   fetal distress and, 15
   fetal hydrocephaly and, 93
   fetal macrosomia and, 36
   in patients with chronic renal disease, 96–97
   in patients with diabetes, 8, 9
   in patients with hypertension, 3–5
   in patients with immune thrombocytopenic purpura, 89, 90
   in patients with uterine myomas, 170
   intrauterine growth retardation and, 56–57
   multiple pregnancy and, 35–36
   obstruction of birth canal and, 36
   of twins, 92
   placenta previa and, 10
   premature rupture of extraembryonic membranes and, 20, 35
Depakene (valproic acid), for convulsions, 62(t)
Depo-Provera. See *Provera (medroxyprogesterone acetate)*.

DES (diethylstilbestrol), effects of exposure to, 144–146
Descensus uteri, 146–147
Dexamethasone (Decadron), for adrenal hyperfunction, 237
　for polycystic ovary syndrome, 211, 221, 223
　for shock, 173
　in lowering of androgen levels, 220
Dextran, for venous thrombosis, 54
Dextrometer, and blood sugar measurements, as basis for insulin dose adjustment, 7, 7(t)
Dextrose, barbiturate clearance with, 77
　for neonatal hypoglycemia, 121, 124, 125, 125(t), 132
　for shock, 173
　in peripheral parenteral nutrition, 267
Diabetes, in pregnancy, 5–9
　and neonatal hypoglycemia, 124
Dialysis, patient management in, pregnancy and, 97
Diaphragm, hernia of, congenital, 137
Diaphragm contraceptive, 232
Diazepam, for alcohol intoxication, 80(t)
　for convulsions, 63
　in alcohol withdrawal syndromes, 81(t), 82
　in drug overdose, 77
　in status epilepticus, 63
Dicyclomine (Bentyl), for urinary incontinence, 149
Diethylstilbestrol (DES), effects of exposure to, 144–146
Digoxin, for pulmonary embolism, 51
　for rheumatic heart disease, in pregnant patient, 59
Dilantin. See *Diphenylhydantoin (Dilantin, phenytoin)*.
Diphenylhydantoin (Dilantin, phenytoin), for convulsions, 61, 62(t), 63
　in newborn, 133(t)
　in status epilepticus, 63
Disseminated intravascular coagulation, fetal death syndrome and, 26
Ditropan (oxybutynin), for urinary incontinence, 149
Diuretic(s), for hypertension, 269
Diverticulum (diverticula), urethral, 149–150
Dopamine, for shock, 51, 173
Down syndrome, 135–136
　maternal age and, 111(t)
Doxycycline (Vibramycin), for chlamydial infection of female genital tract, 165
　for gonorrhea, 156, 159(t)
　for salpingitis (PID), 156, 159(t), 165
　for syphilis, 161(t)
　use of, prior to planned conception, 28
Drug abuse, in pregnancy, 74–77
　and potential teratogenesis, 74(t)
　and seizures in newborn, 132
　screening for, 75(t)
Drug-induced amenorrhea, 214
Drug-induced galactorrhea, 224
Drug-induced seizures, in newborn, 132–133
Drug overdose, 77
Duplication, of uterus, 182
Dysfunctional labor, 35–39, 36(t)
Dysfunctional uterine bleeding, 233–235
Dysmenorrhea, 150–152
Dyspareunia, 174–176
Dysplasia, skeletal, 137
Dystrophy, vulvar, 143–144, 179–180

Ear(s), examination of, in newborn, 134
Eclampsia, 3

Econazole, for infectious vaginitis, 166
Ectopic pregnancy, 34–35
　after sterilization, 241
Elavil (amitriptyline), for headache, 277, 278
Electrocautery, for chronic cervicitis, 179
Electrolyte(s), in intravenous hyperalimentation, 266
　in peripheral parenteral nutrition, 267
Embolism, pulmonary, 50, 51
　thrombotic, 50–55
　　rheumatic heart disease and, 59
Endometriosis, 170–171
Endometrium, carcinoma of, 195–198, 196(t)
Endoscopy, of uterus, for Asherman's syndrome, 238
Enflurane, in analgesia, in second stage of labor, 86
Enovid, for dysfunctional uterine bleeding, 234
Enteral nutrition, 265
Ephedrine, for asthma, in pregnancy, 108
　for hypotension, 85
Epidural analgesia, in labor, 84–86
Epilepsy, 60–64
Epinephrine, in resuscitation of newborn, 119
Ergot preparations, for headache, 277
　in induction of uterine contractions, in uterine atony and hemorrhage, 88
Erythroblastosis fetalis, 41–43
　and neonatal hypoglycemia, 124
Erythromycin, for acne, 273
　for bacterial bronchitis, in pregnant asthmatic patient, 108
　for bacterial rhinosinusitis, 107
　for chlamydial infection of female genital tract, 165
　for gonorrhea, 158(t), 160(t)
　for infectious vaginitis, 141(t), 142
　for legionnaires' disease, 282
　for pneumonia, 279
　for syphilis, 161(t), 162
Esophagitis, reflux, in pregnancy, 98–99
Estrogen, for dysfunctional uterine bleeding, 234
　for dysmenorrhea, 150
　for hypogonadism, in Sheehan's syndrome, 247
　for menopause, 235–236
　for XY gonadal dysgenesis, 244
　in follow-up to operative treatment of testicular feminization, 245
　in oral contraceptives, 226–229
　in prophylaxis against osteoporosis, 235
Ethambutol, for tuberculosis, 65–68, 154
　toxic effects of, 66, 67
Ethanol, for premature labor, 23
　for pruritus vulvae, 144, 181
Ethosuximide (Zarontin), for convulsions, 62(t)
Exchange transfusion, for anemia, 73
　for neonatal hyperbilirubinemia, 127–128
Exenteration, pelvic, for cervical carcinoma, 194–195
Exercise-induced amenorrhea, 212
Extraembryonic membranes, premature rupture of, 19–20, *20*, 35
　and amnionitis, 19–20, 35, 82–83
　oxytocin induction of uterine contractions after, 20, 35, 83
Extremities, examination of, in newborn, 135

Fallopian tube, inflammation of, 155–157
　gonococcal, 157–160, 158(t)–160(t)
　occlusion of, and sterilization, 239–240

Fallopian tube *(Continued)*
  resection of. See *Salpingectomy* and *Salpingo-oophorectomy*.
Fat, in peripheral parenteral nutrition, 267
Feminization syndrome, testicular, 211–212, 244–245
Fenoprofen (Nalfon), for dysmenorrhea, 151(t)
Ferrous sulfate, for iron-deficiency anemia, 73
Fetal alcohol syndrome, 78
Fetal death syndrome, 24–27
Fetal descent, slow, in labor, 38–39
Fetal distress, after premature rupture of extraembryonic membranes, 20
  intrapartum, 13–16, *15*
Fetal growth, retardation of, 55–57
  maternal renal disease and, 97
  twin gestation and, 91–92
Fetal heart rate monitoring, after premature rupture of extraembryonic membranes, 20
  bradycardia on, eclampsia and, 3
  contraction stress test findings on, 17–18, *18*
  distress patterns on, 14
  in hypocontractile labor, 37
  in pregnancy complicated by drug abuse, 75
  nonstress test findings on, 17, *18*
  variability on, 14, *15*
Fetal heart rate testing, 16–18, *18, 19*
Fetal hemolytic disease, 41–43
  and neonatal hypoglycemia, 124
Fetal hydrocephaly, 92–93, 92(t)
Fetal macrosomia, 36
Fetal malnutrition, and neonatal hypoglycemia, 124
Fetus, effect of maternal alcohol abuse on, 78, 78(t)
  effect of maternal drug abuse on, 74–75, 74(t)
  genetic defects in, diagnosis of, 111–113, 111(t)
  sex of, determination of, 112
Fibrinolytic agents, for venous thrombosis, 54
Fibrocystic disease of breast, 255
First stage of labor, analgesia in, 84–85
Fistula, tracheoesophageal, 137
  ureterovaginal, 149
  urethrovaginal, 149
  vesicovaginal, 149, 152–153
Flavoxate (Urispas), for urinary incontinence, 149
Fluid replacement, in management of shock, 173
Foam, spermicidal, 232
Folic acid, for anemia, 73
Fungal infection, of vagina, 141–142, 141(t), 165–166

Galactorrhea, 223–226, 256–257
Gallbladder, inflammation of, in pregnancy, 99, 100
Gallstone disease, in pregnancy, 99, 100, 102
Gantrisin (sulfisoxazole), for urinary tract infection, 32
Gardnerella vaginalis infection, of vagina, 141(t), 142, 166–167
Gastrointestinal tract, disorders of, in pregnancy, 98–102
Gastroschisis, 138
General anesthesia, in cesarean section, 87
Genetic defects, antenatal diagnosis of, 111–113, 111(t)
  chromosomal, 135–136
  mendelian, 136–137
  polygenic-multifactorial, 137–138

Genital tract, examination of, in newborn, 135
  female, hematoma(s) of, postpartum, 93–94
    infections of, 32–34, 64–66, 141–143, 153–167
    sexually transmitted diseases of, 32–34, 157–167
    tuberculosis of, 64–66, 153–155
Gentamicin, for amnionitis, 83
  for pneumonia, 281
  for salpingitis (PID), 156
  in prophylaxis against bacteremia, in pregnant patient with rheumatic heart disease, 59
German measles, in pregnancy, 109–111
Gestation, twin, 90–92
Gestational trophoblastic disease, 201–203, *202*
  hyperthyroidism in, 45
Glucose, diminished serum levels of, in newborn, 121, 123–125, 124(t)
  and seizures, 131–132
  for alcohol-induced coma, 80(t)
  for drug overdose, 77
  for neonatal hypoglycemia, 121, 125, 125(t)
  in intravenous hyperalimentation, 266
Gonad(s), streak, extirpation of, 244
Gonadotropin, chorionic. See *Human chorionic gonadotropin*.
  insufficient release of, 212
  menopausal. See *Human menopausal gonadotropin (Pergonal)*.
Gonorrhea, 157–160, 158(t)–160(t)
Graves' disease, 45
Growth retardation, intrauterine, 55–57
  maternal renal disease and, 97
  twin gestation and, 91–92
Guanethidine, for hypertension, 270(t), 271
Gynergen (ergotamine tartrate), for headache, 277

Hallucinosis, alcoholic, 81, 81(t)
Haloperidol, for alcoholic hallucinosis, 81, 81(t)
  for drug overdose, 77
Hashimoto's disease, 43
Head, examination of, in newborn, 134
Headache, 276–278
Heart, congenital defects of, 137–138
Heart disease, rheumatic, in pregnant patient, 57–60
Heart massage, in resuscitation of newborn, 119
Hematoma(s), pelvic, postpartum, 93–94
Hemodialysis, patient management in, pregnancy and, 97
Hemolytic disease of newborn, 41–43
  and neonatal hypoglycemia, 124
Hemorrhage. See *Bleeding*.
Heparin, for disseminated intravascular coagulation, 26
  for venous thrombosis, 51–54
  in management of ileus, 276
  in peripheral parenteral nutrition, 267
  in prophylaxis against venous thrombosis, 55
    in pregnant patient with rheumatic heart disease, 59–60
Hernia(s), diaphragmatic, congenital, 137
Herpes genitalis, 32–34, 162–164
High-fiber diet, for constipation, 102
Hirsutism, in adrenal disorders, 238
  in polycystic ovary syndrome, 211, 223
Human chorionic gonadotropin, for luteal phase defects, 249
  in induction of ovulation, 219, 220
    in polycystic ovary syndrome, 221

Human menopausal gonadotropin (Pergonal), in induction of ovulation, 220
  in treated anorexia patient, 243
Hyaline membrane disease, 119–123
Hydatidiform mole, 200–201
Hydralazine (Apresoline), for hypertension, 270(t), 271
  in pregnancy, 3, 5
Hydrocephaly, fetal, 92–93, 92(t)
Hydrochlorothiazide, for hypertension, 270(t)
Hydrocortisone, as steroid supplement, in pregnant asthmatic patient, 109
  for amniotic fluid embolism, 50
  for neonatal hypoglycemia, 125
  for Sheehan's syndrome, 246
  for systemic lupus erythematosus, 69
Hydroxyzine (Atarax), for pruritus vulvae, 181
  in improvement of analgesia, in first stage of labor, 84
Hymen, imperforate, 210
Hyperalimentation, 265–267
Hyperbilirubinemia, in newborn, 125–130
Hyperplastic dystrophy, vulvar, 144, 180
Hyperprolactinemia, 223–226
  and hypogonadotropinism, 212
Hypertension, in non-pregnant patient, 267–271, 269(t), 270(t)
  in pregnant patient, 3–5
Hyperthyroidism, 45–49
Hypertonic saline, in induction of uterine contractions, after fetal death, 25, 26
  in abortion, 30
Hypocalcemia, in newborn, 125
  and seizures, 132
Hypocontractile labor, 37–38
Hypoglycemia, in newborn, 121, 123–125, 124(t)
  and seizures, 131–132
Hypogonadotropinism, 212
Hypomagnesemia, in newborn, 125
  and seizures, 132
Hypopituitarism, 217–218, 245–247
Hypothalamic dysfunction, and amenorrhea, 214, 215
  and anovulation, 210–211
Hypothalamic-hypophyseal failure, 217–218
Hypothyroidism, 43–45, 43(t), 224, 225
  in Sheehan's syndrome, 246, 247
Hypovolemic shock, 172(t)
Hysterectomy, and sterilization, 240
  for cervical carcinoma, 194
  for endometrial carcinoma, 197
  for hydatidiform mole, 201
  for ovarian carcinoma, 198
  for tuberculosis of female genital tract, 155
  for uterine myomas, 169
  for uterine prolapse, 147
  vaginal prolapse after, 147–148
Hysteroscopy, for Asherman's syndrome, 238

Ibuprofen (Motrin), for dysmenorrhea, 151(t)
Ileus, 274–276
Imipramine (Tofranil), for headache, 278
  for urinary incontinence, 149
Immune hemolytic disease, fetal, 41–43
  and neonatal hypoglycemia, 124
Immune thrombocytopenic purpura, 89–90
Imperforate hymen, 210
Inborn errors of metabolism, 136–137
Incontinence, urinary, 148–150
Indocin. See *Indomethacin (Indocin)*.

Indomethacin (Indocin), for dysmenorrhea, 151(t)
  for pain of herpes genitalis, 163
  for premature labor, 23
Infectious vaginitis, 141–143, 141(t), 165–167
Infertility, in endometriosis, 171
  in polycystic ovary syndrome, 221, 223
Inflammatory bowel disease, in pregnancy, 100–101
Inflammatory headache, 278
Inguinal lymphadenectomy, for vulvar carcinoma, 190
Inhalation analgesia, in second stage of labor, 85, 86
Insulin, use of, by pregnant diabetic patient, 6–7, 7(t), 9
Insulin-dependent diabetes, 6–9
Intercourse, painful, 174–176
Intestine, atresia of, 138
  inflammatory disease of, in pregnancy, 100–101
  obstruction of, 274–276
  stenotic, 138
Intoxication, alcoholic, 80–81, 80(t)
Intracranial hemorrhage, and seizures in newborn, 131
Intrauterine device, 229–232
Intrauterine growth retardation, 55–57
  maternal renal disease and, 97
  twin gestation and, 91–92
Intravenous analgesia, in second stage of labor, 86
Intravenous hyperalimentation, 265–266
Iodide, deficiency of, and hypothyroidism, 43
  for hyperthyroidism, 48
  for thyroid storm, 48
Iodine, radioactive, in ablation of thyroid gland, 47
Iron-deficiency anemia, 71, 73
Isoniazid, for tuberculosis, 65–68, 154
  toxic effects of, 66, 67
    pyridoxine therapy for, 66, 67
Isoproterenol, for shock, 51
IUD, 229–232

Jaundice, in newborn, 125–130

Kanamycin, for amnionitis, 83
Kenalog (triamcinolone), for acne, 273
  for headache, 278
  for vulvar hyperplastic dystrophy, 144
Ketamine, in analgesia, in second stage of labor, 86
  in general anesthesia, 86, 87
Kidney(s), chronic disease of, in pregnancy, 94–97, 95(t), 96(t)
  polycystic disease of, perinatal, 137
  transplantation of, pregnancy after, 98
Kidney stone(s), in pregnancy, 97

Labor, analgesia in, 84–86
  and delivery. See *Delivery*.
  anesthesia in, 83–86
    in rheumatic heart disease patient, 60
  diagnosis of, 35
  dysfunctional, 35–39, *36*
  fetal distress in, 13–16, *15*
  first stage of, analgesia in, 84–85
  hypocontractile, 37–38

Labor *(Continued)*
  premature, 21–24
    in twin gestation, 91
    risk factors for, 21(t)
    treatment of, patient selection for, 22(t)
  second stage of, analgesia in, 85–86
    arrested, 38–39
    slow fetal descent in, 38–39
Laser surgery, for cervical intraepithelial neoplasia, 193, 204
Legionnaires' disease, 281–282
Lichen sclerosus, vulvar, 143–144, 180
Lidocaine, pudendal nerve block with, in second stage of labor, 86
  subarachnoid (saddle) block with, in second stage of labor, 86
Lip, cleft, 138
Lithium, in prophylaxis against headache, 278
LSD (lysergic acid diethylamide), teratogenic potential of, 74(t)
Lugol's solution, for thyroid storm, 48
Luminal (phenobarbital), for alcohol intoxication, 80(t)
  for convulsions, 62(t), 63
    in newborn, 133(t)
    in status epilepticus, 63
  for neonatal hyperbilirubinemia, 129
  substitution of, for drugs of abuse, 76, 76(t)
Lupus erythematosus, systemic, in pregnancy, 69–70
Luteal phase defects, 28, 247–249
Lymphadenectomy, inguinal/pelvic, for vulvar carcinoma, 190
Lysergic acid diethylamide (LSD), teratogenic potential of, 74(t)

Macrosomia, fetal, 36
Magnesium, diminished serum levels of, in newborn, 125
  and seizures, 132
Magnesium sulfate, for convulsions, 3, 5
  for neonatal hypomagnesemia, 125, 132
  for premature labor, 23
  toxic effects of, calcium gluconate therapy for, 4
Malignant melanoma, of vulva, 191
Malnutrition, fetal, and neonatal hypoglycemia, 124
Mandelamine, for urinary tract infection, 32
Marijuana, teratogenic potential of, 74(t)
Marsupialization, for cyst of Bartholin's gland, 167–168
Mass lesions, of breast, 255–256
Mastalgia, 257–259
Mastectomy, radical, for breast cancer, 261
Meclofenamate (Meclomen), for dysmenorrhea, 151(t)
Meconium, in amniotic fluid, 41
Medroxyprogesterone acetate (Provera), for dysfunctional uterine bleeding, 234
  for hypogonadism, in Sheehan's syndrome, 247
  for hypogonadotropinism, 212
  for menopause, 236
  for ovarian failure, 217
  for polycystic ovary syndrome, 223
  for precocious puberty, 250
  for uterine myomas, 169
  for XY gonadal dysgenesis, 244
  in follow-up to operative treatment, of intrauterine synechiae, 238
    of testicular feminization, 245

Medroxyprogesterone acetate (Provera) *(Continued)*
  in induction of withdrawal bleeding, in diagnosis of cause of amenorrhea, 214
  in treatment of amenorrhea, 215
Mefenamic acid (Ponstel), for dysfunctional uterine bleeding, 235
  for dysmenorrhea, 151(t)
Mefoxin (cefoxitin), for gonorrhea, 158(t)–160(t)
  for salpingitis (PID), 156, 159(t)
Megaloblastic anemia, 71
Melanoma, malignant, of vulva, 191
Membrane(s), extraembryonic, premature rupture of, 19–20, *20*, 35
  and amnionitis, 19–20, 35, 82–83
  oxytocin induction of uterine contractions after, 20, 35, 83
Mendelian disorders, 136–137
  antenatal diagnosis of, 112
Menopause, 235–236
  hypertension after, 271
Menorrhagia, 233–235
Menstrual extraction, 29
Menstruation, absence of, 209–218, 210(t), *216*
  and serum prolactin levels, 225
  cessation of, 235–236
    hypertension after, 271
  excessive, 233–235
  painful, 150–152
Meperidine, for drug withdrawal symptoms, 77
  in analgesia, in first stage of labor, 84
Mestinon (pyridostigmine), for mayasthenia gravis, 104
Metabolism, inborn errors of, 136–137
Methadone maintenance, in pregnant opiate abuser, 76–77
Methaqualone, teratogenic potential of, 74(t)
Methimazole, for hyperthyroidism, 47
  for thyroid storm, 48
Methotrexate, for gestational trophoblastic disease, 203
  for mixed connective tissue disease, 70
Methoxyflurane, in analgesia, in second stage of labor, 86
Methyldopa (Aldomet), for hypertension, 270(t)
  in pregnancy, 5
Methylprednisolone, for asthma, in pregnancy, 108(t)
Methysergide (Sansert), for headache, 277, 278
Metoprolol, for hypertension, 270(t)
Metronidazole, for infectious vaginitis, 141(t), 142, 165, 167
  for salpingitis (PID), 156, 159(t)
Metroplasty, for congenital uterine anomalies, 182–183
Miconazole, for infectious vaginitis, 141(t), 142, 166
Midrin, for headache, 277
Migraine, 276–277
Minocycline, for acne, 273
Minoxidil, for hypertension, 270(t)
Mixed connective tissue disease, in pregnancy, 70
Molar pregnancy, 200–201
Morphine, and pain relief, in hypocontractile labor, 38
  for amniotic fluid embolism, 50
Motrin (ibuprofen), for dysmenorrhea, 151(t)
Mouth, examination of, in newborn, 134
Multiple pregnancy, 35–36
Multiple sclerosis, in pregnancy, 103–104
Muscle contraction headache, 278
Myasthenia gravis, in pregnancy, 104–105

Mycobacterium tuberculosis infection, of female genital tract, 64–66, 153–155
   of pelvis, 153
   of pulmonary tissue, 66–68
Mycoplasmal infection, of vagina, 141(t), 143
Myoma(s), of uterus, 168–170
Myomectomy, uterine, 169
Mysoline (primidone), for convulsions, 62(t)
Myxedema coma, 44
   treatment of, 45

Nadolol, for hypertension, 270(t)
Nalfon (fenoprofen), for dysmenorrhea, 151(t)
Naloxone (Narcan), in reversal of effects of narcotics, in delivery, 84
   in drug abuser, 77
   in newborn, 119
   in offspring of drug abuser, 76
Naproxen (Anaprox, Naprosyn), for dysmenorrhea, 151(t)
Narcan (naloxone), in reversal of effects of narcotics, in delivery, 84
   in drug abuser, 77
   in newborn, 119
   in offspring of drug abuser, 76
Narcotic(s), and analgesia, in first stage of labor, 84
   effects of, naloxone for reversal of, in delivery, 84
      in drug abuser, 77
      in newborn, 119
      in offspring of drug abuser, 76
Neck, examination of, in newborn, 134
Neisseria gonorrhoeae infection, 157–160, 158(t)–160(t)
Neonatal care, 117–138. See also entries under *Newborn.*
Neostigmine, for myasthenia gravis, 104, 105
Nephrolithiasis, in pregnancy, 97
Neural tube defects, 137
   antenatal diagnosis of, 112–113
Neurogenic shock, 172(t)
Neurologic function, examination for, in newborn, 135
Nevatol (trichloroacetic acid), for condyloma acuminatum, 90
Newborn, airway patency in, 117
   anticonvulsant drug dosages for, 133(t)
   convulsions in, 130–133
   effects of narcotics on, naloxone for reversal of, 119
   evaluation of, for congenital abnormalities, 134–138
   examination of, 134–135
   hemolytic disease of, 41–43
      and neonatal hypoglycemia, 124
   hyaline membrane disease in, 119–123
   hyperbilirubinemia in, 125–130
   hypocalcemia in, 125
      and seizures, 132
   hypoglycemia in, 121, 123–125, 124(t)
      and seizures, 131–132
   hypomagnesemia in, 125
      and seizures, 132
   jaundice in, 125–130
   respiratory distress syndrome in, 119–123
   resuscitation of, 117–119, *118*
   seizures in, 130–133
   tracheal suction in, 117, 117(t)

Nipples, discharge form, nonpuerperal, 223–226, 256–257
Nitrofurantoin, for urinary tract infection, 32
Nitrous oxide, and analgesia, in second stage of labor, 86
   and anesthesia, in cesarean section, 87
Nonstress test, 16–17, *18*
   in postterm pregnancy, 40
Norethindrone, for dysfunctional uterine bleeding, 234
Nose, examination of, in newborn, 134
Nutrition, enteral, 265
   parenteral, peripheral, 266–267
Nystatin, for infectious vaginitis, 166

Omentectomy, partial, for ovarian carcinoma, 198
Omphalocele, 138
Oophorectomy, in treatment of breast cancer, 262
   with salpingectomy. See *Salpingo-oophorectomy.*
   with total hysterectomy, for uterine myomas, 169
Opiate(s), teratogenic potential of, 74(t)
Oral contraceptive(s), 226–229
   and amenorrhea, 214
Ortho Novum, for dysfunctional uterine bleeding, 234
Osteoporosis, prophylaxis against, 235
Ovarian failure, 212–213, 217
Ovary, carcinoma of, 198–200
   resection of, in treatment of breast cancer, 262
      with salpingectomy. See *Salpingo-oophorectomy.*
      with total hysterectomy, for uterine myomas, 169
Overflow incontinence, urinary retention with, 149
Ovulation, absence of, hypothalamic dysfunction and, 210–211
   induction of, 218–220
      in polycystic ovary syndrome, 221
      in treated anorexia patient, 243
Oxybutynin (Ditropan), for urinary incontinence, 149
Oxygenation, in management of shock, 172
Oxymetazoline (Afrit), for rhinitis, 107
Oxytocin, in induction of uterine contractions, after fetal death, 25, 26
   after premature rupture of extraembryonic membranes, 20, 35, 83
   in abortion, 30
   in hypocontractile labor, 37–38
   in patient with rheumatic heart disease, 58–59
   in treatment of hydatidiform mole, 200
   in uterine atony and hemorrhage, 88

Paget's disease, of vulva, 189
Palate, cleft, 138
Pancreatitis, acute, in pregnancy, 102–103
Pancuronium (Pavulon), and respiratory support, in respiratory distress syndrome, 122
Papanicolaou smear, abnormal findings on, evaluation of, 203–206, *205*
Paraldehyde, for convulsions, in status epilepticus, 63
Parenteral nutrition, peripheral, 266–267
Parlodel (bromocriptine), for galactorrhea, 257
   for hyperprolactinemia, 226
   for hypogonadotropinism, secondary to hyperprolactinemia, 212

Parlodel (bromocriptine) *(Continued)*
  for luteal phase defects, 249
  for mastalgia, 259
  in induction of ovulation, 220
Partial omentectomy, for ovarian carcinoma, 198
Pavulon (pancuronium), and respiratory support, in respiratory distress syndrome, 122
PBZ (tripelennamine), for rhinitis, 107
PCP (phencyclidine), teratogenic potential of, 74(t)
Pelvic exenteration, for cervical carcinoma, 194–195
Pelvic hematoma(s), postpartum, 93–94
Pelvic inflammatory disease (PID), 155–157
  gonococcal, 157–160, 158(t)–160(t)
Pelvic lymphadenectomy, for vulvar carcinoma, 190
Pelvis, contraction of, 37
  disorders of support in, 146–148
  tuberculosis of, 153
Penicillin(s). See also specific agents, e.g., Ampicillin.
  for legionnaires' disease, 282
  for pneumonia, 281
  for urinary tract infection, 31
Pentobarbital, in treatment of drug withdrawal symptoms, 76
Perforation, uterocervical, IUD use and, 230
Pergonal (human menopausal gonadotropin), in induction of ovulation, 220
  in treated anorexia patient, 243
Periactin (cyproheptadine), for headache, 277, 278
Peripheral parenteral nutrition, 266–267
Pharynx, gonococcal infection of, 157, 158, 158(t)
Phencyclidine (PCP), teratogenic potential of, 74(t)
Phenobarbital (Luminal), for alcohol intoxication, 80(t)
  for convulsions, 62(t), 63
    in newborn, 133(t)
    in status epilepticus, 63
  for neonatal hyperbilirubinemia, 129
  substitution of, for drugs of abuse, 76, 76(t)
Phenylpropanolamine (Propadrine), for urinary incontinence, 149
Phenytoin (Dilantin, diphenylhydantoin), for convulsions, 61, 62(t), 63
  in newborn, 133(t)
  in status epilepticus, 63
Phototherapy, for neonatal hyperbilirubinemia, 128–129
PID (pelvic inflammatory disease), 155–157
  gonococcal, 157–160, 158(t)–160(t)
Pituitary gland, adenomas of, 217–218, 224, 246
  and galactorrhea, 257
  treatment of, 225, 226
  hypofunctioning of, 217–218, 245–247
Placenta, implantation of, in lower uterus, 10
  premature detachment of, 10–11
Placenta previa, 10
Plasmapheresis, for systemic lupus erythematosus, 70
Pneumonia, 278–282
Podophyllum, for condyloma acuminatum, 90
Polycystic kidney disease, perinatal, 137
Polycystic ovary syndrome, 211, 215, 220–223, *222*
Polygenic-multifactorial genetic disorders, 137–138
Ponstel (mefenamic acid), for dysfunctional uterine bleeding, 235
  for dysmenorrhea, 151(t)

Post-pill amenorrhea, 214
Postterm pregnancy, 39–41, *40*
Potassium penicillin G, for gonorrhea, 159(t), 160(t)
  for salpingitis (PID), 159(t)
Prazosin, for hypertension, 270, 270(t)
Precocious puberty, 249–251
Prednisone, for acne, 274
  for asthma, in pregnancy, 108
  for headache, 278
  for immune thrombocytopenic purpura, 89
  for multiple sclerosis, 104
  for myasthenia gravis, 104, 105
  for neonatal hypoglycemia, 125
  for systemic lupus erythematosus, 69, 70
  for systemic vasculitis, 70
Preeclampsia, 3–4, *4*
  chronic renal disease and, 97
Pregnancy, abortion of. See *Abortion.*
  abruptio placentae in, 10–11
  acute cholecystitis in, 99, 100
  acute hypertension in, 3–4
  acute pancreatitis in, 102–103
  after renal transplantation, 98
  alcohol abuse in, 77–82
    risk to fetus in, 78, 78(t)
  amniorrhexis in, 19–20, *20,* 35
    and amnionitis, 19–20, 35, 82–83
    oxytocin induction of uterine contractions after, 20, 35, 83
  amniotic fluid embolism in, 49–50
  and delivery. See *Delivery.*
  and labor. See *Labor.*
  anemia(s) in, 70–74, *72*
  arthritis in, rheumatoid, 69
  asthma in, 106–109, 108(t)
  biliary colic in, 99, 100
  bowel disease in, inflammatory, 100–101
  bronchitis, asthma and, 108–109
  chlamydial infection of cervix in, 164
  cholangitis in, 99, 100
  cholecystitis in, acute, 99, 100
  cholelithiasis in, 99, 100, 102
  chronic hypertension in, 4–5
  chronic renal disease in, 94–97, 95(t), 96(t)
  colic in, biliary, 99, 100
  colitis in, ulcerative, 100
  collagen diseases in, 68–70
  condyloma acuminatum in, 90
  constipation in, 101–102
  convulsions in, 60–64
  Crohn's disease in, 100
  diabetes in, 5–9
    and neonatal hypoglycemia, 124
  drug abuse in, 74–77
    and potential teratogenesis, 74(t)
    and seizures in newborn, 132
  dysfunctional labor in, 35–39, 36(t)
  eclampsia in, 3
  ectopic, 34–35
    after sterilization, 241
  esophagitis in, reflux, 98–99
  fetal death syndrome in, 24–27
  fetal distress in, 13–16, *15*
  fetal hemolytic disease in, 41–43
    and neonatal hypoglycemia, 124
  fetal hydrocephaly in, 92–93, 92(t)
  fetal malnutrition in, and neonatal hypoglycemia, 124
  gallstone disease in, 99, 100, 102
  gastrointestinal disorders in, 98–102
  German measles in, 109–111

Pregnancy *(Continued)*
  gonorrhea in, 158, 158(t), 160, 160(t)
  hydatidiform mole in, 200–201
  hypertension in, 3–5
  hyperthyroidism in, 46–48
  hypothyroidism in, 45
  immune thrombocytopenic purpura in, 89
  inflammatory bowel disease in, 100–101
  in hemodialysis patients, 97
  in IUD user, 230–231
  intrauterine growth retardation in, 55–57
    maternal renal disease and, 97
    twin gestation and, 91–92
  kidney disease in, chronic, 94–97, 95(t), 96(t)
  kidney stones in, 97
  lupus erythematosus in, systemic, 69–70
  mixed connective tissue disease in, 70
  molar, 200–201
  multiple, 35–36
  multiple sclerosis in, 103–104
  myasthenia gravis in, 104–105
  myomas in, uterine, 170
  nephrolithiasis in, 97
  pancreatitis in, acute, 102–103
  placenta previa in, 10
  postterm, 39–41, *40*
  preeclampsia in, 3–4, *4*
  premature labor in, 21–24
  premature rupture of extraembryonic membranes in, 19–20, *20*, 35
    and amnionitis, 19–20, 35, 82–83
    oxytocin induction of uterine contractions after, 20, 35, 83
  pulmonary tuberculosis in, 66–68
  purpura in, thrombocytopenic, immune, 89
  reflux esophagitis in, 98–99
  renal disease in, chronic, 94–97, 95(t), 96(t)
  rheumatic heart disease in, 57–60
  rheumatoid arthritis in, 69
  rhinitis in, 105–107
  rubella in, 109–111
  scleroderma in, 70
  seizures in, 60–64
  syphilis in, 161(t), 162
  systemic lupus erythematosus in, 69–70
  systemic vasculitis in, 70
  third trimester of, bleeding in, 9–11
  thrombocytopenic purpura in, immune, 89
  thromboembolism in, 50–55
    rheumatic heart disease and, 59
  tuberculosis in, pulmonary, 66–68
  twin gestation in, 90–92
  ulcerative colitis in, 100
  uterine myomas in, 170
  vasculitis in, systemic, 70
  venereal warts in, 90
  venous thrombosis in, 50–55
    rheumatic heart disease and, 59
Premarin, for dysfunctional uterine bleeding, 234
  for hypogonadotropinism, 212
  in follow-up to operative treatment of intrauterine synechiae, 238
Premature labor, 21–24
  in twin gestation, 91
  risk factors for, 21(t)
  treatment of, patient selection for, 22(t)
Premature rupture, of extraembryonic membranes, 19–20, *20*, 35
  and amnionitis, 19–20, 35, 82–83
  oxytocin induction of uterine contractions after, 20, 35, 83
Prematurity, and hypoglycemia, 124

Presentation(s), abnormal, 36
  breech, 11–13
Primary amenorrhea, 209–213, 210(t)
Primidone (Mysoline), for convulsions, 62(t)
Probenecid, for cervicitis, 179
  for gonorrhea, 158(t)–160(t)
  for salpingitis (PID), 156, 159(t)
Procaine penicillin G, for cervicitis, 179
  for gonorrhea, 158(t), 159(t)
  for salpingitis (PID), 156, 159(t)
  for syphilis, 161(t)
Procidentia, 146–147
Products of conception, curettage for removal of, in treatment of postpartum hemorrhage, 89
Progestational challenge test, 214
  negative response to, diagnostic significance of, 215, 217–218
  positive response to, diagnostic significance of, 214–215
Progesterone, for luteal phase defects, 28, 249
  in induction of withdrawal bleeding, in diagnosis of cause of amenorrhea, 214
  in initiation of menstruation, in treatment of infertility in polycystic ovary syndrome, 221
  in prevention of premature labor, 22
Prolactin, elevated serum levels of, 223–226
  and hypogonadotropinism, 212
Prolapse, uterine, 146–147
  vaginal, after hysterectomy, 147–148
Propadrine (phenylpropanolamine), for urinary incontinence, 149
Propranolol, for headache, 277
  for hypertension, 270(t)
    in pregnancy, 5
  for hyperthyroidism, 47–48
  for thyroid storm, 49
Propantheline, for pancreatitis, 103
Propylthiouracil, for hyperthyroidism, 47
  for thyroid storm, 48
Prostaglandin(s), in induction of uterine contractions, after fetal death, 25–26
  in abortion, 30
  in uterine atony and hemorrhage, 88
Prostaglandin antagonists, *151*
Prostaglandin synthetase inhibitors, for dysmenorrhea, 150–152, 151(t)
  for premature labor, 23
Protein, in intravenous hyperalimentation, 266
  in peripheral parenteral nutrition, 267
Provera (medroxyprogesterone acetate), for dysfunctional uterine bleeding, 234
  for hypogonadism, in Sheehan's syndrome, 247
  for hypogonadotropinism, 212
  for menopause, 236
  for ovarian failure, 217
  for polycystic ovary syndrome, 223
  for precocious puberty, 250
  for uterine myomas, 169
  for XY gonadal dysgenesis, 244
  in follow-up to operative treatment, of intrauterine synechiae, 238
  of testicular feminization, 245
  in induction of withdrawal bleeding, in diagnosis of cause of amenorrhea, 214
  in treatment of amenorrhea, 215
Pruritus vulvae, 144, 179–181
Pseudoephedrine, for rhinitis, 107
Psittacosis, 280
Puberty, precocious, 249–251
Pudendal nerve block, and analgesia, in second stage of labor, 86
Pulmonary embolism, 50, 51

Pulmonary tuberculosis, in pregnancy, 66–68
Purpura, thrombocytopenic, immune, 89–90
Pyridium, and symptomatic relief in herpes genitalis, 33
Pyridostigmine (Mestinon), for myasthenia gravis, 104
Pyridoxine, for isoniazid toxicity, 66, 67

Q fever, 280

Radical hysterectomy, for cervical carcinoma, 194
  for endometrial carcinoma, 197
Radical mastectomy, for breast cancer, 261
Radical vulvectomy, for vulvar carcinoma, 191
Radioiodine, in ablation of thyroid gland, 47
Radiotherapy, for breast cancer, 261
  for cervical carcinoma, 194
  for endometrial carcinoma, 197
  for metastatic gestational trophoblastic disease, 203
  for ovarian carcinoma, 199
Rectocele, 147
Recurrent abortion, 27–29, 27(t)
Reflux esophagitis, in pregnancy, 98–99
Reserpine, for hypertension, 270(t), 271
Resistant ovary syndrome, 213, 217
Respiratory distress syndrome, 119–123
Respiratory support, in care of newborn, 119
    with respiratory distress syndrome, 121–122
  in management of shock, 172
  in treatment of atelectasis, 283
Resuscitation, of newborn, 117–119, *118*
Retardation, of fetal growth, 55–57
  maternal renal disease and, 97
  twin gestation and, 91–92
Retinoic acid, for acne, 272, 274
Rh₀(D) immune globulin, in prophylaxis against erythroblastosis fetalis, 42–43
Rheumatic heart disease, in pregnancy, 57–60
Rheumatoid arthritis, in pregnancy, 69
Rhinitis, in pregnancy, 105–107
Rhythm method, of birth control, 233
Rifampin, for tuberculosis, 65–68, 155
  toxic effects of, 66, 68
Ringer's lactate, in resuscitation of newborn, 119
Ritodrine (Yutopar), in prevention of premature labor, 22
  in treatment of premature labor, 23–24
Rubella, in pregnancy, 109–111
Rupture, premature, of extraembryonic membranes, 19–20, *20*, 35
  and amnionitis, 19–20, 35, 82–83
  oxytocin induction of uterine contractions after, 20, 35, 83

Saddle block, and analgesia, in second stage of labor, 86
Saline, hypertonic, in induction of uterine contractions, after fetal death, 25, 26
  in abortion, 30
Salpingectomy, for ectopic pregnancy, 35
  for tuberculosis of female genital tract, 155
Salpingitis (PID), 155–157
  gonococcal, 157–160, 158(t)–160(t)
Salpingo-oophorectomy, for ectopic pregnancy, 35
  for endometrial carcinoma, 197

Salpingo-oophorectomy *(Continued)*
  for ovarian carcinoma, 198
  for tuberculosis of female genital tract, 155
Salpingostomy, for ectopic pregnancy, 35
Sansert (methysergide), for headache, 277, 278
Scleroderma, in pregnancy, 70
Secondary amenorrhea, 213–218, *216*
Second stage of labor, analgesia in, 85–86
  arrested, 38–39
Seizure(s), 60–64
  alcohol withdrawal and, 81–82, 81(t)
  drug overdose and, diazepam for, 77
  drugs for control of, 3, 5, 61, 62(t), 63
    in newborn, 133(t)
  in newborn, 130–133
Septic shock, 172(t)
  abortion and, 174
Septum, uterine, 182
  vaginal, 185–186, 210
Sexual intercourse, painful, 174–176
Sexually transmitted diseases, 32–34, 157–167
Sheehan's syndrome, 218, 246, 247
Shock, management of, 171–174, 172(t)
Skeletal dysplasia, 137
Skin, examination of, in newborn, 135
Sodium bicarbonate, in resuscitation of newborn, 119
Sodium iodide, for thyroid storm, 48
Sodium penicillin G, for gonorrhea, 159(t), 160(t)
  for salpingitis (PID), 159(t)
Spectinomycin, for gonorrhea, 158(t)–160(t)
  for salpingitis (PID), 159(t)
Spermicide(s), vaginal, 232
Spironolactone (Aldactone), for hirsutism, in adrenal disorders, 238
  in polycystic ovary syndrome, 211, 223
Splenectomy, in treatment of immune thrombocytopenic purpura, 90
Spontaneous abortion, 27
Squamous cell carcinoma, of vulva, 189–190
SSKI, for thyroid storm, 48
Starvation, and amenorrhea, 241, 242
Status epilepticus, 63
Sterilization, 239–241
Steroid(s). See also specific agents, e.g., *Prednisone*.
  for inflammatory bowel disease, 101
  for systemic lupus erythematosus, 69
  for vulvar hyperplastic dystrophy, 180
Streak gonads, extirpation of, 244
Streptococcal infection, of vagina, 141(t), 143
Streptokinase, for venous thrombosis, 54
Streptomycin, for tuberculosis, 68
Stress incontinence, 148–149
Stress-induced amenorrhea, 214
Struma ovarii, and hyperthyroidism, 46
Subarachnoid block, and analgesia, in second stage of labor, 86
Subtotal thyroidectomy, for hyperthyroidism, 46
Suction curettage, after fetal death, 25, 26
  and abortion, 30
  in removal of hydatidiform mole, 200
Sulfamethoxazole-trimethoprim, for gonorrhea, 158(t)
Sulfasalazine, for inflammatory bowel disease, 101
Sulfisoxazole (Gantrisin), for urinary tract infection, 32
Sulindac (Clinoril), for dysmenorrhea, 151(t)
Suppository, spermicidal, 232
Synechia(e), uterine, 215, 238–239
Syphilis, 160–162, 161(t)
Systemic lupus erythematosus, in pregnancy, 69–70
Systemic vasculitis, in pregnancy, 70

Tegretol (carbamazepine), for convulsions, 62(t)
Terbutaline, for asthma, in pregnancy, 108, 108(t)
Testicular feminization, 211–212, 244–245
Testis (testes), removal of, in treatment of testicular feminization, 245
Testosterone, for vulvar lichen sclerosus, 144, 180
Tetracaine, subarachnoid (saddle) block with, in second stage of labor, 86
Tetracycline, for acne, 273
   for cervicitis, 179
   for chlamydial infection of female genital tract, 165
   for gonorrhea, 158(t)–160(t)
   for infectious vaginitis, 141(t), 142
   for pneumonia, 279
   for psittacosis, 280
   for salpingitis (PID), 156, 159(t), 165
   for syphilis, 161(t)
Theophylline, for asthma, in pregnancy, 107, 108(t)
Therapeutic abortion, 29–30
Thiazide duiretic(s), for hypertension, 269
Thiopental, in induction of general anesthesia, 87
Thrombocytopenia, 89
Thrombocytopenic purpura, immune, 89–90
Thromboembolism, 50–55
   rheumatic heart disease and, 59
Thrombosis, venous, 50–55
   rheumatic heart disease and, 59
Thymectomy, for myasthenia gravis, 105
Thymol, in treatment of herpes genitalis, 33
Thyroidectomy, subtotal, for hyperthyroidism, 46
Thyroid gland, ablation of, with radioactive iodine, 47
   hyperfunctioning of, 45–49
   hypofunctioning of, 43–45, 43(t), 224, 225
   in Sheehan's syndrome, 246, 247
   resection of, 46
Thyroiditis, chronic, 43
Thyroid storm, 48–49
Thyrotoxicosis, 45–49
Thyroxine, for hypothyroidism, 44–45, 225
   in Sheehan's syndrome, 247
   for myxedema coma, 45
Timolol, for hypertension, 270(t)
Tobramycin, for pneumonia, 281
   for salpingitis (PID), 156, 159(t)
Tofranil (imipramine), for headache, 278
   for urinary incontinence, 149
Total hysterectomy, for endometrial carcinoma, 197
   for ovarian carcinoma, 198
   for uterine myomas, 169
Trachea, suction of, in newborn, 117, 117(t)
Tracheoesophageal fistula, 137
Traction headache, 278
Tranquilizer(s), and analgesia, in first stage of labor, 84
Transfusion, for anemia, 73–74
   for neonatal hyperbilirubinemia, 127–128
Transplantation, renal, pregnancy after, 98
Tremulousness, alcohol withdrawal and, 81, 81(t)
   in newborn, 135
Treponema pallidum infection, 160–162, 161(t)
Triamcinolone (Kenalog), for acne, 273
   for headache, 278
   for vulvar hyperplastic dystrophy, 144
Trichloroacetic acid (Nevatol), for condyloma acuminatum, 90
Trichomonas vaginalis infection, of vagina, 141(t), 142, 165

Trimethoprim-sulfamethoxazole, for gonorrhea, 158(t)
Tripelennamine (PBZ), for rhinitis, 107
Trisomy 13, 136
Trisomy 18, 136
Trisomy 21, 135–136
   maternal age and, 111(t)
Tube feeding, 265
Tuberculosis, of female genital tract, 64–66, 153–155
   of pelvis, 153
   of pulmonary tissue, 66–68
Turner syndrome, 136
Twin gestation, 90–92
Twins, delivery of, 92

Ulcerative colitis, in pregnancy, 100
Unicornuate uterus, 182
Ureter, ectopic, 149
Ureterovaginal fistula, 149
Urethra, diverticula of, 149–150
Urethrovaginal fistula, 149
Urinary incontinence, 148–150
Urinary tract infection(s), 30–32
Urine, retention of, with overflow incontinence, 149
Urispas (flavoxate), for urinary incontinence, 149
Urokinase, for venous thrombosis, 54
Uterine adnexa, masses of, 177
Uterine cervix, adenocarcinoma of, 206
   carcinoma of, 191–195
   chlamydial infection of, in pregnancy, 164
   conization of, for intraepithelial neoplasia, 193, 204
   inflammation of, 177–179
   intraepithelial neoplasia of, 192–193, 204, 206
   perforation of, IUD use and, 230
Uterine tube, inflammation of, 155–157
   gonococcal, 157–160, 158(t)–160(t)
   occlusion of, and sterilization, 239–240
   resection of. See *Salpingectomy* and *Salpingo-oophorectomy*.
Uterus, adnexa of, masses of, 177
   arcuate, 182
   atony of, in postpartum hemorrhage, 88
   bicornuate, 182
   bleeding from, dysfunctional, 233–235
      IUD use and, 230
   congenital absence of, 211
   congenital anomalies of, 181–183
   contraceptive device(s) in, 229–232
   contractions of, abnormal, 37–38
      after amniotomy, 37
      ergotrate in induction of, in uterine atony and hemorrhage, 88
      hypertonic saline in induction of, after fetal death, 25, 26
      in abortion, 30
      oxytocin in induction of, after fetal death, 25, 26
         after premature rupture of extraembryonic membranes, 20, 35, 83
         in abortion, 30
         in hypocontractile labor, 37–38
         in patient with rheumatic heart disease, 58–59
         in treatment of hydatidiform mole, 200
         in uterine atony and hemorrhage, 88
      prostaglandin(s) in induction of, after fetal death, 25–26

Uterus (Continued)
  contractions of, prostaglandin(s) in induction of,
      in abortion, 30
      in uterine atony and hemorrhage, 88
  duplication of, 182
  endoscopy of, for Asherman's syndrome, 238
  expulsion of IUD from, 230
  fetal growth in, retardation of, 55–57
      maternal renal disease and, 97
      twin gestation and, 91–92
  hypocontractility of, 37–38
  lower, placental implantation in, 10
  myomas of, 168–170
  pain in, IUD use and, 230
  perforation of, IUD use and, 230
  prolapse of, 146–147
  resection of. See *Hysterectomy*.
  septate, 182
  synechiae in, 215, 238–239
  unicornuate, 182

Vagina, adenosis of, 144–146
  agenesis of, 183–186
  bleeding from, in third trimester of pregnancy, 9–11
  hematoma(s) of, postpartum, 94
  infections of, inflammatory, 141–143, 141(t), 165–167
  longitudinal septum of, 186
  prolapse of, after hysterectomy, 147–148
  septum of, 185–186, 210
  spasm of, 174–176
  spermicides for use in, 232
  surgical construction of, 184–185
  transverse septum of, 185–186, 210
Vaginismus, 174–176
Vaginitis, infectious, 141–143, 141(t), 165–167
Valproic acid (Depakene), for convulsions, 62(t)
Vascular headache, 276–277
Vasculitis, systemic, in pregnancy, 70
Venereal diseases, 32–34, 157–167
Venereal wart(s), 90
Venous thrombosis, 50–55
  rheumatic heart disease and, 59
Ventilation, in care of newborn, 119
      with respiratory distress syndrome, 121–122
  in management of shock, 172
  in treatment of atelectasis, 283

Vesicovaginal fistula, 149, 152–153
Vibramycin (doxycycline), for chlamydial infection of female genital tract, 165
  for gonorrhea, 156, 159(t)
  for salpingitis (PID), 156, 159(t), 165
  for syphilis, 161(t)
  use of, prior to planned conception, 28
Virilization, adrenal tumor and, 213
Vitamin(s), in intravenous hyperalimentation, 266
  in peripheral parenteral nutrition, 267
Vitamin B_{12}, in treatment of anemia, 73
Vitamin K, for reversal of effects of warfarin, 53
Vulva, carcinoma of, 189–191, 190(t)
  dystrophy of, 143–144, 179–180
  hematoma(s) of, postpartum, 94
  lichen sclerosus of, 143–144, 180
  Paget's disease of, 189
  pruritus of, 144, 179–181
Vulvectomy, radical, for vulvar carcinoma, 191

Warfarin, for venous thrombosis, 53–54
  reversal of effects of, vitamin K for, 53
Wart(s), venereal, 90
Weight gain, and amenorrhea, 215
Weight loss, and amenorrhea, 212, 214, 241, 242
Withdrawal syndromes, after abstinence from alcohol, 81–82, 81(t)
  after abstinence from drugs, 76
  in offspring of drug abuser, 75, 75(t), 132

45,X syndrome, 136
XY gonadal dysgenesis, 243–244

Yeast infection, of vagina, 141–142, 141(t)
Yutopar (ritodrine), in prevention of premature labor, 22
  in treatment of premature labor, 23–24

Zarontin (ethosuximide), for convulsions, 62(t)
Zomepirac, for headache, 278
Zovirax (acyclovir), for herpes genitalis, 33, 163

Dear Colleague:

We invite your help to keep

CURRENT THERAPY IN Obstetrics and Gynecology 2

in tune with your needs.

Use the postcard below to tell us what topics and features you especially liked or found particularly useful in this edition. We'd also appreciate your suggestions for future editions—what subjects you would like added or deleted. Thank you for your help.

P.S. Need extra copies of **CURRENT THERAPY IN OBSTETRICS AND GYNECOLOGY 2** for the hospital, office or friends? Please indicate how many copies on the postage paid order card below and we'll be glad to send them to you on 30-day approval.

Available from your bookstore or the publisher

Medical Editor   CURRENT THERAPY IN OBSTETRICS AND GYNECOLOGY 2

Comments: _____

_____

_____

_____

_____

_____

Name _____

Address _____

City_____ State_____ ZIP_____

Use this postcard to order additional copies of **Current Therapy In Obstetrics and Gynecology 2**

YES! Please send me _____ copies of

Quilligan: CURRENT THERAPY IN OBSTETRICS AND GYNECOLOGY 2

About $32.50 • Over 250 pages • Illustrated • Order #7413-5

Bill me plus postage & handling. If not completely satisfied, I may return the book with the invoice within 30 days at no further obligation.

☐ Check enclosed (Save postage & handling)
☐ Charge my credit card (Save postage & handling)
☐ VISA
☐ MASTERCARD   Credit card # ☐☐☐☐☐☐☐☐☐☐☐☐☐☐

Exp. Date ☐☐–☐☐   Interbank # ☐☐☐☐

Signature _____
Add sales tax where applicable

☐ Send me future editions of **CURRENT THERAPY IN OBSTETRICS AND GYNECOLOGY 2** as available.

Name _____

Address _____

City_____ State_____ Zip_____

Prices are US only and subject to change.
483 MO5110

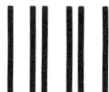

BUSINESS REPLY MAIL
FIRST CLASS   PERMIT NO. 101   PHILADELPHIA, PA

postage will be paid by addressee

W.B. SAUNDERS COMPANY

west washington square
philadelphia, PA 19105

NO POSTAGE
NECESSARY
IF MAILED
IN THE
UNITED STATES

BUSINESS REPLY MAIL
FIRST CLASS   PERMIT NO. 101   PHILADELPHIA, PA

postage will be paid by addressee

W.B. SAUNDERS COMPANY

west washington square
philadelphia, PA 19105

NO POSTAGE
NECESSARY
IF MAILED
IN THE
UNITED STATES